Surface and Dermal Monitoring for Toxic Exposures

Also by Shirley A. Ness
Air Monitoring for Toxic Exposures: An Integrated Approach

Related Titles of Interest from Van Nostrand Reinhold

Aerosol Measurement: Principles, Techniques, and Applications
Klaus Willeke and Paul A. Baron

Air Monitoring Instrumentation: A Manual for Emergency, Investigatory, and Remedial Responders
Carol J. Maslansky and Steven P. Maslansky

Biological Monitoring: An Introduction
Shane S. Que Hee

Hawley's Condensed Chemical Dictionary, Twelfth Edition
Richard J. Lewis, Sr.

Hazardous Chemicals Desk Reference, Third Edition
Richard J. Lewis, Sr.

Industrial Toxicology: Safety and Health Applications in the Workplace
Philip L. Williams and James L. Burson

Physical and Biological Hazards of the Workplace
Peter H. Wald and Gregg M. Stave

Proctor and Hughes' Chemical Hazards of the Workplace, Third Edition
Gloria J. Hathaway, Nick H. Proctor, James P. Hughes, and Michael L. Fischman

Quick Selection Guide to Chemical Protective Clothing, Second Edition
Krister Forsberg and S. Z. Mansdorf

Sax's Dangerous Properties of Industrial Materials, Eighth Edition
Richard J. Lewis, Sr.

SURFACE AND DERMAL MONITORING FOR TOXIC EXPOSURES

SHIRLEY A. NESS

VAN NOSTRAND REINHOLD
An International Thomson Publishing Company

New York • London • Bonn • Boston • Detroit • Madrid • Melbourne • Mexico City
Paris • Singapore • Tokyo • Toronto • Albany NY • Belmont CA • Cincinnati OH

Library of Congress Catalog Card Number 94-10018
ISBN 0-442-01465-1

I(T)P Van Nostrand Reinhold, an International Thomson Publishing Company.
ITP logo is a trademark under license.

Printed in the United States of America

Van Nostrand Reinhold
115 Fifth Avenue
New York, NY 10003

International Thomson Publishing
Berkshire House
168-173 High Holborn
London WC1V 7AA
England

Thomas Nelson Australia
102 Dodds Street
South Melbourne, Victoria 3205
Australia

Nelson Canada
1120 Birchmount Road
Scarborough, Ontario
M1K 5G4, Canada

International Thomson Publishing GmbH
Königswinterer Strasse 418
53227 Bonn
Germany

International Thomson Publishing Asia
221 Henderson Road
#05 10 Henderson Building
Singapore 0315

International Thomson Publishing Japan
Hirakawacho Kyowa Building, 3F
2-2-1 Hirakawa-cho, Chiyoda-ku
Tokyo 102
Japan

16 15 14 13 12 11 10 9 8 7 6 5 4 3 2 1

Library of Congress Cataloging-in-Publication Data

Ness, Shirley A.
Surface and dermal monitoring for toxic exposures/Shirley Ness.
p. cm.
Includes bibliographical references and index.
ISBN 0-442-01465-1
1. Dermatotoxicology—Methodology. 2. Toxicity testing.
I. Title.
RL803.N47 1994
616.5—dc20 94-10018
CIP

Contents

PART III: SURFACE MONITORING

PART IV: DERMAL SAMPLING TECHNIQUES

Preface

It is my hope that compiling information on the wide variety of dermal and surface monitoring methods that have been in use as early as the late 1970s, in addition to the significant number of exposure evaluations that have already been performed, will inspire industrial hygiene and environmental science professionals to apply and improve upon them. The time has come for practicing professionals to join the effort of the government agencies and the academic community so that the number and breadth of exposure evaluations increase. Industrial hygienists are at an advantage in doing these evaluations since they are well versed in monitoring methods and need only to redirect these from airborne exposure evaluations to surface and dermal. A determination of what parts of the body are at greatest risk and the determination of dose are also important.

Many studies are presented in this book. Some samples were collected using experimental methods and others were based on standardized techniques. Most dermal studies are done for agricultural work, but many are also done in industrial workplaces and community residences. The reader is encouraged to remain objective because much experimentation is still necessary and some of these techniques may be applicable to new chemicals and processes not yet studied. New materials are being developed that may prove more useful for contaminants not previously measured.

Comparing studies can be difficult because many use different techniques. Also, the terminology is not standardized. Many common words are used to describe sampling media, such as *cloth,* which has been used to refer to work fabrics, gauze, or cheesecloth. A similar problem exists with cellulose in that *pads* might be referred to as filter paper, blotter paper, or other terms. Many studies have not monitored the hands, but instead the pad exposure data from various body positions have been used to calculate total dermal exposure. Furthermore, the number of pads and relative positions can be different. To some degree this issue is being addressed in the form of standardized methods issued by the Environmental Protection Agency and World Health Organization; however, even these methods have their differences and the current trend is total body dosimetry using disposable suits. Methods of calculating dose vary, from none at all, to simplistic ones, to detailed risk assessments. These approaches are likely to be more refined in the future. Those readers who are interested have the opportunity to make a contribution by performing their own studies and research and sharing this information.

ACKNOWLEDGMENTS

I would like to thank Hank McDermott for his continuing support. He provided me with my first opportunity to have an exhibition of photos on the topic of women in the workplace in 1982 and has contributed his excellent guidance to both of my books. Thanks to Alex Padro of Van Nostrand Reinhold for his enthusiasm and assistance, and to Bernice Pettinato of Beehive Production Services for her patience. Also thanks to the folks at the National Institute of Occupational Safety and Health, including Mark Boeniger, who provided me with so much information. Plus a very special thanks to Will Popendorf for his contributions to the field of dermal monitoring and to this book.

I would like to also extend my gratitude to Ted Zellers, Steve Levine, and Richard Garrison along with their colleagues at the University of Michigan, for providing guidance and for developing new directions in the field of industrial hygiene. Ed Wesly of the school of the Art Institute of Chicago graciously provided a number of the photos used in several chapters, and Renea Joslin supplied original drawings for several figures.

I would also like to acknowledge as constantly in my thoughts Roger Ness and Sandy LeRoy Ness who are members of my family, and, most importantly, Jennifer Joslin, born February 4, 1994.

Lastly, I would like to remind my professional colleagues that *air sampling does not account for skin exposures*.

Surface and Dermal Monitoring for Toxic Exposures

Introduction

Historically, most toxic exposures have been categorized using air monitoring techniques because occupational and environmental standards for chemicals were based on air concentrations. However, air sampling will not measure the total exposure to chemicals capable of penetrating the skin. Skin contamination can occur as a result of fall-out from aerosols, via direct immersion into the chemical, as a result of accidental spills onto the body, through vapor penetration of the skin, or from contact with contaminated surfaces. Such contamination can produce the same types of toxic effects as inhalation exposure if a chemical can significantly penetrate the skin. Surface contamination can be ingested orally, create airborne exposures when surface buildup is disturbed, and be transferred into other areas, including from the workplace to the home. Some compounds, such as arsenic and lead, are highly toxic when orally ingested and are stable enough to remain on surfaces for long periods of time.

Monitoring for surface contamination has been a standard practice in work with radioactive materials since the 1950s, and a similar time span exists for dermal monitoring of pesticide applicators and harvesters. Only since the 1980s have these methods been applied to industrial and residential contamination with any regularity. Most notably, this testing has been applied during the investigation and cleanup of polychlorinated biphenyl releases inside buildings.

The attention continues to increase. Guidelines issued by the Housing and Urban development (HUD) Agency in 1990 require that surface sampling be performed prior to and following lead-paint abatement of public housing. The Lead Exposure Reduction Act of 1993 would expand these requirements to include schools and day-care centers. The Environmental Protection Agency (EPA) and the World Health Organization (WHO) have both issued standardized methods for assessing dermal exposure, and although the focus of these methods is to monitor pesticides, similar methods have been successfully used for amines, PAHs, and other chemicals. In the National Human Exposure Assessment Survey (NHEXSUS) project, the EPA will be surveying the status and trends of human environmental exposures of the national population, taking into account all relevant pathways of exposure including ingestion, dermal absorption, and inhalation. The EPA will be using surface and dermal monitoring methods to estimate exposures to contaminants in house dust.

The concern over dermal exposures is also

being reflected in the Occupational Safety and Health Administration's (OSHA) standard-setting effort. It has proposed in chemical standards set for the construction, maritime, and agricultural sectors that exposure to compounds with a "skin" notation be reduced or prevented to the extent possible through the use of gloves, coveralls, goggles, or other appropriate chemical protective clothing (CPC), engineering controls, or work practices (OSHA, 1992).

In recent substance-specific standards such as glycol ethers and methylene dianiline (MDA), OSHA has required controls to protect workers from dermal exposure. In the glycol ethers standard there are specific requirements for protection from spills, splashes, leaking equipment, and contaminated CPC due to the ability of these compounds to penetrate the skin (OSHA, 1993*a*). Most notably, the definition of employee exposure to glycol ethers has been expanded to include airborne and liquid (dermal) exposure that would occur if the employee were not using respirator protection or CPC.

Similarly, where the contaminant is highly toxic and can be resuspended into the air if allowed to remain on surfaces or can be taken home on workers' clothing, OSHA has increased its requirements for hygiene controls. The 1993 cadmium standard requires that CPC be decontaminated prior to workers entering lunchrooms, contaminated CPC must be placed in sealed containers, clean CPC be provided weekly at a minimum, and that changing and shower rooms be provided, as well as specific methods for cleaning surfaces to minimize resuspended dust (OSHA, 1993*b*).

When used to determine the potential for dermal exposure, methods are often categorized as indirect or direct. Indirect methods are used to estimate the potential for dermal exposure but not whether an exposure has occurred. Such methods involve the use of filters, gauze pads, or swabs to wipe surfaces; the use of instruments to "sniff" surfaces for volatile compounds; and the use of vacuum methods and adhesive tape to lift dust from surfaces. Direct methods measure exposures to the body and include the use of gauze, cellulose, or charcoal pads for dosimetry (Fig. 1); clothing; skin wipes; washing the skin with a solvent; and monitoring for skin color change and fluorescence.

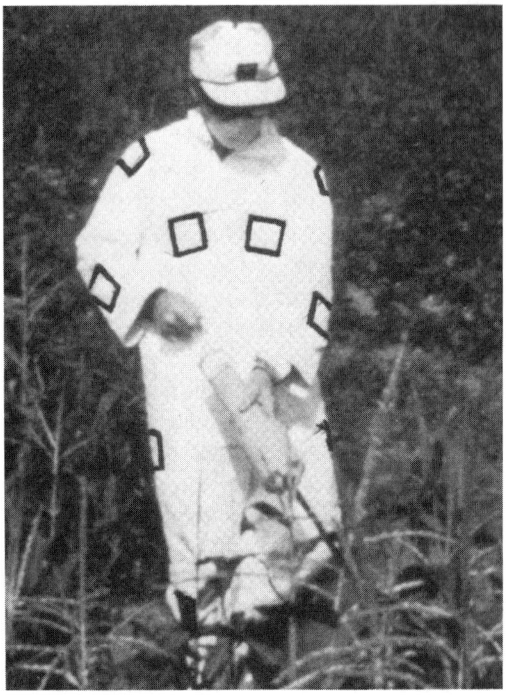

Figure 1. Pesticide worker wearing dosimetry pads. *Source:* From D. A. Kurtz and W. M. Bode. 1985. Application exposure to the home gardener. In R. C. Honeycutt, G. Zweig, and N. N. Ragsdale (eds.), *Dermal Exposure Related to Pesticide Use*. Washington, DC: American Chemical Society, p. 142. Reprinted with permission; copyright © 1985 by the American Chemical Society.

Dermal studies can identify specific body areas that are being exposed, thus making sure the proper CPC is selected. They can also identify activities and work tasks within an operation that pose the highest risk of exposure, and assist in determining the proper types of controls needed. In some instances, dermal sampling will identify compounds to which workers are exposed that are not collected on air samples. For example, with PCBs the ones with higher vapor pressures tend to volatilize while the heavier ones remain on the skin. Therefore, the relative contributions of dermal and respiratory exposure routes can be assessed. Penetration of CPC and clothing by contaminants can be determined, in part, by measuring contamination on the interior of garments as well as of the skin that was to be protected. The effectiveness of decontamination procedures can also be assessed.

Definitions as to what constitutes dermal exposure vary. One which has been used is contact with skin that provides an opportunity for skin absorption as well as nondietary ingestion. Skin contact with contaminants can occur in the following ways:

- Direct contact with settled materials on contaminated surfaces.
- Direct contact with hands and fingers, then transfer of the contaminant to other body parts (face, shoulders, etc.).
- Absorption of contaminants by work clothing, which may act as a "wick" for transfer to the skin. The chemical may also be transferred to the face from other parts of the body, for example, by touching the face with contaminated gloves, or by contaminated fingers.
- Penetration and deposition on CPC by the contaminant.
- The use of CPC that is soiled on the inside, or direct contact with the (contaminated) exterior surfaces during removal.
- Direct contact with aerosols and vapors of contaminants.

However, dermal absorption must take place in order for contact to actually produce an exposure. A central issue is determining when dermal exposure is likely to be the major route of entry compared with other routes of exposure (Fig. 2). It is also important to determine what parts of the body are at greatest risk and to measure dose. The best program is often an integrated approach that uses surface and dermal sampling in conjunction with air and biological monitoring to assess not only the true dose an individual is receiving, but also the sources of exposure.

There are a variety of reasons why surface con-

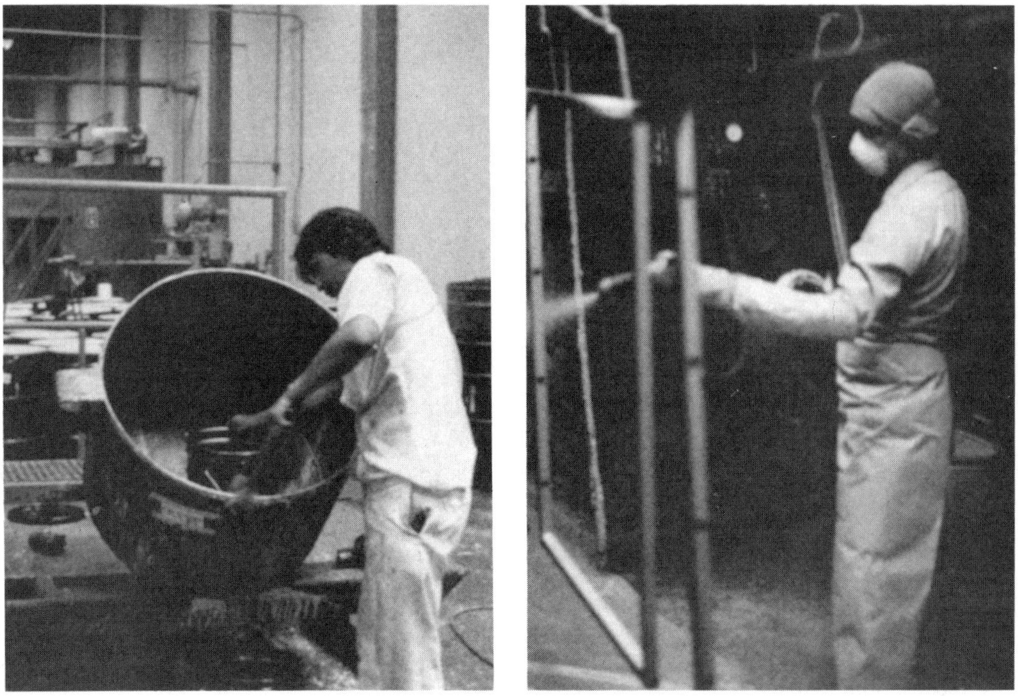

Figure 2. Dermal exposure situations. Cleaning a mixing tank (*left*) with solvents can lead to skin contact with liquids. Working near paint spray robots (*right*) can yield high vapor concentrations that can penetrate the skin. Note that the worker is attempting to protect himself using paper and a hat.

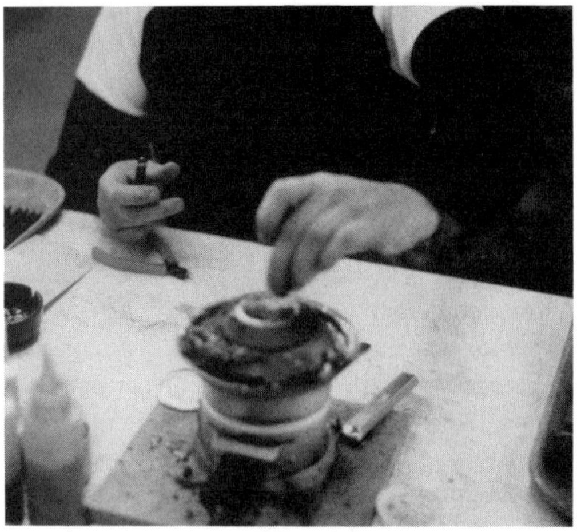

Figure 3. Tinning leads with lead-tin solder in an electronics fabrication shop. Airborne exposures from the pot are frequently low, but the potential for oral exposure is high if eating, drinking, chewing gum, or applying cosmetics is done without washing hands or in the work area.

tamination, especially removable surface contamination, may have to be sampled. Selection of compounds for surface monitoring depends on their ability to cause systemic toxicity via penetration of the skin, dermal irritation, sensitization, cancer, or oral toxicity (Fig. 3). Whenever persistent contaminants are present on surfaces or in the air there is a possibility that workers' skin and clothing may become contaminated, and that these materials be transported to surfaces in their personal vehicles and their homes thus exposing their families. This is thought to be the primary reason blood lead levels of household members residing in homes of workers with occupational lead exposures can be much higher than those of families of non-lead-exposed workers.

SOME EXPOSURE CONCERNS: PAST AND PRESENT

The recognition that dermal absorption could produce serious disease is not a recent phenomenon. The first identified disease related to skin exposure was scrotum cancer in chimney sweeps (Fig. 4) as identified by Percival Pott in 1775. At the time most houses and buildings in England burned coal for heat. The soot contained ash, free carbon, and polycyclic aromatic hydrocarbon (PAH) containing coal tar varying in concentration from 1% at the top of a high boiler chimney to over 40% in the flue of a chimney grate (Waldron, 1983). Although chimney sweep's cancer originally referred only to cancer of the scrotum, it is not the only site affected. When 147 fatal cases of cutaneous cancer in chimney sweeps were tracked from 1911 to 1935, 44 (30%), were on cutaneous sites other than the scrotum (see Table 1).

This exposure concern is not just a historical issue. More importantly, PAH exposures remain a concern in the 1990s. During the energy crisis of the 1980s an increase in the number of compa-

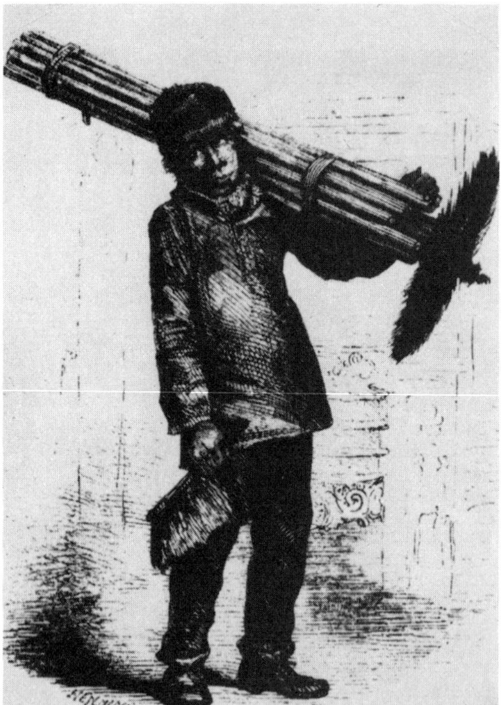

Figure 4. An English chimney sweep in 1851. *Source:* From H. A. Waldron. 1983. A brief history of scrotal cancer. *Brit. J. Ind. Med.* **40:**394.

TABLE 1. Number of Fatal Cases of Cutaneous Cancer in Chimney Sweeps Occurring Between 1911 and 1925

Site	*1911–15*	*1916–20*	*1921–25*	*1926–30*	*1931–35*	*Total*
Scrotum	22 (81.5%)	20 (67%)	25 (67.5%)	17 (65%)	19 (70%)	103 (70%)
Other than scrotum	5 (18.5%)	10 (33%)	12 (32.5%)	9 (35%)	8 (30%)	44 (30%)
Total	27	30	37	26	27	147

Source: From Henry, S. A. 1936. The study of fatal cases of cancer of the scrotum from 1911 to 1935 in relation to occupation, with special reference to chimney sweeping and cotton mule spinning. *J. Ind. Hyg.* **18:**25–57.

nies performing chimney cleaning resulted from the increased use of coal and wood to supplement gas and oil for heating. The first part of cleaning is done by lowering steel brushes inside the chimney. The brushes are then inserted from the hearth. The resulting dust is vacuumed from below. An industrial hygiene evaluation found that dust exposures when cleaning from the top were higher, especially the benzene soluble fraction, which would include PAHs, probably because the smaller size particles rise while the heavier material settles to the hearth (Bagchi and Zimmerman, 1980; see Table 2). The study identified arsenic in addition to PAHs.

In the 1950s, coal gasification facilities were developed in the United States to provide alternative forms of fuel because the availability of crude oil is expected to decrease in the future. Since the skin exposure concerns of PAHs were well known at this point, there was an effort to monitor dermal exposure using medical surveillance and fluorescence techniques at these plants. Coal conversion processes can produce a liquid (liquefaction) as well as the gas (gasification). The skin cancer rate in a small group of U.S. workers employed in coal liquefaction has been reported as between 16 and 37 times greater than expected for the general population (Lloyd and Young, 1983). Steel workers are still exposed to these materials on coke ovens and the 1974 OSHA standard on coke oven emissions addressed the skin hazard by requiring these workers to shower at the end of the day and not wear or take work clothing home.

More recently, other synthetic fuel processes, such as the recovery of shale oil, have received attention. Oil shale is a layered, gray-brown sedimentary rock known as marlstone that was laid down eons ago in freshwater lakes (Table 3). The oil in oil shale is contained in kerogen, a complex

TABLE 2. Air Contaminants Identified in Breathing Zone Samples During Chimney Sweeping (air contaminant concentration [mg/M³])

Location	*Type*	*Coal Tar Pitch Volatiles*	*Benzo-α pyrene*	*Sulfur Dioxide*	*Arsenic*
Cleaning from top	Dry	14.53	0.04	0.06	Not sampled
	After rains	0.68	ND	ND	0.013
	With mist	ND	ND	ND	0.013
Cleaning from hearth	Dry	2.16	ND	ND	Not sampled
	With mist	ND	ND	ND	0.005

Source: From Bagchi, W. J., and R. E. Zimmerman. 1980. An industrial hygiene evaluation of chimney sweeping. *AIHA J.* **41**(4):297–299.
Note: ND = no data.

TABLE 3. Benz(a)pyrene Analyses in Oil Shale and Other Petroleum Products

Product	*3.4-Benz(a)pyrene Content (ppb)*
Raw oil shale	14
TOSCO II process shale	28
TOSCO II effluent (lift pipe particulate from the atmospheric exhaust of crushed raw oil shale)	140
Shale oil coke	129
Raw shale oil (Colorado)	3,100
Hydrotreated shale oil (0.25% nitrogen)	800
Hydrotreated shale oil (0.05% nitrogen)	690
Coal	4,000
Libyan crude oil	1,320

Source: From Coomes, R. M. 1982. Oil shale. The state of the industry and potential health effects. In W. N. Rom and V. E. Archer (eds.), *Health Implications for New Technologies*. Ann Arbor, MI: Ann Arbor Science, pp. 445–456.

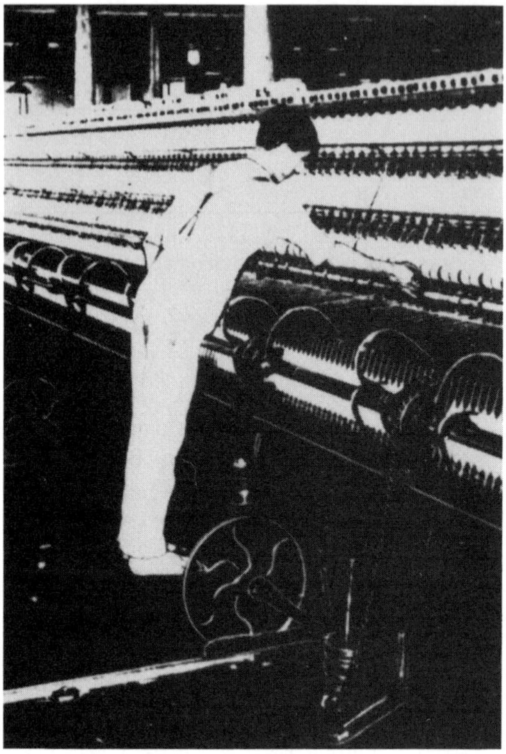

Figure 5. A cotton mule spinner at work in the 1930s. Note how he leans across faller bar to mend a broken thread.
Source: From H. A. Waldron. 1983. A brief history of scrotal cancer. *Brit. J. Ind. Med.* **40**:398.

organic material composed mainly of carbon, hydrogen, oxygen, sulfur, and nitrogen. Cotton mule spinners had a high incidence of scrotal cancer that was attributed to the use of mineral oil derived from oil shale (Fig. 5). Prior to 1848, lubricating oil for mule spindles consisted solely of a vegetable or whale oil, but after that time mineral oil derived from shale or coal replaced sperm oil with tragic consequences (Henry, 1936). The use of this material in Scotland has since ceased.

Many chemical warfare agents were selected based on their ability to penetrate or injure skin and were developed for use in World War I. Mustard gas (bis-beta dichlorodiethyl sulfide) is an oily, liquid vesicant with an odor of garlic, mustard, or horseradish that has a significant ability to penetrate the skin because of its lipid solubility (Scherling, Overholt, and Stahmer, 1943). Signs and symptoms of exposure do not appear until several hours have lapsed, by which time it is too late to ward off the effects of the gas. Nitrogen mustard is a similar agent that is odorless. Lewisite (beta-chlorovinyldichlorarsine), another war gas, is a heavy, oily liquid with an odor resembling geraniums. It is both a skin penetrant and a vesicant, but the irritant effects are felt immediately by the exposed person. Once it gains access to the system, it can cause acute arsenical poisoning.

Chemical warfare agents that can penetrate or injure the skin are just as much of a concern today. Activated charcoal cloth, used in a number of systems proposed for dermal and breath monitoring, was developed in England for use in modern chemical warfare protective clothing and has been used in the British army's chemical warfare suits. A similar design of coverall suit with charcoal impregnated in polyurethane foam was sent to Saudi Arabia for U.S. soldiers in preparation

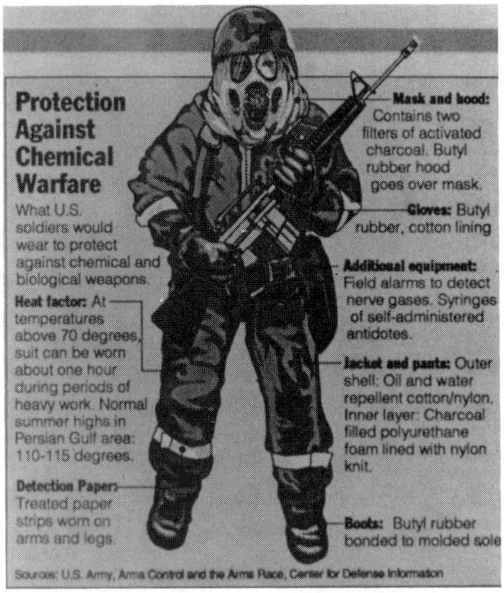

Figure 6. Chemical warfare protective clothing.
Source: From *Chicago Tribune*, 1991.

for the 1991 Gulf crisis (Fig. 6). Chemically treated paper strips on the legs of the U.S. suit are designed to change color in the presence of certain gases and vapors as an early warning system.

In industry the ability of certain chemicals to penetrate the skin was recognized in the early twentieth century. As early as 1928, the Bureau of Mines required the following label on canisters approved for use against hydrocyanic acid gas: "While this canister will give respiratory protection in atmospheres containing 2% hydrocyanic acid gas, it is not safe to encounter such high concentrations because the gas is absorbed through the unprotected skin of the body and in that manner will produce poisoning." Unfortunately the significance of this warning was not always grasped. The following account was published in 1932:

> Three men were wearing gas masks in an atmosphere containing approximately 2% of hydrocyanic acid gas and the masks were giving excellent respiratory protection. After eight or ten minutes, however, the men felt symptoms of marked dizziness, weakness, and throbbing pulse. They immediately left the poisonous atmosphere and were just in time to avoid collapse and unconsciousness. Marked weakness and high pulse rate, together with a headache, persisted for several hours after exposure, and the men were incapacitated for two or three days. (Drinker, 1932)

Since then many other sources of industrial exposure have been identified and evaluated, including carcinogenic amines, heavy metals, and PCBs. Pharmaceutical manufacturing, especially where hormones are involved, is another situation where evaluations have identified dermal effects such as male mammary gland development.

Shortly after parathion, the first acutely toxic synthetic insecticide, became widely used in agriculture, a number of worker poisonings resulted. During the investigations, dermal exposure to pesticides was identified as a significant contributor. In 1954 the first study of dermal exposure to pesticides was performed by attaching cellulose pads to workers' clothing (Batchelor and Walker, 1954). In the early 1960s other studies validated these initial efforts, and techniques have continued to be refined (Durham and Wolfe, 1962).

Sometimes the skin penetrant is directly related to the crop. Recently an advisory was issued to tobacco harvesters by the National Institute of Occupational Safety and Health regarding a nicotine-related illness caused when nicotine from wet tobacco penetrates workers' skin during harvesting. The disease, known as green tobacco sickness, is common because few of these workers wear protective clothing for their skin.

Airborne exposures to the wood preservative (and skin penetrant) tetrachlorophenol (TCP) were measured at both the wood grading and wood puller stations at a sawmill over a two-year period, and levels were found to be low, averaging 8 mg/M^3 (Fenske, Horstman, and Bentley, 1987). This finding was not surprising as the wood spray apparatus had been effectively enclosed and air monitoring was conducted periodically. However, samples of workers' urine continued to have elevated TCP concentrations, averaging 1.13 ppm TCP, corresponding to an average body burden of 1.84 mg/day. This figure was a much greater level than air sampling levels warranted. Dermal exposures were suspected as the source and further evaluation identified the forearms and hands as those parts of the body that were receiving the highest exposures.

While surface contamination from mercury in dental offices and laboratories has long been a concern in settings often considered free of contaminants, modern technology has produced new sources of exposure. Silver-coated paper is used in photo laser machines that are common in many offices (Clark, 1991). After employees in one office experienced dermatitis, air samples for inorganic mercury vapor were collected, and bulk samples of silver paper and paper dust were analyzed for mercury content. Both unprocessed and processed paper were found to contain in excess of 200 μg/g mercury. Dust collected from the floor surrounding the machines did not contain detectable levels of mercury, but dust collected from air supply diffusers, exhaust grills, and a wall behind the photo laser machines contained a trace levels of mercury. Due to the potential for skin absorption of mercury from handling the paper and dust, it was recommended that nitrile gloves be worn while cleaning the machines and handling the silver paper, and that a search be conducted for a source of mercury-free paper.

As noted previously, surface and dermal exposure concerns in the community are becoming increasingly important, especially for heavy metals and pesticides.

BIOLOGICAL MONITORING

There is currently debate as to whether external measurements of dermal exposure or biological monitoring represents the best approach to determining exposure. Biological monitoring measurements of contaminants or their metabolites in bodily fluids (or breath) are considered better measurements of exposure in some cases because they represent an individual's actual absorbed dose. However, the individual must have been exposed to and absorbed the contaminant in order to use these methods to determine dose.

Although in some cases biological monitoring is the only effective means of determining whether skin absorption is a significant concern, including detention of contaminants that do not have reliable sampling methods, it is ineffective for other compounds that are rapidly metabolized in the body. Some chemicals have poor biological warning properties or biological indicators of exposure and therefore are not good choices for biological monitoring (OSHA, 1992). As an example, MDA easily enters the body through the skin, and once absorbed into the body, it is rapidly eliminated so that using a biological measurement, such as urine, may not detect the apparent exposure.

There are two basic types of biological monitoring methods: (1) direct measurement of a chemical or metabolite in a biological media, and (2) indirect measurement by quantifying subclinical biological change related to the chemical. Since most chemicals capable of causing systemic effects are generally transported by the blood, the blood is often considered the most useful biological medium to monitor as it generally provides an accurate, although indirect, measurement of the level of most toxic agents in target organs or tissues. Chemicals that enter the blood can be found at different concentrations depending on whether the site of entry is measured or what blood vessel is sampled. Therefore, blood collected from an area where dermal exposure has occurred will have higher levels of a contaminant than blood from another location. Examples of chemicals for which blood tests are done are lead, perchloroethylene, nitrobenzene, organophosphate pesticides, and styrene. Chemicals can concentrate in red blood cell plasma, or serum, depending on the contaminant, or can be found in equal concentrations in both.

Another option involves the measurement of concentrations of parent chemical(s) and/or corresponding metabolites in the urine. Urine sampling is noninvasive and relatively easy to analyze. Urine is suitable for monitoring hydrophilic chemicals, metals, and metabolites. There are three types of urine samples: (1) collection of all urine voided during a 24-hour period; (2) collection of a single sample, often called spot collection; and (3) pooling of several spot samples over the course of a day. The 24-hour sample is the most desirable, since the levels best represent actual exposures; however, this sample is the most difficult to obtain.

Selecting the right biological monitoring method is also a challenge. Biomonitoring depends on the pharmacokinetics of the compound rather than its physical chemicals and therefore detection requires knowledge of the compound. Since biological monitoring is typically done following the exposure (workday) and sometimes requires several days to properly assess the dose, the relative contributions of different work activities cannot be assessed.

Biological monitoring cannot identify the source of exposure, which often can be done using surface and/or air sampling methods. The results of an appropriate biological monitoring study provide an integrated exposure picture. Biological monitoring is a chemical-specific approach because it is very difficult to extrapolate results to the other compounds due to differences in absorption, metabolism, and excretion profiles. Table 4 lists the advantages and disadvantages of dermal dosimetry and biological monitoring.

One technique that has been used to identify whether exposure was primarily dermal or respiratory relies on biological sampling and the use of special CPC (Hayes, Funckes, and Hartwell, 1964). Workers are divided into groups, some wearing rubber and plastic clothing to prevent skin contamination, but allowed to breathe the air so respiratory exposure can occur. Other workers have air-line respirators but wear ordinary clothing so that dermal exposure can occur. Urine or blood samples are collected and the results compared for the two groups. It is doubtful that this technique could be used now because of awareness of the potential danger.

TABLE 4. Advantages and Disadvantages of Estimating Occupational Exposure with Dermal Dosimetry and Biological Monitoring

	Advantages	*Disadvantages*
Dermal dosimetry	Routes and areas of exposure clearly defined. Routine experimental design and execution. Generic database may be created.	Dermal and respiratory absorption must be estimated. Extrapolation from pad to body surface area must be made. Not all exposure scenarios are amenable.
Biological monitoring	Actual dose may be measured. Unnecessary to adjust for value of garment/protective clothing. Integrates all routes of exposure.	Limited methods without potential interferences or cross-specificity. Pharmacokinetics must be known. Routes of exposure cannot be distinguished. Potential problems when using invasive techniques required for specimen collection. Requires more intervention to collect completely. Requires controlled dose database to interpret.

Source: Adapted from EPA, 1992.

WORK TO BE DONE

As the following chapters demonstrate, there are many methods and variations of individual methods for measuring dermal exposure. Work must be done not only in validating methods but also in determining whether comparisons can be made of sampling results collected with different methods. For example, can a gauze pad taped to the back of the hand compare to a cotton glove sample, or can a wipe sample be compared with a sample of vacuumed surface dust?

Dermal exposure warnings for workers are not often available. For example, most container labels and some material safety data sheets for chemicals with an OSHA or threshold limit value (TLV) skin designation fail to include a warning that skin penetration can occur.

Since dermal exposure limits have not been established, in most cases it is not known how much of a chemical can safely contact the skin. Currently the approach is to perform a risk assessment to develop safe exposure estimates. For the workplace the premises used for dermal risk assessments vary widely and need to be standardized. The assumptions used in risk assessment on which safe levels of dermal exposure were calculated can be relatively simplistic. These need to be upgraded to take into account clothing permeation and leakage at sleeves and other variables. Examples include the assumptions of 100% absorption for the skin and that normal work clothing provides 100% protection.

Currently there are no correlations between PELs for airborne exposure and the corresponding exposure that could occur either to the vapor/mist at PEL levels or to the most likely amount to be received in a typical dermal exposure scenario. For example, it has been calculated for PCBs, which have very low vapor pressures and are unlikely to produce significant airborne levels unless heated, spilled, sprayed, or misted, that an 8-hour inhalation exposure at the OSHA PEL of 1 mg/M^3 would produce a dose of 8 mg/day (8,000 μg/day) while the dose from one drop of 70% Askarel on the skin would produce a dermal exposure of 54,000 μg/day (Gillen and Schneider, 1992).

It is known that vapors can penetrate the skin, although the specific airborne concentrations that present a hazard to skin are unknown. In the case of benzene, it has been extrapolated from published studies that whole, unclothed human body exposure to the dose from approximately 900 ppm may be equivalent to the dose from breathing 1 ppm over 8 hours (Buteau, Nocco, and McDermott, 1991). This type of information would be useful for setting limits for Level A (total encapsulating suit) protection as well as making estimates for the contribution of airborne vapors to inhalation dose.

More research needs to be done on the function of the skin barrier or how various chemical molecules penetrate this barrier. There is a great need for systematic modeling of the skin response when it is exposed to industrial chemicals, whether in vapor, aerosol, liquid, or solid form at the site of contact (Thomas, 1986). As a result of many studies in dermal absorption, a closer look is being taken at actual does, and experimentally derived coefficients are being developed to more closely describe actual absorption through the skin.

More information on the rates at which chemicals are absorbed through the skin must be developed. An agreed upon experimental parameter must be established as it is unrealistic to expect human or intensive in vivo animal testing data to be established for the many chemicals in use in a short period of time. Although rates of absorption based on in vitro studies and rates determined from mathematical models for skin absorption are available for some industrial chemicals (EPA, 1992), these data are based on exposure of the skin to high concentrations of the test agent (Cummins et al., 1992). Additional work is needed to verify or determine absorption rates for industrial chemicals at the comparatively low exposure levels that typically occur in the work environment. Even lower levels of exposure are expected at the community level.

Studies need to determine the likelihood of excretion through the skin via sweating or other mechanisms of absorbed chemicals. The impact on analytical results in sampling surveys may require adjustments. The types of chemicals most likely to be excreted through the skin must be identified as well.

Furthermore, standards need to be developed to determine "safe" levels of exposure for materials present on surfaces or collected on gauze pads. If an airborne PEL is allowable for a substance, it hardly makes sense to expect dermal and surface contamination to be zero (Cummins et al., 1992). The presence of material on surfaces when none is present in the air suggests the primary concern is dermal or oral exposure, depending on the toxicity characteristics of the material. At a minimum, surface and dermal contamination criteria need to be developed for high hazard dermal penetrants such as carcinogens and highly toxic compounds.

Evaluation of suitable skin cleaning methods for compounds of significant dermal concern is needed since soap and water have been shown to be ineffective in a number of instances.

Researchers need to agree on a uniform terminology. In many cases, the term *cloth* is used interchangeably with *gauze* (for pads) and in other cases it has a different meaning. The same problem exists with the term *filter*.

Development of new systems designed to expedite the changing of dermal exposure pads and/or to hold the pads in locations that would provide a more realistic estimate of exposure to the face are two areas that deserve further work (Davis, 1980). More research also needs to be done in comparing exposure assessments by bag rinses and absorbent gloves. The comparison should include handling all different types of concentrated formulations and application of both sprays and dusts.

An understanding of the actual amount of contaminants absorbed into materials versus what gets into the skin is needed. This is true for dermal collectors such as pads as well as clothing (and the various types of fabrics and construction). The extrapolation of dermal testing data without the concomitant knowledge of the toxicologic activity of the absorbed contaminant does not provide a complete assessment of the risk. Therefore, experimentally derived information must be integrated with field derived measurements.

Currently many dermal monitoring studies focus on providing results in terms of an exposure rate; however, corrections for exposure duration are particularly important in the case of chronic exposures to cumulative materials. As an example, pyrene, a PAH, has a biological half-life of >24 hours (Jongeneelen et al, 1988).

Chemicals that are exposed to the environment can undergo many changes. Bioavailability of materials adsorbed onto soil has been recognized and many studies are in progress, although their focus has been chlorinated materials (PCBs, tetrachlorodibenzodioxins). Just as residue decay studies for pesticides have identified that the materials present often include degradation materials, other materials that commonly contaminate surfaces in the workplace are also exposed to environmental factors (heat, light, humidity, process variables), which can affect their stability over time (Renman, Sango, and Skarping, 1986). More research needs to be done in this area to assure sampling of correct materials.

CPC effectiveness, especially of gloves, needs to be evaluated in the actual workplace operation where it will be used as well as in the laboratory. Lab tests can determine which glove materials are most effective for specific contaminants, but not how they will stand up under humidity, high temperatures, and pressure required to perform various tasks (Gunderson et al., 1989). Therefore, more studies are needed that reflect actual field conditions including exposures to mixtures rather than pure substances.

Surface sampling techniques need to be standardized (EPA, 1985). Sampling of contaminated equipment and structural materials is the foundation upon which decontamination strategies are built and the means by which the effectiveness of strategies are evaluated. Surface sampling generally employs a variation of wet and dry wiping techniques as a means of assessing the nature and extent of contamination, but suffers from variable collection efficiency.

Problems also exist for standardizing hand wiping and house dust collection techniques in order to facilitate comparison of results across studies (Que Hee et al., 1985).

In cases where the contaminant of interest is very expensive to sample and analyze (e.g., dioxin), methods should be developed with other less costly sampling parameters and testing techniques that can indicate with acceptable accuracy the presence and level of the contaminant of interest (EPA, 1985).

There is a wide choice of materials and approaches for sampling professionals. In some cases, materials have already been evaluated for collection of certain contaminants. Reviewing the various dermal and surface studies described in the tables in Chapters 4 and 5 as well as Appendixes A–D can assist in this determination. In many other cases, evaluation has not been done prior to field use; therefore, effectiveness assessment of the sampling media will need to be performed to include the impact of various environmental conditions expected, especially for outdoor studies.

REFERENCES

Bagchi, N. I., and R. E. Zimmerman. 1980. An industrial hygiene evaluation of chimney sweeping. *AIHA J.* **41:**297–299.

Batchelor, G. S., and K. C. Walker. 1954. Health hazards involved in the use of parathion in fruit orchards of North Central Washington. *AMA Arch. Indust. Hyg.* **10:**522–529.

Buteau, G. H., R. A. Nocco and H. J. McDermott. 1991. Protecting against dermal absorption of airborne benzene vapor. *American Industrial Hygiene Conference Abstract*, Salt Lake City, UT.

Clark, N. J. 1991. Mercury exposure from silver coated paper used in photo laser machines. *Appl. Occup. Env. Hyg.* **619:**754.

Cohen, J. B., and A. G. Ruston. 1912. *Smoke, A Study of Town Air.* London.

Cummins, K., D. Morton, D. Lee, E. Cook, and R. Curtis. 1992. Exposure to acrylamide in chemical sewer grouting operations. *Appl. Occup. Env. Hyg.* **7**(6):385–391.

Davis, J. E. 1980. Minimizing occupational exposure to pesticides: Personal monitoring. *Residue Reviews* **75:**34–49.

Drinker, P. 1932. Hydrocyanic acid gas poisoning by absorption through the skin. *J. Ind. Hyg.* **14:**1–2.

Durham, W. F., and H. R. Wolfe. 1962. Measurement of the exposure of workers to pesticides. *Bull. WHO* **26:**75–91.

EPA. 1985. *Guide for Decontaminating Building, Structures and Equipment at Superfund Sites*. Washington, DC: EPA, EPA 600/2-85-028.

EPA. 1992. *Dermal Exposure Assessment: Practices and Principles*. Washington, DC: EPA.

Fenske, R. A., S. W. Horstman, and R. K. Bentley. 1987. Assessment of dermal exposure to chlorophenols in timber mills. *Appl. Ind. Hyg.* **2:**143–147.

Gillen, M., and S. Schneider. 1992. *Testimony on Behalf of the Occupational Health Foundation on OSHA's Reopening of the Proposed Rule for PPE in General Industry*. Washington, DC: OHF.

Glaser, R. A., and J. E. Arnold. 1989. Investigation of charcoal cloth as a sorbent for integrated sampling of solvent vapors in mixed-expired breath using a new stainless steel sampler. *AIHA J.* **50**(2):112–121.

Gunderson, E. C., B. A. Kingsley, C. L. Witham, and D. C. Bomberger. 1989. A practical study in laboratory and workplace permeation testing. *Appl. Ind. Hyg.* **4**(12):324–329.

Hayes, G. R., A. J. Funckes, and W. V. Hartwell. 1964. Dermal exposure of human volunteers to parathion. *Arch. Env. Health* **8:**829–833.

Henry, S. A. 1936. The study of fatal cases of cancer of the scrotum from 1911 to 1935 in relation to occupation, with special reference to chimney sweeping and cotton mule spinning. *J. Ind. Hyg.* **18:**25–29.

Honeycutt, R. C. 1986. NACA overview of assessment of mixer-loader applicator exposure to pesticides. *Toxicol. Letters* **33:**175–182.

Jongeneelen, F. J., R. B. M. Anzion, P. T. J. Scheepers, R. P. Bos, P. T. Henderson, E. H. Nijenhuis, S. J. Veenstra, R. M. E. Brouns, and A. Winkes. 1988. 1-Hydroxypyrene in urine as a biological indicator of exposure to polycyclic aromatic hydrocarbons in several work environments. *Ann. Occup. Hyg.* **32:**35–43.

Leitch, A. 1922. Note on chimney sweeps' cancer. *Brit. Med. J.* **2:**112–113.

Lloyd, J. W. 1980. Historical perspective of polycyclic aromatic hydrocarbon carcinogenesis: Implications for the transition to regenerative energy. In W. Rom and V. E. Archer (eds.), *Health Implications of New Energy Technologies*. Ann Arbor, MI: Ann Arbor Science, pp. 301–306.

Lloyd, J. W., and R. J. Young. 1983. Health and safety hazards associated with production of synthetic fuels—an introduction. *Ann ACGIH* **4:**115–118.

Nigg, H. N., J. H. Stamper, and R. M. Queen. 1986. Dicofol exposure to Florida citrus applicators: Effects of protective clothing. *Arch. Env. Contam. Toxicol.* **15:**121–134.

OSHA. 1992. *Occupational Exposure to 4,4'-Methylenedianiline (MDA)*. Final Rule. Preamble. Washington, DC: Dept. of Labor.

OSHA. 1993*a*. *Occupational Exposure to Cadmium*. Final Rule CFR 1910.1027. Washington, DC: Dept. of Labor.

OSHA. 1993*b*. *Occupational Exposure to 2-Methoxyethanol, 2-Ethoxyethanol and Their Acetates (Glycol Ethers)*. 58FR15526. Washington, DC: Dept. of Labor.

Que Hee, S. S., B. Peace, C. S. Cleark, J. R. Boyle, R. L. Bornschein, and P. B. Hammond. 1985. Evolution of efficient methods to sample lead sources such as house dust and hand dust, in the homes of children. *Env. Res.* **38:**77–95.

Rapport, S. 1988. Biological considerations for designing sampling strategies. In *Advances in Air Sampling*. Chelsea, MI: Lewis Pubs., Inc., pp. 84–93.

Renman, L., C. Sango, and G. Skarping. 1986. Determination of isocyanate and aromatic amine emissions from thermally degraded polyurethanes in foundries. *AIHA J.* **47:**621–628.

Rom, W. N., J. S. Lee, and B. F. Craft. 1981. Occupational and environmental health problems of the developing oil shale industry: A review. *Am. J. Ind. Med.* **2:**247–260.

Scherling, S. S., B. M. Overholt, and K. H. Stahmer. 1943. Treatment of burns due to chemical warfare agents. *Bull. U.S. Army Med. Dept.* **69:**52–62.

Thomas, T. A. 1986. Skin absorption: A potential contributing factor to the BEI. *Appl. Ind. Hyg.* **1**(2):87–90.

Waldron, H. A. 1983. A brief history of scrotal cancer. *Brit. J. Ind. Med.* **40:**390–401.

PART I

Chemical Hazards

CHAPTER 1

Identifying Chemicals as Hazards

While no formal mechanism exists to list chemicals as surface hazards, there are a number of approaches that have been used to categorize chemicals as dermal hazards. These include lists created in Europe and the United States. There are some commonalities among these lists, but there are also differences. It has been noted by several researchers that there are inconsistencies in the criteria used for identifying chemicals as skin permeants by various agencies and organizations, especially when individual chemicals are compared. Only a limited number of compounds with exposure limits are also regarded as skin hazards. This is true for exposure standards worldwide.

It should be noted that although some materials are capable of causing irritation, dermatitis, and sensitization in workers, only permeation is considered relevant when various government agencies or organizations categorize a chemical as a skin concern, although the development of a dermatological condition can significantly increase the potential for dermal absorption. However, this does not mean that other chemicals that can have adverse effects on the skin should be ignored. Also, where there is a significant potential for oral ingestion to occur, chemicals posing this hazard should also be identified. Microbials and radiation also pose skin hazards and should be evaluated if present. Since the most common occupational disease is dermatitis, it is useful to review these conditions and some of their common causative agents as listed in Table 1-1.

DERMAL ABSORPTION

Since most skin problems result from direct contact with a chemical substance, it is often difficult to identify a single causative substance when many chemicals are in a mixture or when multiple substances are present in an area, such as occurs during an industrial process.

To be considered a potential skin permeation hazard, chemicals do not have to be in the pure concentrated state. For example, in its proposed glycol ethers standard, the Occupational Safety and Health Administration (OSHA) has specified that operations using liquid mixtures containing less than 1% will not be exempted from the standard if there is reason to believe an airborne concentration meets or exceeds the action levels or PELs, or could present a hazard through dermal contact.

Exposures are further modified by a variety of

TABLE 1-1. Types of Occupational Dermatoses

Type	*Chemical Categories*	*Characteristics*
Inflammatory eczematous	Primary irritant Sensitizer Photosensitizer	Erythema, edema, papules, vesicles or bullae, crust, scale, and desquammation.
Chronic eczematous	Alkalis Liquids and dusts Solvents Soaps and detergents	Erythema, lichenification, scaling, dryness, and fissuring.
Folliculitis and acne form dermatoses including chloracne	Insoluble oils Greases Tars Waxes Chlorinated compounds	Chloracne with plugged sebaceous follicles and nodular and suppurative lesions. Chloracne also shows multiple cystic lesions that contain straw-colored material.
Pigmentary disturbances	Coal tars Monobenzyl ether of hydroquinone Tertiary butyl catechol Tertiary amyl phenol Tertiary butyl phenol	Increase or decrease of pigment in the epidermis.
Neoplastic	Certain petroleum products Coal tar	Keratoses, papilomata, epitheliomas, carcinomas.
Ulcerative	Arsenic trioxide Calcium compounds Cement Chromic acid	Loss of tissue on a cutaneous or mucous membrane surface leading to necrosis.
Granulomatous	Asbestos Beryllium Silica	Chronic indolent focal inflammations.
Miscellaneous	Chloroprene Vinyl chloride polymization Certain chlorinated hydrocarbons	Alopecia. Sclerodermoid changes. Porphyria cutanea tarda.

factors including a chemical's specific physical properties and the length of time it remains on the skin. For example, chemicals with good warning properties, such as irritation, are unlikely to remain on the skin because the discomfort will cause the subjects to wash their skin.

When selecting chemicals for surface or dermal sampling, it should be remembered that most criteria identifying chemicals as concerns do not consider the potential for a chemical to be a skin sensitizer, injure the skin, or cause skin cancer. These properties can also be reasons for selecting chemicals to sample.

ACGIH/OSHA Criteria

The American Conference of Governmental Industrial Hygienists (ACGIH) uses the skin notation to refer to the potential significant contribution by a chemical to exposure by the cutaneous route, including mucous membranes and the eyes, either by contact with vapors or by direct skin contact with the substance (liquid or dust). ACGIH has a policy of using a dermal lethal dose to 50% (LD_{50}) (of rabbits) of 1 g/kg as a general cutoff for determining when to classify a substance as sufficiently absorbable to present a hazard via the percutaneous route; that is, substances having a single dose dermal LD_{50} of less than 1 g/kg receive a skin notation, and those with a dermal LD_{50} above this cutoff do not. If a repeated dose (chronic) dermal study produces significant systemic effects, this finding is also considered relevant. In general, available data that suggest that chemicals with the potential for absorption via the hands/forearms during the workday could be significant and would most likely receive designation of this skin notation. Substances having a skin notation and a low threshold limit value-time weighted average (TLV-TWA) may present special problems for operations involving high airborne concentrations, due to the need to protect all skin areas as well as the inhalation route.

Historically, the majority of OSHA's chemical standards have been created by adopting ACGIH's TLVs, which generally include adopting a skin notation along with it. However, when OSHA has done its own evaluation to assign a skin notation, it has used a slightly different criteria and assigns only in instances where a substance can be percutaneously absorbed in quantities sufficient to cause systemic poisoning. OSHA also uses criteria that are defined through dermal LD_{50}s. OSHA's logic for establishing these skin notations is derived from definitions contained in an appendix of the Hazard Communication Standard 1910.1200. These definitions provide criteria for determining if chemicals are highly toxic or toxic by dermal exposure. According to OSHA, a chemical is *highly* toxic via skin absorption if it has a median LD_{50} of 200 mg/kg or less when administered by continuous contact for 24 hours (or less if death occurs within 24 hours) with the bare skin of albino rabbits weighing between 2 kg and 3 kg each. It is considered toxic via skin absorption if it has a median LD_{50} of more than 200 mg/kg but not more than 1,000 mg/kg of body weight under the same circumstances as the prior test. In both instances a skin notation would be assigned. In addition, as noted, in certain cases where available data (for any species) indicate that dermal contact results in a systemic dose that is equivalent to or greater than the dose that would be permitted by the permissible exposure limit (PEL) via inhalation, OSHA has assigned a skin notation.

In the future, the criteria for a skin designation is likely to be more complicated than that which has been used previously. In September 1991 OSHA asked the Toxic Substances Control Act (TSCA) Interagency Testing Committee to evaluate the need for dermal absorption testing for 658 chemicals. So far, of 99 that have been reviewed, 58 have been designated for testing. TSCA requires the Environmental Protection Agency (EPA) to either begin rulemaking to test the chemicals or to publish its reasons for not doing so within 12 months of these requests.

Criteria Based on Pesticides

Field reentry intervals are required by the EPA (in 40 *CFR* 158.140) for highly toxic pesticides that have use types likely to result in high dermal and inhalation exposure to people entering pesticide-treated fields. For estimating penetration of pesticides through the skin, pesticide manufacturers who are required to submit data can either assume 100% absorption or provide testing data to indicate that absorption is less than 100%. The EPA has also set a criterion for pesticide toxicity based on the dermal LD_{50}, which designates chemicals with an LD_{50} of 200 mg/kg or less for dermal testing. The California Department of Food and Agriculture (CDFA) has also established field reentry toxicology criteria as follows: LD_{50} less than 2,000 mg/kg for dermal testing; highly irritating to skin; being a sensitizer; and involving a potential risk of a chronic health effect.

The World Health Organization (WHO) has also established criteria for the classification of pesticides. It differs from the EPA in that it incorporates the physical state of the pesticide, liquid or solid. The dermal LD_{50}s are set accordingly. The criteria are intended to be applied to the formulation as sold rather than just the pure substance.

The European Economic Community (EEC) criteria is similar to those established by WHO. It also differentiates between the physical state of the pesticide, liquid or solid. These criteria in turn have been adopted by various countries that be-

TABLE 1-2. Dermal Toxicity Classifications

	EPA Rat Dermal LD_{50} (mg/kg)	*EEC Rat Dermal LD_{50} (mg/kg)*			*WHO Rat Dermal LD_{50} (mg/kg)*	
	All	*Solids*	*Liquids*		*Solids*	*Liquids*
Highly Toxic	0–200	0–10	0–50	Extremely hazardous	0–10	0–40
Toxic	>200–2,000	>10–100	>50–400	Highly hazardous	>10–100	>40–400
Moderate	>2,000–20,000			Moderately hazardous	>100–1,000	>400–4,000
Harmful		>100–1,000	>400–4,000	Slightly hazardous	>1,000	>4,000
Low	>20,000					

long to the EEC. See Table 1-2 for the dermal toxicity classifications of the EPA, WHO, and EEC.

Other Dermal Criteria

Sampling professionals who are not acquainted with the experimental criteria used to test chemicals for skin absorption can identify chemicals for dermal sampling by following the previous criteria or by reviewing the literature for pertinent studies. In some cases, review articles exist that identify chemicals as dermal permeants. Because this type of data is frequently used by organizations to identify chemicals, it is often more current and will provide information on chemicals not currently classified as skin permeants. In the future, it is likely that simplistic criteria such as relying on acute LD_{50}s will be abandoned in favor of more sophisticated criteria such as permeability constants, flux, and short-term absorption rates.

A completely different criterion for that is not LD_{50}-based for identifying chemicals posing a dermal absorption concern has been defined on the basis of the flux predicted from physical properties of the chemical (Fiserova-Bergerova, Pierce, and Droz, 1990). Critical flux is defined as a hypothetical penetration rate through the stratum corneum, which causes the biological levels to increase above those reached during inhalation exposure to a TLV-TWA. Critical flux is determined by comparing the dermal uptake rate under specified exposure conditions with the pulmonary uptake rate during exposure to the TLV-TWA at a steady rate.

A critical effect for a skin notation can be (1) the appearance of the chemical in a biological specimen obtained from dermally exposed subjects; (2) the increase of biological level of the chemical above the no-effect level; (3) biochemical changes; and (4) acute or chronic systemic toxic effect.

The effect of dermal absorption has been evaluated at two biologically significant levels: (1) the dermal absorption potential is considered significant if the dermal penetration rate of nonvolatile chemicals exceeds 30% of the pulmonary uptake rate during an occupational inhalation exposure to the TLV-TWA, or if dermal absorption of volatile chemicals increases the arterial blood concentration 30% above the concentration most likely reached during occupational inhalation exposure to the TLV-TWA; and (2) the potential for systemic toxicity induced by dermal exposure is considered significant if the biological levels triple compared with the biological levels resulting from inhalation exposure to a TLV-TWA. It is recommended that only chemicals in the second category, which have the potential for systemic toxicity, be assigned a skin notation. Compounds that are considered skin permeants by the various criteria discussed so far are listed in Table 1-3.

(Text continues on page 27.)

TABLE 1-3. Compounds Considered Skin Permeants

Compound	ACGIH	OSHA	EPA	OTHER
Acetic acid				• (1)
Acetone				• (1)
Acetonitrile				• (1)
Acetylsalicylic acid				• (1)
Acrylamide	•	•	• (2)	• (11)
Acrylic acid	•	•		
Acrylonitrile	•			• (11)
Adiponitrile	•			
Aldrin	•	•		• (11,20)
Allyl alcohol	•	•		• (1,11)
2-Aminopyridine				• (1)
n-Amyl acetate				• (1)
Aniline and homologues	•	•		• (1,11)
Anisidine	•	•		
Atrazine				• (1)
Azinphos-methyl	•	•		• (20)
Azodrin				• (20)
Baygon				• (20)
Benzene	•			• (1,9,11,12)
Benzidine	•			
Biphenyl				• (1)
Bromoform		•		
1,3-Butadiene				• (1)
2-Butoxyethanol	•	•		• (17)
n-Butyl alcohol	•	•		• (1)
sec-Butyl alcohol				• (1)
n-Butyl acetate				• (1)
n-Butyl acrylate				• (1)
n-Butylamine	•			• (1,11)
tert-Butyl chromate	•	•		
o-sec-Butylphenol	•	•		
p-tert-Butyltoluene				• (1)
Caffeine				•
Captafol	•			
Carbaryl				• (11,15,20)
Carbon disulfide	•	•		• (1,11)
Carbon tetrachloride	•			• (1,11)
Catechol	•	•		
Chlordane	•	•		• (11)
Chlorinated camphene	•	•		
Chlorinated naphthalenes				• (11)
Chloroacetyl chloride	•			
o-Chlorobenzylidene malononitrile	•	•		
Chlorodiphenyl (42% and 54% chlorine)	•	•	•	
2-Chloroethanol				• (11)
bis(2-Chloroethyl)ether				• (11)
Chloroform				• (1)
Chloropicrin				• (1)
β-Chloroprene	•	•		• (11)
Chlorpyrifos	•	•		
Chromium				• (14)
Cresol isomers	•	•		• (1,11)
Cumene	•	•		• (1)
Cyanides	•			• (11)

TABLE 1-3. *continued*

Compound	*ACGIH*	*OSHA*	*EPA*	*OTHER*
Cyclohexanol	•	•		• (1)
Cyclohexanone	•	•		• (1)
Cyclonite	•	•		
2,4-D				• (20)
DDT		•		
Decaborane	•	•		
Demeton	•	•		• (11)
Diazinon	•	•		• (11)
2-N-Dibutylaminoethanol	•			
Dibutyl phenyl phosphate	•			
o-Dichlorobenzene	•			• (1)
3,3′-Dichlorobenzidine	•			
1,4-Dichloro-2-butene	•			
Dichloroethane				• (1)
Dichloroethyl ether	•	•		• (1)
Dichloropropene	•	•		
Dichlorvos	•	•		• (11)
Dicrotophos	•	•		
Dicyclopentadiene				• (1)
Dieldrin	•	•		• (1,11,20)
Diethanolamine				• (1)
Diethylamine	•			
2-Diethylaminoethanol	•	•		• (1)
Diethylene triamine	•			• (1)
Diethyl ketone				• (1)
Diisopropylamine	•	•		• (1)
N,N-Dimethyl acetamide	•	•		• (11)
Dimethylaniline	•	•		• (1,11)
Dimethyl 1,2-dibromo-2,2-dichloroethyl phosphate		•		
Dimethylformamide	•	•		• (11)
1,1-Dimethylhydrazine	•	•		• (11)
Dimethyl phthalate				• (1)
Dimethyl sulfoxide (DMSO)	•	•		• (11)
Dinitrobenzene	•	•		• (11)
Dinitro-o-cresol	•	•		• (11)
Dinitrotoluene	•	•		• (11)
Dioxane	•	•		• (1,11)
Dioxathion	•	•		
Dioxin				• (3)
Diphenylamine				• (1)
Dipropylene glycol methyl ether	•	•		
Diquat	•			• (20)
Disulfoton		•		
Diuron				• (1)
DMAC				• (1)
DMF				• (1)
Endosulfan	•	•		
Endrin	•	•		• (11)
Enflurane				• (1)
Epichlorohydrin	•	•		• (11)
EPN	•	•		• (11)
Ethanolamine				• (1)
Ethion	•	•		• (20)
2-Ethoxyethanol	•	•		• (1,11)

TABLE 1-3. *continued*

Compound	*ACGIH*	*OSHA*	*EPA*	*OTHER*
2-Ethoxyethyl acetate	•	•		
Ethyl acetate				• (1)
Ethyl acrylate		•		• (11)
Ethyl alcohol				• (1)
Ethyl amine				• (1)
Ethyl benzene				• (1)
Ethyl bromide	•			
Ethyl butyl amine				• (1)
Ethylene chlorohydrin	•	•		
Ethylene diamine	•			
Ethylene dibromide	•			• (11)
Ethylene glycol				• (1)
Ethylene glycol, monobutyl ether				• (11)
Ethylene glycol, monoethyl ether acetate				• (11)
Ethylene glycol, monomethyl ether acetate				• (11)
Ethylene glycol dinitrate	•	•		
Ethylene imine				• (11)
Ethyl ether				• (1)
Ethyl formate				• (1)
Ethyl mercaptan				• (1)
N-Ethylmorpholine	•	•		
Fenamiphos	•	•		
Fenthion	•	•		
Fonofos	•	•		
Formaldehyde				• (1)
Formamide	•			• (1)
Formic acid				• (1)
Furfural		•		• (1,11)
Furfuryl alcohol	•	•		
Glycerin				• (1)
Halothane				• (1)
Heptachlor	•	•		• (11)
Heptachlor epoxide	•			
Heptane				• (1)
Hexachlorobenzene	•			
Hexachlorobutadiene	•			
Hexachloroethane	•	•		• (1,11)
Hexachloronaphthalene	•	•		
Hexafluoroacetone	•	•		
Hexamethyl phosphoramide	•			
Hexane				• (1)
Hexylene glycol				• (1)
Hydrazine	•	•		• (1,11)
Hydrogen cyanide	•	•		• (11)
2-Hydroxypropyl acrylate	•	•		
Isoamyl alcohol				• (1)
Isobutyl alcohol				• (1)
Isooctyl alcohol	•	•		
Isophorone diisocyanate		•		
Isopropyl alcohol				• (1)
Isopropylamine				• (1)
N-Isopropylaniline	•	•		
Lindane	•	•		• (1,11,20)
Malathion	•	•		• (11,20)
Manganese cyclopentadienyl tricarbonyl	•	•		

TABLE 1-3. *continued*

Compound	*ACGIH*	*OSHA*	*EPA*	*OTHER*
Mercury (aryl and inorganic compounds)		•		
Mercury (alkyl organic compounds)		•		
Mercury vapor	•	•		• (11,16)
Mesityl oxide				• (1)
Methacrylic acid		•		
Methoxychlor				• (1)
2-Methoxyethanol	•	•		• (1,11)
2-Methoxyethyl acetate	•	•		
4-Methoxyphenol				• (1)
Methyl acetate				• (1)
Methyl acrylate	•	•		• (11)
Methylacrylonitrile	•	•		
Methyl alcohol	•	•		• (1,11)
Methylamine				• (1)
Methyl n-amyl ketone				• (1)
n-Methyl aniline	•			• (1,11)
Methyl bromide	•	•		• (11)
Methyl n-butyl ketone	•			• (1)
Methyl chloride	•			• (1)
o-Methylcyclohexanone	•	•		• (11)
2-Methylcyclopentadienyl manganese tricarbonyl	•	•		
Methyl demeton	•	•		• (11)
Methylene chloride				• (1)
4,4′-Methylene bis (2-chloroaniline)	•	•		
Methylene dianiline	•			
Methyl ethyl ketone				• (1)
Methyl hydrazine	•	•		
Methyl iodide	•	•		• (1,11)
Methyl isoamyl ketone				• (1)
Methyl isobutyl ketone				• (1)
Methyl isobutyl carbinol	•	•		• (11)
Methyl isocyanate	•	•		• (11)
Methyl parathion	•			• (11)
Methyl propyl ketone				• (1)
Metribuzin				• (1)
Mevinphos	•			• (11)
Monocrotophos	•			
Monomethyl aniline		•		
Morpholine	•	•		• (1,11)
Naled	•			
Naphthalene				• (1)
Nicotine		•		• (11)
p-Nitroaniline	•	•		• (1,11)
Nitrobenzene	•	•		• (11,18)
p-Nitrochlorobenzene	•	•		• (11)
4-Nitrodiphenyl	•			
Nitroglycerin	•	•		• (11)
Nitroglycol				• (11)
Nitromethane				• (1)
N-Nitrosodimethylamine	•			
Nitrotoluene	•	•		• (1,11)
Octachloronaphthalene	•	•		
PAHs				• (4,5)
Paraquat		•		• (11)

TABLE 1-3. *continued*

Compound	*ACGIH*	*OSHA*	*EPA*	*OTHER*
PCBs				• (6,7,8,11,13)
Parathion, ethyl	•	•	•	• (11,15,20)
Pentachlorophenol	•	•		• (1,11)
Pentaerythritol				• (1)
Phenol	•	•		• (11,19)
Phenothiazine	•	•		
Phenylene diamine				• (1,11)
Phenyl ether				• (1)
Phenylhydrazine	•	•		• (11)
Phenyl mercaptan				• (1)
Phorate	•	•		
Phosdrin		•		
Picric acid		•		• (11)
Propargyl alcohol	•	•		• (11)
Propoxur				• (1)
Propyl acetate				• (1)
n-Propyl alcohol	•			• (1)
Propylene dichloride				• (1)
Propylene imine	•	•		
Ronnel				• (1)
Sodium azide		•		
Sodium fluoroacetate	•	•		• (11)
Sodium perfluoroacetate	•			
Strychnine				• (1)
Styrene	•			• (1)
Sulfotep	•	•		
2,3,7,8-TCDD			•	
TEPP	•	•		
1,1,2,2-Tetrachloroethane	•	•		• (1,11)
Tetrachloronaphthalene	•	•		
Tetraethyl lead	•	•		• (11)
Tetramethyl lead	•	•		• (11)
Tetramethyl succinonitrile	•	•		
Tetryl		•		• (11)
Thallium	•	•		• (11)
Thiocarb				• (15)
Thioglycolic acid	•	•		• (1)
Tin (organic compounds)	•	•		
Toluene	•			• (1,11)
Toluidine	•			
o-, m-, p-Toluidine	•	•		• (1)(o-,p-) • (11)(o-)
Toxaphene				• (11)
Tributyl phosphate				• (1)
Trichloroacetic acid				• (1)
1,2,4-Trichlorobenzene				• (1)
1,1,1-Trichloroethane				• (1)
1,1,2-Trichloroethane	•	•		• (1,11)
Trichloroethylene				• (1,10)
Trichloronaphthalene	•	•		
1,2,3-Trichloropropane	•			
Triethylamine				• (1)
Trimethyl benzene				• (1)
2,4,6-Trinitrotoluene	•	•		• (11)

TABLE 1-3. *continued*

Compound	*ACGIH*	*OSHA*	*EPA*	*OTHER*
Triorthocresyl phosphate	•	•		
Vinyl cyclohexene dioxide	•	•		
Xylene				• (1,11)
m-Xylene α,α′-diamine	•	•		
Xylidine	•	•		• (11)

1. V. Fiserova-Bergerova, J. T. Pierce, and P. O. Droz. 1990. Dermal absorption potential of industrial chemicals: Criteria for skin notation. *Am J. Ind. Med.* **17:**617–635.
2. Environmental Protection Agency. 1987. *Acrylamide Grouting Exposure Assessment*. EPA 560/5-87-009. Washington, DC.
3. F. S. Kelada. 1990. Occupational intake by dermal exposure to polychlorinated dibenzo-p-dioxins and polychlorinated dibenzofurans in pulp mill industry. *AIHA J.* **51**(9):519–521.
4. WHO, IARC. 1985. IARC monographs on the evaluation of the carcinogenic risk of chemicals to humans. Polynuclear aromatic compounds. Part 4. Bitmus, coal-tars and derived products, shale-oils and soots. *IARC* **35:**39–159.
5. M. S. Wolff, R. Herbert, M. Marcus, M. Rivera, P. J. Landrigan, and L. R. Andrews. 1989. Polycyclic aromatic hydrocarbon (PAH) residues on skin in relation to air levels among roofers. *Arch. Env. Health* **44**(3):157–163.
6. M. Nishizumi. 1976. Radiographic evidence for absorption of polychlorinated biphenyls through the skin. *Ind. Health* **14:**41–51.
7. M. Maroni, A. Colombi, S. Cantoni, E. Ferioli, and V. Foa. 1981. Occupational exposure to chlorinated biphenyls in electrical workers. I. Environmental and blood polychlorinated biphenyls concentrations. *Brit. J. Ind. Med.* **38:**49–54.
8. P. J. Lees, M. Corn, and P. N. Breysse. 1987. Evidence for dermal absorption as the major route of body entry during exposure of transformer maintenance and repairment to PCBs. *AIHA J.* **48:**257–264.
9. J. Hanke, T. Dutkiewica, and J. Piotrowski. 1961. The absorption of benzene through the skin in men. *Med. Pracy* **12:**413–426.
10. R. D. Stewart and H. C. Dodd. Absorption of carbon tetrachloride, trichloroethylene, tetrachloroethylene, methylene chloride, and 1,1,1-trichloroethane through human skin. *AIHA J.* **25:** 438–443.
11. P. Grandjean. 1990. *Skin Penetration: Hazardous Chemicals at Work*. New York: Taylor & Francis.
12. A. S. Susten, B. L. Dames, J. R. Burg, and R. W. Niemeler. 1985. Percutaneous penetration of benzene in hairless mice: An estimate of dermal absorption during tire-building operations. *Am. J. Ind. Med.* **7:**323–335.
13. R. C. Wester, D. A. W. Bucks, H. I. Maibach, and J. Anderson. 1983. Polychlorinated biphenyls (PCBs): Dermal absorption, systemic elimination, and dermal wash efficiency. *J. Tox. Env. Health* **12:**511–519.
14. R. E. Bagdon and R. E. Hazen. 1991. Skin permeation and cutaneous hypersensitivity as a basis for making risk assessments of chromium as a soil contaminant. *Env. Health Perspective* **92:**111–119.
15. J. B. Knaak and B. W. Wilson. 1985. Dermal dose-cholinesterase response and percutaneous absorption studies with several cholinesterase inhibitors. In *Dermal Exposure Related to Pesticide Use*. Washington, DC: American Chemical Society.
16. J. B. Hursh, T. W. Clarkson, E. F. Miles, and L. A. Goldsmith. 1989. Percutaneous absorption of mercury vapor by man. *Arch. Env. Health* **44**(2):120–127.
17. G. Johanson, A. Boman, and B. Dynesius. 1988. Percutaneous absorption of 2-butoxyethanol in man. *Scand. J. Work Env. Health* **14:**101–109.
18. J. Piotrowski. 1967. Further investigations on the evaluation of exposure to nitrobenzene. *Brit. J. Ind. Med.* **24:**60–65.
19. J. Piotrowski. 1971. Evaluation of exposure to phenol: Absorption of phenol vapour in the lungs and through the skin and excretion of phenol in urine. *Brit. J. Ind. Med.* **28:**172–178.
20. R. J. Feldmann and H. I. Maibach. 1974. Percutaneous penetration of some pesticides and herbicides in man. *Toxicol. Appl. Pharm.* **28:**126–132.

DERMAL CONTACT EFFECTS

Skin Irritation

Most occupational dermatitis is caused by primary irritant chemicals. These agents cause dermatitis by directly acting on the surface of normal skin if they are left in contact for a sufficient length of time. Strong or concentrated materials such as sulfuric acid, sodium hydroxide, or methyl bromide produce an observable effect within a few minutes depending on their concentration. Conversely, weak or marginal irritants such as acetone and detergents may require several days and several exposures before a recognizable change occurs. The degree of irritation can vary, and, in some cases, the impact of a corrosive chemical such as concentrated sodium hydroxide can be very severe, causing significant burns to the skin's surface. Amines comprise a class of irritants for which surface sampling is commonly performed because they can stick and remain on surfaces. Some amines can also be sensitizers. Table 1-4 is a listing of skin irritants.

The mechanism by which chemicals produce skin damage varies according to the specific properties of the chemical. Lipid solvents disturb the water-holding quality of the skin cells, allowing the skin to dry out and producing a scaly dermatitis.

TABLE 1-4. Chemicals That Are Skin Irritants

Acrolein
Allyl alcohol
Allyl glycidyl ether
Ammonia
Ammonium chloride fume
n-Butyl acetate
Caprolactam, dust and vapor
Chlorine
Chloroacetyl chloride
o-Chlorobenzylidene malononitrile
Diethylamine
Diethylenetriamine
Ethyl benzene
Glutaraldehyde
2-Hydroxypropyl acrylate
Methyl 2-cyanoacrylate
Phosphoric acid
Potassium hydroxide
Sodium bisulfite
Sodium hydroxide
Thioglycolic acid
1,2,4-Trichlorobenzene
Triethylamine
Tetrasodium borate salts

Skin Sensitization

Cutaneous sensitizers pose greater concerns than primary irritants as a skin hazard in that once sensitized, many persons cannot tolerate further exposure to the chemical. Most sensitizers do not produce demonstrable cutaneous changes on first contact however, the sensitizer induces certain specific cellular changes in the skin so that after a period of incubation (five to seven days or more) further contact with the same or a closely related agent on the same or other parts of the body produces an acute skin response such as erythema, edema, and vesiculation. Sensitization reactions are frequently more severe and more persistent than irritation reactions. Some sensitizing chemicals are epoxy monomers and their amine hardeners, formaldehyde, and tetramethylthiuram disulfide. In some cases, compounds producing an allergic sensitization of the skin have also produced sensitization in the lungs. This effect is thought to be produced by isocyanates. Table 1-5 lists other chemicals that are skin sensitizers.

Photosensitivity and Vitiligo

Photosensitivity is the capacity of a chemical to be stimulated to activity by light or to react to light. The exposed skin displays a markedly enhanced sunburn response with sufficient ultraviolet (UV) stimulation. Eventually, hyperpigmentation of exposed skin areas results. These chemicals cause two different effects: phototoxic (a nonallergenic reaction) and photoallergenic materials (Table 1-6). Several derivatives of coal tar, such as anthracene,

TABLE 1-5. Chemicals That Are Skin Sensitizers

Alprenolol[a]	1-Fluoro-2,4-dinitrobenzene[b]	Phenyl glycidyl ether
Ammonicated mercury	Formalin (aqueous)	Picric acid
Bacampicillin[a]	Hydrazine[d,e]	Poison ivy
Benzocaine	Isophorone diisocyanate	Potassium dichromate
Captafol	Malathion[f]	Potassium ferricyanide[c]
Cobalt metal, fume and dust	Mercaptobenzothiazole	Quinidine[a]
Cyclomethycaine sulfate	Methylene diisocyanate	Subtilisins
Dibucaine HCl	Neomycin sulfate	Thimerosal
Diglycidyl ether of bisphenol A	Nickel	Thiram
2,4-Dinitro-1-fluorobenzene[b]	p-Phenylenediamine	Toluene-2,4-diisocyanate
Ethylenediamine	Parabens mixture	Woolwax alcohol
Ferric ammonium citrate[c]	Phenothiazine	

[a] E. V. Sargent and D. Kirk. 1988. Establishing airborne exposure control limits in the pharmaceutical industry. *AIHA J.* **49:**309–313.
[b] E. Schultheiss. 1959. Hypersensitiveness to hydrazine. *Bernfsdermatosen* **7:**131. (In German.)
[c] W. von Keilig and U. Speer. 1983. Occupational allergic dermatitis from hydrazine. *Dermatosen Beruf Umwelt* **31:**25. (In German.)
[d] T. H. Milby and W. L. Epstein. 1964. Allergic contact sensitivity to malathion. *Arch. Env. Health* **9:**434.
[e] J. S. Thompson and O. P. Edmonds. 1980. Safety aspects of handling the potent allergen FDND. *Ann. Occup. Hyg.* **23:**27–33.
[f] NIOSH Health Hazard Evaluation. May 1981. *Cyanotype Printing in an Artist's Workshop. Bucyrus*, OH. Cincinnati, OH: NIOSH, HETA 81-171-880.

TABLE 1-6. Phototoxic and Photoallergic Chemicals

Phototoxic Compounds	*Photoallergic Chemicals*
Acridine	Bithional
Anthracene	4-Chloro-2-hydroxybenzoic acid N-m-butylamide
Chlorothalonil	Chloropromazine
Chlorothiazides	Fentichlor
Coal tar	Griseofulvin
Cyanophos	Halogenated salicylanilides
Dichlorovos	6-Methylcoumarin
Dyes (acridine orange)	Promethazine
Maneb	
Paraquat	
Phenanthrene	
Phenothiazines (chlorpromazine)	
Porphyrins	
Psoralens	
Pyridine	
Salithion	
Sulfonamides	
Sulfonylureas	
Tetracyclines	

Source: After Marzulli, F. N., and H. I. Maibach (eds.). 1991. *Dermatoxicology*, 4th ed. New York: Hemisphere Publ. Corp., Div. Taylor & Francis.

phenanthrene, and pitch, possess this activity, as well as creosote.

Phototoxicity, like primary irritation, can affect anyone; however, heavily pigmented skin is more resistant. Phototoxic skin reactions are produced by certain classes of chemicals that increase the sensitivity of the skin to UV radiation, resulting in erythema, hyperpigmentation, and sometimes blistering. Among the most common phototoxins are the psoralens or furocoumarins contained in perfumes, in wild plants (stinking mayweed and giant hogweed), and in common vegetables such as celery, carrots, dill, parsley, and Persian limes. When infected by a common fungus known as pink rot, celery becomes a potent phototoxin. Outbreaks of phototoxic dermatitis have been seen in both celery harvesters and celery canners.

Vitiligo, the loss of pigment in the skin, is the opposite of photosensitization. Exposures occur most commonly with phenol-based germicidal agents, antioxidants used in rubber processing, materials or chemicals used in the manufacture of phenolic resins, and photographic processing chemicals such as hydroquinone. Often the depigmentation is permanent as many of these chemicals kill the melanocytes in the tissue. In one plant an individual who often smoked cigarettes without washing his hands was assigned the task of adding scoops of p-tertiary butyl catechol to batches of polyester resin during which he did not always use gloves (Horio, Tanaka, and Komura, 1977). After some months he noticed that there was depigmentation on his hands, arms, and lower lip.

Skin Cancer

The primary chemicals associated with skin cancer are polycyclic aromatic hydrocarbons (PAHs) such as those found in coke oven batteries, coal tar, used motor oils, and many other similar materials. The main types of skin cancer related to these chemicals are basal cell carcinoma and squamous cell carcinoma (NIOSH, 1983). For light-skinned individuals who spend a lot of time outdoors exposed to the sun, there is an increased likelihood of basal cell carcinomas regardless of exposure to chemicals. However, if exposed to both they may have an increased susceptibility. Some genetic conditions (e.g., xeroderma pigmentosum) also increase the risk for developing basal cell carcinoma.

Squamous cell carcinomas have numerous predisposing factors including chronic sun exposure in fair complexioned people. Other factors include exposure to arsenic compounds, organic hydrocarbons such as pitch and tar, chewing betel nut and tobacco, chronic ulcers, and radiation or thermal injury. A condition that, while not in itself malignant, may progress to squamous cell carcinoma is actinic keratosis. It occurs at skin surfaces previously damaged by the sun. Hence, occupational groups with chronic sun exposure have a higher risk than similar workers in sun-sheltered jobs to developing skin malignancies.

Other Chemical Concerns

Some chemicals cannot be classified under any of these categories. Metallic salts of arsenic, mercury, zinc, and chromium precipitate skin protein, and if the concentration of these materials is sufficient, ulceration of the skin occurs. Beryllium can produce contact dermatitis in which a variety of rashes may develop after an incubation period of 10 to 14 days. Accidental implantation of a metal sliver in the skin may produce a beryllium ulcer, which may become chronic. Chloracne is an extreme form of acne produced by exposure to a variety of chlorinated aromatic compounds, and is often accompanied by serious systemic toxicity. Compounds known to cause chloracne include chloronaphthalenes, polychlorinated biphenyls, polychlorinated dibenzofurans, chlorobenzenes, dichlorobenzonitrile, and polychlorinated dibenzo-p-dioxin. The clinical features of chloracne consist of cysts, comedones (blackheads), pustules, and abscesses that heal with eventual scarring. Comedones resulting from follicular hyperkeratosis may predominate and may involve nearly every hair follicule.

TABLE 1-7. Oral Toxicity Classifications

	EPA Rat Dermal LD_{50} (mg/kg)	EEC Rat Dermal LD_{50} (mg/kg)			WHO Rat Dermal LD_{50} (mg/kg)	
	All	Solids	Liquids		Solids	Liquids
Highly toxic	0–50	0–5	0–25	Extremely hazardous	0–5	0–20
Toxic	>50–500	>5–50	>25–200	Highly hazardous	>5–50	>20–200
Moderate	>500–5,000			Moderately hazardous	>50–500	>200–2,000
Harmful		>50–500	>200–2,000	Slightly hazardous	>500	2,000
Low	>5,000					

Microbials and Radiation

Microorganisms and radioactive dusts pose skin as well as surface concerns due to their potential to become airborne if dust is resuspended. Microbials pose a unique concern in that they often get into heating, ventilating, and air conditioning systems, and once a reservoir is established, they can be blown into various parts of buildings.

ORAL TOXICITY

Just as there are several different criteria for dermal absorption, so are there for oral toxicity. In general, compounds with oral LD_{50}s (to rats) of 500 mg/kg and less are candidates, but those with higher LD_{50}s (meaning less toxic) must be evaluated on a case-by-case basis. Similar to their dermal toxicity criteria, the EPA, EEC, and WHO have criteria for oral toxicity of pesticides (Table 1-7).

Cadmium is an example of a chemical that is hazardous if ingested orally. It can be toxic even though only 3–7% of ingested cadmium will be absorbed by the digestive system. Toxicity increases with nutritional deficiencies of calcium, iron, or protein to as high as 20% (Elinder, 1985). However, like many chemicals it poses a greater hazard if inhaled because 25–50% of inhaled cadmium is absorbed (Friberg, 1985).

REFERENCES

Elinder, C. G. 1985. Cadmium: Uses, occurrence and intake. In L. Friberg et al. (eds.), *Cadmium and Health*. Boca Raton, FL: CRC Press.

Fiserova-Bergerova, V., J. T. Pierce, and P. O. Droz. 1990. Dermal absorption potential of industrial chemicals: Criteria for skin notation. *Am. J. Ind. Med.* **17:**617–635.

Friberg, L. T. 1985. The rationale of biological monitoring of chemicals—with special reference to metals. *AIHA J.* **46:**633–642.

Horio, T., K. Tanaka, and J. Komura. 1977. Depigmentation due to para tertiary butyl catechol. *Int. Arch. Occup. Env. Health* **39:**127–133.

Marzulli, F. N., and H. I. Maibach. 1974. The use of graded concentrations in studying skin sensitizers: Experimental contact sensitization in man. *Food Cosmet. Toxicol.* **12:**219–227.

NIOSH. August 1983. *Health Hazard Evaluation Report*. Markland Lock & Dam. Markland, KY. HETA 82-185-1353. Cincinnati, OH: NIOSH.

Nordberg, G. F., and M. Nordberg. 1988. Biological monitoring of cadmium. In T. W. Clarkson et al. (eds.), *Biological Monitoring of Toxic Metals*. New York: Plenum Press, pp. 151–168.

CHAPTER 2

Factors Affecting Chemical Permeation

The focus of skin exposure determinations is often the permeability characteristics of the contaminant, but other factors relating to the anatomy and the environment are also important. The importance of dermal exposure often depends on its contribution relative to other routes of exposure. Some factors increase the rate or extent of dermal absorption of a compound without impacting pulmonary or oral uptake, which increases the relative contribution of the dermal pathway to total dose. Therefore, performing dermal exposure evaluations is much more complicated than just identifying those chemicals with high permeation rates.

The structure and condition of the skin as well as the specific characteristics of a contaminant determine whether a harmful exposure takes place. The skin surface area and skin site exposed, duration and frequency of exposure, contaminant absorption rate and fraction absorbed through the skin, concentration of the contaminant, its physical state and the mixture in which it is contained are all important factors that affect dermal exposure. Individual and job-specific factors include skin hydration from sweating, preexisting dermatitis, abrasions, the effectiveness of chemical protective clothing (if worn) and wearing contaminated work clothing for extended periods of time (see Chapter 4). In addition, the absence or presence of adequate chemical warning properties is important, such as visual stains on the skin or irritation that would make a person more likely to wash the skin promptly, thus limiting the exposure period.

THE SKIN

Commonly called the acid mantle of the skin, a waxy type of mixture composed of sebum, breakdown products of keratin, and sweat coats the outer surface of the skin. It is believed that this coating protects against the penetration of water and water-soluble chemicals, but this protection is minimal and the layer is easily removed by soaps, solvents, and alkaline compounds. The pH of normal skin is variable but usually is between 4.5 and 5.5 (slightly acidic), which inhibits the growth of many microbes. Figure 2-1 illustrates the structure of the skin.

The skin itself is composed of two layers: (1) the epidermis, a layer about 100 μm thick, and (2) the dermis, a layer about 500–3,000 μm thick. The outermost layer of the epidermis, the multilayered stratum corneum, is about 10–40 μm thick and is considered the first and main

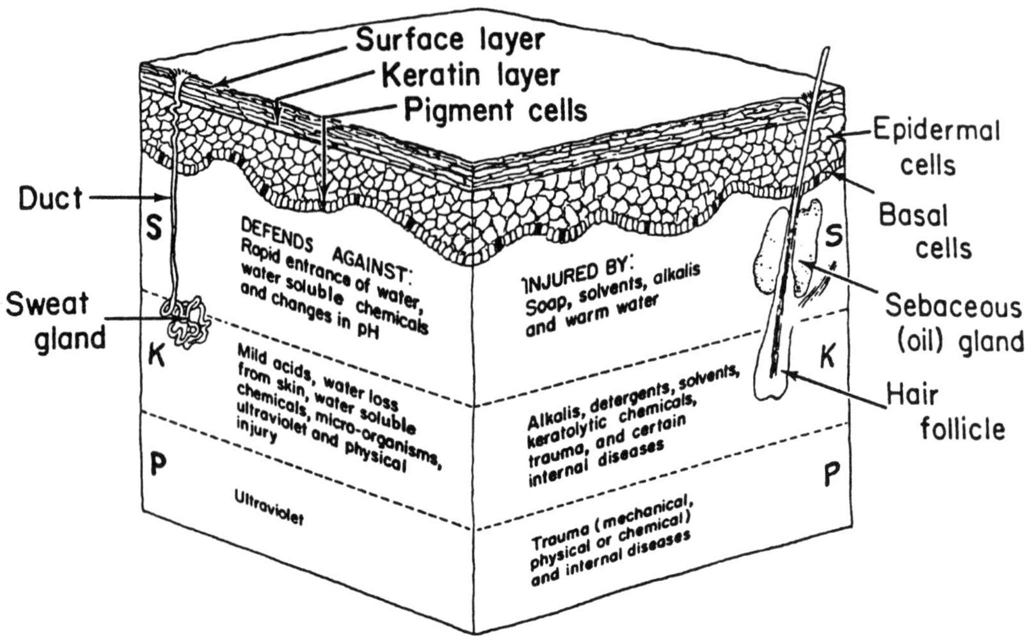

Figure 2-1. Structure of the skin.
Source: From NIOSH. 1973. *The Industrial Environment, Its Evaluation and Control*. Cincinnati: NIOSH.

diffusion barrier for most compounds. This layer contains about 40% protein, 40% water, and 15–20% lipids. It is composed of dead, partially desiccated and keratinized epidermal cells that continually slough off, exposing new skin cells. Below this layer lies the viable epidermis, a region without a blood supply, containing at its base the basal cell layer whose cells divide and multiply, moving outward to replace the outer epidermis as it wears away. This layer generates about one new cell layer per day, which results in the stratum corneum becoming totally replaced once every two to three weeks.

Dermis forms the main bulk of the skin and is composed of elastic and collagen tissue that provides the skin with its resiliency. It contains sweat glands with ducts that deliver sweat to the surface of the skin; hair follicles that encase hairs; sebaceous or oil glands that excrete their products, including sebum, through the hair follicle openings on the skin; blood vessels; and nerves. The blood vessels are composed of an embedded capillary system that transports chemicals penetrating through the upper skin layers to the body's main circulatory system.

In the lowermost region of the epidermal layer are the basal cells that divide to produce the epidermal cells. Within the basal cell layer are melanocyte cells that produce pigment in the form of melanin granules. Melanin is a protective screen against sunlight because the granules absorb photons of light. Sunlight and certain chemicals stimulate pigment formation and other chemicals inhibit formation.

Absorption and Exposure Site

Skin can absorb chemicals directly through the epidermal cells and through the hair and sweat follicles. The stratum corneum has an affinity for both water-soluble (hydrophilic) and lipid-soluble (hydrophobic) compounds, which is sometimes referred to as bifunctional solubility. This affinity is due to the mosaic, filament-matrix ultrastructure of the intracellular keratin that allows for layers of both aqueous (protein-water) and lipid membranes (Scheuplein, 1976). These layers provide separate pathways for the cellular diffusion of hydrophilic and hydrophobic molecules through the epidermis (Michaels, Chandrasekaran, and Shaw, 1975).

An alternative to transport of a compound through cellular pathways in the stratum corneum is penetration via skin appendages, such as hair follicles, sebaceous glands, and sweat glands. Chemicals that get in through these structures would bypass the stratum corneum reaching the dermis directly, however, since they occupy less than 1% of the human skin surface, their role as transport channels is often negligible (EPA, 1992). It is thought that for slowly diffusing chemicals this mode may be a contributing or even dominant pathway of dermal permeation, especially during the period immediately following skin exposure (Scheuplein and Blank, 1971). As an example, due to the high follicular density of the scalp, it may be a significant absorption route for certain organic chemicals if encountered during swimming or showering.

The specific skin site that is exposed will also influence the degree of exposure. Certain areas such as the scrotum are more permeable than other areas of the body primarily due to differences in stratum corneum thickness (Table 2-1). However, site-specific variations in permeability may also be related to the lipid content of the stratum corneum at that site with higher content favoring increased absorption (Elias et al., 1981). In addition, the effects of regional variation appear to be modified by whether the compound involved is hydrophilic or lipophilic, which may be related to the different mechanisms by which these compounds penetrate the skin (Marzulli, 1962). Table 2-2 lists anatomical regions and the amount of parathion and malathion that would be absorbed by a specific anatomical area if each one received the same dose, providing a comparison of the differences in permeability for each area.

As noted, contaminants that permeate the skin can enter the systemic circulation via the capillaries in the dermis. However, before reaching the capillaries, these compounds can also be depleted by evaporation from the surface of the skin; reversible or irreversible binding with the stratum corneum; metabolism in the viable epidermis; or by temporarily partitioning into the protein or lipid phases of the various dermal strata. In the case of irreversible binding, the percutaneous absorption of a compound may be limited. For example, the regular sloughing of dead cells by the skin aids in the elimination of compounds, such as mercury, that bind to the stratum corneum. In other cases, binding could create a reservoir of the compound in the tissue, reducing the rate and amount of chemical enter-

TABLE 2-1. Regional Variation in Stratum Corneum Thickness in Humans

Skin Area	*Stratum Corneum Thickness (μm)*
Abdomen	15.0
Volar forearm	16.0
Back	10.5
Forehead	13.0
Scrotum	5.0
Back of Hand	49.0
Palm	400.0
Sole	600.0

Source: From EPA. 1992. *Dermal Exposure Assessment: Principles and Applications*. Washington, DC: Office of Health and Environmental Assessment. EPA 600/8-91-011B.

TABLE 2-2. Effect of Anatomical Region on In Vivo Percutaneous Absorption of Pesticides in Humans

Anatomical Region	*Parathion Dose Absorbed (%)*	*Malathion Dose Absorbed (%)*
Forearm	8.6	6.8
Palm	11.8	5.8
Foot, ball	13.5	6.8
Abdomen	18.5	9.4
Hand, dorsum	21.0	12.5
Forehead	36.3	23.2
Axilla	64.0	28.7
Jaw angle	33.9	69.9
Fossa cubitalis	28.4	
Scalp	32.1	
Ear canal	46.6	
Scrotum	101.6	

Source: From Wester, R. C., and H. I. Maibach. 1989. Regional Variation in percutaneous absorption. In R. Bronaugh and H. I. Maibach (eds.). *Percutaneous Absorption*. New York: Marcel Dekker, pp. 335–342.

ing the systemic circulation (EPA, 1992). High concentrations of chromium were measured in the severely damaged skin of a patient who continued to have a high body burden despite reduction of blood concentrations through treatment. It was theorized that the skin had become a depot from which chromium continued to enter the blood, explaining how a secondary increase in blood concentration of chromium occurred after a blood exchange transfusion had been completed (Kelly et al., 1982).

The skin contains many of the same enzymes as the liver; thus, contaminant metabolism by the skin could affect absorption, making metabolism an important factor in determining both the rate and amount of percutaneous absorption. The metabolizing potential of the skin has been estimated to be about 2% of the liver, with most of the enzyme activity localized in the epidermal layer (Pannatier et al., 1978). The metabolic activity of the epidermis, in turn, depends on the distribution and activity of specific enzyme systems and on the rate of chemical diffusion. The slower a chemical is absorbed through the skin, the greater the opportunity for some metabolism to occur. Rates of chemical transport could increase if metabolic reaction products are toxic to skin cells. Human skin may also contain enzyme detoxification systems similar to an enzyme identified in rat skin that detoxifies certain polycyclic aromatic hydrocarbons (PAHs) (Bentley et al., 1976).

A chemical that is metabolized faster than it is absorbed into the skin may be reduced in concentration (and toxic effect) as it moves through the skin compared to a chemical that is not metabolized. Similarly, the amount of parent chemical that enters the systemic circulation may be reduced because it is converted to other metabolites instead. Toxicity is not necessarily reduced. Parathion is degraded to paraoxon in the environment and in the body, a compound which is more toxic than its parent compound. Similarly, other organophosphates also degrade to more toxic oxons including ethyl parathion, azinphosmethyl, methidathion, and phosalone. Large errors in estimating absorption are possible with chemicals like organothiophosphates, which can either be activated (transformed to their oxons) or detoxified (hydrolyzed) by these enzymes during their transit through the skin (Popendorf and Leffingwell, 1982).

There is some evidence to suggest that certain chemicals can be eliminated through the skin either as a result of sweating or simply over time if they are absorbed slowly and tend to be retained in the skin. In one study of workers using an epoxy resin and amine hardener, exposure to the amine was easy to identify because it discolored when exposed to the air. As a result of their exposure to the amine, workers had persistently stained hands. To minimize this condition workers were provided with protective gloves and with white cotton gloves to wear under the protective gloves to assist in identifying breakthrough. When staining occurred to the interiors of the cotton gloves as well as the exteriors, it was determined that the workers' hands were excreting the amine while sweating, which was intensified by the use of the protective gloves (Gunderson et al., 1989). In another study using fluorescence methods to detect PAH exposure of workers in coal gasification facilities, a high fluorescence was detected on the skin of some workers before starting work. The cause was thought to be excretion of the PAHs through skin during their time away from work (Hill, 1984).

However, a moisture balance is important for the skin because increased levels of moisture including sweat or a lack of moisture (dry skin) will both increase skin absorption of chemicals (NIOSH, 1977). The stratum corneum binds a certain amount of water, normally 5–15%, and if the skin is occluded the water content can increase to as much as 50% causing permeability to increase by a factor of five for some compounds (most likely non-water-soluble and nonpolar) (Bird, 1981). It has been estimated that up to 500 mL of perspiration passes through the human skin during a single day (up to 1,000 mL with hard work and hot conditions) (Easter and Nigg, 1992). Ninety-nine percent of sweat is water, with the balance consisting of products from the body's metabolic function such as urea, lactic acid, amino acids, sugar, alkali and sulfates/phosphates (Fishberg and Bierman, 1932). The pH of perspiration is about 5.4 when freshly secreted, but it can turn alkaline with time, and in extreme cases an individual's pH may be as low as 4.0 (Raheel, 1991). Dry skin results from the loss of lipids creating a porous tissue (Scheuplein and Blank, 1971).

Skin-specific Factors

Any skin condition that compromises the capability of the stratum corneum to serve as a permeability barrier, including psoriasis, eczema, rashes, or dermatitis, may also result in increased percutaneous absorption in affected individuals (Brown, Bishop, and Rowan, 1984). Damage to the skin may occur from cuts, wounds, abrasions, or other insults such as sunburn. Chemicals such as corrosives that damage the integrity of the skin enhance its permeability to other chemicals.

Other factors that affect the degree of hazard presented by dermal exposure include individual specific individual differences, age, and gender. In addition to the basic structures, there are a wide range of skin variations both between and within individuals due to such factors as hairiness, ease of sweating, wrinkling, calluses, and smoothness (Wester and Maibach, 1983). Infants and children are at an increased risk for dermal exposure to toxic compounds because of their greater surface-to-volume ratio, immature detoxification pathways, and rapidly developing nervous systems. Although gender-related permeability differences have not been measured directly in humans, animal data that demonstrate gender differences have been noted in toxicity studies (Table 2-3). As an example, skin LD_{50}s are frequently different when both sexes of a species are dosed. There are also differences in the structure of fat cells located under the dermis. Whereas the collagen fibers of the network form a system of vertical structure in female skin, diagonal cross-striation of collagen fibers are additionally encountered in the male skin. The fibers arch upwardly into the dermis (Muller and Nurnberger, 1972).

In general, the larger the exposed surface area, the more contaminant that can be absorbed through the skin. Surface area is affected by age and body weight; children have less total surface area than adults. The relative sizes of surface areas also undergo changes with age. In general, the percentage of total surface area of the head, face, and neck decreases for the population with age. The percentage of total surface area of the lower extremities, such as thighs, increases with age, and the differences in percentages represented by different body regions between sexes changes over time, the thigh hav-

TABLE 2-3. Effect of Gender and Body Site on the Permeability of Rat Skin

	Male			*Female*		
	Permeability Constant (cm/hr + SD)	*Lag Time (hr + SD)*	*No. of Tests*	*Permeability Constant (cm/hr + SD)*	*Lag Time (hr + SD)*	*No. of Tests*
Water						
Back	0.00049 ± 0.00004	2.4 ± 0.1	7	0.00093 ± 0.00011	2.0 ± 0.1	4
Abdomen	0.00131 ± 0.00021	1.7 ± 0.2	4			
Urea						
Back	0.00016 ± 0.00005	15.0 ± 1.8	6	0.00048 ± 0.00013	11.1 ± 0.6	3
Abdomen	0.00188 ± 0.00055	16.5 ± 4.3	4			
Cortisone						
Back	0.00017 ± 0.00004	33.4 ± 4.4	8	0.00047 ± 0.00011	20.0 ± 2.6	3
Abdomen	0.00122 ± 0.00006	32.9 ± 2.4	4			

Source: From Bronaugh, R. L., and H. I. Maibach. 1983. In vitro percutaneous absorption. In F. N. Marzulli and H. I. Maibach (eds.), *Dermatoxicology*. Washington, DC: Hemisphere Press, pp. 117–129.

ing a higher percentage in the female and the stomach in the male because of the differing tendencies to store fat in these areas (Fujimoto and Watanabe, 1969). The amount of surface area available for exposure to particulate chemicals and soil is also affected by the type of clothing worn. A person wearing a long- sleeved shirt and pants has less exposed skin surface than one wearing shorts and a short-sleeved shirt.

CHEMICAL CHARACTERISTICS

It is well known that chemicals can penetrate the skin at different rates ranging from fast to extremely slow. The dermal penetration rate of exposures to 50 $\mu g/M^3$ of mercury vapor is about 0.072 $\eta g/cm^2/hr$ (Hursh et al., 1989), while contact with liquid aniline (saturated layer) yields absorption rates on the order of 0.2–0.7 $mg/cm^2/hr$ (Piotrowski, 1957). However, even though the absorption rate for aniline is much faster, if a whole-body exposure to aniline occurred, dermal absorption would account for approximately 2.6% of the exposure while respiratory intake would account for the rest.

Important factors that influence the permeation of chemicals through the skin include the compound's solubility, molecular size, concentration gradient on the skin, polarity, pH and other permeability characteristics that are measured experimentally. Skin absorption for specific chemicals is described experimentally using a number of different chemical-specific parameters, the most important being flux, permeability constants, diffusion coefficient, partition coefficients, and metabolic constants. These are defined as follows:

Flux: the amount of chemical absorbed across a defined surface area of the skin over unit time ($mg/cm^2/hr$). Flux is equal to the dermal permeability coefficient (K_p) multiplied by the concentration of the chemical. Flux and concentration are interdependent. The flux of pure liquid forms of chemicals is expected to be greater than that of a compound in the vapor phase.

Metabolic Constants: describe the rate of loss of chemical from a lumped body compartment, although they have been determined for whole animals and representative tissue. The primary metabolic constants are the maximum velocity (V_{max}) and the membrane partition coefficient (K_m).

Permeability coefficient: a flux value (K_p), normalized for concentration, that represents the rate at which a chemical crosses the stratum corneum (cm/hr). This constant is generally determined at steady state or near steady state and infinite dose, and it varies with the thickness of the skin, specifically the stratum corneum. Sometimes a chemical specific permeability coefficient is indicated as K_p*. In many studies used to generate K_p values, the extent of skin absorption was estimated by measuring the loss of compound from the skin surface. However, if loss processes are occurring, an overestimation of the extent and rate of skin absorption may be made (EPA, 1992).

Diffusion coefficient: describes diffusion for molecules within the membrane (D_m). It is needed to calculate the permeability constant and the flux. Most diffusion coefficients in liquids are on the order of 10^{-5} cm^2/sec to 10^{-6} cm^2/sec. Diffusion coefficients in liquids are about ten thousand times slower than those in dilute gases. Therefore diffusion often limits the overall rate of processes occurring in liquids (EPA, 1992).

Partition coefficient: vehicle specific relationships between a chemical and its relative presence within two competing media (such as between water and n-octanol in the octanol/water partition coefficient). Partition coefficients are expressed as the ratio of the amounts in each medium at steady state. Chemicals that have a greater partition coefficient for the skin will generally achieve higher concentrations in the skin, and as a result will also appear in the systemic circulation to a greater extent than chemicals that have lower partition coefficients. There are a variety of partition coefficients describing relationships between various boundaries such as muscle/air, fat/air, liver/air, blood/air, and various media. Descriptions for some commonly used partition coefficients follow. A comparison of partition coefficients in vari-

TABLE 2-4. Partition Coefficients for Some Organic Solvents

Chemical	*Muscle/Air*	*Fat/Air*	*Liver/Air*	*Blood/Air*
Styrene	46.7	3476	140.7	40.2
m-Xylene	41.9	1859	92.0	46.0
Toluene	27.7	1021	82.8	18.0
Perchloroethylene	20.0	1638	69.9	19.9
Benzene	10.3	499	17.8	17.8
Halothane	4.5	182	7.6	5.3
Hexane	2.9	159	12.0	2.3

Source: From McDougal, J. N. 1991 Physiologically based pharmacokinetic modeling. In F. N. Marzulli and H. I. Maibach (eds.), *Dermatotoxicology*, 3d ed. New York: Hemisphere Publishing Co.

ous tissue and air that describes the potential for dermal absorption of certain organic vapors is shown in Table 2-4.

Fat/Air Partition Coefficient: the relationship between lipid solubility (and thus permeability into skin) and vapor phase transport (and thus relative volatilization rate and vapor pressure) for organic compounds. A compound with a high fat/air partition coefficient would have a high lipid solubility and/or low potential to enter into the vapor phase, while a compound with a low fat/air partition coefficient would have a low lipid solubility and/or a high potential to volatilize and remain in the vapor phase. It is often compared with the octanol/water partition coefficient.

Membrane Partition Coefficient: the stratum corneum/vehicle partition coefficient (K_m). This constant is determined by dividing the solubility of the chemical in the stratum corneum by its solubility in the vehicle.

Octanol/Water Partition Coefficient: the relative solubility of a compound in an organic and a water phase ($K_{o/w}$) or its logarithmic form (log $K_{o/w}$). It is sometimes used as an estimator of a fat/water coefficient. However, discrepancies have been noted in the relationship between skin permeability and lipophilicity as expressed by the log $K_{o/w}$ for some compounds such as phenols (Jetzer et al., 1986). Therefore for some compounds this index may not always properly reflect the lipophilicity, and thus, may be an inconsistent predictor of skin permeability.

Organic Carbon/Water Partition Coefficient: the value (K_{oc}) gives an indication of the likelihood that a chemical will bind to the organic carbon in the soil or sediment rather than remaining in solution. The higher the value the more likely a chemical will bind to soil.

Both human and animal studies are used to determine the skin absorption characteristics of chemicals. Percutaneous absorption in vivo is usually determined by measuring radioactivity in excreta following the topical application of a labeled compound. The material under study is labeled with C^{14} or tritium and following application, the total amount of radioactivity excreted in urine or urine plus feces is determined. The radioactivity in the excreta can be a mixture of the parent compound and any metabolites. The amount of radioactivity retained in the body or excreted through expiration or sweat can be determined by measuring the amount of radioactivity excreted following an intravenous injection; the fraction determined by intravenous dose is then used to correct the amount of radioactivity found after topical administration (Wester and Maibach, 1983).

Another in vivo method of measuring absorption is the detection of plasma radioactivity following topical administration. This method may be difficult to apply because penetrant concentrations in blood after topical administration are often very low (Wester and Maibach, 1983). Determining the loss of material from the surface as it penetrates the skin is another way to measure in vivo absorption. It is assumed that the difference between applied dose and residual dose is the amount of penetrant absorbed. The difficulties inherent in skin recovery, volatility of penetrant, and errors associated with using the difference between amount applied and amount left make this method less quantitative. Biological or pharmacological responses, such as vasodilation, have also been used to estimate absorption for a limited number of compounds (Stroughton, Clendenning, and Kruse, 1960). Table 2-5 compares the in vivo absorption in humans following topical administration for selected compounds.

Animal methods include measurements of dermal lethal dose to 50% (LD_{50}s) in rats, rabbits or guinea pigs, and subchronic studies designed to permit the determination of the no-observed-effect level and toxic effects associated with continuous or repeated exposure to a test substance for a period of 90 days. Animals are also used to derive experimental values for estimating absorption of chemicals similar to those determined in humans. Since human skin is generally a better barrier to absorption of chemicals than animal skin, extrapolation of animal data to humans must be done carefully. However, due to the uncertainties involved it may be best to consider animal data as a conservative estimate of human absorption and not attempt to use any factors to lower (divide) these values.

It has been suggested that the absorption characteristics of a chemical be taken into account in order to determine what the actual dose an exposure would produce. Currently most studies determine only exposure, the amount of material coming in contact with the skin that is *available* for absorption rather than absorbed dose, which is the amount of the material contacting the skin that then becomes absorbed into the body. *Deposited dose* is often used to refer to that mass of material deposited on the surface of the skin. *Absorbed dose* takes into consideration only the amount of contaminant that actually penetrates the skin (or other body barrier) and reaches the bloodstream, thus being

TABLE 2-5. In Vivo Absorption in Humans of Selected Chemicals with Topical Administration

	Absorption Rate (%dose/hr)								
Compound	*0–12 hr.*	*12–24 hr.*	*24–48 hr.*	*48–72 hr.*	*72–96 hr.*	*96–120 hr.*	*% of Dose*	*SD*	*No. of Subjects*
Acetylsalicylic acid	0.141	0.438	0.334	0.147	0.076	0.060	21.81	3.11	3
Benzoic acid	3.036	0.340	0.055	0.000	0.000	0.000	42.62	16.45	6
Butter yellow	0.215	0.685	0.289	0.083	0.054	0.022	21.57	4.88	4
Caffeine	0.559	1.384	0.855	0.109	0.032	0.014	47.56	20.99	12
Chloramphenical	0.007	0.019	0.021	0.022	0.015	0.012	2.04	2.46	6
Colchicine	0.036	0.038	0.033	0.040	0.025	0.004	3.69	2.50	6
Dinitrochlorobenzene	3.450	0.565	0.134	0.045	0.018	0.009	53.14	12.41	4
Diethyltoluamide	0.773	0.331	0.084	0.036	0.016	0.012	16.71	5.10	4
Hexachlorophene	0.029	0.031	0.020	0.028	0.034	0.030	3.10	1.09	7
Hippuric acid	0.005	0.003	0.001	0.001	0.001	0.001	0.21	0.09	7
Malathion	0.313	0.170	0.044	0.017	0.011	0.006	7.84	2.71	7
Methylcholanthrene	0.062	0.329	0.258	0.127	0.064	0.045	16.81	5.16	3
Nicotinic acid	0.000	0.002	0.001	0.001	0.002	0.007	0.34	0.09	3
Nicotinamide	0.019	0.168	0.177	0.088	0.052	0.031	11.08	6.17	7
Nitrobenzene	0.022	0.022	0.013	0.013	0.011	0.006	1.53	0.84	6
p-Aminobenzoic acid	0.159	0.648	0.444	0.196	0.058	0.044	28.37	2.43	13
Phenol	0.254	0.091	0.010	0.601	0.000	0.000	4.40	2.43	3
Potassium thiocyanate	0.051	0.060	0.078	0.097	0.100	0.093	10.15	6.60	6
Salicylic acid	0.116	0.535	0.356	0.156	0.080	0.033	22.78	13.25	17
Thiourea	0.046	0.035	0.010	0.008	0.007	0.007	0.88	0.22	3
Urea	0.008	0.021	0.051	0.073	0.075	0.034	5.99	1.91	4

Source: From Feldmann, R. J., and H. I. Maibach. 1969. Absorption of some organic compounds through the skin in man. *J. Invest. Dermatol.* **54**:339–404.

able to be transported to target organs. The elimination rates of chemicals must also be taken into account when estimating exposures because some compounds may be a concern even at low levels. Compounds with long half-lives in the body (e.g., benzidine) tend to increase overall body burden with daily exposures such as could occur in the workplace. In one study utilizing urine samples, benzidine levels found in consecutive days of the week displayed a steep rising trend. The exposure was due to contamination of clothing and skin (Ader, Piotrowski, and Zaremba, 1958).

Molecular Size and Chemical Structure

Except for compounds with a molecular weight of 400 g/mole and more, the molecular size and weight of a compound appear to have less of an effect on the rate or extent of percutaneous absorption than lipophilicity. Changes in chemical structure across a series of homologous compounds have the potential to alter the permeability of these compounds. For example, the addition of two hydrogen molecules to a double bond in the A ring of testosterone to yield dihydrotestosterone results in a 30-fold decrease in the relative absorption of the latter compound over the former. Benzoic acid is a good skin penetrant, while nicotinic acid, a related organic acid with a nitrogen added to a similar ring structure, is water soluble, insoluble in lipids, higher melting, and a poor skin penetrant. Since marked changes in percutaneous absorption can result from small structural differences, it is very difficult to use an experimentally derived value for one compound to estimate the permeability of another (EPA, 1992). Table 2-6 indicates permeability data for various chemicals with similar structures.

TABLE 2-6. Permeability Data for Various Homologous Series

Chemical	*Formula*	K_p *(cm/hr)*
C_4 series		
Ethyl ether	C–C–O–C–C	15–17
2-Butanone	C–C–C–C ‖ O	4–5
1-Butanol	C–C–C–C–OH	2–4
2-Ethoxy ethanol	C–C–O–C–C–OH	0.2–0.3
2,3-Butane diol	C–C– C–C | | OH OH	0.05
Alcohols		
Ethanol	C–C–OH	1.0
Pentanol	C–C–C–C–C–OH	6.0
Octanol	C–C–C–C–C–C–C–C–OH	52.0

Source: From Scheuplein, R.J., and I. H. Blank. 1971. Permeability of the skin. *Physiol. Rev.* **51:**702–747.

Effect of Physical Form: Vapor, Liquid, and Dust

The physical form of the chemical, be it a dust, liquid or vapor, primarily affects the concentration at the skin surface. Since concentrations are far greater in the pure liquid than in the vapor form, penetration into the skin from exposure to the liquid phase of a chemical will be greater than that from the vapor phase. Other factors such as loss of liquid contaminant from skin due to volatility of the material as well as condensation of vapor on the skin are also concerns when estimating the potential for absorption of chemicals. Dust loadings can be disturbed (lowered) by physical and air movements.

Chemical specific properties also apply; tetrachloroethylene will absorb through the skin if applied as a liquid whereas permeability by its vapor is much poorer (Stewart and Dodd, 1964). On the other hand, nitrobenzene passes directly through the skin in the vapor state. The rate of absorption is proportional to air concentration and ranges from 1 mg/hr to 9 mg/hr at 5 mg/M^3 and 20 mg/M^3, respectively (Piotrowski, 1967). Many chemicals, due to their low vapor pressure (VP), cannot achieve adequate vapor concentrations to pose a dermal exposure hazard, but pose a significant hazard in the liquid form. Also, chemicals with low VPs, such as 4,4'-methylene bis (2-chloroaniline) (MOCA) and 4,4'-methylene dianiline (MDA), can remain on surfaces longer. For example the VP of

MOCA is less than 0.000036 mmHg at 100°C, so most exposures will occur when workers directly contact MOCA or surfaces contaminated with the material (Clapp et al., 1991).

In certain instances absorption decreases as concentration increases. The rate of systemic absorption via the skin at a high concentration (90%) of aniline in air is comparable with the rate of absorption in the respiratory tract; at low concentrations the skin absorption is even greater. While concentration is important, so is volume. Even liquid mixtures containing less than 1% of a contaminant could release vapor concentrations at hazardous levels if a large volume were released due to a spill or tank rupture.

Solubility

The best penetrants are those that are soluble in both lipids and water, traversing the skin via both the lipid and aqueous pathways, whereas compounds that are largely soluble in one medium or the other are not as good at penetrating the skin (EPA, 1992). Solubility of a substance both in water and in lipids is reflected by a not-too-high coefficient of fat/water distribution. Examples are dimethylsulfoxide (DMSO), benzoic acid, and caffeine. Compounds naturally diffuse across the path of least resistance to them, so that those that are only water soluble traverse the skin largely via the aqueous pathway, whereas those that are fat soluble penetrate via the lipid pathway. The aqueous pathway is more resistant to permeation and even concentrated solutions of water-soluble compounds have slow human skin permeability constants that are unlikely to exceed 0.001 cm/hr. The lipid pathway is more facile than the aqueous pathway, and concentrated fat-soluble liquids have a higher rate of penetration. Since the blood is a relatively lipophilic medium, these compounds may be taken up by the cutaneous capillaries faster than water soluble compounds.

The capacity of a substance to penetrate the skin is also at least partially dependent on polarity and pH. As a rule, polar compounds are generally poorly absorbed through the skin, whereas nonpolar compounds are more readily absorbed. As polarity increases, fat solubility decreases (EPA, 1992). Examples are inorganic salts or weak organic acids and bases, whose state and extent of ionization depend on the pH of the environment. Weak organic acids or bases in their nonionized form are much more soluble in lipids and are absorbed more readily through the skin than in their ionized form. Therefore, changes in pH can affect the penetration of an ionizable compound. When a chemical exists in both nonionic and ionic forms, the nonionic (and therefore more lipophilic) form is the better skin penetrant (Michaels, Chandrasekaran, and Shaw, 1975). For metals, permeability may be higher for salts than for the elemental material. About 7% of Hg^{2+} is absorbed from food, but less than 0.01% of ingested elemental mercury is absorbed (WHO, 1980).

The mixture a chemical is contained in (carrier solvent) also impacts permeation. Where two or more compounds that traverse the skin by the same route are present, competition may decrease the skin sites available for diffusion. The carrier solvent in a mixture can also affect the skin permeation rate either by retaining a chemical or by facilitating its penetration. Compounds like dimethyl sulfate, DMSO, and peanut oil will allow a poorly absorbed chemical to be absorbed much faster through the skin.

ENVIRONMENTAL FACTORS

Processes that play a role in the evaporation of compounds from the skin include wind, humidity, temperature, and vapor pressure (Reifenrath and Spencer, 1989). Factors that increase evaporation of a compound from the skin surface (high wind speed and temperature, low humidity) will accelerate the loss of compound from the skin and reduce the dose available for absorption.

Skin absorption of organic compounds increases with increasing temperature. Frequently, in the absence of skin damage, a 10-fold increase in temperature results in a doubling of skin permeability. However, this increase may be different for different chemicals (EPA, 1992). Elevated temperatures enhance the cutaneous absorption of aniline, and absorption increases by 20% with a temperature rise from 25°C to 30°C (Dutkiewicz, 1961).

A similar phenomenon was observed with nitrobenzene. The maximum absorption rate resulting from the application of enough liquid to create a saturated layer at the skin surface was dependent on skin temperature. At the lowest temperature tested the rate was 0.2 mg/cm^2/hr, and at the highest skin temperature it rose to 3 mg/cm^2/hr (Salmova and Piotrowski, 1960).

As noted in a previous section, increased moisture on the skin will increase skin absorption of chemicals. Even moisture in the air can increase skin absorption. Increased air humidity (from 35% to 75%) led to a rise of the absorption of aniline by 30% (Dutkiewicz, 1961). Well-hydrated skin tends to be more permeable than relatively dry skin. As a rule, hydration increases the permeability of skin for most compounds. For example, when the relative humidity was increased from 35% to 67%, the rate of absorption of nitrobenzene increased by about 40% (Piotrowski, 1967). However, the degree to which temperature and relative humidity affect blood flow to the skin is limited, and for most organic chemicals that have good solubility in the blood, diffusion through the skin is the limiting factor rather than removal from the skin by the blood (McDougal et al., 1990). Table 2-7 summarizes some general concepts which

TABLE 2-7. General Concepts of Skin Permeation by Chemicals

1. Percutaneous absorption is exclusively a diffusion process, in which active transport mechanisms play no role.

2. The main barrier to percutaneous absorption is the stratum corneum.

3. The entire stratum corneum acts as a limiting barrier, whose function can be described by a multilayer model, provided that undamaged stratification pertains.

4. The reciprocal function of the barrier is the reservoir function of the stratum corneum, that is, the accumulation of substances on and within the barrier. The reservoir function imparts unique pharmacokinetics and is essential for the effectiveness of external therapy and is responsible for the course and type of percutaneous intoxication.

5. The state of the stratum corneum determines the absorption rate: if this layer is damaged, the barrier is lowered and the percutaneous absorption is generally raised considerably.

6. In normal stratum corneum, the surface area of application and the localization play a dominant role; if the exposure (liquid, dust) concentrations are low, the absorption rate is directly proportional to these concentrations and thus to the size of the area exposed. High absorption rates pertain in hydrated areas. At the higher concentrations the flux is no longer proportional to the quantity applied.

7. The flux increases with increasing solubility and mobility (diffusion coefficient) of the penetrating agent in the layers of the stratum corneum.

8. Up to a molecular weight of at least 500, the molecular size plays no role in the absorption rate. Decisive physicochemical parameters are the partition coefficient (for substances with moderate lipophilicity penetrate best) and the (preferably simultaneous) solubility in lipid and aqueous phases.

9. For relatively rapidly penetrating substances, the preferred route is directly through the cells of the stratum corneum. The early onset of penetration may nevertheless be via the follicles and sweat glands.

10. Following exposure (liquids, dusts), flux through epidermal tissue is more rapid than through the stratum corneum. The resultant concentrations in the epidermis are lower than those in the straum corneum; the concentrations in the upper layers of the epidermis are higher than those in the innermost layer.

11. The flow through dermal tissue is more rapid than through epidermal tissue. The resultant concentrations in the dermis are lower; near the basal layer (upper capillary bed), concentrations are higher than in the lower dermal layers.

12. Factors such as metabolism, binding to proteins, and accumulation in subcutaneous fat tissue may play a role, although they generally have little influence on the total percutaneous absorption rates.

13. Those quantities of foreign materials reaching the epidermis and dermis following topical application are practically totally absorbed by the blood and lymph system.

Source: From Schaefer, H., A. Zesch, and G. Stuttgen. 1982. *Skin Permeability*. New York: Springer-Verlag.

apply to the skin permeation of chemical contaminants.

Chemicals adsorbed to soil and dusts may behave differently than when in the pure state. Skin temperature and exposed surface area, soil pH, and soil moisture content have all been proposed as factors that can affect the desorption of organic compounds from soil and subsequent uptake across the skin (Skowronski, Turkall, and Abdel-Rahman, 1989).

STANDARD PHYSICAL PARAMETERS

Because there are so many variables involved with exposure estimates, several models have been developed to estimate surface areas of the body. Standardized physical parameters are used to calculate the exposures to subjects in dermal monitoring studies due to the difficulties in making individual measurements of body parts. Average values of total surface area of body parts for a population can be used for cases in which only a certain area of the body is at risk of exposure. In tables of standard physical parameters, individual surface areas of the various body regions have been calculated using previously determined anatomic proportions assumed to be representative for the (U.S.) population (Spear et al., 1977). The table most used has been developed by the EPA using available direct measurement data to generate equations that estimated surface area of body parts as a function of height and weight (EPA, 1985). These equations were then applied to the U.S. population, using height and weight distribution data obtained from the National Health and Nutrition Examination Survey II (NCHS, 1983). Due to certain concerns with the methods of calculation, the sizes of men's heads and women's heads and hands may not be as accurate as for the other body parts.

Table 2-8 lists standard physical parameters for men and women. Surface areas can also be calculated using the following formula (Dubois and Dubois, 1916):

$$\text{Total body surface area} = 0.007184(BW)^{0.425} \times (nt)^{0.725}$$

where BW = body weight (kg) and nt = body height (meters). However using a more detailed approach to estimate the surface area exposed can be helpful, since with dermal exposure to contaminants there is a greater likelihood that only certain areas of the body are at risk of exposure (Fig. 2-2; Table 2-9).

TABLE 2-8. Standard Physical Parameters

Parameter	*Men*	*Women*
Body weight	70 kg	60 kg
Breathing rate		
Heavy work	1.8 M^3/hr	1.5 M^3/hr
Light work	1.2 M^3/hr	1.0 M^3/hr
Skin penetration[a]	10% for liquids or sprays, 1% for granulars and dusts	10% for liquids or sprays, 1% for granulars and dusts
Lung absorption	100%	100%
Daily urine volume	1.4 L/day	1.4 L/day
Surface area exposed[b]	0.294 M^2	0.294 M^2

Source: From Jensen, J. K. 1984. The assumptions used for exposure assessments. In M. Siewierski (ed.), *Determination and Assessment of Pesticide Exposure*. Studies in Environmental Science 24. Amsterdam: Elsevier, pp. 148–152.

[a]Unless specific information for a particular chemical is available.

[b]Based on head, neck, "V" of chest, hands, and forearms.

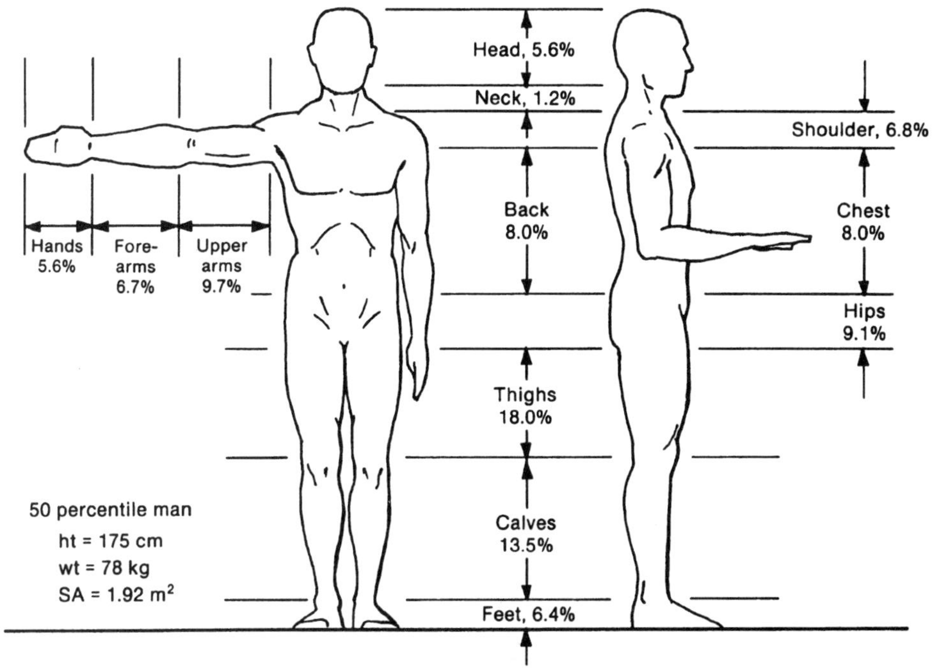

Figure 2-2. Total surface area for humans.
Source: From W. J. Popendorf and J. T. Leffingwell. 1982. Regulating OP pesticide residues for farmworker protection. *Res. Rev.* **82**:125.

TABLE 2-9. Surface Area by Body Part for Adults (M^2)

	Men			*Women*		
Body Part	*Mean (SD)*	*Min.–Max.*	*n*	*Mean (SD)*	*Min.–Max.*	*n*
Head	0.118 (0.0160)	0.090–0.161	29	0.110 (0.00625)	0.0953–0.127	54
Trunk	0.569 (0.0140)	0.306–0.893	29	0.542 (0.0712)	0.437–0.867	54
Upper extremities	0.319 (0.0461)	0.169–0.429	48	0.276 (0.0241)	0.215–0.333	57
Arms	0.229 (0.0374)	0.109–0.292	32	0.210 (0.0129)	0.193–0.235	13
Upper arms	0.143 (0.0143)	0.122–0.156	6			
Forearms	0.114 (0.0127)	0.0945–0.136	6			
Hands	0.084 (0.0127)	0.0596–0.113	32	0.0746 (0.00510)	0.0639–0.0824	12
Lower extremities	0.636 (0.0994)	0.283–0.868	48	0.626 (0.0676)	0.492–0.809	57
Legs	0.505 (0.0685)	0.221–0.656	32	0.488 (0.0515)	0.423–0.585	13
Thighs	0.198 (0.1470)	0.128–0.403	32	0.258 (0.0333)	0.258–0.360	13
Lower legs	0.207 (0.0379)	0.093–0.296	32	0.194 (0.0240)	0.165–0.229	13
Feet	0.112 (0.0177)	0.0611–0.156	32	0.0975 (0.00903)	0.0834–0.115	13
Total	1.94 (0.00374)[a]	1.66–2.28[b]	48	1.69 (0.00374)[a]	1.45–2.09[b]	58

Source: Adapted from *Development of Statistical Distributions or Ranges of Standard Factors Used in Exposure Assessments*. Washington, DC: Office of Health and Environmental Assessment, Exposure Assessment Group, EPA/600/8-85-010.
Note: SD = standard deviation and n = number of observations.
[a]Median (standard error for the 5th to 95th percentile of each body part).
[b]Percentiles (5th–95th).

While oral doses are based on the weight of the exposed individual (mg/kg), skin exposure should be related to total body surface area exposed. It has actually been suggested that all doses should be based on surface area rather than weight because interspecies variation would be reduced (for purposes of comparing animal tests to humans) as well as would human variations (Klassen and Doull, 1980).

REFERENCES

Ader, D., J. Piotrowski, and Z. Zaremba. 1958. Chemical evaluation of industrial exposure to benzidine. II. Attempt to evaluate the absorption of benzidine in industrial conditions. *Med. Pracy* **9:**207–217.

Bentley, P., H. Schuassmann, P. Sims, and F. Oesch. 1976. Epoxides derived from various polycyclic hydrocarbons as substrates of homogeneous and microsome bound epoxide hydratase. *Dur. J. Biochem.* **69:**97–103.

Bird, M. G. 1981. Industrial solvents: Some factors affecting their passage through the skin. *Ann. Occup. Hyg.* **24:**235–244.

Brown, H. S., D. R. Bishop, and C. A. Rowan. 1984. The role of skin absorption as a route of exposure for volatile organic compounds (VOCs) in drinking water. *Am. J. Public Health* **74**(5):479–484.

Clapp, D. E, G. M. Piacitelli, D. D. Zaebst, and E. Ward. 1991. Assessing exposure to 4,4'-methylene bis(2-chloroaniline) (MBOCA) in the workplace. *Appl. Occup. Env. Hyg.* **6**(2):125–130.

Dubois, D., and E. F. Dubois. 1916. Clinical calorimetry, tenth paper: A formula to estimate the approximate surface area if height and weight be known. *Arch. Int. Med.* **17:**863–871.

Dutkiewicz, T. 1961. Aniline vapors absorption in men. *Med. Pracy* **12:**1–15.

Easter, E. P. and H. N. Nigg. 1992. Pesticide protective clothing. *Res. Rev.* **129:**1–16.

Elias, P. M., E. R. Cooper, A. Korc, and B. E. Brown. 1981. Percutaneous transport in relation to stratum corneum structure and lipid composition. *J. Invest. Dermatol.* **76:**297–301.

EPA. 1985. *Development of Statistical Distributions or Ranges of Standard Factors Used in Exposure Assessments*. Washington, DC: Office of Health and Environmental Assessment, Exposure Assessment Group, EPA/600/8-85-010.

EPA. 1992. *Dermal Exposure Assessment: Principles and Applications*. Washington, DC: Office of Health and Environmental Assessment, EPA 600/8-91-011B.

Fishberg, E. H., and W. Bierman. 1932. Acid base balance in sweat. *J. Biol. Chem.* **97:**433–441.

Fujimoto, S., and T. Watanabe. 1969. Studies on the body surface area of Japanese. *Acta Med. Nagasaki* **13:**1–13.

Gunderson, E. C., B. A. Kingsley, C. Witham, and D. C. Bomberger. 1989. A practical study in laboratory and workplace permeation testing. *Appl. Ind. Hyg.* **4**(12):324–329.

Hill, R. H. 1984. Ultraviolet detection of synthetic oil contamination of skin. *AIHA J.* **45**(7):474–484.

Hursh, J. B., T. W. Clarkson, E. F. Miles, and L. A. Goldsmith. 1989. Percutaneous absorption of mercury vapor by man. *Arch. Env. Health* **44**(2):120–127.

Jetzer, W. E., A. S. Huq, N. F. Ho, G. L. Flynn, N. Duraiswamy, and L. Condie, Jr. 1986. Permeation of mouse skin and silicone rubber membranes by phenols: Relationship to in vitro partitioning. *J. Pharm. Sci.* **75**(11):1098–1103.

Kelly, W. F., P. Ackrill, J. P. Day, M. O-Hara, C. T. Tye, I. Burton, C. Orton, and M. Harris. 1982. Cutaneous absorption of trivalent chromium: Tissue levels and treatment by exchange transfusion. *Brit. J. Ind. Med.* **39:**397–400.

Klassen, C. D. and J. D. Doull. 1980. Evaluation of safety: Toxicologic evaluation. In J. Doull, C. D. Lkaassen, and M. O. Amdur (eds.), *Casarett and Doull's Toxicology: The Basic Science of Poisons*. New York: Macmillan.

McDougal, J. N., G. W. Jepson, H. J. Clewell, M. L. Gargas, and M. E. Andersen. 1990. Dermal absorption of organic chemical vapors in rats and humans. *Fund. Appl. Tox.* **14:**299–308.

Marzulli, F. N. 1962. Barriers to skin penetration. *J. Invest. Dermatol.* **39:**393–397.

Michaels, A. S., S. K. Chandrasekaran, and J. E. Shaw. 1975. Drug permeation through human skin: Theory and in vitro experimental measurement. *Am. Inst. Chem. Eng. J.* **21**(5):985–996.

Muller, G., and F. Nurnberger. 1972. Anatomische grundlagen der sogenannten zellulitis. *Arch. Dermatol. Forsch.* **244:**171–172. (As described in H. Schaefer, A. Zesch, and G. Stuttgen, 1982, *Skin Permeability*, New York: Springer-Verlag.)

NCHS. 1983. *National Health and Nutrition Examination Survey 1976–1988*, Hyattsville, MD: NCHS.

NIOSH. 1977. *Exposure Tests for Organic Compounds in Industrial Toxicology*. Pub. No. 77-144. Cincinnati: NIOSH.

Pannatier, A., B. Jenner, B. Testa, and J. C. Etter. 1978. The skin as a drug-metabolizing organ. *Drug. Metab. Rev.* **8:**319–343.

Piotrowski, J. K. 1957. Quantitative estimation of aniline absorption through the skin in man. *J. Hyg. Epid. Microbiol. and Immunol.* **1:**1–23.

Piotrowski, J. K. 1967. Further investigations on the

evaluation of exposure to nitrobenzene. *Brit. J. Industr. Med.* **24:**60–65.

Popendorf, W. J. and J. T. Leffingwell. 1982. Regulating OP pesticide residues for farmworker protection. *Res. Rev.* **82:**125.

Raheel, M. 1991. Pesticide transmission in fabrics: Effect of perspiration. *Bull. Env. Contam. Tox.* **46:**845–851.

Reifenrath, W. G. and T. S. Spencer. 1989. Evaporation and penetration from skin. In R. L. Bronaugh, and H. I. Maibach, (eds)., *Percutaneous Absorption*. New York: Marcel Dekker, pp. 313–334.

Salmova, J., and J. Piotrowski. 1960. Attempt on the quantitative estimation of the nitrobenzene resorption in experimental conditions. *Med. Pracy* **11:**1–14.

Scheuplein, R. J. 1976. Percutaneous absorption after twenty-five years: Or "old wine in new wine skins." *J. Invest. Dermatol.* **67:**31–38.

Scheuplein, R. J. and I. H. Blank. 1971. Permeability of the skin. *Physiol. Rev.* **51:**702–747.

Skowronski, G. A., R. M. Turkall, and M. S. Abdel-Rahman. 1989. Effects of soil on percutaneous absorption of toluene in male rats. *J. Tox. Env. Health* **26:**373–384.

Spear, R. D., W. J. Popendorf, J. T. Leffingwell, T. H. Milby, J. E. Davies, and W. F. Spencer. 1977. Fieldworkers' response to weathered residues of parathion. *J. Occup. Med.* **19:**406–410.

Stewart, R. D., and H. C. Dodd. 1964. Absorption of carbon tetrachloride, trichloroethylene, tetrachloroethylene, methylene chloride and 1,1,1-trichloroethane through human skin. *AIHA J.* **25:**438–443.

Stroughton, R. B., W. E. Clendenning, and D. Kruse. 1960. Percutaneous absorption of nicotinic acid and derivatives. *J. Invest. Dermatol.* **35:**337–341.

Wester, R. C., and H. I. Maibach. 1983. Percutaneous pharmacokinetics: Ten steps to percutaneous absorption. *Drug Metab. Rev.* **14:**169–205.

WHO Study Group. 1980. Inorganic mercury. In *WHO Study Group: Recommended Health-Based Limits in Occupational Exposure to Heavy Metals*. Tech. Rep. Series 647. Geneva: WHO, pp. 102–114.

CHAPTER 3

Chemical Protective Clothing

SELECTION

Selection of chemical protective clothing (CPC) is based on chemical resistance, the areas of the body most likely to be exposed (configuration), and cost. Selection may also be based on the availability of sizes, ease of donning, sturdiness of construction, need to accommodate other selected equipment such as self-contained breathing apparatus (SCBAs), and whether or not mobility is restricted or heat stress is likely to occur (comfort). These same factors are important in determining whether leaks, permeation of the materials, penetration or tears, degradation or decontamination, and ability to reuse are issues.

There is no material that will protect against all chemicals or combinations of chemicals including mixtures, and there is no polymer currently available that is an effective barrier with any prolonged chemical exposure. Figure 3-1 shows structures of common CPC polymers. The range of materials available differs significantly in terms of strength, resistance to physical hazards, and ability to use in extreme environmental conditions. Garments can offer different levels of chemical resistance. For example, vapor permeation resistance is provided by vapor protective suits; liquid and particulate resistance is provided by liquid splash and particulate protective garments, respectively. The type of operation is another factor to consider in CPC selection and can introduce variables such as temperature, period of use, and physical form of the contaminant. The following guidelines should be taken into account:

1. Assess the type of exposure—vapor, splash, dust—and which portions of the body are likely to be exposed.
2. Review chemical toxicities.
3. If there is more than one chemical involved, compare solubility properties.
4. Review permeation literature for various polymers.

CPC should be the last line of defense to protect against accidental contact from spills and splashes. Engineering and work practice controls are the preferred methods to eliminate or minimize contact and should be implemented and evaluated prior to using CPC.

CPC is manufactured by three processes: solvent dip, latex, or milling (Perkins, 1987). In the solvent dip process, most commonly used for gloves, a form is dipped into a polymer-solvent

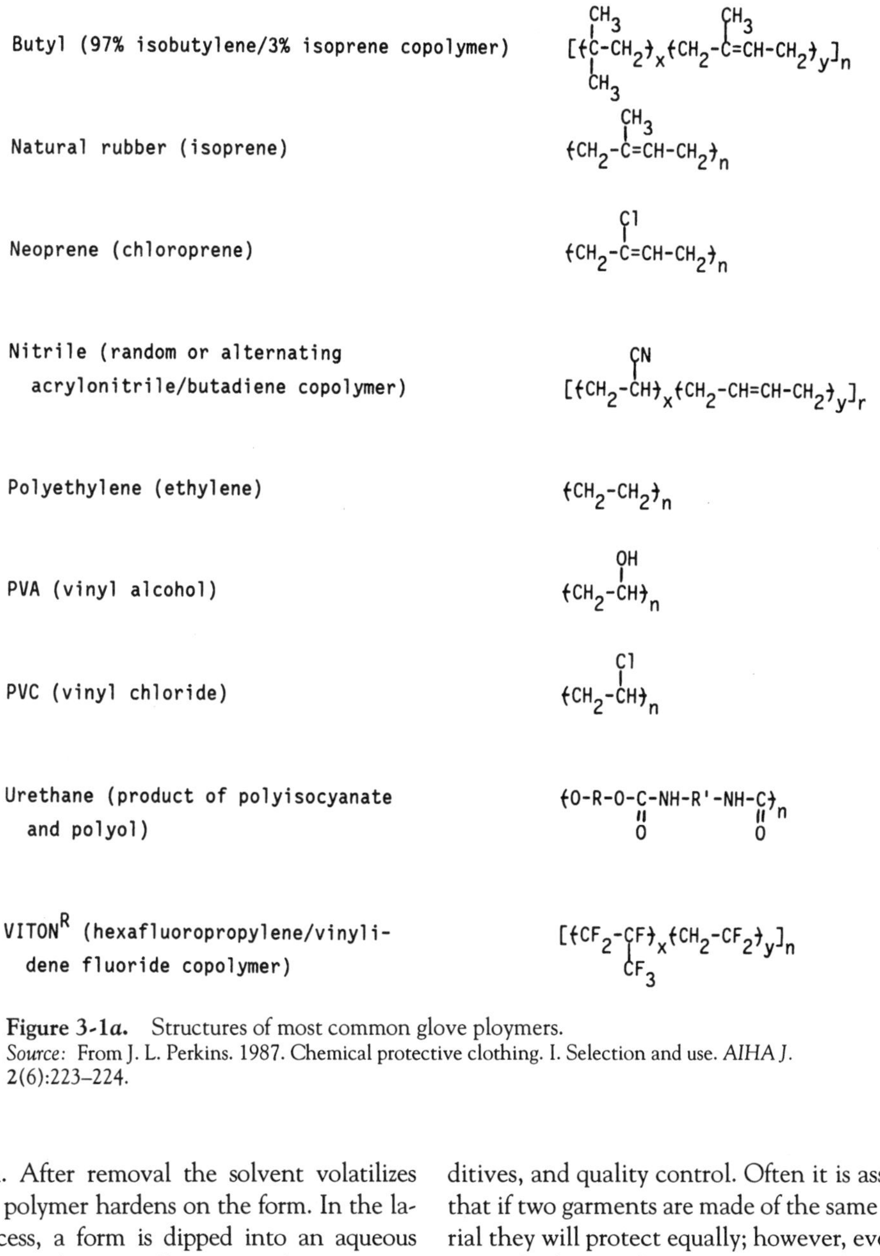

Figure 3-1*a*. Structures of most common glove ploymers.
Source: From J. L. Perkins. 1987. Chemical protective clothing. I. Selection and use. *AIHA J.* 2(6):223–224.

solution. After removal the solvent volatilizes and the polymer hardens on the form. In the latex process, a form is dipped into an aqueous polymer emulsion. Milling is used most commonly for larger pieces of CPC such as suits and jackets. A polymeric resin that has been softened using heat and pressure or a solvent is rolled into sheets or laminated to another material such as a woven fabric. Each manufacturer's polymer formulation differs slightly, as do test methods.

Factors affecting the comparison of permeation results include the manufacturer's source of polymer resin, the manufacturing process, additives, and quality control. Often it is assumed that if two garments are made of the same material they will protect equally; however, even the same thickness of a generic material, such as neoprene or nitrile, supplied by different manufacturers may provide significantly different levels of protection because of variations in the manufacturing surface, and the existence of interfaces with different materials. In general, effective protective materials should have relatively long breakthrough times and low permeation rates. For more information on terminology, see Table 3-1.

Suits and coatings	
Chlorobutyl (butyl rubber with chlorine atoms substituted randomly for hydrogens)	See butyl rubber
EVA/PE (blend of 14% ethylene/vinyl acetate copolymer; 86% polyethylene)	$[(CH_2-CH_2)_x(CH_2-CH(O-C(=O)-CH_3))_y]_n ; (CH_2-CH_2)_n$
FEP, fluorinated ethylene-propylene resin (teflon[R], hexafluoropropylene/tetrafluoroethylene copolymer)	$[(CF_2-CF(CF_3))_x(CF_2-CF_2)_y]_n$
SARAN[R] (SARANEX[R], 85% vinylidene chloride/15% vinyl chloride copolymer)	$[(CH_2-CCl_2)_x(CH_2-CHCl)_y]_n$
Tyvek (polyethylene)	See polyethylene
Face shield polymers	
CR-39 (diethylene glycol-bis allylcarbonate)	$[O(CH_2-CH_2-O-C(=O)-O-CH_2-CH-CH_2)_2]_n$
Polycarbonate (condensation product of bisphenol-A and phosgene)	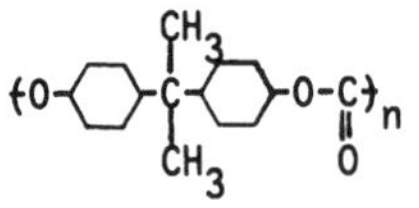
Woven fabrics	
Duraguard (polypropylene)	$(CH_2-CH(CH_3))_n$
Nomex (aramid fiber, polyamide)	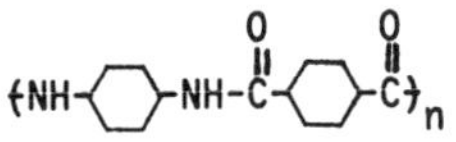
Nylon (polyamide, condensation product of diamine and dicarboxylic acid, e.g., nylon 66)	$(NH-R-NH-O-C(=O)-R'-C(=O)-O)_n$
Polyester (condensation product of dicarboxilic acid and glycol, for example; terepthtalic acid and ethylene glycol)	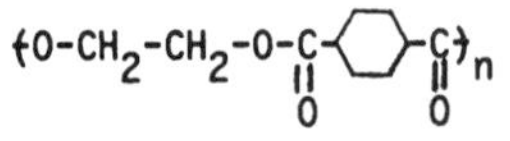

Figure 3-1*b*. Structures of other commonly used CPC polymers.
Source: From J. L. Perkins. 1987. Chemical protective clothing. I. Selection and use. *AIHA J.* 2(6):223–224.

TABLE 3-1. CPC Terminology

Breakthrough time	The elapsed time between initial contact of the chemical on the CPC surface and the analytical detection of the chemical on the inside of the material. Because this depends on the sensitivity of the instrument, problems arise when comparing one breakthrough time to another when the analytical methods are different. The greater the sensitivity of an instrument, the shorter the breakthrough time. Ways to increase sensitivity are by selecting a more sensitive analytical method (one that can concentrate period samples), by increasing the exposed material surface area, or by decreasing the collection volume. Breakthrough times of greater than 1 hour are usually considered an indication of acceptable performance.
Permeation	The process by which a chemical dissolves in or moves through a material on a molecular basis and is defined as the rate at which a chemical passes through the CPC material. Permeation generally increases until it reaches a steady state rate. The rate of permeation is a function of several factors such as chemical concentration, material thickness, humidity, temperature, and pressure. Permeation data provided by manufacturers should include the following: chemical name, breakthrough time, permeation rate, system sensitivity (allows a comparison of test results from different laboratories), and a citation that the data were obtained in accordance with ASTM Standard Test Method F739-85.
Degradation	A deleterious change in one or more physical properties of a protective clothing material due to contact with a liquid chemical. Degradation involves physical changes in one or more properties of the material as the result of a chemical exposure, use, or ambient conditions such as sunlight. The most common observations of material degradation are discoloration, swelling or stiffness, softening, hardening, shrinkage, loss of physical strength, or other deterioration.
Penetration	The movement of chemicals through zippers, seams, pinholes, rips, or other imperfections (thin spots due to uneven coatings) in a protective clothing material. Open-face zippers offer the greatest amount of penetration while the traditional lapped zipper provides the best protection. Liquid penetration data should include a pass or fail determination for each chemical listed, and a citation regarding ASTM Standard Test Method F903-86. Particulate penetration data should show some measure of material efficiency in preventing particulate penetration in terms of particulate type or size and percentage held out. There are no standard tests for this area, so testing criteria may vary among manufacturers.

Liquids spilled on protective clothing such as aprons or coveralls are often wiped off within a few minutes. Therefore, the materials of construction can be less impermeable than those for other CPC as long as exposures are limited to splashes. Although in some cases breakthrough time can be safely increased if intermittent contact is expected, in other cases breakthrough times for intermittent exposure are similar to continuous contact; therefore, it should not be assumed that CPC can be worn longer in these instances without proper testing. Breakthrough times for intermittent exposure can be estimated during testing of the candidate CPC by using intermittent chemical contact to simulate expected use.

As noted, the emphasis in CPC selection is usually on the permeability of a material to a specific chemical. However, this is only the first step. In addition to requesting information on permeation testing from manufacturers, it is useful to request copies of the instruction manuals provided with the clothing, and to obtain and inspect sample garments. Breakthrough time data used in the selection of CPC should be manufacturer and product specific. Comparisons between manufacturers may be significantly affected and therefore breakthrough time values for the same polymer from different sources can show notable variations. For example, a 0.56 mm Edmont 37–155 nitrile glove and a 0.36 mm North LA-142G nitrile glove are reported in manufacturers' literature to yield breakthrough times for perchloroethylene of 5.0 and 1.3 hours, respectively.

The type of work and the work environment will determine if a material must be durable enough not to tear or puncture when brushing against rough surfaces, or degrade when exposed to heat. Therefore it may also be useful to request physical testing information. Physical resistance data for various CPC materials are shown in Table 3-2.

An improper style, regardless of how impermeable the material is, can promote exposure. Collecting samples with a short glove without a gauntlet can result in spillage inside of gloves. Many gloves have an uncoated cotton knit wristlet to allow them to fit snug and spillage onto these absorbent wristlets will permanently contaminate the glove and (in most instances) expose the skin. For more loosely fitting gloves spillage into the interiors is also a problem.

Other exposures during the use of CPC are usually due to multiple chemical exposures to a polymer that was selected to protect against a single contaminant, overuse, or lack of decontamination practices in the field; even when CPC is removed, an exposure might not be recognized if an odor is unnoticeable or the skin's appearance is unchanged. Under these conditions, detecting a permeated chemical is difficult unless sensory or visual effects result, such as itching, burning, or discoloration.

CPC generally has no identification on it as to the polymer type. Therefore, in the field it is easy for workers to be confused and assume one type is as good as another. Labeling and identification systems, whether colorimetric or printed text or symbolic, need to be developed. (See Table 3-3 for an example of a proposed colorimetric system.)

Proper work practices must also be in place and used. The most likely source of contamination to workers who do not double glove is the exterior of the gloves and other CPC they are wearing, such as boots. Handling the exteriors of contaminated gloves will contaminate the hands; if the gloves are later redonned, the contamination is then transferred to the interior of the glove. If the soiled interiors are disregarded because it is assumed that harmless oil, grease, or dirt is responsible rather than the contaminant, then the opportunities for exposure increase. Workers have also been known to modify the way CPC is worn over what is recommended by turning glove gauntlets down, exposing the lining, or wearing shirt or jacket sleeves over the gauntlet. Workers have also been known to modify CPC itself, cutting ventilation holes in the backs of gloves because they make the hands

TABLE 3-2. Summary of Physical Resistance Data for CPC Generic Materials

Generic Material	*Abrade*	*Cut*	*Tear*	*Puncture*	*Heat*	*Ozone*	*Flexibility*
Butyl	F	G	G	G	E	E	G
CPC	E	G	G	G	G	E	G
Natural rubber	E	E	E	E	F	P	E
NBR	E	E	G	E	G	F	E
Neoprene	E	E	G	G	G	E	G
Nitrile	E	E	G	E	G	F	E
Nitrile-PVC	G	G	G	G	F	E	G
Polyethylene	F	F	F	P	F	F	G
Polyurethane	E	G	G	G	G	G	E
PVA	F	F	G	F	G	E	P
PVC	G	P	G	G	P	E	F
SBR	E	G	F	F	G	F	G
Viton	G	G	G	G	G	E	G

Source: From NIOSH. 1990. *A Guide for Evaluating the Performance of Chemical Protective Clothing*. Cincinnati, OH: NIOSH.
Note: These are general ratings for the generic polymer and could vary significantly for the material in a specific product. E = Excellent, G = Good, F = Fair, P = Poor.

TABLE 3-3. Recommended Color Coding for Polymers Used in Chemical Protective Clothing

Type of Polymer	*Color Assigned*[a]
Butyl	Light blue
Natural rubber	Light beige
Neoprene	Light green
Nitrile	Light yellow
Polyethylene	Light gray
Polyvinyl alcohol (PVA)	Light red
Polyvinyl chloride (PVC)	Light orange
Urethane	Light purple
Viton	2 Blue strips

Source: From Gillen, M., and S. Schneider. 1992. *Testimony on Behalf of the Occupational Health Foundation on OSHA's Reopening of the Proposed Rule for Personal Protective Equipment for General Industry*. Washington, DC: Occupational Health Foundation.

[a]All colors should be clearly identifiable by the user and clearly distinguishable from one another. They should be light in shade to make it easier to observe contamination inside the glove. The colors should be resistant to chipping, scaling, peeling, blistering, fading, and sunlight. In lieu of the entire glove or article being of the appropriate color, a 1-inch color stripe at wrist level for gloves, or at the collar or waist for garments, should be used.

sweat; since CPC presents evaporative cooling of the skin, the skin temperature and moisture underneath increase along with the permeability of the skin. See Table 3-4 for CPC selection guidelines.

Only qualified individuals trained in selection, use, and maintenance procedures should be responsible for a CPC program. Correct CPC for each job should be identified in written work procedures that may require more than one change if several different chemicals must be used. Workers should be informed of cleaning requirements including the need to clean daily or more often if necessary. Where possible, CPC should be assigned to individual workers for their exclusive use. Each item should be permanently marked to identify the user. The date of issuance should be recorded for discard purposes. Available sizes should reflect the demographics of the workers, including small females and very large males.

LABORATORY VERSUS FIELD TESTING

Proper CPC selection using laboratory data is the first step in preventing exposures, and field testing is the second. Sample garments should be field tested prior to providing them to personnel for work in hazardous atmospheres. Many of the sampling methods used are the same as those implemented to measure dermal exposure, including wipes, rinses, gauze pads, fluorescence, and detectors that change color. Field testing is the key to making decontamination and reuse decisions. Breakthrough times can decrease over time for CPC that is reused, even with an effective decontamination program. As shown in Table 3-5, breakthrough times were halved for nitrile gloves decontaminated with aeration and detergent washing after exposure to chlorinated solvents.

When the CPC being used has not been tested under the expected conditions, it may fail to provide adequate protection. In this situation, the wearer should observe the CPC during use and treat any noticeable change, such as color, stiffness, or a chemical odor inside, as a failure until proven otherwise by testing. If the work must continue, new CPC should be worn for a shorter exposure time, or CPC of a different polymeric material should be selected.

Laboratory tests usually measure breakthrough time, degradation, and penetration. Most laboratory breakthrough testing is done with the pure concentrated chemical over an extended period of time in a two-chambered test cell with the clothing material (20 cm^2) acting as a barrier between the chambers. The challenge chemical or mixture is placed in the chamber toward which the outside of the clothing material faces and the downstream chamber is monitored for the challenge chemical. This method of testing CPC materials while in continuous contact with a chemical is considered the worst-case condition that produces the quickest breakthrough time. The main function of degradation testing is as a screening test. Weight change and visual examination are the principal methods used to detect degradation.

TABLE 3-4. CPC Selection

Chemical identification	It is important to know all of the components of each chemical mixture used. The presence of less toxic chemicals may decrease the protection provided against the more toxic ones.
Chemical state and properties	The physical state and chemical properties of the chemicals used in the workplace are important. If a chemical is present as a vapor and the vapor exposure can be harmful then this would dictate the need for whole body protection.
Chemical contact sequence	Determine if the chemical contact is limited to an occasional accidental splash, with the opportunity available to quickly change the CPC. Determine if the CPC is in continuous contact with the chemical for long periods of time.
Potential CPC use/reuse pattern	If CPC is to be removed after a short exposure time and then donned for another subsequent exposure time, determine if the worker can be exposed as the result of handling, doffing, and donning the contaminated CPC.
Environmental conditions	What is the temperature of the environment in which chemical contact may occur? With each 10°C rise in temperature, the permeation rate roughly doubles and breakthrough time significantly decreases. If there is a potential for contact with an open flame or high temperatures, most CPC products cannot be used as they are flammable.
Contact location	Determine what parts of the body the chemical can potentially contact. Some types of garments, such as boots, are available in only a few generic materials, which limits the number of chemicals they will protect against.
Resistance to physical stress	If the CPC is to be used in a workplace where abrasions, cuts, punctures, or tears will occur, it must be made of special materials or have certain backings such as canvas.
CPC interference with task	If the work includes delicate tasks, such as handling very small parts that require high manual dexterity, CPC may interfere. If CPC catches on moving equipment it may cause an injury. The work rate may be high enough to cause heat stress if large areas of the body are covered with a vapor barrier of CPC.

Source: From NIOSH. 1990. A *Guide for Evaluating the Performance of Chemical Protective Clothing*. Cincinnati, OH: NIOSH.

TABLE 3-5. Permeation Results for New and Preexposed Specimens with Aeration and Detergent Washing as the Decontamination Method

	Breakthrough Time (min)				*Permeation Rate (μg/cm².min)*			
Systems	*New* M	*New* SD	*Decon* M	*Decon* SD	*New* M	*New* SD	*Decon* M	*Decon* SD
Neoprene/toluene	10	1.0	8	0.0	2500	115	2400	270
Neoprene/trichloroethane	22	2.0	15	3.4	2500	50	2500	114
PVC (Best)/perchloroethylene	12	1.1	15	3.0	500	23	300	46
PVC (Edmont)/methylene chloride	8	2.8	8	3.2	1300	83	1200	50
Nitrile (Best)/perchloroethylene	10	0	5	2	500	66	500	67
Nitrile (Edmont)/trichloroethane	110	7.1	67	4.0	150	20	160	18
Butyl/trichloroethane	82	8.4	59	3.7	160	8	170	10

Source: From Vahdat, N., and R. Delaney. 1989. Decontamination of chemical protective clothing. *AIHA J.* 50(3):152–156.
Note: M = mean and SD = standard deviation

Materials that show extensive weight gain, swelling, stiffening, softening, discoloration, or deterioration (such as cracking, delamination, stickiness, or bubbling) for a particular chemical are likely to fail in the field. Lab penetration tests assess only liquid penetration resistance; therefore, they are not applicable for measuring the vapor penetration associated with liquid contact of the material (Mansdorf and Berardenelli, 1988).

There is some disagreement as to whether the laboratory methods most often used to evaluate CPC reflect field use conditions. For example, the use of CPC generally produces an elevated skin temperature under the garment. However, very few breakthrough tests take this temperature into consideration; consequently, it has been recommended that current standardized permeation test methods be upgraded to reflect field conditions (Gillen and Schneider, 1992). This upgrade would include extending the test period from 8 to 16 hours to reflect the extended shifts often worked as well as the effects of residual contamination generally not removed after and prior to CPC reuse. Also considered would be the use of skin temperature (37°C) rather than room temperature (20°C) and sweat would be simulated using a solution containing electrolytes such as Ringer's saline instead of deionized water.

CPC tests are usually done using pure compounds; however, real life exposures are most often to mixtures, whether they are due to the use of a formulation or mixture or impact of the environment, such as contacting more than one contaminated surface over the course of a workday. Many formulations including paints, adhesives, and other mixtures contain solvents in addition to other more hazardous constituents such as methylenedianiline. Very few data are available for chemical mixtures and published permeation data of CPC tested against pure chemicals do not necessarily correlate with test data for those same chemicals in mixtures, making it difficult to reliably predict breakthrough times for chemical mixtures. If the components of a mixture have similar structure or polarity, then the permeation will be the sum of their concentrations, but if their solubility characteristics are significantly different, then the better penetrant will act as a solvent to increase the penetration of the other chemical. This action is a significant concern if the second chemical is highly toxic (Perkins, 1987).

In cases of mixtures and unknowns, if clothing must be used without test data, garments with materials that demonstrate the best chemical resistance against the widest range of substances should be worn. The worst-case data for any component of the mixture should be used to select the candidate CPC. Other situations may involve unidentified substances. Similarly, one way to compensate for the effects of a mixture is to drastically reduce the period of time a pair of gloves can be used and to require disposal rather than decontamination. In some instances, a new pair of gloves may be required for a specific task, or replacing gloves at specified intervals during the workday may be necessary.

All CPC materials contain some type of additives such as plasticizers or fillers whose concentrations can vary by type of glove as well as in different sites on individual gloves. A common plasticizer is bis(2-ethyl hexyl) phthalate, a suspected carcinogen and teratogen. Some solvents have the potential to extract chemical additives from gloves and/or to solubilize the glove material under the conditions of evaluation, exposing the wearer to these additives. Perchloroethylene has been shown to dissolve the plasticizers in polyvinyl chloride. Although this effect does not occur with all chemicals, it is a matter of concern and should be evaluated.

Impermeable Suits

Vapor protective suits (Fig. 3-2) require additional testing to that normally performed for CPC such as gloves and boots because if the suit fails to function it could lead to a life-threatening situation. These suits also provide liquid splash and particulate protection, whereas clothing intended only for that kind of protection does not provide vapor protection. Many garments may be labeled as totally encapsulating but they do not

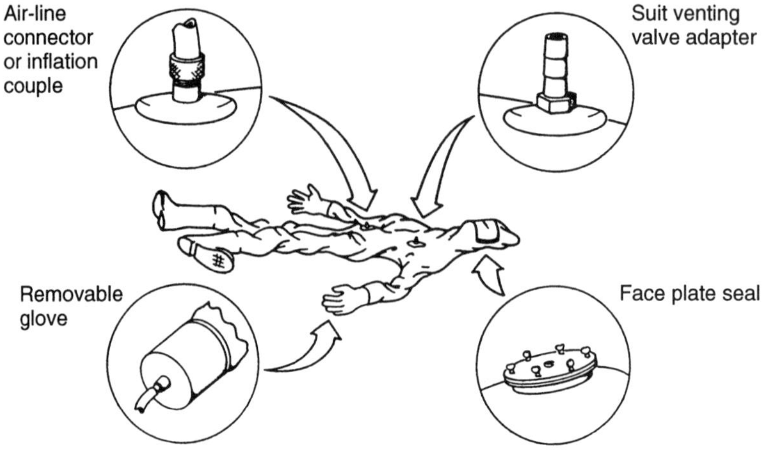

Figure 3-2. Methods for pressure testing vapor protective suits.
Source: From J. O. Stull and D. F. White. 1992. A review of overall integrity and material performance tests for the selection of chemical protective clothing. *AIHA J.* **53**:456.

provide gas-tight integrity due to inadequate seams or closures. Often the gloves, boots, face shield, and exhalation valves on vapor protective suits are composed of materials differing from the suit itself, and, therefore, it is important that each of these elements be tested. Gas-tight integrity can only be determined by performing a pressure or inflation test and a leak-detection test using procedures set out by the American Society of Testing and Materials Standard Practice F1052 (1987).

It is important not to confuse the type of protection afforded by splash suits with that of vapor protective suits. Splash suits must cover the entire body when combined with the respirator, gloves, and boots; however, simply applying duct or electrical tape to a splash suit does not make it impervious to vapors. For example, in an acid suit with detachable gloves, a plastic cuff fits inside the sleeve and the glove is inserted between this cuff and the sleeve. The cuff is then pushed down toward the wrist where the sleeve narrows. The cuff-glove seam is then taped. For acids without appreciable vapor pressures, such as sulfuric acid, this suit will provide protection because the airborne acid is in the form of an aerosol consisting of droplets as opposed to a vapor consisting of individual molecules. In comparison, hydrofluoric acid readily off-gases hydrogen fluoride gas, so the selection of this type of suit must be considered with great care.

Common reasons for whole body suits to fail testing are material pinholes, incompletely closed zippers, defects in material seams, and poor component interfaces (e.g., glove to sleeve attachment) (Stull and White, 1992). A common manufacturing defect is the use of cloth-based, open-teeth zippers as garment closures. Also many splash suits have exposed edges or inner surfaces with one-sided polymer coatings that can allow liquid transfer to seams, which can then permit access to the suit interior through wicking.

Suits of materials such as Tyvek protect only against dusts and do not have to cover the entire body, depending on the hazard of the specific particulate present. Since these are designed to be worn in low skin hazard situations, testing is not required. In general, some form of gloves, boots, and face protection are also necessary.

Gloves

Selecting the right glove size and style means a comfortable, safe fit, and helps ensure that workers will wear their gloves. Gloves that are too large reduce dexterity and can get caught in machinery while those that are too small are binding and cause the hand to tire more quickly. Cuff designs range from pinked and rolled to snug-fit knit wrists. Gauntlet cuffs offer the benefits of a safety cuff, plus a flared design that fits over the sleeve (if it is large enough). The gauntlet length needed is determined by the depth to which the hand and arm will be immersed in solution and the extent of splash protection required. In cold weather the use of insulated clothing for working outside requires a gauntlet large enough to fit over the sleeve.

Gloves of the same manufacturer can also have variation, such as differences in thickness, formulation, and drying time. It is not uncommon for gloves to have some variation in polymer thickness, otherwise known as thin spots, due to variation in the manufacturing process. Two gloves made of the same polymer but subject to different manufacturing processes will have differing permeation and other characteristics, owing either to the process or to the differences in starting materials. Gloves can also be made of more than one polymer. One study of glove permeation used gloves made of different materials that were visually different in both the palm and gauntlet areas. Significantly different breakthrough times were found for the palm and gauntlet areas (Abernathy and Genova, 1991).

In some instances, the gloves themselves can cause skin problems, such as itching, sweating, and rashes. Possible causes for these reactions include additives in the glove material, powders sometimes used on the interiors, and occlusion effects. Some workers use a medicated powder in gloves to help absorb perspiration not knowing that the powder contains additives such as eucalyptus that can be irritating to the skin. One option is to wear a thin cotton glove as a liner under the protective glove to absorb sweat. Liner gloves should be changed at least twice daily and workers with hand dermatitis need to change liners even more frequently.

Liquid contamination is much less likely to be wiped off gloves than are splashes to other CPC. Consequently, concentrated materials are allowed to remain in contact. Because gloves need to be worn more snugly than most CPC in order not to interfere with dexterity, they are especially prone to temperature buildup. Not only will solvents permeate faster, but the glove material may undergo some chemical/physical transformation such as cracking or change of elasticity. When gloves are worn in a typical work situation, a temperature differential of about 13°C exists between the skin and the atmosphere providing the ambient air is at room temperature (Jencen and Hardy, 1988). With each 10°C rise in temperature, the permeation rate roughly doubles and breakthrough time significantly decreases (Comyn, 1985).

Boots

The need to offer protective boots in a variety of polymers similar to gloves has only recently been recognized. However, boots are far more likely than other protective garb to come into contact with concentrated materials, especially during spill cleanup. Yet boots (Fig. 3-3) are rarely ever decontaminated in routine workplace situations and are the piece of work clothing most frequently worn home. Overboots can be worn with or without normal work shoes inside; however, they must be properly sized and have protective soles. Soles are the most common part of the work boots to be decontaminated; however, this is often inadequate and will allow residues to build up in the rest of the boot.

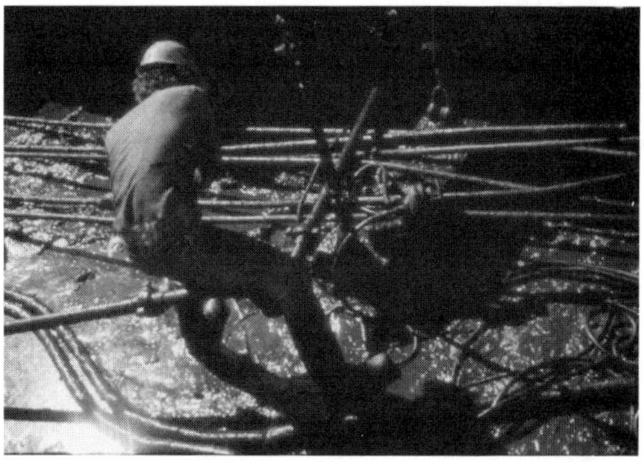

Figure 3-3. Worker wearing boots in a pool of $BaCl^2$ drilling mud. Boots are rarely decontaminated in routine workplace situations and are the most common piece of work clothing worn home.

REFERENCES

Abernathy, R. N., and S. A. Genova. 1991. Measurements of hypergolic fuels and oxidants' permeation through commercial protective materials—Part II: Nitrogen tetroxide, monomethyl hydrazine, and anhydrous hydrazine. *AIHA J.* **52**(1):20–29.

Comyn, J. (ed.). 1985. *Polymer Permeability*. New York: Elsevier Applied Science Publishers.

Gillen, M., and S. Schneider. 1992. *Testimony on Behalf of the Occupational Health Foundation on OSHA's Reopening of the Proposed Rule for PPE in General Industry*. Washington, DC: Occupational Health Foundation.

Gunderson, E. C., B. A. Kingsley, C. L. Witham, and D. C. Bomberger. 1989. A practical study in laboratory and workplace permeation testing. *Appl. Ind. Hyg.* **4**(12):324–329.

Jencen, D. A., and J. K. Hardy. 1988. Method for the evaluation of the permeation characteristics of protective glove materials. *AIHA J.* **49**(6):293–300.

Mansdorf, S. Z., and S. P. Berardenelli. 1988. Chemical protective clothing standard test method development. Part I: Penetration test method. *AIHA J.* **49**(1):21–25.

Perkins, J. L. 1987. Chemical protective clothing: I. Selection and use. *Appl. Ind. Hyg.* **2**(6):222–230.

Stull, J. O., and D. F. White. 1992. A review of overall integrity and material performance tests for the selection of chemical protective clothing. *AIHA J.* **53**(7):455–462.

Vahdat, N. 1987. Permeation of polymeric materials by toluene. *AIHA J.* **48:**155–159.

PART II

Developing Strategies for Sampling

CHAPTER 4

Assessment of Workplace Exposures

Workers are exposed to a variety of physical states and concentrations of chemicals including concentrated and dilute liquids, vapors in confined spaces and contaminated soil, and sludge on hazardous waste sites. Exposures do not have to be to large volumes to have a significant dermal effect. Many small exposures over a consistent period can build up over time, especially for chemicals that tend to have long half-lives in the body. If a laboratory chemist using carbon disulfide splashes small amounts on her hands from a pipette that squirts while filling vials for gas chromatography analysis, over time an antabuse effect can develop. While the emphasis of this book is on sampling to detect surface and dermal contamination, it should not be forgotten that eliminating the source of exposure through workplace controls should always be the first effort.

The events leading up to a skin problem are not always obvious. In a facility manufacturing gas and electric ranges, several employees were suffering from skin disorders including ulcers (NIOSH, June 1989). Eighty-seven employees worked in the enamel department where the primary responsibility was painting the individual range parts prior to assembling the units.

Porcelain enamel paints were applied to range parts by either a dipping or flow coat process. The porcelain enamels contained chromium in the trivalent state. Oxidizers were added to the enamels, creating the potential for Cr^{+3} to change to Cr^{+6}. The skin problems were found mainly among the ground coat line workers who were responsible for hanging parts on hooks to enter a curing oven. Most workers did not wear protective rubber gloves. It was determined that holes had developed in the heating coils of the curing oven, producing open flames. The open flames had caused burn-off from the parts, depositing sharp bits of metal slag on hooks used to hang parts. Samples taken from these hooks indicated Cr^{+6} concentrations of 0.09–2.41 μg/mg. Sharp edges on the hooks allowed the chromium to get beneath the skin surface of the workers' hands causing the ulcerations.

Dermal exposures to workers can be categorized as either primary or secondary (Lees, Corn, and Breysse, 1987). Primary exposures occur as a result of direct involvement with the operation and include contact with process generated contamination, equipment and materials used in the work area, or exposures generated as a result of work activities. The secondary exposures, which are more difficult to identify, occur when workers in turn contaminate surfaces remote from the original work area, such as lunchrooms, office areas, washrooms, and their personal vehicles. Primary exposures will be limited to the workers themselves and are easier to control because the exposure population is already identified. The other exposures may involve workers and numerous others who are not involved in the work activities themselves, and are much more difficult to anticipate and control. The contamination is spread from the work site primarily on workers skin, clothing, portable tools, and equipment.

DETERMINANTS OF THE POTENTIAL FOR AND DEGREE OF CONTAMINATION

Environmental Factors

Environmental factors include temperature, humidity, and wind. Seasonal differences in exposures have been determined, indicating that warmer months are frequently the periods of higher exposure. Seasonal production variations that are common in the workplace can also be a contributing factor. Sciarini and Meigs (1961) found that benzidine levels in the urine of dyestuff workers were 230 ±158 μg/L in the cool season and elevated to 674 ±534 μg/L in the warm season. Electrical linemen's exposure to pentachlorophenol while climbing utility poles were increased in the summer (as measured in their leather gloves) and were consistent with increased amounts of pentachlorophenol leaching from the poles in warmer weather (Thind, Karmali, and House, 1991).

Depending on the operation, if performed outdoors, concentration and spread of materials can be impacted by the wind speed and direction as well as humidity. In cold weather, heavy outer garments may reduce the potential for chemical exposures to the forearms and other parts of the body. In some jobs during the summer, such as harvesting, workers may work shirtless and wear shorts because of high temperatures and humidity. However, even unexposed areas are a concern, since perspiration-soaked clothing can allow penetration of higher levels of chemicals than dry material because the perspiration lowers the liquid holding capacity of the fabric, allowing contaminants to move more freely. When impervious chemical protective clothing (CPC) is worn, perspiration is also increased. Therefore it is important to monitor exposed areas where there is sweat buildup on the skin, since there is likely to be an increased absorption of chemicals. In a study of pesticide permeation (Raheel, 1991), cotton fibers and blends were found to allow lower levels of penetration compared to 100% synthetic fiber woven fabrics such as nylon, acrylic, and polyester. Similarly, when surfaces such as industrial equipment, tools, switches, or benches are wet and touched by workers, a greater contamination transfer occurs than when they are dry.

Skin Conditions

Work that promotes disease or damage to skin increases the risk of percutaneous absorption. Common skin diseases are psoriasis, eczema, rashes, and dermatitis. Damage to the skin can be from mechanical injuries such as knife cuts, punctures, or slips and falls resulting in cuts, wounds, or abrasions (Fig. 4-1). Even sunburn can increase the skin's permeability. Chemicals, such as acids and caustics, which produce skin damage on contact, can make the skin more susceptible to skin permeants, while other chemicals, such as ethylamine, are both corrosive and capable of entering the skin; with increased contact its penetration increases.

Occlusion, wherein contaminants are trapped next to the skin by coverings such as barrier creams, bandages, clothing, or CPC, will enhance the likelihood of the material penetrating or irritating the skin but will cause the exposure to last longer by restricting evaporation of the chemical and removal by other mechanisms. Occlusion increases the skin temperature and hydration, and can increase absorption through hair follicles for chemicals that normally will not penetrate the epidermis (Scheuplein, 1978). It may increase skin absorption of some compounds by a factor of 5 to 10 (Scheuplein and Bronaugh, 1983).

In operations where greases, heavy oils, and tars are present, workers may be tempted to use

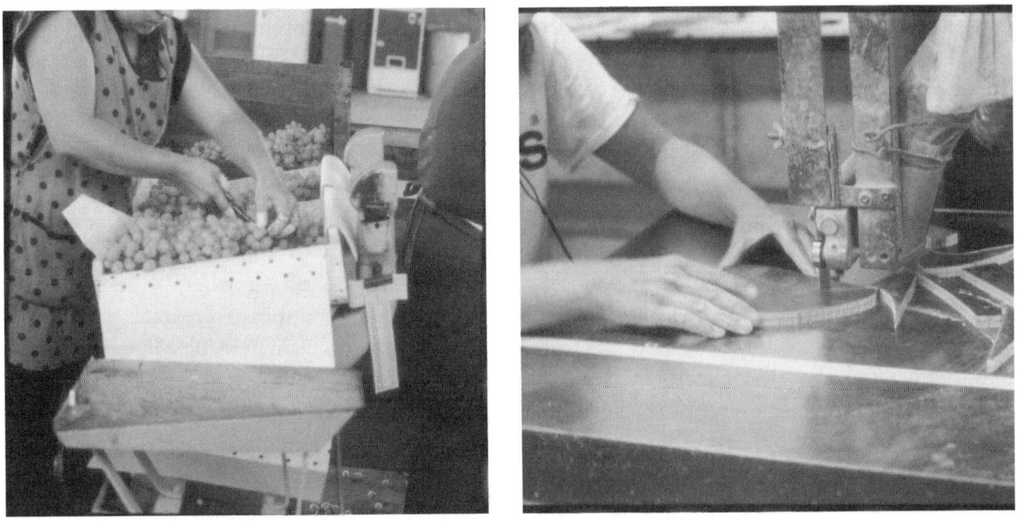

Figure 4-1. *Left:* Grape trimming workers are frequently cut with the sharp, pointed shears used for trimming. Note bandages on the fingers. The unwashed grapes can have pesticide residues on them. *Right:* Jobs involving mechanical stress can increase the potential for permeation.

solvents for skin cleaning. Organic solvents such as naphtha, gasoline, and kerosene should not be used to clean hands because they may facilitate skin penetration of contaminants and are also sources of exposures. In some cases they contain hazardous components such as benzene that are also capable of entering the skin. When exposed to skin drying solvents, workers often compensate by using lotions and creams. Lotions and creams containing skin penetrating oils such as lanolin can also increase absorption of contaminants. A waterless skin cleanser followed by soap and water should be used instead.

Alkaline hand cleansers can remove the natural protective oils from the skin, allowing the hands to become dry, cracked, and irritated. To some extent there is a trade-off between effectiveness to remove oil and grime and mildness to the hands. The cleansers' ability to clean effectively depends on their alkalinity, which allows them to soaponify the oil, which can then be washed away. The more alkaline a cleanser is, the more effectively it can remove the oil grime from the hands, but also the more likely it is to be irritating to the hands by removing the natural oils from the skin. Additionally, if the alkalinity is well buffered so that the cleanser will remain alkaline, it will both clean better and be more likely to cause skin problems (NIOSH, December 1976). The use of strong cleansers, especially those containing abrasives, should be reserved for when soap and water cleansing is not sufficient; they should not be used routinely.

Barrier creams have been around for some time and are often promoted in lieu of protective gloves. However, without strict hygiene, regardless of the claims of the manufacturer, barrier creams will not protect against exposure. When they are applied over permeable chemicals they will occlude the material and enhance absorption. Barrier cream is often called protective cream. A typical claim for barrier creams is: "Helps protect skin against many sticky, staining, and irritating industrial substances." A typical disclaimer is: "Not for use with harsh acids or alkalis, or with toxic substances." All barrier creams require that skin be washed and dried prior to each application, a practice which can prove difficult in many operations.

A test on a barrier cream containing 10% silicone indicated it had no significant influence on decreasing the rate of percutaneous absorption of m-xylene (Lauwerys et al., 1978). It was suggested that since silicone creams are hydrophobic, they are mainly active in preventing absorption of polar compounds and not liposoluble solvents. Another barrier cream containing glycerol was also tested and did not significantly reduce the amount of m-xylene absorbed through the skin of volunteers.

An evaluation of the effectiveness of a barrier cream specifically formulated for protection against amine hardeners was performed by applying the cream to the interiors of protective gloves prior to permeation testing by metaphenylene diamine (MPDA). The breakthrough times for MPDA in gloves with cream coatings were not significantly different from those without cream, which suggested that the effectiveness of the cream with or without the gloves was very limited (Gunderson et al., 1989). Another study indicated that barrier creams provided insufficient protection against skin contamination by coal liquefaction products containing polyaromatic hydrocarbons (PAHs) and concluded that they should not be used in place of other means of protection (Weil and Condra, 1960). Finally, barrier creams are not designed for use in situations where there is a considerable amount of mechanical stress to the skin nor are they a replacement for gloves.

Good personal hygiene practices are required to remove harmful skin contaminants, especially skin carcinogens and penetrants. Employers should provide showering and washing facilities in readily accessible locations. (Such provisions can be a problem, however, at remote sites.) Workers should thoroughly wash their hair during showers and should pay particular attention to cleaning skin creases, fingernails, and hairlines. While on the surface this type of control may seem simple, enforcement is extremely difficult. Many workers are reluctant to be thorough because they want to avoid redoing their hair styles or makeup.

Dermal testing can be useful for reinforcing the need for workers to properly remove skin contamination. For example, in a radiator repair shop, washing with liquid detergent and water was generally effective when wipes collected before and after washing were examined (6,788 $\mu g/M^2$ average versus 593 $\mu g/M^2$, respectively. However, one worker still had 2,439 $\mu g/M^2$ present after hand washing, which indicates how variable personal hygiene is.

Quick drench showers should be conveniently located in the immediate work area for emergencies. They should be able to rapidly drench a worker with a forceful flow of water in order to effectively remove skin permeants, thereby minimizing dermal absorption. It is also important to locate these showers in areas such as storage rooms and unloading sites where workers would not normally wear full body protective clothing yet might be accidentally splashed or where a large volume release might occur.

Personal Habits

Oral ingestion is commonly linked with personal habits in the workplace and is frequently the result of hand contact with chemicals and transfer to the mouth during such activities as smoking, eating (see Table 4-1), and the application of cos-

TABLE 4-1. Potential Contamination of Food Items and Hands by Workers Thinning Apples in Parathion-Sprayed Orchards (expressed as parathion recovered [mg])

	1 Hr Exposure 24 Hr After Spraying			*1 Hr Exposure 48 Hr After Spraying*			*5 Hr Exposure 24 Hr After Spraying*		
Item	*No. Reps.*	*Range*	*Avg.*	*No. Reps.*	*Range*	*Avg.*	*No. Reps.*	*Range*	*Avg.*
Half-sandwiches	6	0.022–0.029	0.026	6	0.021–0.027	0.024	7	0.010–0.037	0.021
Cookies	6	0.007–0.008	0.008	9	0.005–0.007	0.006	12	0.004–0.011	0.007
Pickles	6	0.004–0.006	0.005	9	0.004–0.006	0.005	12	0.001–0.008	0.004
Lunch break[a]			0.190			0.172			0.155
Hands	4	3.4–4.0	3.7	6	2.4–2.6	2.5	16	3.4–7.9	5.7

Source: From Armstrong, J. F., H. R. Wolfe, S. W. Comer, and D. C. Staiff. 1973. Oral exposure of workers to parathion through contamination of food items. *Bull. Env. Contam. Toxicol.* 10(6):321–327.

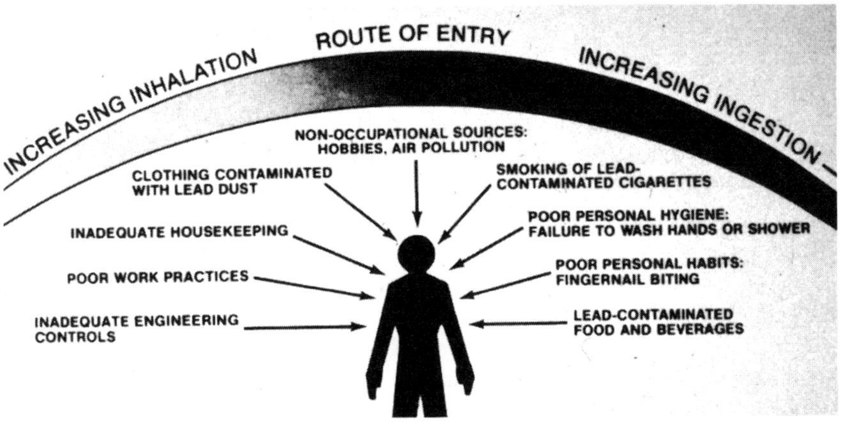

Figure 4-2. Impact of work practices on the route of entry for lead exposure among battery plant workers.

metics. Contaminated surfaces can transfer chemicals to food or other material such as chewing tobacco, gum, and cigarettes. Applying cosmetics in work areas can also lead to skin and eye contamination. Personal habits such as chewing on pencils, chewing snuff or gum, or licking the fingers to turn or sort through papers can also promote opportunities for oral exposure.

The importance of oral exposures is demonstrated by a study of arsenic exposure at a smelter. Air sampling results were compared to arsenic in urine. On average, 74% of the calculated inhaled dose was excreted as inorganic arsenic or its metabolites. However, in one case the urinary excretion of arsenic corresponded to approximately 300%. The source was determined to be the snuff this person chewed throughout the workday. As Figure 4-2 illustrates, smoking, poor personal hygiene, and eating contaminated food in the workplace favor increased oral exposures, and poor housekeeping, contaminated clothing, and work practices will produce resuspended dust and increase inhalation exposures (see also Table 4-2).

TABLE 4-2. Geometric Mean Blood Lead Levels by Smoking and Work Practices Among Battery Workers

Behavior Present		*Yes*	*No*
Current smoker	GM (N)	57 (15)	46[a] (23)
Always washes hands before eating	GM (N)	48 (34)	71[a] (4)
Always showers before leaving work	GM (N)	48 (29)	59 (9)
Always changes clothes before leaving work	GM (N)	All	All
Always wears respirator while working	GM (N)	45 (14)	54 (24)

Source: NIOSH. September 1989. *Health Hazard Evaluation Report*. Technical Assistance to the Jamaican Ministry of Health, Kingston, Jamaica. HETA 87-371-1986. Cincinnati, OH: NIOSH.
Notes: GM = Geometric mean blood lead in µg/dl; (N) = Number of workers.
[a] $p < 0.05$, t-test for difference in geometric means.

Being right- or left-handed can determine which side of the body has the greatest exposure for jobs where the source of exposure is held in the hand such as spraying pesticides and paints. In a study on maleic hydrazide exposure during tobacco picking the left chest and stomach region of the workers had higher residues than the right chest and stomach. This was due to the harvesters being right-handed, thus picking the tobacco leaves with their right hand and holding the leaves against the left side of the body with the left arm (Herman, Hunt, and Sheets, 1985).

In a facility using 4,4′-methylene bis chloroaniline (MOCA) in a mold-making process, two secretaries showed low but detectable levels of MOCA in their urine (Klingner, 1992). The cause was determined to be contamination on paperwork that followed jobs and therefore circulated around the plant. When the secretaries processed the paperwork, their hands were exposed. This exposure was probably enhanced by the common habit of frequently licking a finger to leaf through papers.

Smoking increases exposures to toxic materials contained in the tobacco and combustion products. Smoking is also a consideration when biological monitoring is integrated into studies due to the wide variety of contaminants present in cigarette smoke. Metals such as arsenic, lead, and cadmium that contaminate a cigarette are likely to increase exposures while organic compounds may break down during the burning process and be converted into a greater or lesser hazard. One way of determining if cigarette contamination is an issue is to collect butts and have them analyzed. In one study this was done for polychlorinated biphenyls (PCBs) and *significant* amounts were found (Lees, Corn, and Breysse, 1987).

Workers were asked to carry cigarettes in a shirt pocket and smoke them during airblast spraying of pesticides (Wolfe et al., 1975). A high contamination resulted when cigarettes were handled with moist, contaminated hands (Table 4-3). The highest levels were transferred to cigarettes after their hands became contaminated from handling a pesticide drum. Even after hands were thoroughly washed with soap and water, detectable levels of parathion were transferred to the cigarette. It was calculated that if in a one-day period a worker smoked a pack of 20 cigarettes, all of which were contaminated with 235.6 μg of parathion (the highest level identified in the study, which resulted from handling drums contaminated with concentrated material), a dose of 4.7 mg would result. This dose would be sufficient to cause cholinesterase depression in a 60 kg adult.

Workers in remote areas may be less likely to practice good hygiene than those in factories whose work activities are more closely monitored. In a study on exposure to a mixture of 2,4,5-T and 2,4-D during spray application, it was determined that poor work habits contributed significantly to exposures (Kolmodin-Hedman et al., 1979). The workers wore the same clothes all week without laundering them. Two of them lived in a house trailer in the spray area and took their rest breaks in this trailer where the odor of the herbicide was noted. All workers were smokers and worked all day without washing their hands. Other habits included removing hats or visors with contaminated hands and putting them back on, wiping off sweat with a contaminated rag, rolling sleeves up, and pushing hats up off of the head.

Effect of Work Operations

There are many factors that can impact the effect of work operations on exposure. These include operating parameters related to the equipment such as speed, maintenance schedule, controls, and specified good operating work practices, as well as personal factors related to the workers such as work habits and experience. Job activities

TABLE 4-3. Cigarette Surface Contamination Versus Penetration to the Tobacco During Normal Handling up to Lighting of Cigarette

		μg Parathion per Cigarette			
Condition	*No. of Cigarette Exposures*	*Paper*	*Tobacco*	*Total*	*Percent of Total in Tobacco*
Dry hands	8	1.0	0.5	1.5	33.4
Moist hands	9	1.2	1.5	2.7	55.6

Source: From Wolfe H. R., J. F. Armstrong, D. C. Staiff, and S. W. Comer. 1975. Potential exposure of workers to parathion through contamination of cigarettes. *Bull. Env. Contam. Toxicol.* 13(3):369–376.

that can result in dermal exposure include splashes when working with or near liquids, wiping with contaminated rags, contact with contaminated tools or surfaces, and immersing parts in cleaning solvents manually rather than with a remote apparatus such as a hoist. When dermal exposures to auto body workers were studied, it was determined that the predominant skin exposure activity was the wiping of auto body surfaces with solvent-soaked rags prior to painting with a variety of solvent mixtures without using hand protection (Daniell et al., 1992). Another process where rags are frequently used is metalworking. However, oily work cloths from these operations should not be used to wipe off the skin, as metal particles may cause skin abrasions and get imbedded, which can lead to infection, and the oil itself can cause dermatitis.

Another factor is work experience. In one study it was shown that among electrical lineman responsible for climbing utility poles, those with less experience had higher dermal exposures to pentachlorophenol, the material used to preserve the poles (Thind, Karmali, and House, 1991). It was determined that linemen with less work experience were required to do more pole climbing than their fellow linemen with more seniority.

The type of operation can also influence which areas of the body are most likely to be exposed. Standing at a conveyor belt to grade treated lumber can require body movements such as leaning forward over the lumber, exposing the groin and thigh areas (front of the trousers) (Kleinman et al., 1986). During pesticide spray applications, if the spray is directed upward into the trees, the upper part of the body receives the greatest exposure; if the spray is directed at young crops, the rebound from the ground concentrates on the lower extremities (Wolfe, Durham, and Batchelor, 1961). Hydraulic sprayers tend to deposit more overspray on the arms, while when telescoping extension poles are used most of the material lands on the arms and legs (Haverty et al., 1983). All of these examples point out how the operating parameters can have a significant impact on the potential for skin contamination. These include the spray pump pressure (the higher the pressure, the greater the exposure), the height of the area being sprayed, and the type of apparatus. Table 4-4 lists practices that can increase dermal exposure for workers.

Exposures have been shown to be proportional to both the period of time worked and the rate at which work is performed, also referred to as the amount of material handled. Jobs in which the work is machine paced are closely related to work time, while work rate is the driving factor when the pace depends on the worker. For crop harvesting, work rate significantly affects exposure because it determines the number of contacts with residues; the more productivity, the higher the exposure (Nigg and Stamper, 1985). Skin deposition of tetrachlorphenol during work in timber mills is directly related to the speed with which workers pull and sort treated lumber, which in turn is related to the speed of the conveyor belt (Fenske, Horstman, and Bentley, 1987). When the belt stops so the workers can take breaks, the lumber often soaks in the treatment liquid, increasing exposures when the work starts up (Kleinman et al., 1986). All of these factors can increase the frequency of contact with contaminated materials. Frequency of exposure is important not only in determining total dose but also the exposure periods to solvents such as 2-butoxy ethanol, which will dry out the skin over time, therefore allowing greater penetration.

Poor operating practices can undermine the most carefully engineered situation. For example, ventilated glove boxes are commonly used for highly toxic compounds, such as beryllium, and will contain airborne material. However, surface and airborne contamination outside the box can still occur if the operator has to transfer pieces manually from one box to another. It can also happen if the seams of the gloves are not inspected regularly and they develop cracks.

Defective, poorly maintained equipment can also increase exposures. Leakage can result from cracked joints, corroded tanks, broken gaskets, and worn valve packings. Repairing contaminated equipment, such as pumps, can result in dermal exposure unless the equipment is cleaned before repair starts and handled with hoists and impermeable gloves while contaminated. Periodic inspections and maintenance of process equipment to minimize these events is therefore

TABLE 4-4. Work Practice Observations Illustrating Possible Sources of Dermal Exposure

Direct handling (without gloves) of contaminated transformer parts
Direct handling of contaminated tools, pumps, hoses, and test equipment
Failure to wear protective clothing
Failure to clean tools before returning them to tool boxes
Failure to clean pumps, hoses, and test equipment after each use
Improper storage of respirators in contaminated areas and with contaminated personal protective equipment
Improper glove and coverall removal techniques
Reuse of contaminated personal protective equipment
Failure to remove contaminated protective clothing upon leaving contaminated areas
Failure to wash hands, forearms, and face before smoking, eating, or drinking outside of contaminated areas (has dermal/oral component)
Cigarette smoking during work in contaminated areas (has dermal/oral component)
Eating and drinking in contaminated areas (has dermal/oral component)
Failure to use showers and clean/dirty locker rooms provided
Wearing work clothes and shoes home
Laundering work clothes at home
Dry sweeping—dust clouds land on clothing
Hopper treating potatoes with Captan dust-searching inside for stones and loosening jam-ups
Climbing on top of loaded trucks—coke dust, treated seed potatoes to install tarps
Dust falling from a conveyor holding pesticide treated seed potatoes
Entering truck beds to cover or unload contaminated cargo
Turned down gauntlets on gloves, exposing the lining
Ventilation holes cut into the backs of gloves/jacket cuffs outside of gloves
Wet fronts of shirts
Conveyor line work requiring workers to lean toward and stretch over contaminated materials in order to perform tasks

Sources: Data from Lees, P. S. J., M. Corn, and P. N. Breysse. 1987. Evidence for dermal absorption as the major route of body entry during exposure of transformer maintenance and repairmen to PCBs. *AIHA J.* **48**(3):257–264. Stevens, E. R., and J. E. Davis. 1981. Potential exposure of workers during seed potato treatment with Captan. *Bull. Env. Contam. Toxicol.* **26**:681–688. Kleinman, G. D., S. W. Horstman, D. A. Kalman, J. McKenzie, and D. Stansel. 1986. Industrial hygiene, chemical and biological assessments of exposures to a chlorinated phenolic sapstain control agent. *AIHA J.* **47**(12):731–741.

an important workplace control and can allow for repairs before failures occur.

In a plant using MOCA in its operation, two maintenance workers who did not work in the MOCA area had high urine levels of the chemical (Klingner, 1992). The source of their exposures was the tools used to perform weekly maintenance on the MOCA-handling equipment. These tools were stored unmarked in the tool bin and the workers used them for other purposes without wearing gloves. The solution was to decontaminate all the tools and dedicate those used for MOCA equipment to that area only. To provide further safety, the MOCA tools were painted red so they were easily differentiated from other equipment.

Contaminated tools should be decontaminated or stored inside marked containers, closets, or cabinets. Plastic handles are prone to absorption of many types of contaminants so tools with nonabsorbent handles should be selected for situations where decontamination is required. Another option is to cover absorbing work surfaces with a disposable cover, such as aluminum foil, during tasks.

Controls

Engineering, work practice, and housekeeping controls can have a significant impact on dermal exposures. Pumping of liquids (e.g., from drums) can eliminate worker contact from pouring. A control often recommended for skin penetrants such as 2-methoxy and 2-ethoxy ethanol is to restrict their use to a regulated area. A regulated area should be segregated with barriers and identified with readily observable signs at all entrances and accessways. Frequently these signs also contain reminders as to the CPC and good hygiene practices required when working in these areas. Entry to regulated areas should be restricted to authorized people only.

Grinding fluids used in metalworking operations, especially synthetic mixtures, can produce significant dermal exposures if controls are not in place. In metalworking operations examples of controls include daily monitoring of the coolant for biocide and microbial content, along with weekly laboratory analysis of coolant characteristics. Proportionate pumps can be installed in each of the central coolant systems to help maintain the proper coolant concentrations. Splash guards along with the installation of pneumatic cylinders to lift the guards so that the coolant will not drip on the operators' arms, will also help to minimize dermal exposures.

Good housekeeping in the workplace is important in controlling exposures and minimizing the spread of contaminants. Dust that has accumulated on surfaces can be reintroduced into the air, thereby increasing airborne exposures. Dust accumulated on chairs or work surfaces can cause unnecessary contamination of the employees' protective and personal clothing.

Lead contamination in nonproduction areas of radiator and battery shops is not uncommon (Goldfield et al., 1991). Lead can build up in production areas, and as a result of doors opening, ventilation systems that pull air into office areas, and traffic, lead migrates into the office and other nonproduction areas. In a study of several radiator shops that included surface wipes in both work and nonproduction areas, lead contamination was found to be pervasive in all the nonproduction areas including the shop office (up to 84,500 $\mu g/M^2$) (Piacitelli and Rice, 1993). Therefore, not only were the workers and office staff exposed, but also customers and families who would visit the shops.

A regular housekeeping program should be established to ensure that all surfaces are regularly cleaned and decontaminated and all unnecessary tools, objects, and waste are removed. Vacuuming is one of the most effective cleaning methods provided the vacuum is outfitted with the proper filter. Wet mopping can be used in areas where vacuuming is not feasible. Regular visual inspections should be performed for verification as well as for the detection of leaks and spills. Spills should be cleaned up promptly and the surfaces decontaminated. Surfaces to be cleaned include those that may cause inadvertent dermal contact, such as drinking fountains, tools, and control panels that may be touched by unprotected hands.

One way of controlling contamination from airborne materials deposited on surfaces is to keep lunchrooms under a positive pressure filtered air supply. Also, the location of lunch facilities is important, that is, keeping distance between them and the production areas. Eating facilities should be cleaned at the end of each work shift to reduce the potential for both oral and skin exposures. This is especially important if the facilities are located near the process areas.

Work Clothing and CPC

One inherent assumption often made is that clothing prevents dermal contact and, subsequently, absorption of contaminants; however, this is not always true. As noted in a previous section, contaminated work clothing can be a source of continuing exposure (see, for example, Fig. 4-3). It is not uncommon for work clothing such as coveralls or jumpsuits to be worn for up to a week

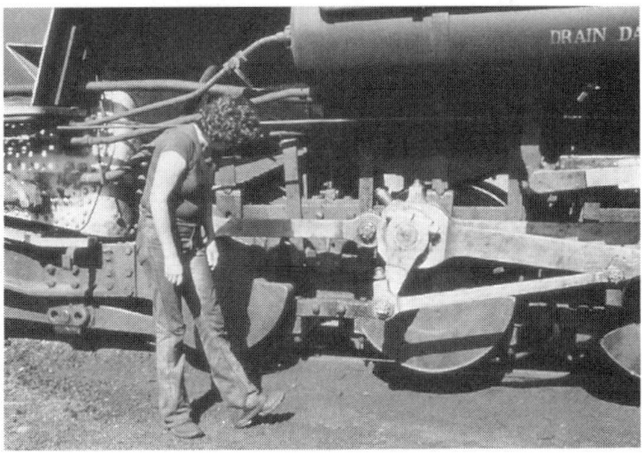

Figure 4-3. Contaminated clothing on a railroad worker.

or longer without cleaning; thus, the employee continues to be exposed even if he or she showers before leaving work each day. It is especially important for underclothing to be changed frequently and washed thoroughly before reuse because it is in direct contact with bare skin. It has been demonstrated repeatedly (Ader et al., 1958) that a positive correlation exists between benzidine concentrations on the skin, underwear, and clothes of workers and its concentration in the urine. Furthermore, when a daily change of underwear and working denims and after-work bath were introduced, the urinary level of benzidine was reduced by a factor of 2 to 3.

Contaminated work clothing (Fig. 4-4) has also been responsible for incidences of disease in worker's families. Cases associated with beryllium, lead, and asbestos are common in the literature (Table 4-5). High exposures were associated with laundering the contaminated clothing. Fortunately, employer-provided work clothing, locker rooms, and showers have decreased these exposures significantly, but such provisions are not available everywhere (Andersen et al., 1979; Grandjean and Bach, 1986).

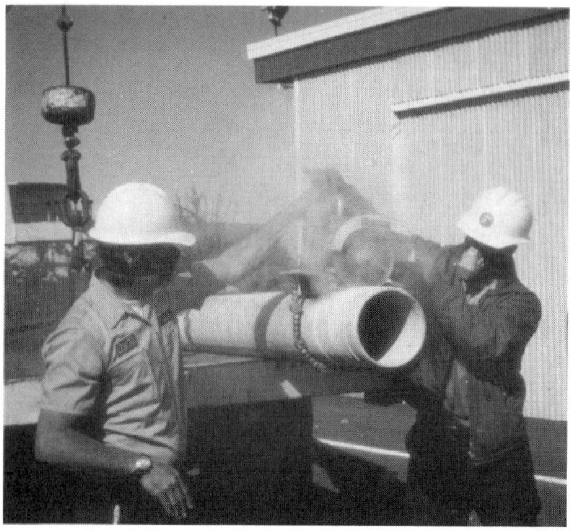

Figure 4-4. Dust flying onto workers' clothing during the cutting of asbestos/concrete pipe for community water systems.

Shoes are the most likely piece of personal clothing to be reused by workers. Leather work boots and gloves that are never cleaned can be a source of continuing exposure for months. Staining also decreases the likelihood that shoes

TABLE 4-5. Cases of Beryllium Disease from Contact with Contaminated Clothing

No.	*Age Group*	*Sex*	*Duration of Contact*	*Onset of Symptoms*	*Latency*	*Lung Biopsy or Autopsy*	*Be Analysis of Lung Tissue*
1	50–60	F	5 years	1944	No	+	+
2	30–40	F	1 year	1947	5 years	+	+
3	40–50	F	6 months	1948	5 years	+	+
4	50–60	F	9 years	1946	1 year	+	+
5	50–60	F	5 years	1948	4 years	+	+
6	30–40	F	11 years	1956	No	+	+
7	30–40	F	1 year	1957	14 years	+	+
8	50–60	F	7 years	1953	5 years	+	–
9	20–30	M	2 years	1949	4 years	+	Not done
10	10–20	F	2 months	1947	No	+	Not done
11	30–40	F	9 years	1943	No	+	Not done
12	40–50	F	12 years	1946	No	+	Not done
13	50–60	F	7 years	1945	No	+	Not done
14	50–60	F	3 years	1954	6 years	Not done	Not done
15	10–20	F	2 years	1954	9 years	Not done	Not done
16	40–50	F	7 years	1955	3 years	Not done	Not done
17	40–50	F	2 months	1949	1 year	Not done	Not done
18	50–60	F	13 years	1954	No	Not done	Not done
19	50–60	F	6 years	1947	No	Not done	Not done

Source: From Mitchell, R. N., and B. C. Eutslev. 1967. A study of beryllium surface contamination and resuspension. In *Surface Contamination*, G. W. Royster and B. R. Fish (eds.), New York: Pergamon Press, pp. 349–353.

will be used anywhere other than the workplace, allowing contamination to build up over time. Overboots are often perceived to be needed only if there is heavy liquid contamination present.

When a worker with consistently high urine levels from exposure to an aromatic amine was removed from a regulated job area, it was a surprise when he continued to have elevated urine levels, so further evaluation was done (Klingner, 1992). Wipe samples showed that the worker's shoes were heavily contaminated. Skin wipes showed that the worker contaminated his hands while putting the shoes on before work and then covered the contamination with his gloves. At the end of the shift the worker washed his hands and then removed his work clothing and shoes, thus recontaminating his hands with the chemical. A more serious exposure resulted when a painter who accidentally poured methanol on his clothing and shoes, and did not clean or change them, went blind within a few days, suggesting the primary source of exposure was through his skin (Lazariev, 1954).

Even in situations where clothing is exchanged on a daily basis exposures can occur. Fluorescence tracer monitoring has been used to demonstrate that a substantial portion of exposure can get beneath clothing, especially near the sleeves and neck openings of the garments, particularly for workers wearing coveralls (Fenske, 1990). The following garments were worn during the testing period: 50/50 cotton-polyester work shirts, coveralls of a 65/35 cotton/polyester fabric, or Tyvek coveralls. Most workers also had on cotton T-shirts under their clothing. Exposure clearly occurred beneath areas covered by both the T-shirt and the work shirt, with tracer deposition decreasing with increasing distance from the neck opening. The work shirt group had the greatest exposure, with the cotton/polyester coverall group next, and the Tyvek group third. Hand exposures occurred even though workers wore chemical protective gloves as they did not double glove (i.e., wear liner gloves underneath) and they handled the contaminated exteriors of their gloves at breaks. It was concluded that a significant portion of exposure beneath protective clothing occurs through the sleeves and neck openings of the garments rather than through penetration of the material. One possibility is to have employees wear light-colored uniforms, if appropriate, so it is easier to tell when skin contact with chemicals occurs.

Extensive research has been done to identify laundering variables that enhance the removal of pesticides from contaminated reusable clothing, since it has been demonstrated that routine laundering techniques do not remove all of these contaminants. Even when a laundry service is provided by employers, the employees generally wear their underclothes home. In a Danish study of smelter workers, workers had their personal underwear and socks washed at home while the company sent other work clothes to a commercial laundry (Table 4-6). Twelve pairs of socks from these men were examined. Workers with higher levels of lead in socks worked in the areas with higher airborne levels. The number of days worn (without laundering) was not as important in affecting lead

TABLE 4-6. Lead Contents of Socks (g/pair) worn by Secondary Lead Smelter Workers

Air Concentration[a]	*Number of Workers*	*Sock Concentration Median (Range)*	*Number of Days Worn Median (Range)*
<0.1 mg/M^3	5	0.28 (0.13–1.62)	8 (2–8)
>0.1 mg/M^3	7	1.26 (0.06–2.19)	14 (8–30)

Source: Grandjean, P., and E. Bach. 1986. Indirect exposures: The significance of bystanders at home and at work. *AIHA J.* **47**(12):822. (See also Danish Agency of Environmental Protection. 1983. *Indirect and Direct Occupational Lead Exposure* by E. Bach, J. M. Christiansen, P. Grandjean, and E. Olsen. Env. Proj. No. 50. Copenhagen [in Danish].)

[a]0.1 mg/M^3 was the PEL in Denmark for airborne lead.

concentrations in socks as were the airborne concentrations (Danish Agency of Environmental Protection, 1983). The airborne fume most likely settled out onto the floor and was resuspended as the workers walked about their work areas.

Contaminated CPC such as gloves, coveralls, boots, shoes, and respirators are all potential sources of contaminant transfer as they are most often reused and stored in the workplace. Contamination transfer often occurs when donning or removing contaminated gloves because workers are rarely taught what precautions to use in order to not contaminate themselves during doffing procedures (e.g., to clean off the exteriors of gloves prior to removal). A common practice is for workers to turn down the gauntlet on gloves while working, exposing both their forearm and the interior of the glove to contamination (Fig. 4-5).

If CPC is stored in a tool box, contamination from tools can spread to the CPC. The CPC in turn contaminates the workplace when the worker touches other items such as hard hat brims, handrails, door knobs, or control panels. Workers who use lunchrooms and offices without decontaminating can spread the contamination further.

Poorly fitting CPC including gloves, suits, and respirators can enhance exposures because the worker may have a false sense of protection. When gauze pads were mounted on the skin under Tyvek suits to monitor for 3,3′-dichlorobenzidine, contamination was found on the pads. It was suspected that the source of this exposure came during donning/doffing the suits rather than from permeation (NIOSH, May 1986). During a grouting operation it was noted that the grouting solution would splash back at the worker, resulting in the outer clothing becoming covered with acrylamide. Even though the individual was wearing rain gear, the acrylamide solution was observed entering the inside sleeves of the rain jacket and wetting the arms (Hills and Griefe, 1986).

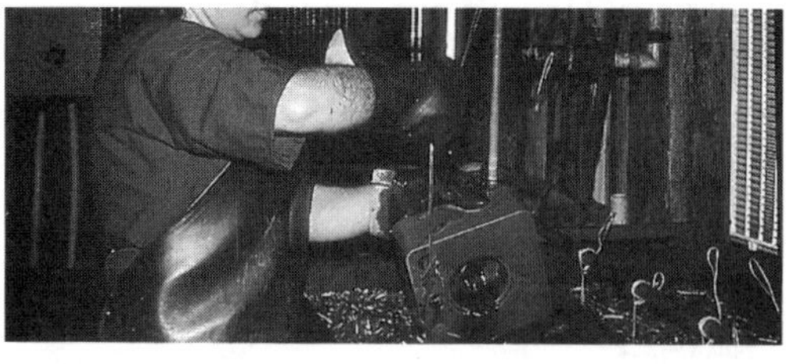

Figure 4-5. Turned-back cuff on glove of elecroplater. Note chromic acid stain on cuff. Although the apron protects the worker's front, his arms are exposed.

METHODS USED TO MONITOR WORKPLACE EXPOSURES

Site Inspections

Exposure assessments in which skin contact is considered important often start with an evaluation of the chemicals. As an example, a study was conducted in the tire and rubber manufacturing industry to determine if there was an association of skin cancer with the process (Bourguet, Checkoway, and Hulka, 1987). The jobs were grouped into occupational titles combining jobs from different parts of the industry that involve a similar operation (type of machinery and/or process); similar stock or product (different materials for the same product or the same materials for different products); or both similar operation and stock/product. For the next step two industrial hygienists who were familiar with the manufacturing facility rated each occupational title for skin contact with rubber stock, carbon black, extender oils, lubricating oils, and solvents. Company-specific ratings to describe the amount of exposure and the frequency of exposure were assigned. This information was then used by epidemiologists to review the lifetime job history of the workers. It may also be useful for prioritizing situations in which skin contact should be studied.

A walk through of work areas is often done prior to conducting any sampling. Subjective assessments of personal and work area hygiene are made. Often the first step in identifying whether specific compounds associated with skin problems are present is to collect a bulk sample and have it analyzed. Typical analytes are solvents, metals, amines, PAHs, and microbials. For each job where skin contamination is a problem, a specific note is made of those parts of the skin regularly contaminated due to machine design or employee work habits such as being right- or left-handed.

Sampling methods should always take into consideration the potential for the worker to be exposed through handling contaminated equipment, wearing contaminated clothing for several days, or driving a contaminated car prior to the work shift beginning. In one study of workers paving roads sprayed with a binder containing asphalt/coal tars, it was found that their hands were contaminated before they started work (Jongeneelen et al., 1988). In addition to those factors noted that can lead to contamination, it was also determined that the hands were chapped and the materials could impregnate in this skin over several days of exposures.

Surfaces frequently touched by production workers, such as drum lids, control panels, equipment, tools, switches, benches, or personal items, are commonly contaminated and good to sample as primary exposures. Cross-contamination from work surfaces is common in production offices on desks where people sit and fill out paperwork and on doorknobs and light switches, which are good to sample as sources of secondary exposures. Cafeteria tabletops and office desktops are most commonly sampled using wipes. Where workers change into and out of their work clothing, the clean side and the dirty side of the room need to be carefully monitored for cross-contamination.

Vehicle door handles, shift knobs, and steering wheels often build up contamination and therefore are commonly wiped. Seats can be vacuumed. Workers' clothes and shoes (which they wear home) have also been wiped, sniffed, vacuumed, and cut up and analyzed. Other surfaces in the workplace that are commonly wiped include the exterior of gloves and hard hats and the inside of respirator face pieces. Direct reading methods, such as wipes that change color or spot tests, are useful in training employees to modify their work practices because they are made immediately aware of the contamination. Table 4-7 lists typical surfaces wiped in workplace studies.

TABLE 4-7. Typical Surfaces Wiped in Workplace Studies

Production Areas
- Work benches and tabletops
- Stacks of production material
- Tools
- Unfinished and finished product surfaces
- Floors
- Exit doors
- Doors, cabinets, drawers, and work cart handles
- Parts baskets
- Equipment surfaces such as capacitors
- Washing machine control panels and lift handles
- Light switches
- Equipment switches

Conveyors
- Conveyor belts
- Tunnel walls
- Light fixtures
- Floors

Support Areas
- Tables used to clean respirators
- Changing room floors and benches
- Work shirt collars
- Street shoes (in change room)
- Work boots
- Lunch tables
- Vending machines
- Water fountains (mouthpiece)
- Coffee pots
- Shower stalls
- Refrigerator handles

Vehicle Interiors, Both Work and Personal
- Dashboard
- Window exteriors
- Floor under gas pedal
- Seats
- Steering wheel
- Door handles
- Brake pedal

Helicopter and Airplane Interiors
- Seats
- Controls
- Door latches
- Pilot's helmet
- Passenger headsets

Living and Eating Facilities (especially in field locations)
- Sinks
- Refrigerator door handles
- Freezer door handles
- Dining tabletops
- Water cooler base and spigots
- Lunch cooler tops
- Vending machine tops

Medical Evaluations

Medical evaluations also monitor workplace exposures. The following is a description of the recommended content for physical examinations for workers exposed to arsenic, a skin carcinogen (NIOSH, 1983). Note that it includes an inspection of the skin.

Preplacement Physical Examinations

The medical and work history questions should include background on photosensitivity and skin irritations or sensitivity. In addition to the regular preplacement physical examination and appropriate laboratory tests, all skin areas should be thoroughly examined. Warts, pigmented nevi, scars, and all other abnormal skin lesions should be recorded on a body outline form showing both front and back views. Inquiry should be made as to how any scar was obtained, since skin tumors or cancers may have been removed by electrocautery or excision on an outpatient basis. The size of all lesions should be measured and recorded so that any future change in size can be noted. A careful examination of the scrotum should be included. In addition, if the worker has not received a chest X-ray within a year's time, a preplacement chest X-ray should be taken.

Periodic Physical Examinations

Chest X-rays should be repeated on an annual basis or whenever the physician believes they are necessary. The examining physician should be trained in the identification of skin lesions that could be precancerous or cancerous, such as melanomas.

In addition to the regular physical examinations and appropriate laboratory tests, the skin should be examined at three- to six-month intervals, using the body outline form previously described. At these times the education of the worker can be continued and reinforced. Eventually, with conscientious workers, periodic skin examinations can probably be extended to once yearly.

Workers should also be encouraged to conduct periodic self-examinations of their skin, and any unexplained or changed rash, sore, wart, or mole should receive medical attention. Dermatitis, which can facilitate absorption, should be tended to immediately. All cuts and scratches should be washed and covered by an appropriate dressing, which should be changed as often as necessary to keep the injury free of oil and dirt. Any cut or scratch that appears to be infected, that is suspected to contain a piece of metal or other foreign body, or that does not seem to be healing properly should be brought to medical attention.

Record Keeping

It is just as important for an employer to keep records demonstrating efforts to prevent and minimize dermal exposure as it is to keep air sampling records. At a minimum, an estimate of the frequency and extent of skin contamination from chemicals posing a significant skin hazard, such as PAHs, should be recorded annually for each employee. Also performing tests will demonstrate that control measures are working, so the presence of these controls is not an excuse to not sample the skin or surfaces. A monitoring program to identify exposures and ascertain the effectiveness of controls will protect employees.

Sampling records (according to OSHA) should include, as a minimum, the names and social security numbers of those employees who were samples; the number, duration, and results of each of the samples collected, including a description of the sampling strategy that makes this representative sampling for all the employees in a given operation; a description of the operation involving exposure to the contaminant(s); date(s) on which monitoring was performed; the type of CPC, including gloves and suits used by the employee; and a description of the sampling and analytical methods. If an industrial hygiene consultant performs the monitoring, this information is likely to be contained in the consultant's report. Monitoring should be repeated whenever there is a change in the production process, chemical present, control equipment, personnel, or work practices, since such a change may result in new or additional exposures.

SURFACE MONITORING FOR WORKPLACE CONCERNS*

Contaminant	*Activity*	*Surface Methods*	*Other Monitoring*	*Reference*
Heavy metals Organics/semivolatiles PCBs 2,3,7,8-TCDD	Cleanup and closure of a dioxin incineration facility	Wipes of sheet metal walls, concrete foundations, and wood framework to determine the level and extent of contamination in the buildings	Bulk samples of floor dust	Perdek et al., 1991
Lead Mercury PCBs	Municipal water supply facility with contamination from prior uses	Wipes for PCBs Direct reading measurements on surfaces for mercury	Concrete chip and core Area air sampling Paint chips (lead)	Van Vynck and Shortsleeves, 1991
Acrylamide	Grouting sewers to plug leaks	Wipe samples of work surfaces including van	Personal breathing zone air samples Area air samples Dermal pad samples Hand rinses Wipes of CPC Urine	EPA, 1990
Acrylamide	Manufacturing plants	Wet wipes with MCE filters of reactor vessels, lab counter tops, door handles, and cafeteria tabletops	Personal breathing zone air samples Area air samples	Hills and Greife, 1986
Acrylamide	Sewer line grouting repair	Wipe samples with filters of control panel in van, on exterior of work gloves, and mixing tank	Personal breathing zone air samples Area air samples Rinse of glove interiors	Hills and Greife, 1986
Acrylamide	Sewer line grouting repair	Wipe samples using filters on work surfaces in vans	Personal breathing zone air samples Area air samples Skin wipes Hand rinses	Cummins et al., 1992
Asbestos	Abatement project	Transparent adhesive tape samples collected for decontamination effectiveness of equipment used in abatement projects; residual contamination in clean rooms and showers		Beaulieu, 1991

*For surface studies on amines, metals, PCBs and TCDD, and agriculture, see the Appendixes.

Contaminant	*Activity*	*Surface Methods*	*Other Monitoring*	*Reference*
Asbestos	Manufacture of brake linings	Vacuum sampling with personal sampling pump and 25 mm MCE filter cassette of employees' car seats Settled dust samples	Personal breathing zone air samples Clothing samples	NIOSH, March 1990 (HETA 87-126-2019)
Asbestos	Bakery with insulation on baking ovens suspected of containing asbestos	Vacuum sampling with personal sampling pump and 25 mm MCE filter cassette from the top of an electrical box, above thermostat, top of ovens, and ledge	Personal breathing zone air samples for aldehydes, VOCs, and dusts Area air sampling for aldehydes, ammonia, VOCs, and asbestos fibers	NIOSH, 1989*b* (HETA 87-379-1977)
Asbestos	Salt mining	Vacuum sampling with personal sampling pump and 25 mm MCE filter cassette of dust from office and steam cylinder	Personal breathing zone air samples for nitrogen oxides and diesel particulates Area air samples for CTPV, PAHs, and carbon monoxide	NIOSH, October 1991*a* (HETA 88-389-2147)
Asbestos	Salt mining	Vacuum sampling with personal sampling pump and 25 mm MCE filter cassette of dust from control rooms, hoist house ledge, turbine drive, and floor	Personal breathing zone air samples for nitrogen oxides and diesel particulates Area air samples for CTPV, PAHs, and carbon monoxide	NIOSH, October 1991*b* (HETA 88-390-2148)
Asbestos	Vehicle maintenance shop	Vacuum sampling with personal sampling pump and 25 mm MCE filter cassette of dust on outside of truck cab and floor near wheel of brake job	Area air samples Bulk samples of insulation	NIOSH, 1989 (HETA 88-372-1953)
Asbestos	Power station where workers had stations outside an asbestos abatement containment	Settled dust vacuumed into filter cassette with personal air sampling pump	Personal breathing zone air samples Area air samples Bulk samples of insulated wire	NIOSH, November 1989 (HETA 89-262-1994)
3,4-Benzpyrene	Coal hydrogenation plant with processes suspected of releasing a mist	Whatman No. 1 filters placed on a music stand at 12 representative areas to collect fallout to determine source of freckles on workers' skin	Area air samples Skin examination	Ketcham and Norton, 1960

Contaminant	*Activity*	*Surface Methods*	*Other Monitoring*	*Reference*
Benzo(a)pyrene	Steel mill rolling plant, coke oven, blast furnace, and electric furnace areas	Settled dust samples in these areas to compare with levels of suspended dust	Area air samples	Tanimura, 1968
Cyanide	Jewelry manufacture	Wipe samples of a (50 sq. in.) area in glove box interior and exterior and storage cabinet using silver membrane filters	Personal breathing zone air samples Area air samples CPC wipes	NIOSH, March 1987 (HETA 86-30-1785)
Decomposition products of white pine tar rosin	Manufacture of telecommunications switchboard systems where a wave soldering machine was used to process flexible plastic circuit boards	Wipe samples of circuit boards	Personal breathing zone air sample for fluoride and isopropanol Area air samples for fluoride and isopropanol Bulk sample of soldering flux	NIOSH, February 1981 (HHE 80-151-821)
Diethylamino-ethanol (DEAE)	Office building in a pharmaceutical packaging facility	Whatman filter wipes from skylight in office and desktop	Area air sample for DEAE, hydrazine, and organic vapors Bulk samples of boiler condensate, water, and additive	NIOSH, 1981 (HETA 81-247-958)
DEAE	Manufacturing facility of circuit boards and electrical equipment for commercial and defense uses where steam is treated with DEAE and an illness outbreak has occurred and odors are present	Whatman smear tabs used to wipe for DEAE on tabletops, table supports, and floor	Area air sampling for organic vapors, metals, DEAE, and cyclohexylamine Bulk boiler water	NIOSH, December 1989 (HETA 89-57-2003)
Diethylstilbestrol (DES)	Manufacturing of diethylstilbestrol	Wipe samples in finishing area (roof, floor) and of the lunchroom drink dispenser to assess the potential exposures of male workers with breast symptoms	Personal breathing zone air samples Area air samples Urine (spot samples)	Shmunes and Burton, 1981
DES	Facility producing DES where there were concerns of breast enlargement in male employees	Wipe samples on roof over finish room, floor, and on drink dispenser in lunchroom	Personal breathing zone air samples Area air samples Urine	NIOSH, June 1973 (HHE 71-9-50)

Contaminant	*Activity*	*Surface Methods*	*Other Monitoring*	*Reference*
Dinitrochlorobenzene (DNCB)	Manufacture of oryzalin (4-di-n-propylamine-3,5-dinitro-1-trifluoromethyl-benzene)	Whatman smear tabs used to wipe for DNCB on desk and top of storage cabinet	Personal breathing zone air samples for DNCB and oryzalin	NIOSH, November 1985 (HETA 80-35-1635)
Dinitrotoluene (DNT)	Synthesis of dinitrotoluene (operations, maintenance, and quality control staffs)	Wetted gauze pads used to wipe equipment, valves, door handles, desks, logbook cover, knobs, and switches in the work area	Personal breathing zone air samples Urine Skin wipes CPC wipes	Levine et al., 1985
Dipropylene glycol monomethyl ether	Printing facility	Whatman filter wipes of work bench	Personal breathing zone air samples Area air samples Skin and CPC wipes Bulk samples of washing solution	NIOSH, August 1983*a* (HETA 81-304-1361)
2,4-Ditertbutyl phenol	Manufacture of cylindrical hydraulic pumps with rubber coated interiors	Wetted cotton balls used to wipe surfaces of rubber used in manufacturing to determine source of employees' vitiligo	Bulk samples of formulated stock rubber	O'Malley et al., 1988
2,4-Ditertbutyl phenol	Pump manufacture involving injection molding of rubber products	Cotton swabs wetted with ethanol used to wipe rubber products for unknown contaminants to determine source of employees' vitiligo	Bulk samples of spray adhesive, cured and uncured rubber	NIOSH, December 1986 (HETA 86-018-1758)
Ethylene thiourea (ETU)	Manufacture of molded rubber products, rubber coated fabric, and liquid rubber adhesives	Wipe samples of windows, work surfaces, light switches, and equipment with Whatman smear tabs	Personal breathing zone air samples Area air samples Skin and CPC wipes Blood	NIOSH, 1978 (HHE 77-67-499)
Explosives Pentaerythritol Styphnic acid Trinitroresorcinol Nitrocellulose Nitroglycerin Trinitrotoluene Dinitrotoluene N-Tetranitro-N-methylaniline (tetryl) Cyclotrimethyl-enetrinitramine (RDX)	Closure of Frankford military arsenal	Surface samples with Q-tips (acetone) (5 circles 5 cm in diameter per m^2) used for initial and repeat sampling to verify decontamination	Samples of sump liquid	EPA, 1985

Contaminant	*Activity*	*Surface Methods*	*Other Monitoring*	*Reference*
Formaldehyde Paraformaldehyde	Research and development laboratory with contamination from bird droppings above suspended ceiling (histoplasma capsulatum)	Wipe samples using impregnated filters on office and laboratory surfaces for paraformaldehyde contamination after fumigation of air handling unit	Area samples for formaldehyde	NIOSH, January 1984 (HETA 83-312-1400)
Hexachlorocyclopentadiene Octachlorocyclopentene	Sanitary wastewater treatment plant that experienced major chemical contamination	Whatman filters, wetted, used to wipe a ($100\ cm^2$) area on a typewriter, desk, window sill, and table to determine if decontamination was effective inside the administration building, which was very close to the contaminated treatment facility	Area air samples	NIOSH, August 1978 (TA 77-39)
Hydrogen peroxide	Manufacture of picture tubes for TVs where employees were experiencing hair discoloration	Wipes with strips of litmus paper in work areas including on screens and canopies	Personal breathing zone air samples for metals and solvents Area air samples for metals and solvents Skin and hair wipes Checks of bulk solutions with wipes	NIOSH, May 1980 (HHE 79-105-687)
Isodecanes Polymethacrylate amines	Toner used in platemaking operation	Wipe samples using dry and wet filters in the work area	Personal breathing zone air samples Hand wipes Bulk samples of toner	NIOSH, January 1980*a* (HHE 78-77-659)
Mercury	Dental clinic	Bachrach Mercury Sniffer used to sniff surfaces: countertops, carpet, and floor	Personal breathing zone air samples Ambient air monitoring	NIOSH, November 1976 (TA 76-108)
Mercury	Dental clinic	Bachrach Mercury Sniffer used to sniff carpets	Breathing zone air samples for mercury General area air samples for nitrous oxide	NIOSH, July 1982*b* (HETA 82-70-1148)
Mercury	Dental clinic	Bachrach Mercury Sniffer used to sniff: carpets, table, under floor mat, countertops, cabinet, chair seat, mop, and floors	Breathing zone air samples General area air samples Urine	NIOSH, April 1977 (HHE 77-21-381)

Contaminant	*Activity*	*Surface Methods*	*Other Monitoring*	*Reference*
Mercury	Dental clinic	Bachrach Mercury Sniffer used to sniff surfaces: carpet and tile floors, before and after scuffing, sink, and trash can	Personal breathing zone air samples Area air samples	NIOSH, May 1981 (HETA 81-63-869)
Mercury	Dental clinic	Wipe samples for mercury on surfaces Bachrach Mercury Sniffer used to sniff surfaces: sink trap, instruments, wall, shoe soles, dental chair, carpeting, and baseboard where visible droplets of mercury were present	Personal breathing zone air samples Air area samples	NIOSH, June 1978 (TA 78-35)
Mercury	Dental clinic	Bachrach Mercury Sniffer used to sniff surfaces: floor, lab shelves, and stand under the wiggle bug	Personal breathing zone air samples	NIOSH, October 1978 (TA 78-45)
Mercury	Dental clinic	Bachrach Mercury Sniffer used to sniff surfaces: amalgamator, radiator, chair seat, drawer, floor, cuspidor drain	Personal breathing zone air samples Area air samples	NIOSH, 1976 (TA 76-45)
Mercury	Dental office	Direct reading instrument used to sniff floors, sinks, column, and the interior of a vacuum to identify surface contamination	Personal breathing zone air samples during normal operations and vacuuming Area air samples during normal operations and vacuuming	NIOSH, February 1988 (HETA 87-147-1873)
Mercury	Dental clinic	Bachrach Mercury Sniffer used to sniff surfaces: countertops, shelves, carpet, couch, and mops	Ambient air samples	NIOSH, April 1979 (HHE 79-47-582)
Mercury	Dental office	Bachrach Mercury Sniffer to "map" mercury contamination on floor in patient area	Personal breathing zone air samples for mercury and nitrous oxide Area air sampling for mercury	NIOSH, 1970 (HHE 79-107-632)

Contaminant	*Activity*	*Surface Methods*	*Other Monitoring*	*Reference*
Mercury	Dental office	Bachrach Mercury Sniffer used in areas where mercury silver dental fillings are prepared	Personal breathing zone air samples	NIOSH, May 1976 (HHE 76-6-294)
Mercury	Dental office	Monitoring of surfaces (counters, cracks, heating ducts, floors, carpet) and dust inside carpet sweeper using a Bachrach Mercury Sniffer	Personal breathing zone air samples Area air sampling	NIOSH, February 1985 (HETA 84-90-1533)
Mercury	Dental office	Monitoring of surfaces (amalgamator, doorway, floors, carpet) and dust inside a vacuum cleaner using a Jerome Gold Film Mercury Vapor Analyzer	Personal breathing zone air samples Area air sampling	NIOSH, August 1989*a* (HETA 87-265-1975)
Mercury	Hospital	Monitoring of surfaces (sinks, centrifuge, drawers, cabinet, floor, workbench, air conditioner) in areas where there had been breakage of mercury containing instruments with a Bachrach Mercury Sniffer	Personal breathing zone air samples	NIOSH, June 1980 (TA 79-19)
Mercury	Thermometer manufacturing facility	Sampling with a direct reading instrument to pinpoint localized sources of mercury and areas of potential contamination	Personal breathing zone air samples Area air samples Urine	NIOSH, February 1986 (HETA 83-465-1674)
Mercury	Thermometer manufacturing facility	Bachrach Mercury Sniffer used to sniff workbenches and trash	Breathing zone air monitoring Area air monitoring Clothing monitoring	NIOSH, July 1976 (HETA 76-49-312)
Mercury	Thermometer manufacturing facility	Bachrach Mercury Sniffer used to sniff work tables and floors at workstations and lunch station	Breathing zone air samples	NIOSH, December 1982 (HETA 82-364-1243)

Contaminant	*Activity*	*Surface Methods*	*Other Monitoring*	*Reference*
Mercury	Scientific glassware manufacturing plant	Direct reading instrument used to sniff work tables and floors	Breathing zone air samples Urine	Danziger and Possick, 1973
Mercury	Altimeter testing area of an aircraft instrument manufacturing facility	Monitoring of surfaces (cracks, workbenches, floors) in areas with a Bachrach Mercury Sniffer	Monitoring for combustible gases and vapors	NIOSH, 1981 (HHE 78-22-732)
Mercury	R&D laboratory of a facility manufacturing industrial chemicals, pharmaceutical intermediates, and urethanes	Monitoring of surfaces (sinks, countertops, lab hoods, floors) in areas where there had been breakage of mercury containing instruments with a direct reading instrument	Breathing zone air monitoring for acetone	NIOSH, September 1986*a* (HETA 85-131-1731)
Mercury	Microfiche filming operation in building with mercury contamination from a prior operation	Sampling with a direct reading instrument on surfaces (under sinks, floors) to pinpoint localized sources of mercury and areas of potential contamination	Area air monitoring indoors and ambient levels outdoors Urine	NIOSH, July 1988 (HETA 87-431-1916)
Mestranol Norethindrone	Manufacturing of oral contraceptives: granulation, pelletizing, and packaging	Glass fiber filters used to wipe workbench, employees' clothing, and changing room surfaces	Personal breathing zone air samples Area air samples Blood Clothing wipes	Harrington et al., 1978
Methylene diisocyanate (MDI)	Hand casing MDI-based polyurethane to produce parts	Surface wipes of work surfaces with Perma-Tec color-change isocyanate pads	Hand wipes Urine	Klingner, 1993
Mixex Lindane 2,3,7,8-TCDD	Manufacturing facility	Settled dust samples collected with vacuuming technique and personal air sampling pump to determine the effectiveness of decontamination		NIOSH, June 1978 (TA 78-35)
NIAX Catalyst ESN Components: bis (2-Dimethyl amino) ethyl ether Dimethylamino-propionitrile	Manufacture of molded flexible polyurethane foam seat cushions for autos and pickup trucks	Whatman filters used to wipe drum tops, conveyor belts, process equipment, seat cushions, rollers, and stirring rod in mixing drum	Personal breathing zone air samples Area air samples	NIOSH, December 1978 (HHE 78-68-546)

Contaminant	*Activity*	*Surface Methods*	*Other Monitoring*	*Reference*
Nicotine	Tobacco harvesting	Wipe samples with cotton cloth of moisture that had gathered on tobacco leaves during an evaluation of the effectiveness of CPC in preventing green tobacco sickness in workers	Urine	Gehlbach, Williams, and Freeman, 1979
Nor-nitrogen mustard chloride	Chemical plant	Rayon cloth (10 × 10 cm) used to wipe surfaces in the weighing room, reactor hall, and corridors during weighing and charging operations	Personal breathing zone air samples	Thulin, 1993
Oil Metals Particulates	Employees assembling speedometers in a car component factory with irritant dermatitis	Swabs of ionizer head and top of compressed air line	Area air samples Bulk samples Solvent wash of compressed air gun	Zsigmond, 1985
PAHs (cyclohexane solubles)	Maintenance work on electrostatic precipitators in coke plant	Wipe samples of electrode and insulator surfaces	Personal breathing zone air samples Skin and CPC wipes Bulk samples of precipitator particulates	NIOSH, October 1985 (HETA 82-309-1630)
PAHs	Manufacture of faucets (die/punch, drop forge)	Wipe samples of the die/punch area, conveyor belt and back side of the drop-forge assembly to be used for potential testing of carcinogenicity and mutagenicity of released air contaminants	Personal breathing zone air samples Area air samples	NIOSH, April 1980 (HHE 79-37-684)
Particulates (Fibrous glass)	Passenger service area of an airline where agents have dry skin and itching dermatitis	Wipes of settled dust on the arrival desk, check-in counters, and agent's office.	High volume area air samples Bulk air samples	NIOSH, August 1983c (HETA 82-100-1349)
Pentachlorophenol, sodium salt 2,3,4,6-Tetrachlorophenol	Spray application, grading and pulling spray-treated lumber in a timber mill	Filter disks (42.5 mm) placed on surface of lumber for 1 minute to determine the effect of time on the chemical's binding to lumber	Area air samples Urine Fluorescence tracer with skin evaluation under UV light	Bentley, Horstman, and Morgan, 1989

Contaminant	*Activity*	*Surface Methods*	*Other Monitoring*	*Reference*
Rozol	Research institute on animal behavior	Wipe samples for rodenticide collected on lab surfaces to determine source of abnormal incidence of cancer, breast and ovarian cysts among employees	Area air samples	NIOSH, 1980 (HETA 80-92-769)
Sodium cyanide		Wipe samples of 55 gallon container exteriors and interiors to determine if labels were correct	Personal breathing zone air samples for organic vapors and total dust Area air samples for organic vapors and carbon monoxide	NIOSH, December 1979 (HHE 79-103-640)
Tetrachlorophenol	Grading and pulling spray-treated lumber in a timber mill	Gauze (12 ply) pads used to wipe over a 6 sq. in. area of treated wood to determine dislodgeable residues Gauze (12 ply) pads taped to boards prior to spray treatment to determine total spray deposition	Fluorescent tracer treatment and video imaging of skin Urine Cotton gloves	Fenske, Horstman, and Bentley, 1987
Triethylene glycol diacrylate	Production of UV sensitive photography plates	Wipe samples on surfaces to determine if TDA has been dripping from overhead piping		NIOSH, January 1980*b* (HHE 80-5-651)
Tris 2,3-dibromopropyl phosphate Aluminum trihydrate	Fabrication of seat covers and interior carpets for automobiles	Wipe samples with MCE filters of tabletops in work areas	Personal breathing zone air samples Skin wipes	NIOSH, June 1977 (HHE 77-39-400)
Zeranol	Formulation, pelletizing, and packaging	Gauze pads wetted and wiped over a 100 cm^2 area on work surfaces, ventilation duct interiors, and walls	Personal breathing zone air samples General area air samples Dermal pads on hands Work clothing	NIOSH, March 1985 (HETA 82-257-1571)
Zeranol	Manufacturing plant involving formulation, pelletizing, and packaging of an animal growth promoter	Gauze pads wetted and wiped over a 25 cm^2 area inside lunchrooms, ventilation system, and work surfaces to evaluate the potential for exposures and the development of breast symptoms in both male and female workers	Personal breathing zone air samples Gauze dermal pads Blood Work garments	Aw et al., 1989

DERMAL MONITORING FOR WORKPLACE CONCERNS*

Contaminant	*Activity*	*Dermal Methods*	*Other Monitoring*	*Reference*
Acid ions	Cleanup of chemical manufacturing site	Wipe samples of boots and gloves to verify the effectiveness of decontamination procedures	Personal breathing zone air samples for acids and solvents Area air samples for acids and solvents	NIOSH, August 1983*b* (HETA 83-417-1357)
Acrylamide	Grouting sewers to plug leaks	Cellulose pads attached to outside of workers' clothing at 10 different sites Bag hand rinses Wipes of respirator interiors and exteriors, and exteriors of work gloves	Personal breathing zone air samples Area air samples Wipe samples of work surfaces including van Urine	EPA, 1990
Acrylamide	Grouting sewers to plug leaks	Wipe samples with filters of forearms and necks of workers Hand rinse with 50 mL of deionized water of predominant hand	Personal breathing zone air samples Area air samples Wipe samples on van work surfaces	Cummins et al., 1992
Acrylamide	Sewer line grouting repair	Rinse of glove interiors and exteriors	Personal breathing zone air samples Area air samples Wipe samples with filters of van and mixing tank to identify surface contamination	Hills and Greife, 1986
Acrylonitrile	Fire in a chemical synthesis facility	Patch samples cut from turnout gear and analyzed		NIOSH, September 1983 (HETA 83-157-1373)
Asbestos	Manufacture of brake linings	Vacuum sampling with personal sampling pump and 25 mm MCE filter cassette of workers' personal clothing: shirts and pants	Personal breathing zone air samples Car interiors Settled dust samples	NIOSH, March 1990 (HETA 87-126-2019)
Asbestos	Manufacture of brake shoes	Vacuum sampling with personal sampling pump and 25 mm MCE filter cassette of workers' personal clothing: shirts and pants	Personal breathing zone air samples	NIOSH, September 1986 (HETA 84-262-1734)
Beclomethasone	Synthesis and processing into aerosol containers for inhalational use	Skin swabs of workers	Air samples	Phillips, 1982

*For dermal studies with metals, PCBs and TCDD, amines, and pesticides, see the Appendixes.

Contaminant	*Activity*	*Dermal Methods*	*Other Monitoring*	*Reference*
3,4-Benzpyrene	Coal hydrogenation plant with processes suspected of spraying employees	Examination of employees' skin for fluorescence under UV (253.7 ηm) light	Area air samples Fallout samples using filter paper on a music stand	Ketcham and Norton, 1960
3,4-Benzpyrene	Pitch (coal-tar) producing plant	Underwear and working clothes of workers analyzed before and after laundering		Kandus, Masek, and Jach, 1972
Cyanide	Jewelry manufacture	Wipe samples of glove exteriors using silver membrane filters	Personal breathing zone air samples Area air samples Surface wipes	NIOSH, March 1987 (HETA 86-30-1785)
Dimethylpolysiloxane (DMPS)	Cracker and cookie baking facility	Wipe samples with Whatman smear tabs on faces of exposed and non-exposed workers to determine source of eye irritation	Personal breathing zone air samples for DMPS, aldehydes, and alcohols Area air samples for DMPS, aldehydes, and alcohols	NIOSH, May 1982 (HETA 81-396-1118)
Dinitrotoluene (DNT)	Synthesis of dinitrotoluene (operations, maintenance, and quality control staffs)	Skin wipes with cotton gauze and isopropanol of operations and lab workers' hands and forehead or face following specific tasks	Personal breathing zone air samples Urine Work surface and CPC wipes	Levine et al., 1985
Dipropylene glycol monomethyl ether	Printing facility	Wipe samples with Whatman filters of hand and glove of worker	Personal breathing zone air samples Area air samples Bulk samples of washing solution Surface wipes	NIOSH, August 1983*a* (HETA 81-304-1361)
2-Ethylhexanoic acid	Wood preservation operations in sawmills: through dipping and spray irrigation	Pads (10 × 10 cm) of filter papers taped to the inside and outside of work clothing at the back, chest, thigh, and forearm	Personal breathing zone air samples Urine	Kroger, Liesivuori, and Manninen, 1990
Ethylene thiourea (ETU)	Manufacture of molded rubber products, rubber coated fabric, and liquid rubber adhesives	Wipe samples of employees' hands, arms, shirt shoulders, and glove exteriors with Whatman smear tabs	Personal breathing zone air samples Area air samples Surface wipes Blood	NIOSH, 1978 (HHE 77-67-499)
Hydrogen peroxide	Manufacture of picture tubes for TVs where employees were experiencing hair discoloration	Wipes with strips of litmus paper on workers' hands, eyebrows, and hair	Personal breathing zone air samples for metals and solvents Area air samples for metals and solvents Surface wipes pH checks of bulk solutions with litmus	NIOSH, May 1980 (HHE 79-105-687)

Contaminant	*Activity*	*Dermal Methods*	*Other Monitoring*	*Reference*
Mercury Pyridine Hydrofluoric acid	Fire in a chemical warehouse where firefighters developed dermatitis	Wipe samples from a fireman's boot and analysis of a turnout coat both worn at the fire	Area air sampling Bulk samples of runoff water	NIOSH, January 1988 (HETA 85-375-1861)
Methylene diisocyanate (MDI)	Hand casing MDI-based polyurethane to produce parts	Wipes of hands with Perma-Tec color-change isocyanate pads	Surface wipes Urine	Klingner, 1993
Nitrobenzene Pyridene Thiophene	Laboratory for smell tests	Skin wipes on both hands of smell testers before and after washing to determine source of their symptoms	Personal breathing zone air samples	NIOSH, February 1983 (HETA 82-338-1266)
PAHs (cyclohexane solubles)	Maintenance work on electrostatic precipitators in coke plant	Wipes of hands and gloves of workers	Personal breathing zone air samples Surface wipes Bulk samples of precipitator particulates	NIOSH, October 1985 (HETA 82-309-1630)
PAHs	Road paving when binders of asphalt/coal tars are used	Polypropylene pads ($1.77\ cm^2$) mounted with self-adhesive tape to the skin on the neck, elbow, wrist, and under work clothing at shoulder and ankle Handwash using sunflower oil	Personal breathing zone air samples Urine (preshift and end of shift)	Jongeneelen et al., 1988
PAHs	Synthetic fuel (coal derived) pilot plant	Skin of workers with the potential for skin contact with process materials monitored for fluorescence with Spill Spotter (UV based instrument) calibrated with 1 ppm B(α)P, and forehead, neck, cheeks, and back of hand monitored quantitatively pre- and postshift and postshower Skin of workers also monitored qualitatively with black light lamp on face		Hill, 1984

Contaminant	*Activity*	*Dermal Methods*	*Other Monitoring*	*Reference*
PAHs	Coal liquefaction pilot plant: dry cleaning and laundering of workers' clothing	Laundered clothing examined using UV light inspection	Bulk samples of dry cleaning solvent	Shepard, 1981
PAHs (benzene solubles)	Processing of high sulfur, high ash coal into liquids (naphtha, fuel oil)	Facial skin wipes with acetone or isopropanol (pre- and postshower) Skin wash with cyclohexane aerosol spray apparatus with collection cup UV light photography of workers' skin fluorescence	Personal breathing zone air samples	Cheng, 1981
Pentachlorophenol (PCP)	Electrical linemen climbing treated utility poles	Leather gloves analyzed	Urine	Thind, Karmali, and House, 1991
PCP	National monument with PCP treated walls	Skin wipes of palm of right hand of employees with Whatman smear tabs	Area air samples in offices Surface wipes in offices Bulk sample of crystals scraped off wall Urine	NIOSH, January 1985 (HETA 83-090-1326)
PCP, sodium salt 2,3,4,6-Tetrachlorophenol (TCP)	Spray application, grading and pulling spray-treated lumber in a timber mill	Fluorescent tracer (disodium fluorescein) added to spray mix and visualization of workers' skin and clothing performed under UV lamps to motivate workers to improve work practices	Surface samples on lumber Area air samples Urine (postshift, spot)	Bentley, Horstman, and Morgan, 1989
Phosdrin	Pesticide manufacture	Wipes of gloves used for drumming, sampling, and in lab with Whatman smear tabs	Personal breathing zone air samples Blood Surface wipes	NIOSH, January 1985 (HETA 78-4-1511)
Stainless steel and carbon graphite fibers	Manufacture of electrostatic brushes	Pre- and postshift wipe samples from workers' exposed skin using MCE filters	Personal breathing zone air samples Area air samples	NIOSH, August 1984 (HETA 82-289-1496)

Contaminant	*Activity*	*Dermal Methods*	*Other Monitoring*	*Reference*
TCP	Grading and pulling spray-treated lumber in a timber mill	Fluorescent tracer (4-methyl-7-diethylaminocoumarin) added to treating formulation and skin examination under UV with video imaging system of head, hands, forearms, torso, upper and lower legs Cotton gloves Skin wipes	Wipe samples of wood Gauze pads taped to boards prior to spray treatment Urine	Fenske, Horstman, and Bentley, 1987
Tris 2,3-dibromopropyl phosphate Aluminum trihydrate	Fabrication of seat covers and interior carpets for automobiles	Cotton gloves Wipe samples of employees' hands	Personal breathing zone air samples Wipes of work surfaces	NIOSH, June 1977 (HHE 77-39-400)
Vapona	Pesticide manufacture	Wipes of gloves used for drumming, sampling, and in lab with Whatman smear tabs	Personal breathing zone air samples Blood Surface wipes	NIOSH, 1984 (HETA 78-4-1511)
Zeranol	Formulation, pelletizing, and packaging	Cotton gauze pads ($25\ cm^2$) with a wide-mesh canvas cover on top and aluminum foil backing attached to palm of dominant hand in formulation area using elastic straps; placed on nondominant hand in packaging area Work clothing from upper body analyzed	Personal breathing zone air samples General area air samples Wipe samples of work surfaces	NIOSH, March 1985 (HETA 82-257-1571)
Zeranol	Manufacturing plant involving formulation, pelletizing, and packaging of an animal growth promoter	Cotton gauze pads ($25\ cm^2$) with aluminum foil backings attached by plastic straps to the palms of workers to evaluate the potential for exposures and the development of breast symptoms in both male and female workers Work garment surfaces	Personal breathing zone air samples Surface wipes Work garments Blood	Aw et al., 1989

REFERENCES

Ader, D., J. Piotrowski, and Z. Zaremba. 1958. Chemical evaluation of industrial exposure to benzidine. II. Attempt to evaluate the absorption of benzidine in industrial conditions. *Med. Prac.* 9:207–217.

Anderson, H. A., R. Lilis, S. M. Daum, and I. J. Selikoff. 1979. Asbestosis among household contacts of asbestos factory workers. *Ann. N.Y. Acad. Sci.* **330**:387–399.

Aw, T. C., A. B. Smith, R. L. Stephenson, and C. J. Glueck. 1989. Occupational exposure to zeranol, an animal growth promoter. *Brit. J. Ind. Med.* **46**: 341–346.

Batchelor, G. S., and K. C. Walker. 1954. Health hazards involved in use of parathion in fruit orchards of north central Washington. *Arch. Ind. Hyg. Occup. Med.* **10**:522–529.

Beaulieu, H. J. 1991. Asbestos contamination of abatement equipment surfaces. *Appl. Occup. Env. Hyg.* **6**(7):583–587.

Bentley, R. K., S. W. Horstman, and M. Morgan. 1989. Reduction of sawmill worker exposure to chlorophenols. *Appl. Ind. Hyg.* **4**(3):69–74.

Bourguet, C. C., H. Checkoway, and B. S. Hulka. 1987. A case control study of skin cancer in the tire and rubber manufacturing industry. *Am. J. Ind. Med.* **11**:461–473.

Cheng, R. 1981. The industrial hygiene occupational medicine program for the SRC-II project. *Proceedings of a Workshop on Industrial Hygiene and Occupational Medicine in Coal Conversion Projects*. DOE/CONF-801143, 1981, pp. 65–68.

Cummins, K., D. Morton, D. Lee, E. Cook, and R. Curtis. 1992. Exposure to acrylamide in chemical sewer grouting operations. *Appl. Occup. Env. Hyg.* **7**(6):385–391.

Daniell, W., A. Stebbins, D. Kalman, J. F. O'Donnell, and S. W. Horstman. 1992. The contributions to solvent uptake by skin and inhalation exposure. *AIHA J.* **53**(2):124–129.

Danish Agency of Environmental Protection. 1983. *Indirect and Direct Occupational Lead Exposure* by E. Bach, J. M. Christiansen, P. Grandjean, and E. Olsen. Env. Proj. No. 50. Copenhagen (in Danish). Described in P. Grandjean and E. Bach. 1986. Indirect exposures: The significance of bystanders at work and at home. *AIHA J.* **47**:819–824.

Danziger, S. J., and P. A. Possick. 1973. Metallic mercury exposure in scientific glassware manufacturing plants. *J. Occup. Med.* **15**(1):15–20.

Devine, J. M., G. B. Kinoshita, R. P. Peterson, and G. L. Picard. 1986. Farm worker exposure to terbufos (phosphorodithioic acid, S-(tert-butylthio) methyl O,O-(diethyl ester) during planting operations of corn. *Arch. Env. Contam. Toxicol.* **15**:113–119.

EPA. 1985. *Guide for Decontaminating Building, Structures and Equipment at Superfund Sites*. Washington, DC: EPA, 600/2-85-028.

EPA. 1990. *Acrylamide Grouting Study*. Washington, DC: EPA, 560/5-87-009.

Fenske, R. A. 1990. Nonuniform dermal deposition patterns during occupational exposure to malathion. *Arch. Env. Contam.* **19**:332–337.

Fenske, R. A., S. J. Hamburger, and C. L. Guyton. 1987. Occupational exposure to fosetyl-Al fungicide during spraying of ornamentals in greenhouses. *Arch. Env. Contam. Toxicol.* **16**:615–621.

Fenske, R. A., S. W. Horstman, and R. K. Bentley. 1987. Assessment of dermal exposure to chlorophenols in timber mills. *Appl. Ind. Hyg.* **2**(4):143–147.

Frank, R., R. A. Campbell, and G. J. Sirons. 1985. Forestry workers involved in aerial application of 2,4-dichlorophenoxy acetic acid (2,4-D): Exposure and urinary secretion. *Arch. Env. Contam. Toxicol.* **14**:427–435.

Gehlbach, S. H., W. A. Williams, and J. I. Freeman. 1979. Protective clothing as a means of reducing nicotine absorption in tobacco harvesters. *Arch. Env. Health* **34**(Mar./Apr.): 111–114.

Goldfield, J., J. W. Sheehy, B. J. Gunter, and W. J. Daniels. 1991. Cost-effective radiator repair ventilation control. *Appl. Occup. Env. Hyg.* **6**(11):959–965.

Grandjean, P., and E. Bach. 1986. Indirect exposures: The significance of bystanders at work and at home. *AIHA J.* **47**:819–824.

Gunderson, E. C., B. A. Kingsley, C. L. Witham, and D. C. Bomberger. 1989. A practical study in laboratory and workplace permeation testing. *Appl. Ind. Hyg.* **4**(12):324–329.

Harrington, J. M., R. O. Rivera, and L. K. Lowry. 1978. Occupational exposure to synthetic estrogens—the need to establish safety standards. *AIHA J.* **39**:139–143.

Harrington, J. M., G. F. Stein, R. O. Rivera, and A. V. deMorales. 1978. The occupational hazards of formulating oral contraceptives—A survey of plant employees. *Arch. Env. Health* **33**(Jan./Feb.):12–15.

Haverty, M. I., M. Page, P. J. Shea, J. B. Hoy, and R. W. Hall. 1983. Drift and worker exposure resulting from two methods of applying insecticides to pine bark. *Bull. Env. Contam. Toxicol.* **30**:223–228.

Herman, N. D., T. W. Hunt, and T. J. Sheets. 1985. Hand harvester exposure to maleic hydrazide (MH) in flue-cured tobacco. *Bull. Env. Contam. Toxicol.* **34**:469–475.

Hill, R. H. 1984. Ultraviolet detection of synthetic oil contamination of skin. *AIHA J.* **45**(7):474–484.

Hills, B. W., and A. L. Greife. 1986. Evaluation of occupational acrylamide exposures. *Appl. Ind. Hyg.* **1**(3):148–151.

Iwata, Y. 1980. Minimizing occupational exposure to pesticides: Reentry field data—a recapitulation. *Res. Rev.* **75**:127–147.

Jongeneelen, F. J., P. T. J. Scheepers, A. Groenendijk,

L. A. G. J. M. Van Aerts, R. B. M. Anzion, R. P. Bos, and S. J. Veenstra. 1988. Airborne concentrations, skin contamination, and urinary metabolite excretion of polycyclic aromatic hydrocarbons among paving workers exposed to coal tar derived road tars. *AIHA J.* **49**(12):600–607.

Kandus, J., V. Masek, and Z. Jach. 1972. The 3,4-benzpyrene content of working clothes and underwear of workers in a pitch-producing plant. *Zentralblatt fur Arbeitsmedizin und Arbeitsschutz* **22:**138.

Kauppinen, T., and L. Lindroos. 1985. Chlorophenol exposure in sawmills. *AIHA J.* **46**(1):34–38.

Ketcham, N. H., and W. Norton. 1960. The hazards to health in the hydrogenation of coal—III. The industrial hygiene studies. *Arch. Env. Health* **1:**194–207.

Kleinman, G. D., S. W. Horstman, D. A. Kalman, J. McKenzie, and D. Stansel. 1986. Industrial hygiene, chemical and biological assessments of exposures to a chlorinated phenolic sapstain control agent. *AIHA J.* **47**(12):731–741.

Klingner, T. 1992. *New Developments in Surface Contamination Monitoring for Aromatic Amines.* Proceedings on a conference on advanced composites. Cincinnati, OH: ACGIH, pp. 43–46.

Klingner, T. 1993. *Biological Monitoring for Methylene Dianiline to Assess Dermal Exposures to Methylene Diisocyanate (MDI)—Implications for Health Effects and Control Strategies.* American Industrial Hygiene Conference, New Orleans, LA.

Kolmodin-Hedman, B., K. Erne, M. Hakansson, and A. Engqvist. 1979. Testing of professional exposure to phenoxy acids (in Swedish). As described in M. L. Leng, J. C. Ramsey, W. H. Braun, and T. L. Lavy. 1982. Review of studies with 2,4,5-trichlorophenoxyacetic acid in humans including applicators under field conditions. In *Pesticide Residues and Exposure,* Washington, DC: American Chemical Society, pp. 133–156.

Kroger, S., J. Liesivuori, and A. Manninen. 1990. Evaluation of workers' exposure to 2-ethylhexanoic acid (2-EHA) in Finnish sawmills. *Int. Arch. Occup. Env. Health* **62:**213–216.

Lauwerys, R. R., T. Dath, J. Lachapelle, J. Buchet, and H. Roels. 1978. The influence of two barrier creams on the percutaneous absorption of m-xylene in man. *J. Occup. Med.* **20**(10):17–20.

Lazariew, N. W. 1954. *Noxious Substances in Industry.* Warsaw: Panstwowe Wydawnictwo Techniczne (in Polish). As reported in B. Dutkiewicz, J. Konczalik, and W. Karwacki. 1980. Skin absorption and per os administration of methanol in men. *Int. Arch. Occup. Env. Health* **47:**81–88.

Lees, P. S. J., M. Corn, and P. N. Breysse. 1987. Evidence for dermal absorption as the major route of body entry during exposure of transformer maintenance and repairmen to PCBs. *AIHA J.* **48**(3):257–264.

Levine, R. J., M. J. Turner, Y. S. Crume, M. E. Dale, T. B. Starr, and D. E. Rickert. 1985. Assessing exposure to dinitrotoluene using a biological monitor. *J. Occup. Med.* **27**(9): 627–638.

Maddy, K. T., R. G. Wang, and C. K. Winter. 1983. *Dermal Exposure Monitoring of Mixers, Loaders, and Applicators of Pesticides in California.* HS-1069. Sacramento, CA: Worker Health and Safety Unit, State of California, pp. 1–7.

Nigg, H. N., and J. H. Stamper. 1985. Field studies: Methods overview. In *Dermal Exposure Related to Pesticide Use.* Washington, DC: American Chemical Society, pp. 95–108.

NIOSH, Technical Assistance Report. June 1973. *Chemetron Chemical, Organics Division, Newport, TN.* HHE 71-9-50. Cincinnati, OH: NIOSH.

NIOSH, Health Hazard Evaluation Report. November 1975. *Gates Rubber Co., Denver, CO.* HHE 74-73-233. Cincinnati, OH: NIOSH.

NIOSH, Hazard Evaluation and Technical Assistance Report. 1976. *U.S. Public Health Service Dental Clinic, 77 Warren St., Boston, MA.* TA 76-45. Cincinnati, OH: NIOSH.

NIOSH, Health Hazard Evaluation Report. May 1976. *J. A. Devine, D. D. S., Cheyenne, WY.* HHE 76-6-294. Cincinnati, OH: NIOSH.

NIOSH, Health Hazard Evaluation Report. July 1976. *Jay Instruments and Specialty Co., Cincinnati, OH.* HHE 76-49-312. Cincinnati, OH: NIOSH.

NIOSH, Health Hazard Evaluation Report. November 1976. *Children's Dental Services, Batavia and Cincinnati, OH.* TA 76-108. Cincinnati, OH: NIOSH.

NIOSH, Health Hazard Evaluation Report. December 1976. *Comprehensive Thiram Investigation.* HHE-75-THIRAM-352. Cincinnati, OH: NIOSH.

NIOSH, Health Hazard Evaluation Report. June 1977. Fisher Body No. 2 Plant, Grand Rapids, MI. HHE 77-39-400. Cincinnati, OH: NIOSH.

NIOSH, Health Hazard Evaluation Report. April 1977. *H. O. Strickler, D.D.S., Littlestown, PA.* HHE 77-21-381. Cincinnati, OH: NIOSH.

NIOSH, Health Hazard Evaluation Report. 1978. *St. Clair Rubber Co., Marysville, MI.* HHE 77-67-499. Cincinnati, OH: NIOSH.

NIOSH, Hazard Evaluation and Technical Assistance Report. June 1978. *PHS Indian Health Center, Fort Washakie, WY.* TA 78-35. Cincinnati, OH: NIOSH.

NIOSH, Hazard Evaluation and Technical Assistance Report. August 1978. *Morris Forman Wastewater Treatment Plant, Metropolitan Sewer District, Louisville, KY.* TA 77-39. Cincinnati, OH: NIOSH.

NIOSH, Hazard Evaluation and Technical Assistance Report. October 1978. *U.S. Public Health Service Outpatient Dental Clinic, Cincinnati, OH.* TA 78-45. Cincinnati, OH: NIOSH.

NIOSH, Health Hazard Evaluation Report. December 1978. *Lear Siegler, Inc., Marblehead, MA.* HHE 78-68-546. Cincinnati, OH: NIOSH.

NIOSH, Health Hazard Evaluation Report. 1979. *Survey of Dental Offices*. HHE-79-107-632. Cincinnati, OH: NIOSH.

NIOSH, Health Hazard Evaluation Report. April 1979. *Gladnick Dental Clinic, Wilmington, DE*. HHE 79-47-582. Cincinnati, OH: NIOSH.

NIOSH, Health Hazard Evaluation Report. December 1979. *St. Charles Furniture Corp., Wright City, MO*. HHE 79-103-640. Cincinnati, OH: NIOSH.

NIOSH, Hazard Evaluation and Technical Assistance Report. 1980. *Rutgers University, Newark, NJ*. HETA 80-92-769. Cincinnati, OH: NIOSH.

NIOSH, Health Hazard Evaluation Report. January 1980*a*. *R. L. Polk Company, Cincinnati, OH*. HHE 78-77-659. Cincinnati, OH: NIOSH.

NIOSH, Health Hazard Evaluation Report. January 1980*b*. *Dupont Photo Products Department, Cheesquake Rd., Parlin, NJ*. HHE 80-5-651. Cincinnati, OH: NIOSH.

NIOSH, Health Hazard Evaluation Report. 1980*a*. *Acme Parts Manufacturing Co*. HHE 78-22-732. Cincinnati, OH: NIOSH.

NIOSH, Health Hazard Evaluation Report. 1980*b*. *Boehringer Ingelheim, Ltd., Ridgefield, CT*. HETA 81-247-958. Cincinnati, OH: NIOSH.

NIOSH, Health Hazard Evaluation Report. April 1980. *Sterling Faucet Co., Sabraton, W. Va*. HHE 79-37-684. Cincinnati, OH: NIOSH.

NIOSH, Health Hazard Evaluation Report. May 1980. *RCA Corp., Marion, IN*. HHE 79-105-687. Cincinnati, OH: NIOSH.

NIOSH, Technical Assistance Report. June 1980. *Good Samaritan Hospital, Cincinnati, OH*. TA 79-19. Cincinnati, OH: NIOSH.

NIOSH, Health Hazard Evaluation Report. February 1981. *Western Electric Co., Westminster, CO*. HHE 80-151-821. Cincinnati, OH: NIOSH.

NIOSH, Health Hazard Evaluation Report. May 1981. *Clermont County Children's Dental Clinic, Batavia, OH*. HETA 81-63-869. Cincinnati, OH: NIOSH.

NIOSH, Health Hazard Evaluation Report. May 1982. *Keebler Co., Cincinnati, OH*. HETA 81-396-1118. Cincinnati, OH: NIOSH.

NIOSH, Health Hazard Evaluation Report. July 1982*a*. *Shell Chemical Company, Denver, CO*. HHE 80-137-1145. Cincinnati, OH: NIOSH.

NIOSH, Health Hazard Evaluation Report. July 1982*b*. *West Gate Dental Clinic, Cheyenne, WY*. HETA 82-70-1148. Cincinnati, OH: NIOSH.

NIOSH, Health Hazard Evaluation Report. December 1982. *Ohio Thermometer Co., Springfield, OH*. HETA 82-364-1243. Cincinnati, OH: NIOSH.

NIOSH, Health Hazard Evaluation Report. 1983. *Hopkins Agricultural Chemical Company, Atlanta, IL*. HETA 81-465-1323. Cincinnati, OH: NIOSH.

NIOSH, Health Hazard Evaluation Report. February 1983. *Center for Molecular Nutrition and Sensory Disorders, Washington, DC*. HETA 82-338-1266. Cincinnati, OH: NIOSH.

NIOSH, Health Hazard Evaluation Report. August 1983*a*. *Robertson Paper Box Company, Monteville, CT*. HETA 81-304-1361. Cincinnati, OH: NIOSH.

NIOSH, Health Hazard Evaluation Report. August 1983*b*. *U.S. Environmental Protection Agency, Triangle Chemical Site, Bridge City, TX*. HETA 83-417-1357. Cincinnati, OH: NIOSH.

NIOSH, Health Hazard Evaluation Report. August 1983*c*. *British Airways, Kennedy Airpot, Jamaica, NY*. HETA 82-100-1349. Cincinnati, OH: NIOSH.

NIOSH, Health Hazard Evaluation Report. September 1983. *Fire Department, Stamford, CT*. HETA 83-157-1373. Cincinnati, OH: NIOSH.

NIOSH. 1983. *Industrial Hygiene Surveys of Occupational Exposure to Wood Preservative Chemicals*. Cincinnati, OH: U.S. Dept. of Health and Human Services.

NIOSH, Health Hazard Evaluation Report. January 1984. *Champion Technology Center, Hamilton, OH*. HETA 83-312-1400. Cincinnati, OH: NIOSH.

NIOSH, Health Hazard Evaluation Report. August 1984. *Schlegel Corp., Rochester, NY*. HETA 82-289-1496. Cincinnati, OH: NIOSH.

NIOSH, Health Hazard Evaluation Report. January 1985a. *Shell Chemical Co., Axis, Al*. HETA 78-4-1511. Cincinnati, OH: NIOSH.

NIOSH, Health Hazard Evaluation Report. January 1985*b*. *Fort Stanwix National Monument, Rome, NY*. HETA 83-090-1326. Cincinnati, OH: NIOSH.

NIOSH, Health Hazard Evaluation Report. February 1985. *J. Butler, D.D.S., Wellston, OH*. HETA 84-90-1533. Cincinnati, OH: NIOSH.

NIOSH, Health Hazard Evaluation Report. March 1985. *Manufacturing Chemists, Inc., Indianapolis, IN*. HETA 82-257-1571. Cincinnati, OH: NIOSH.

NIOSH, Health Hazard Evaluation Report. June 1985. *Harshaw/Filtrol, Louisville, KY*. HETA 84-128-1601. Cincinnati, OH: NIOSH.

NIOSH, Health Hazard Evaluation Report. October 1985. *Inland Steel, East Chicago, IN*. HETA 82-309-1630. Cincinnati, OH: NIOSH.

NIOSH, Health Hazard Evaluation Report. November 1985. *Bofors-Nobel/Lakeway Corp., Muskegon, MI*. HETA 80-35-1635. Cincinnati, OH: NIOSH.

NIOSH, Health Hazard Evaluation Report. February 1986. *Staco, Inc., Poultney, VT*. HETA 83-465-1674. Cincinnati, OH: NIOSH.

NIOSH, Health Hazard Evaluation Report. May 1986. *Hilton-Davis Chemical Company*. HETA 84-058-1700. Cincinnati, OH: NIOSH.

NIOSH, Health Hazard Evaluation Report. September 1986*a*. *Hexcel Corp., Dublin, CA*. HETA 85-131-1731. Cincinnati, OH: NIOSH.

NIOSH, Health Hazard Evaluation Report. September 1986*b*. *Friction Division Products, Trenton, NJ*. HETA 84-262-1734. Cincinnati, OH: NIOSH.

NIOSH, Health Hazard Evaluation Report. December 1986. *Robbins, and Myers, Inc., Moyno Products Division, Springfield, OH.* HETA 86-018-1758. Cincinnati, OH: NIOSH.

NIOSH, Health Hazard Evaluation Report. March 1987. *Vimar Corp., Boulder, CO.* HETA 86-30-1785. Cincinnati, OH: NIOSH.

NIOSH, Health Hazard Evaluation Report. January 1988. *International Association of Fire Fighters (IAFF), Los Angeles, CA.* HETA 85-375-1861. Cincinnati, OH: NIOSH.

NIOSH, Hazard Evaluation and Technical Assistance Report. February 1988. *Rothan and Rothan, D.D.S., Cincinnati, OH.* HETA 87-147-1873. Cincinnati, OH: NIOSH.

NIOSH, Health Hazard Evaluation Report. July 1988. *Bolles Opera House, West Chicago, IL.* HETA 87-431-1916. Cincinnati, OH: NIOSH.

NIOSH, Health Hazard Evaluation Report. June 1989. *Glennwood Range, Delaware, OH.* HETA 88-266-1970. Cincinnati, OH: NIOSH.

NIOSH, Health Hazard Evaluation Report. 1989. *Barbados Ministry of Health, Bridgetown, Barbados.* HETA 88-372-1953. Cincinnati, OH: NIOSH.

NIOSH, Health Hazard Evaluation Report. August 1989*a*. *Joseph T. Luttmer, D.D.S., Cincinnati, OH.* HETA 87-265-1975. Cincinnati, OH: NIOSH.

NIOSH, Health Hazard Evaluation Report. August 1989*b*. *Keebler Co., Atlanta, GA.* HETA 87-379-1977. Cincinnati, OH: NIOSH.

NIOSH, Health Hazard Evaluation Report. November 1989. *Chapman Corporation, Albright Power Station, Albright, WV.* HETA 89-262-1994. Cincinnati, OH: NIOSH.

NIOSH, Health Hazard Evaluation Report. December 1989. *Cincinnati Electronics Corp., Cincinnati, OH.* HETA 89-57-2003. Cincinnati, OH: NIOSH.

NIOSH, Health Hazard Evaluation Report. March 1990. *Chrysler Chemical Division, Trenton, MI.* HETA 87-126-2019. Cincinnati, OH: NIOSH.

NIOSH, Health Hazard Evaluation Report. October 1991*a*. *International Salt Company, Avery Island, LA.* HETA 88-389-2147.

NIOSH, Health Hazard Evaluation Report. October 1991*b*. *American Salt Company, Lyons, KA.* RDHETA 88-390-2148. Cincinnati, OH: NIOSH.

NIOSH, Hazard Evaluation and Technical Assistance Report. January 1992. *New England Lead Burning Co. (NELCO), Eaton Metals, Salt Lake City, UT.* HETA 91-290-2174. Cincinnati, OH: NIOSH.

O'Malley, M. A., C. G. T. Mathias, M. Priddy, D. Molina, A. A. Grote, and W. E. Halperin. 1988. Occupational vitiligo due to unsuspected presence of phenolic antioxidant byproducts in commercial bulk rubber. *J. Occup. Med.* **30**(6):512–516.

Perdek, J. M., F. J. Freestone, D. Sandifer, and A. Sherman. 1991. Closure of a dioxin incineration facility. *Chemosphere* **23**(8/10):1295–1305.

Phillips, B. L. D. 1982. Effects of beclomethasone exposure in industry. *J. Soc. Occup. Med.* **32:**196–200.

Piacitelli, G., and C. Rice. 1993. Lead contamination in radiator repair shops. *Appl. Occup. Env. Hyg.* **8**(5):434–438.

Piotrowski, J. K. 1967. Quantitative estimation of aniline absorption through the skin in man. *J. Hyg. Epidemiol., Microbiol. and Immunol.* **1:**1–23.

Piotrowski, J. K. 1971. Evaluation of exposure to phenol: Absorption of phenol vapor in the lungs and through the skin and excretion of phenol in urine. *Brit. J. Ind. Med.* **28:**172–178.

Raheel, M. 1991. Pesticide transmission in fabrics: Effect of perspiration. *Bull. Env. Contam. Toxicol.* **46:**837–844.

Scheuplein, R. J. 1978. The skin as a barrier. In A. Jarrett (ed.), *The Physiology and Pathophysiology of the Skin*, vol. 5. London: Academic Press, pp. 1669–1692.

Scheuplein, R. J., and R. L. Bronaugh. 1983. Percutaneous absorption. In L. A. Goldsmith (ed.), *Biochemistry and Physiology of the Skin.* Oxford, England: Oxford University Press, pp. 1255–1295.

Shepard, C. G. 1981. Occupational health aspects related to coal liquefaction. *J. Soc. Occup. Med.* **31:**9–15.

Shmunes, E., and D. J. Burton. 1981. Urinary monitoring for diethylstilbestrol in male chemical workers. *JOM* **23**(3):179–182.

Sciarini, L. H., and J. W. Meigs. 1961. The biotransformation of benzidine. II. Studies in mouse and man. *Arch. Environ. Health* **2:**423–430.

Serat, W. F., A. J. VanLoon, and W. H. Serat. 1982. Loss of pesticides from patches used in the field as pesticide collectors. *Arch. Env. Contam. Toxicol.* **11:**227–234.

Tanimura, H. 1968. Benzo(a)pyrene in an iron and steel works. *Arch. Env. Health* **17:**172–177.

Thind, K. S., S. Karmali, and R. A. House. 1991. Occupational exposure of electrical utility linemen to pentachlorophenol. *AIHA J.* **52**(12):547–552.

Thulin, H. 1993. Determination of nor-nitrogen mustard hydrochloride in air and on surfaces by using filter or wipe sampling and derivatization-gas chromatographic procedure. *AIHA J.* **54**(2): 76–81.

Vahter, M., L. Friberg, and B. Rahnster. 1985. Airborne arsenic and urinary excretion of metabolites of inorganic arsenic among smelter workers. *Int. Arch. Occup. Env. Health* **56:**271–279.

Van Vynck, L., and K. Shortsleeves. 1991. *Decontamination of Polychlorinated Biphenyl, Mercury, and Lead from a Municipal Water Supply Facility: A Case Study.* American Industrial Hygiene Conference, Abstract, Salt Lake City, UT.

Weeks, R. W., and B. J. Dean. 1978. Decontamination of aromatic amine cancer-suspect agents on concrete, metal, or painted surfaces. *AIHA J.* **39:**758–762.

Weil, C. S., and N. I. Condra. 1960. The hazards to health in the hydrogenation of coal—II. Carcinogenic effect of materials on the skin of mice. *Arch. Env. Health* **1**:21/187–27/193.

Wojeck, G. A., J. F. Price, H. N. Nigg, and J. H. Stamper. 1983. Worker exposure to paraquat and diquat. *Arch. Env. Contam. Toxicol.* **12**:65–70.

Wolfe, H. R., W. F. Durham, and J. F. Armstrong. 1963. Health hazards of the pesticides endrin and dieldrin. *Arch. Env. Health* **6**:458–464.

Wolfe, H. R., W. F. Durham, and G. S. Batchelor. 1961. Health hazards of some dinitro compounds: Effects associated with agricultural usage in Washington state. *Arch. Env. Health* **3**:468–475.

Wolfe, H. R., D. C. Staiff, and J. F. Armstrong. 1978. Exposure of formulating plant workers to ethion and malathion. *Bull. Env. Contam. Toxicol.* **20**:778–781.

Wolfe, H. R., K. C. Walker, J. W. Elliott, and W. F. Durham. 1959. Evaluation of the health hazards involved in house-spraying with DDT. *Bull. World Health Organ.* **20**:1–14.

Wolfe, H. R., J. F. Armstrong, D. C. Staiff, and S. W. Comer. 1975. Potential exposure of workers to parathion through contamination of cigarettes. *Bull. Env. Contam. Toxicol.* **13**(3):369–376.

Zsigmond, A. 1985. Sudden onset irritant dermatitis in a car component factory. *J. Soc. Occup. Med.* **35**:62–64.

CHAPTER 5

Assessment of Community Exposures

The concern for dermal exposure does not end in the workplace. Environmental contaminants, such as lead and pesticides, can build up on surfaces such as carpets, walls, and counters inside homes and buildings regularly used by the community—schools, day care centers, and public office buildings—and may be associated with a number of different environmental media including water, soil, sediment, and consumer products. Contamination migrating from hazardous waste sites is also a concern. Workers wearing contaminated clothing may expose their families by close contact, contamination of furniture and rugs, contamination of other family clothing in the laundry, and contamination of family vehicles. Finally, hobbies and home industries can also contaminate residences.

These concerns have been recognized by both the Environmental Protection Agency (EPA) in its national project (NHEXSUS) described in the Introduction, and by the National Institute of Occupational Safety and Health (NIOSH), which, under legislation enacted in 1992, has been designated as the lead agency to determine the extent of contamination in homes from toxic material transported on workers' clothing and other materials (HR 2042, PL 102-522; 2205 HR 1035, 1126). NIOSH has organized a surveillance program to monitor trends in the incidence and prevalence of lead poisoning in order to draw public attention to the problem as well as to target work sites for interventions to reduce lead exposure.

The Adult Blood Lead Epidemiology and Surveillance (ABLES) program draws on reports of high blood levels that medical labs transmit to health departments or other agencies in a number of states. In the first quarter of 1993, 4,447 cases of elevated blood lead levels in adults were reported in 16 states (*Morbidity and Mortality Weekly Report*, June 11, 1993). It has been recognized that parents' exposure in the workplace can be a source of exposure to the children at home either through lead brought home on personal items or through exposing the children to the workplace. When elevated blood lead levels are identified in the parents, further information is gathered on children and other at-risk persons in the home. As an example, a follow-up investigation of two siblings in Colorabo with blood lead levels of 38 μg/dL and 36 μg/dL found that the children were in a day care center set up at their parents' workplace, a radiator shop. In addition, the parents regularly wore their work clothing home. Further testing on the parents indicated the father had a blood lead level of 52 μg/dL and the mother, 20 μg/dL.

In August, 1989, a Detroit-area 4-year-old was diagnosed with a rare form of childhood mercury poisoning 10 days after the inside of his home was painted with 17 gallons of interior latex paint (CDC, 1990). The boy became irritable, suffered uncontrollable tremors, and lost his ability to walk; the skin of his fingers and toes turned pink and peeled. Mercury compounds have been used by paint manufacturers as additives in latex (water-based) paint to protect the paint from mildew and bacteria during production and storage. The most commonly used mercurial compound was phenylmercuric acetate. A sample of paint from the boy's home contained mercury concentrations ranging from 930 mg/L to 955 mg/L, exceeding the EPA recommended limit of 300 mg/L for mercury in interior latex paint. Since then the use of mercury as a preservative in indoor paints has been banned. In this instance the source of exposure was airborne inhalation. Mercury is a surface contaminant that can generate significant airborne levels. While air sampling can assist in identifying overall exposure levels, surface sampling with a direct reading instrument can identify the areas where mercury is present. Fresh paint can be easy to identify, although spills of mercury in dental offices can be much more difficult.

Populations potentially exposed to contaminated groundwater or surface water include people served by a water supply system that draws its water supply from a contaminated source. Such a population may be dermally exposed while swimming in pools or during bathing and washing. Increased water temperature may produce increased dermal absorption, but it may also increase the volatilization rate of volatile organic compounds (VOCs) from tap water, thereby making these compounds more available for respiratory uptake. Contamination from consumer items and services may also be a concern of volatile exposure. Residual dry cleaning solvent on clothing can build up in closets and rooms of residences that often have less ventilation than public buildings and workplaces.

Office buildings, day care centers, and schools often have more concerns in common with the community than with the workplace. For one thing, both of these places, like a residence, are perceived to be chemical-free environments. Also, standards applied to the interiors of offices usually are much lower than those applied to the workplace. Many people choose office work because they prefer a "chemical-free" environment. Offices often allow members of the general public in many areas of the buildings, so these areas must meet standards applying to the general public. Day care centers and schools must meet the same standards that apply to residences.

However, many offices and schools contain chemical processes, such as those required for graphic arts, specialized printing machines and small medical facilities, and food facilities that are regularly treated with insecticides. Measurement of airborne and surface contaminants following building treatment can help evaluate risks to occupants and aid in establishing office reentry guidelines. Upholstered furniture, desks, and carpets are often contaminated during these procedures.

POTENTIAL HAZARDS

Hobbies and Cottage Industries

Sometimes hazardous operations are carried out in the home in connection with certain hobbies, artwork, or cottage industries. Pottery making, silk screening, and jewelry making are examples. One artist who made handmade quilts in her residence developed mucous membrane irritation; burning and itching sensations on her arms, face, and hands; facial and finger edema; difficulty focusing her eyes; a sore mouth; headache; and nausea, which were temporally associated with a cyanotype printing process she had performed on fabrics for her quilts in the basement of her residence (NIOSH, May 1981). This process, which she had learned about in a magazine article, uses ferric ammonium citrate, potassium ferricyanide, and potassium dichromate. The first two chemicals are known sensitizers, and potassium dichromate contains Cr^{+6}, a carcinogen.

Following the directions in the article, the artist mixed the chemicals at a workbench and performed the rinse with potassium dichromate in a washbasin in her basement. She then rinsed the fabrics in 5 gallons of room temperature water, wearing rubber gloves at all times when the chemicals and solutions were handled. An evaluation of the basement by an industrial hygienist identified lingering contamination of Cr^{+6} on the workbench where chemicals had been mixed, on the boards where the fabric was placed during exposure to the sun, on the glass used to sandwich the fabric, and on the bottom panel of the washbasin where the fabric was fixed in the potassium dichromate solution.

Lead-related cottage industries (backyard lead smelting of batteries) have produced lead poisoning in both developed and undeveloped countries. For example, it is estimated that about one third of the spent lead-acid batteries in Jamaica are used by backyard recyclers or by small battery repair shops, where the lead is frequently smelted as well (Matte et al., 1991).

Indoor Dusts

Sources of house dust are highly variable and indicate it may contain residues from food and skin scales, other organic residue from the human and animal occupants of the house; fibers from clothing and household furnishings; fibers and minerals from building materials; organic matter from cleaning compounds, waxes, and other consumer products; fragments of vegetation and humus; and mineral particles, such as clay and sand (EPA, 1988). A study conducted in six U.S. cities found between 37% and 86% of house dust was inorganic (of which about two-thirds was silica and clay), less than 1% to 5% was grease, and the remainder consisted of other organics. One study of lead in house dust, which compared the dustfall average (9.3 µg/M^2/day) and accumulated dust (166 µm/M^2/day) levels, concluded that most of the lead is carried into the house with "dust particles adhering to shoes" (Diemel et al., 1981).

The dust to which residents are exposed can be considered as a weighted average across the surface area where that person has contact, with weights roughly proportional to the time the person spends in different areas of the home. This consideration is particularly important when estimating exposures of children because they spend more time in contact with floors (which are more likely to have the highest concentrations) than adults. Small children spend much of their time on the floor and are very likely to come into contact with yard dirt and lawns. The greatest source of exposure for young children often occurs when dust-laden fingers or objects are put into the mouth allowing a portion of the contamination to be swallowed. It has been estimated that children less than 5 years of age ingest 2.5 times more soil from around the home than adults, although they have only 20% of the body weight (Hawley, 1985). It has also been proposed that indoor exposure to pesticide vapors from carpet treatments and residues is a more significant exposure for children, even in ventilated rooms, because of a gradient of airborne residues that results in higher concentrations in the breathing zone of a child playing on the carpet (Fenske et al., 1990). Pesticides and other organics with lower vapor pressure or higher polarity are expected to partition more to dust than air, making house dust a potential major reservoir of persistent pesticides, such as chlordane, and PAH compounds, such as benzo(a)pyrene.

Pesticides

Studies have shown that residential outdoor air levels of pesticides are generally an order of magnitude lower than indoor levels (Nigg et al., 1990; EPA, 1990). The Nonoccupational Pesticide Exposure Study (NOPES) monitored 32 pesticides in two representative U.S. cities. Jacksonville, FL, was selected as an area of high pesticide usage, and the Springfield, MA, area was selected to represent low to moderate pesticide usage. Indoor, outdoor, and personal samples were collected over high and low usage seasons, including some dermal-contact samples. This study indicated that a number of widely used home and garden pesticides were detectable in the indoor air in these two major urban areas. Some pesticides can persist in the indoor environment for months or years after application or track-in. This condition is especially true for termiticides, because they are usually very persistent compounds such as chlordane. Insecticides and fungicides are applied indoors or tracked in from the outdoors and become embedded in carpets for extended periods, protected from sunlight, rain, temperature extremes, and most microbial action that might otherwise degrade them. Indoor applications include pesticide foggers (or flea bombs); pet products such as flea collars, dips, and shampoos; spot or crack and crevice treatments; vapor strips for flying insects; moth repellents; disinfectants; and indoor plant treatments. Typical active ingredients found in these indoor products include chlorpyrifos, propoxur, diazinon, malathion, DDVP, and pyrethroids. Outdoor applications include homeowner- or commercially-applied lawn products; garden pesticides; and fungicide-treated lumber for decks and landscaping. Commonly used active ingredients for these applications include chlorophenoxy herbicides such as 2,4-D, organophosphate insecticides such as diazinon, malathion, and chlorpyrifos, and carbamate insecticides such as carbaryl.

In recognition of the increasing concerns in pesticide contamination of residences, the EPA is in the process of revising the existing Subdivision K—Exposure Reentry Protection—to incorporate residential exposure studies. Pesticide manufacturers wanting to register chemicals for sale inside and outside residences are likely to be required to perform residential exposure studies as part of their product testing requirements.

Metals

Lead and cadmium in house dust have been extensively studied due to contamination concerns from fallout of nearby industries such as smelters and foundries. While airborne lead from smelters is considered the most significant source of environmental contamination, the most important route of exposures in communities is ingestion of lead-contaminated soil and housedust, especially by children (Roels et al., 1980). Children of smelter workers may also be exposed to lead dust brought home on the parent's work clothing. This concern extends to other types of workers as well, such as electric cable splicers working for large power companies (Rinehart and Yanagisawa, 1993). Even when workers are provided with showering and changing facilities along with separate lockers to store personal clothing, it is still possible for workers to contaminate their homes with metals such as lead due to wearing work shoes home, walking across contaminated parking areas, or driving vehicles that have fallout from plant emissions on them. However, it is important to note that the Occupational Safety and Health Administration's (OSHA) lead standard for general industry only requires employers to launder workers' clothing if airborne exposures exceed the permissible exposure limit (PEL).

Lead in house dust comes from a variety of outdoor and indoor sources. These vary from house-to-house and region-to-region. Natural weathering and other processes have eroded away portions of the paint of many houses and structures, depositing it in the soil. Sanding, abrasive blasting, and chemical removal of the lead-based paint during urban housing renovation and rehabilitation produce small particles. When not properly contained, these particulates may contaminate the soil and contribute to high lead concentrations in urban dust. Once the soil becomes contaminated, weathering and the additional mechanical action from the movement of adults, children, and pets further break down the lead-containing dust. Wind, vehicular traffic, and pedestrians transport the dust throughout the neighborhoods and into residences. Factors that correlate with the lead concentration in the dust include soil and size of exposed soil area; house age, types of housing materials and presence of deteriorated or damaged paint; distance from roads, road type, and presence of street dust; renovation, remodeling, and abatement activities; distance from commercial garages and smelting/mining operations; dust fall rates and suspended particles indoors; carpet wear and existence of a fireplace; and type of occupation and hobbies of occupants (Fergusson and Kim, 1991). For more information on the evaluation of metals in residences, especially lead-containing paint, see Appendix B.

Contaminated Soil

There is a significant seasonal and geographic variation in exposures during gardening and playing outdoors. In warmer climates, people who actively garden or play outdoors might have contact with soil almost every day. However, in cooler climates, outdoor activities involving soil contact may occur only during about half of the year. If contaminated soil is located outside the residential property, contact may only occur a few days per year. Dermal exposure to soil can occur at the hands, legs, arms, neck, and head, with approximately 26% and 30% of the total surface area exposed for adults and children, respectively (McKone and Layton, 1986). Clothing will limit exposure in the case of contaminated soil. Dermal absorption from soils appears to be more significant than direct ingestion for those chemicals that have a percent absorbed exceeding about 10% (EPA, 1992). Chemicals from the soil may also affect the water composition in the skin either by causing occlusion, which would increase the water content, or by dehydrating the skin by absorbing water.

The mobility of a chemical in soil is a complex process and is considered to be much less than the mobility of chemicals in water and air. It is complicated by the fact that soil is a very heterogeneous media and differs in various parts of the country. Dermal exposure scenarios should be related to soil-specific characteristics including particle size distributions and soil type to accurately determine exposure levels for a given toxicant.

Bioavailability Issues

To be absorbed from soil, a chemical must be bioavailable. Bioavailability is the state of being capable of being absorbed and available to interact with the metabolic processes of an organism. Bioavailability is typically a function of chemical properties, the physical state of the material to which an organism is exposed, and the ability of the individual organism to physiologically take up the chemical. To be bioavailable via the dermal route, the chemical must desorb from the soil and come into contact with the absorption barrier, the skin.

Differences in bioavailability between soils can be correlated with differences in the composition of the soils (Skowronski, Turkall, and Abdel-Rahman, 1988). Factors determining the amount of material which is actually absorbed from soil depend on characteristics such as particle size and organic carbon content that affect partitioning of the chemical between soil and skin as well as those related to the chemical itself. Depending on the amount of soil applied, a large percentage of the applied dose may have to diffuse through the soil layer before reaching the skin. Volatilization, friction, and washing may remove some fraction of the applied dose before it can reach the skin. Soil decreased the bioavailability of benzene when male rats were treated topically with benzene adsorbed to either a sandy or a clay soil (Skowronski, Turkall and Abdel-Rahman, 1988; see Table 5-1). The benzene had a greater affinity for the clay soil than the sandy soil, and thus was not as available for absorption.

Fugitive Dust

Residential areas as well as neighboring industries can be exposed to contaminated soil blowing from nearby contaminated sites. One manufacturing facility was concerned about fugitive dust coming from a nearby (200 to 300 yards to the west) zinc recycling company,

TABLE 5-1. Soil Properties

	Cohansey	*Woodbury*
Sand (%)	90	50
Silt (%)	8	28
Clay (%)	2	22
Organic matter (%)	4.4	1.6
Particle size, mm (%)		
0.05–0.1	22.2	17.0
0.1–0.25	76.3	65.3
0.25–0.5	1.2	13.6
0.5–1.0	0.2	3.4
1.0–2.0	0.1	0.7
>2.0	0	0.1

Source: Skowronski, G. A., R. M. Turkall, and M. S. Abdel-Rahman. 1988. Soil adsorption alters bioavailability of benzene in dermally exposed male rats. *AIHA J.* **49**(10):506–511.

which functioned as a zinc smelter prior to the 1980s (Decker, 1992). The company was reclaiming zinc from an electric arc furnace fume, a waste by-product from the steel industry. Although the primary recycled product is zinc, lead contamination of the electric arc fume is a significant hazard. The process was not enclosed within a building, with the exception of the gas compressors and control room, and there were no identified sources of lead or other metals from any other sources. Surface samples were collected at the manufacturing location and results showed notable concentrations ranging from 108 μg/ft^2 on an office trailer desk to 432 μg/ft^2 on top of a gas compressor. The source of lead was the contaminated soil and dust spreading through the air from one site to the other. The wind spread the fine soil and it was pulled inside of the buildings via air intakes, open doors and windows, and foot traffic.

Contaminated Water

Since hydration of the skin tends to increase the absorption of topically applied compounds, there is an increased potential for percutaneous absorption of environmental pollutants in situations such as bathing, swimming, or showering where the skin is well hydrated (EPA, 1992). Exposure assessments of swimming and bathing generally assume that 75% to 100% of the skin surface is exposed (Wester and Maibach, 1989). Concerning VOCs, many in warm, hot, or aerated water would volatilize; those remaining in solution would pass through the skin at an enhanced rate due to their lipid solubility and enhanced blood flow to skin at higher temperatures; and soaps added to wash water would bind with those VOCs remaining insolution.

The importance of dermal contact with water can be evaluated by comparing the possible exposure occurring during normal water contact relative to that occurring as a result of ingestion. Water contact occurs most frequently during showering, bathing, and washing. Assuming the average size adult takes a 10 minute bath or shower, the absorbed dose in mg/day can be estimated as follows:

$$\text{Dermal dose} = (C)(K_p)\,(ET)(A)$$

where

- C = contaminant concentration in water (mg/cm^3)
- K_p = permeability coefficient (cm/hr)
- ET = exposure time (min/day)
- A = exposed skin area (cm^2)

This is often compared to the oral dose in mg/day, which can be estimated by:

$$\text{Oral dose} = (C)(IR)(AF)(S)$$

where

- C = contaminant concentration in water (mg/cm^3)
- IR = adult average ingestion rate (L/day)
- AF = the fraction of the administered dose which is absorbed

SAMPLING METHODS USED IN THE ASSESSMENT OF COMMUNITY EXPOSURES

The most common sampling methods used for residences are vacuum devices for carpets, or dislodgeable residue devices such as the PUF roller. Wipe samples are often used on smooth surfaces such as floors and window sills, and hand washes and skin wipes are the most common dermal techniques. Premoistened glass fiber filters are often used to wipe for pesticides. Moistened towels have been used for wipes of interior surfaces as well. Adhesive tape will also lift dust from surfaces for visual examination. Small test areas can be hand vacuumed using a cut section of Tygon tubing as a nozzle on a mixed cellulose ester filter in a plastic cassette attached to a small portable air sampling pump. Dust samples have also been collected from family-used vacuum cleaner bags. Specially adapted and standard vacuum cleaners have also been used to collect samples directly, and in some cases the dust is sieved to remove larger size particles (Fig. 5-1). Lastly, the EPA developed a vacuum cleaner just for sampling house dust (EPA, 1988). Vacuum methods are dry, whereas many wipe methods

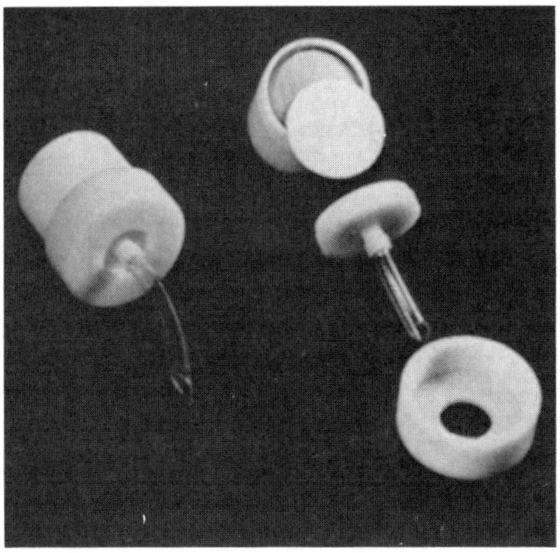
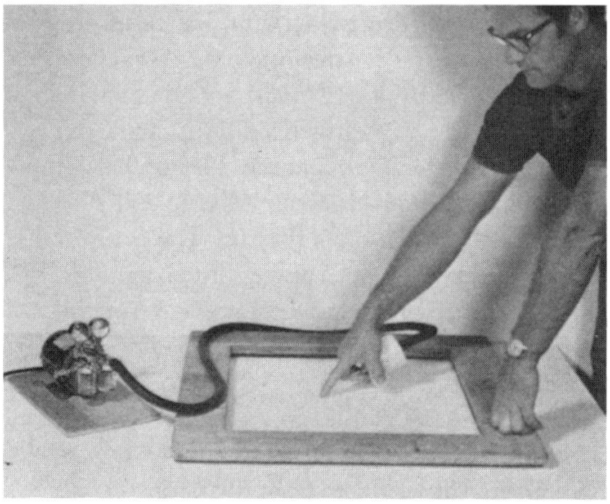

Figure 5-1. *Left:* Dust sampler. *Right:* Dust sampling procedure.
Source: Reprinted with permission from R.I. Solomon and J. W. Hartford. 1976. Lead and cadmium dusts and soils in a small urban community. *Env. Sci. and Tech.* 10:774. Copyright © 1976 by the American Chemical Society.

utilize solvents or premoistened media and may better mimic a child's exposure because their palms are usually wet and sticky.

Surface contamination as a result of immediate spray fallout following application in an office or residence is often measured as well as residual contamination several days later. Aluminum foil and glass plates have been used for spray fallout while wipes are commonly used for residual contamination (dislodgeable residues). Specialized methodologies have been developed to assess human exposure to pollutants resuspended by wind from outdoor surface contamination sites. Soil erosion is affected by soil characteristics and wind. For community exposures, in some cases, analysis of the media is supplemented by environmental fate and transport models.

Residential sampling is most commonly performed in the living room or family room. The most common types of surfaces likely to be monitored are wood floors and window sills, linoleum, carpet, and concrete. However, prior to sampling activity patterns need to be determined. Then selections for sampling may be made as follows: a high traffic area such as near the entrance of the house, an area frequented by children such as in front of the television set, and a less-used area such as under a coffee table. Activities in the house can determine the major sources of exposure as well as the routes of exposure. Some activities will resuspend deposited house dust, which can then be inhaled, while others will promote oral exposure. In addition, the major activity area of a child, the presence of lead-based paint, and the intactness of such surfaces, age and activity of the child, caretaker-child interactions, distance from roads, house cleanliness, ventilation, hermiticity of the home, playmate activities, and family schedules are some factors that should contribute to the selection of sampling locations (Que Hee et al., 1985). X-Ray fluorescence data are commonly used as a guide in homes that have lead containing paint on the walls. Dust fall in homes is usually collected in an out-of-the-way place subject to minimum disturbance such as the top of a refrigerator. Other typical surfaces wiped in residential studies include carpets, floors, window sills and wells, baseboards, swing sets, televisions, and fireplace mantles.

The accumulation of dust in rugs can be expected to vary with the type of carpet, the frequency and manner of cleaning, the sources of dust inside and outside the home, and the behavior of the occupants (EPA, 1988). The addition of a power-driven agitator increases the amount of dust and rug fiber pickup by a vacuum cleaner by a factor of 2 to 6. An upright vacuum cleaner, with a power-driven agitator, can be expected to remove approximately 35% to 55% of the accumulated dust from a plush rug and 70% to 80% of the dust from a flat rug. The canister or tank cleaner, without a power-driven agitator, can be expected to remove about 10% of the dust from a plush rug and 40% to 50% of the dust in a flat rug.

When area air samples are taken in conjunction with house dust studies, the samples are often collected at distances from the floor that are likely to be in the breathing zone of a small child. One study estimated the lowest and average potential breathing zones of a small child to be located at 12.5 cm and 75 cm from the floor, respectively (Lewis et al., 1991).

The biological meaning of levels of contaminants such as lead found in house dust from floors and on the hands of children in these houses will depend on the situation (Que Hee et al., 1985). Thus, a child may prefer one area of a house to another and may suck a preferred finger or part of the hand. Good sampling strategies are necessary to maximize the likelihood of detecting a suspected contaminant once hygienic and preferred area considerations are taken into account. Some studies have also included blood lead sampling and hand wipes for lead. Five factors have been identified that significantly influence the probability of a child experiencing an excess in blood level as a result of lead-contaminated house dust and soil: (1) ambient (outdoor) air concentrations, (2) lead concentration of the soil, (3) age of the child, (4) cleanliness of the home, and (5) occupation of the parents (Yankel, von Lindern, and Walter, 1977).

Typical surfaces wiped in office and school building studies include:

Office Building Interiors

- Baseboard moldings
- Book shelves
- Bookcase top and shelves
- Ceilings
- VDT top
- Chair arms
- Coat rack
- Counters
- Desktops
- Door facings
- Electrical boxes
- Exit lights
- Emergency lighting
- File cabinets
- Fire extinguishers
- Fire sprinkler pipe
- Floors, concrete and linoleum
- Keyboard top
- Lecterns
- Ledges including on balconies and doors
- Light fixtures, especially fluorescent
- Metal cabinets
- Office tables
- Perimeter heating units
- Stair railings
- Refrigerator tops
- Sprinkler pipe
- Suspended ceilings
- Stairwell treads
- Storage locker
- Tables
- Telephones
- Tops of room dividers
- Vending machines
- Walls
- Wall clock
- Wall partition tops
- Water pipe
- Window shades (especially venetian blinds)
- Window sills
- Work counter

Ventilation Systems

- Fan housing interiors
- Supply duct interiors and exteriors
- Louvers of air supply and return vents
- Duct exteriors, including tops
- Fan interior
- Top of fan housing
- Supply air grill
- Power supply boxes
- Risers
- Boiler stacks

SURFACE MONITORING FOR COMMUNITY CONCERNS*

Contaminant	*Activity*	*Surface Methods*	*Other Monitoring*	*Reference*
Allethrin	Fogger application inside residences	Aluminum sheets with gauze pads (12 ply) (57.76 cm^2) adjacent to each sheet during application to determine aerosol distribution of pesticide on floors in rooms	Dosimeter clothing worn during exercise on carpet after application	Ross et al., 1991
Asbestos	Treasury (public) building	Vacuum sampling with personal sampling pump and 25 mm MCE filter cassette of dust from shelves, inside HVAC unit and window sill	Area air samples Bulk samples of insulation	NIOSH, March 1989 (HETA 88-372-1953)
Asbestos	Office building	Settled dust samples of filing cabinets, boxes, window shades, and other surfaces vacuumed with a personal air sampling pump for surface contamination to determine the likelihood of a history of airborne asbestos	Area air samples Bulk samples	NIOSH, September 1987 (HETA 86-434-1833)
Asbestos	High rise office building undergoing abatement where pressure differentials in containment allowed a release of fibers	Wipes on surfaces of both abated and unabated floors to determine extent of contamination	Area air samples	Birkner et al., 1991
Asbestos	Hospital	Vacuum sampling with personal sampling pump and 25 mm MCE filter cassette of dust from window sill and balcony ledge	Area air samples Bulk samples of insulation	NIOSH, March 1989 (HETA 88-372-1953)
Asbestos	School	Vacuum sampling with personal sampling pump and 25 mm MCE filter cassette of dust from window sills and lectern	Area air samples Bulks samples of insulation	NIOSH, March 1989 (HETA 88-372-1953)

*For studies on amines, metals, PCBs, TCDD and pesticides, see the Appendixes.

Contaminant	*Activity*	*Surface Methods*	*Other Monitoring*	*Reference*
Asbestos	One story office building with a parking garage on the roof where occupants were concerned that vibration from the roof might be disturbing sprayed-on insulation	Dry wipes using Whatman filter paper on the surfaces inside the office	Area air samples inside offices	NIOSH, August 1981*a* (HETA 81-309-936)
Asbestos	Three floor office building with asbestos-containing insulation sprayed on the structural beams and underside of the steel floor decks	Vacuum sampling with personal sampling pump and 25 mm MCE filter cassette of dust from smooth interior surfaces (filing cabinets, carpet, top of electrical boxes, top of doors, window shades, light fixtures in offices)	Area air samples inside offices	NIOSH, September 1987 (HETA 86-434-1833)
Bendiocarb	Broadcast spray application of pesticides onto floors of offices for pest control	Aluminum plates to measure aerosol deposition on and above floors Wet gauze wipes of office furniture	Area air samples	Currie et al., 1990
Chlordane Chlorpyrifos Diazinon PCBs	High school with carpet and indoor contamination from subslab injection of chlordane, interior pesticide treatment, and fluorescent light ballast burnouts	Gauze pads (2 × 2 in) wetted with hexane used to wipe (0.25 M^2) floors and walls in hallways and rooms and desktops, textbook covers, book shelves, and storage lockers	Area air samples Blood Bulk samples of carpet	NIOSH, 1991*a* (HETA 89-183-2101)
Chlordane PCBs	Follow-up sampling to verify effectiveness of interior decontamination of high school with pesticide and fluorescent light ballast burnouts	Gauze pads (2 × 2 in) wetted with hexane used to wipe (0.25 M^2) walls, window ledges, desktops, food prep counters, lunch tables, and transformer	Area air samples	NIOSH, 1991*a* (HETA 89-183-2101)
Chlordane	Clinic treated with insecticide	Wipe samples of wall surfaces with Whatman smear tabs	General area air samples Bulk samples of soil and wall block fill Blood	NIOSH, January 1988 (HETA 83-258-1859)

Contaminant	*Activity*	*Surface Methods*	*Other Monitoring*	*Reference*
Chlordane	University library that had a spill released into the space above its false ceiling	Wet wipe samples with Whatman smear tabs of walls, floor, desktops, light fixtures, and shelves	Area air samples Bulk samples of documents	NIOSH, July 1984*b* (HHE 83-444-1491)
Chlordane	Occupants in structures treated for termites using either subsurface injection or topical application to the interior floor and/or exterior soil	Whatman No. 50 filters used to wipe one 6 in. stroke on fireplace, window sill, and floor joist	Area air samples inside buildings Bulk soil and wood chips	NIOSH, January 1984*b* (HETA 83-424-1403)
Chlorpyrifos	Fogger use inside residences	Aluminum sheets and gauze pads (12 ply) (57.76 cm^2) adjacent to each other during actual fogging to determine total deposition of pesticide on floors in rooms	Dosimeter clothing during exercise	Ross et al., 1991
Chlorpyrifos	Broadcast spray application of pesticides onto floors of offices for pest control	Aluminum plates to measure aerosol deposition on and above floors Wet gauze wipes of office furniture	Area air samples	Currie et al., 1990
Chlorpyrifos	Use of home foggers	Dislodgeable residues on carpet sampled using CDFA roller over a piece of bed sheet		Ross et al., 1991
Chlorpyrifos	Application inside residences using hand held nozzle and pressurized tank for flea control	Aluminum foil (10 × 10 cm) placed on top of carpet prior to spraying to measure total deposition Wipe samples with gauze at eight different time intervals following application to determine dislodgeable residues on carpets	Area air samples	Fenske et al., 1990
Chlorpyrifos	Broadcast application for flea control in a 3-room apartment with windows open in one room, doors open in a second, and no ventilation in the third	Aerosol deposition samples collected on aluminum foil placed on surfaces to be treated Wipe samples of carpet using gauze pad wetted with water	Area air sampling at 0.5, 1.5, and 2 hr intervals after application	Fenske et al., 1991

Contaminant	*Activity*	*Surface Methods*	*Other Monitoring*	*Reference*
Chlorpyrifos	Broadcast application for flea control in a 3-room apartment with doors open in one room, doors and windows closed in the other two	Aerosol deposition samples collected on aluminum foil placed on untreated surfaces Wipe samples of carpet with gauze pads wetted with isopropanol	Area air sampling at 0.5, 1.5, and 2 hr intervals after application	Fenske et al., 1991
Chlorpyrifos	Broadcast application for flea control in a residence with doors and windows closed	Aerosol deposition samples collected on aluminum foil placed on untreated surfaces Wipe samples of carpet and vinyl asbestos tile with gauze pads wetted with isopropanol	Area air sampling at 0.5, 1.5, and 2 hr intervals after application	Fenske et al., 1991
Chlorpyrifos	Broadcast and total release applications inside school dormitory to compare differences in ventilated and nonventilated rooms	Gauze pads on top of carpet for aerosol deposition collection Gauze wipes of room surfaces	Area air samples	Lu and Fenske, 1991
Chlorpyrifos Diazinon	Indoor air quality in junior high school following subslab injection and direct in-room application of pesticides	Wipe samples of high dermal contact surfaces	Area air samples Blood Bulk samples of carpet	NIOSH, 1991*a* (HHE 89-183-2101)
Chlorpyrifos Diazinon	Compressed air sprayer and aerosol spray application in dormitory rooms	Rinses of pie plates placed prior to application to measure aerosol deposition Cotton ball wet wipes of stainless steel and formica pieces placed in center of room during spraying to measure dislodgeable residues	Area air samples	Wright, Leidy, and Dupree, 1984
Chlorpyrifos Diazinon	Savings and loan where employees developed symptoms following insecticide application	Whatman filter wetted with toluene used to wipe desktops, work surface and floor in office and teller's station	Area air samples in lobby and offices	NIOSH, July 1984*a* (HETA 83-363-1480)

Contaminant	*Activity*	*Surface Methods*	*Other Monitoring*	*Reference*
DDVP	Insecticide treatment inside residences using an aerosol spray can and water emulsion spray (0.5%)	Gauze pads (2 × 2 in.) placed on the floor, wall, ceiling, cabinet, table, and closet during spraying and for 24 hour intervals (days 2, 3, 4, 5 after treatment)	Modified respirator with prefilters Blood (pre- and postshift and 12 hr postshift) Urine (pre- and during the shift; 12 hr post shift) Dermal monitoring with pads	Das et al., 1983
Diazinon	Broadcast spray application of pesticides onto floors of offices for pest control	Aluminum plates to measure aerosol deposition on and above floors Wet gauze wipes of office furniture	Area air samples	Currie et al., 1990
Diazinon	Insecticide control in buildings	Aluminum pie plates located on floors, countertops, and suspended from floors to collect residue to compare concentrations of aerosol deposition produced by spray and fogging		Wright and Jackson, 1974
Dichlorovos	Residences with interiors sprayed for insect control by commercial pesticide companies	8-ply gauze pads (10.2 × 10.2 cm) of chromatography paper (0.16 mm) with glassine backing placed on top of kitchen appliances, table, and floor prior to application to determine aerosol deposition	Area air sampling Blood (of residents after habitation pre- and posttreatment) Urine (of residents after habitation both pre- and posttreatment)	Gold and Holcslaw, 1985
β-Estradiol Estradiol benzoate Estrone Progesterone Proprionate Testosterone	College building with offices and animal research lab	Gauze wetted with isopropanol water used to wipe an (1/25th M^2) area on surfaces of first three floors and in rooms where hormones were mixed or injected into animals (4th and 5th floors) Follow-up wipes in some areas and a classroom used as a control building	Area air samples in corner rooms and hallways on first three floors and in rooms where hormones were mixed or injected into animals (4th and 5th)	NIOSH, March 1984 (HETA 81-314-1435)

Contaminant	*Activity*	*Surface Methods*	*Other Monitoring*	*Reference*
Fiberglass	Primary school with HVAC problems	Dust samples vacuumed using a personal air sampling pump from cabinet tops, window ledge, and interior of vent diffuser to identify source of skin irritation and flushing in occupants	Area air sampling for fibers and VOCs Bulk sample of fiberglass insulation	NIOSH, September 1991 (HETA 91-143-2136)
Fiberglass	Office building with computer facilities and employee complaints of skin itching and localized rashes.	Transparent tape used to sample windowsills and computer paper for fibers MCE filters used to wipe computer room surfaces Dustfall samples collected by allowing filter cassettes to stand open and by vacuuming surfaces using a personal air sampling pump	General area air samples Skin samples for fibers	NIOSH, April 1984 (HETA 83-409-1450)
Fiberglass	Three story office where employee processes insurance claims and where rashes and itching has developed shortly after installation of fiberglass insulation above suspended ceiling	Wipe samples from horizontal surfaces in offices (file cabinets, desks, air conditioner, and table)	High volume air samples Bulk samples of insulation	NIOSH, January 1982 (HETA 81-58-1037)
Fiberglass	Office building with indoor air concerns	Wipe samples from building surfaces: VDT screen, window ledge, and air conditioning vents	Area air samples for 54 gases and vapors and fiberglass dust Bulk sample of cooling tower additive	NIOSH, July 1981 (HHE 80-118-928)
Fibers Particulate	Office building where employees developed symptoms at the same time two new copy machines were installed	Wipe samples from the air supply and exhaust diffusers in the copy room and in offices nearby	Area air samples for PAHs, dusts, ozone, and organic vapors	NIOSH, August 1981*b* (HETA 81-333-935)
Fibers Particulate	Three story office building recently remodeled in which employees developed skin rash and itching	Wipe samples from building surfaces (HVAC ventilation duct, cabinets)	General area air samples for amines and with detector tubes to screen for 51 different contaminants Bulk samples of dust	NIOSH, September 1981 (HHE 80-176-955)

Contaminant	*Activity*	*Surface Methods*	*Other Monitoring*	*Reference*
Fibers Particulate	Office building where dust buildup is a chronic problem	Transparent adhesive tape samples of VDTs, HVAC diffusers, pipe insulation, and payroll processing machinery in offices	Area air samples for total and respirable dust	NIOSH, February 1984 (HETA 83-214-1424)
Fibers Particulate	Administration building of school where employees have symptoms of eye, skin, and mucuous membrane irritation, tiredness, and itchiness	Personal air sampling pumps used to vacuum surfaces of paper from old files and collect dust in filter cassettes	Area air samples for organic vaporsand formaldehyde	NIOSH, July 1979 (TA 79-12)
Fibers	Primary school	Vacuum sampling with personal sampling pump and 25 mm MCE filter cassette of horizontal surfaces such as cabinet tops, window ledge, and inside of an HVAC diffuser	Area air samples for fiberglass, VOCs, and formaldehyde Bulk sample of fiberglass insulation	NIOSH, September 1991 (HETA 91-143-2136)
Fibers	Office building with asbestos containing insulation sprayed on the structural beams and roof decking	Vacuum sampling with personal sampling pump and 25 mm MCE filter cassette from top of hat rack, desks, file cabinets, top of suspended ceiling, air supply unit, pictures, bookcase, and windowsill	Area air samples for fibers Bulk samples of insulation	NIOSH, September 1983 (HETA 83-358-1362)
Isofenphos	Residence with contaminated living area as a result of contamination of ventilation ducts during subslab application for termites	Wetted gauze used to wipe inside ducts, on furnace, ventilation registers, as well as general surfaces in house outside ventilation system to determine extent of contamination and inside ventilation system to verify effectiveness of decontamination	Area air sampling	Veckman, 1991

Contaminant	*Activity*	*Surface Methods*	*Other Monitoring*	*Reference*
Man-made mineral fibers (MMMF)	Dust in nonresidential buildings with man-made mineral fiber ceiling boards	Stickly gelatinous foils used to sample dust settled on horizontal nontextile surfaces such as tables and cupboard tops	Area air sampling inside each room	Schneider et al., 1990
Mercury	Dental school clinic	Bachrach Mercury Sniffer used to sniff surfaces: drawers, floors, carpet, countertops, floor pads; some surfaces also sniffed before and after being wiped	Personal breathing zone air samples Area air samples Skin and clothing sniffs	NIOSH, March 1978 (TA 78-9)
Mercury	Dental school clinic	Bachrach Mercury Sniffer used to sniff surfaces: drawers, countertops, headrest in patients' chair, stool; some surfaces also sniffed before and after being wiped	Personal breathing zone air samples for mercury and nitrous oxide Area air samples for mercury and nitrous oxide	NIOSH, February 1978 (TA 78-62)
Mercury	Closure of Frankford military arsenal	Surface sampling with direct reading instrument Initial and repeat sampling to verify decontamination for mercury	Area air samples for lead, cadmium, and chromium	EPA, 1985
Mercury	Residence that had interior walls painted with a latex paint containing a preservative	Dust from vacuum cleaner bags collected and sieved in 60-mesh	Area air samples Bulk samples of liquid paint	Beusterien et al., 1991
Mirex Lindane PCBs 2,3,7,8-TCDD	Manufacturing plant contaminated from nearby chemical landfill; testing for effectiveness of decontamination	Dust vacuumed with air sampling pump and filter cassette off surfaces (50 sq. in. area) from structural members, ventilation system, and other surfaces		NIOSH, 1980*a* (HETA 80-087-771)
Mirex Lindane 2,3,7,8-TCDD	Manufacturing plant contaminated with dust from nearby landfill; testing for effectiveness of decontamination	Dust vacuumed with air sampling pump and filter cassette off surfaces (50 sq. in. area) from structural members, windowsills, and other surfaces		NIOSH, 1980*b* (HETA 80-107-772)

Contaminant	*Activity*	*Surface Methods*	*Other Monitoring*	*Reference*
Mirex Lindane	Manufacturing plant that had just built a new plant next to an old plant previously decontaminated due to being in close proximity to a chemical disposal site	Dust samples vacuumed using personal breathing zone pump and filter cassette over 100 cm² from structural members and a window ledge in the old plant from the center of the conveyor system in the new plant to determine if any additional contamination had occurred		NIOSH, May 1981 (HETA 81-213-886)
Pentachlorophenol (PCP)	Gift shop and offices of a national monument with PCP treated walls	Whatman smear tabs, wetted, used to wipe book store counter, walls, and desk	Area air samples in offices Skin wipes Bulk sample of crystals scraped off wall Urine	NIOSH, September 1983 (HETA 83-90-1326)
PCP Tetrachlorophenol	Montana residents in treated log homes	Whatman smear tabs, wetted, used to wipe wood surfaces in living rooms, bedrooms, kitchens,and dining rooms in homes	Area air samples Bulk samples of treating chemicals Skin wipes Urine	NIOSH, April 1986 (HETA 84-53, 425-1680)
Pesticides	Residences	High volume vacuum samples of carpet and area rug surfaces in specific areas (3800 cm²) PUF roller samples on carpets adjacent to areas vacuumed (800 cm²) Bare hand presses on carpet	Area air samples Hand washes Soil samples outside main doorway	Lewis et al., 1991
Pesticides	Residences	High volume surface vacuum samples (18 × 54 in.) from rugs and bare floors of dust and vapor	Area air samples indoors and outdoors Personal breathing zone air samples Tap water sample Cotton gloves	Budd, Roberts, and Ruby, 1990
Pesticides	Residences	Vacuum cleaner dust from a month's cleaning	Blood	Starr et al., 1974

Contaminant	*Activity*	*Surface Methods*	*Other Monitoring*	*Reference*
Pesticides	Migrant camp housing with residences suspected of being contaminated	Settled floor dust vacuumed inside a template (0.5 × 0.5 m) with a small pump onto an AE glass fiber filter cassette on noncarpet surfaces away from major traffic aisles		Morse, McLellan, and Christophersen, 1982
Pesticides (30)	Residential study to evaluate exposures indoors to children in nine homes	HVS3 vacuum samples over a 3,800 cm^2 area of carpet for house dust from a high traffic area, an area frequented by children, and a less-used area on carpet PUF roller (wet) samples adjacent to vacuumed areas Bare hand press adjacent to PUF area, rinse with 2-propanol	Rinses of children's hands 24 hr area air samples in living or family rooms 12.5–74 cm above floor Soil samples from entry way	Lewis, Fortmann, and Camann, 1994
2,4,7-Trinitro-fluorene-9-one (TNF)	Photocopiers with photoconductors that have TNF, a mutagenic compound, on the surface to determine if toner contamination occurs—since TNF makes direct contact with toner during image development IBM facility with 2 IBM 3800s.	Dry Whatman 41 wipe filters used to wipe copier surfaces including near vacuum, toner transfer, copier door, vacuum box, and near drum	Area air samples for TNF, carbon black, and PAHs in three locations: control panel, toner collection bag, and paper/toner cutting cyclone Personal breathing zone air samples during toner addition and toner bag change Bulk sample from filter bag	NIOSH, December 1981 (HETA 81-125-1029, HETA 81-352-1029)
TNF	Photocopiers with photoconductors that have TNF, a mutagenic compound, on the surface to determine if toner contamination occurs—since TNF makes direct contact with toner during image development National Library of Medicine with one 3800	Dry Whatman 41 filters used to wipe on machine cover above fuser section	Area air sample at control panel and above fuser section	NIOSH, December 1981 (HETA 81-125-1029, HETA 81-352-1029)

Contaminant	*Activity*	*Surface Methods*	*Other Monitoring*	*Reference*
TNF	Photocopiers with photoconductors that have TNF, a mutagenic compound, on the surface to determine if toner contamination occurs—since TNF makes direct contact with toner during image development National Institute for Health with 5 3800s in one room	Dry Whatman 41 filters used to wipe on machine cover above fuser section and a spill of used toner	Area air samples at operator position Bulk sample of spent and fresh toner	NIOSH, December 1981 (HETA 81-125-1029, HETA 81-352-1029)
TNF	Photocopiers with photoconductors that have TNF, a mutagenic compound, on the surface to determine if toner contamination occurs—since TNF makes direct contact with toner during image development Computer center with two 3800s	Dry Whatman 41 filters used to wipe on machine cover above fresh toner bag	Area air samples at the control panel and above the fresh toner bag	NIOSH, December 1981 (HETA 81-125-1029, HETA 81-352-1029)
Urethane particles	School district where isocyanate foam insulation had been sprayed to roof and inside exterior walls as well as other sealing measures instituted to decrease energy usage	Wipe samples with Whatman smear tabs of horizontal surfaces in buildings	Area air sample for by-products of foam system, metals, aldehydes, and organic vapors Bulk sample of plaster	NIOSH, January 1984*a* (HETA 83-172-1409)

DERMAL MONITORING FOR COMMUNITY CONCERNS*

Contaminant	*Activity*	*Dermal Methods*	*Other Monitoring*	*Reference*
Captan Malathion Methoxychlor	Home gardener after spraying with an aspirator sprayer attached to a garden hose	Hand rinse with 30 mL hexane poured over them twice up to 7 days after last usage		Kazen et al., 1974
Carbaryl dust (5%), WP, aqueous suspension	Home gardener exposure: Mixing-loading Dust application with shaker can or dust pump; spray application with hand-held pressurized sprayer to sweet corn and green beans	Gauze (10 × 10 cm) pads taped to Tyvek coveralls at shoulders, back (upper), chest (upper), forearms, thighs, lower leg (cuff), and skin of forearm; pad on tongue of shoe (inside) and exterior of shoe; a single pad of denim over gauze attached at calf outside Tyvek Hand wash with 200 mL ethanol containing 0.03% sodium hydroxide	Disposable dust respirator	Kurtz and Bode, 1985
Chlordane	Evaluation of exposure of general population to residual pesticide contamination in environment following ban in 1986 on use	Cotton puffs wetted with ethanol used to wipe skin of antebrachium on a monthly basis	Blood	Hirai and Tomokuni, 1993
Crude oil	Cleanup of Exxon Valdez oil spill on water	Luminoscope (UV) readings of skin of workers hands and arms pre- and postshift (before and after cleanup)	Personal breathing zone samples for PNAs, VOCs oil mist, and nitrogen dioxide Bulk samples of crude oil	NIOSH, 1991*b* (HETA 89-200-2111)
DDVP	Insecticide treatment inside residences using an aerosol spray can and water emulsion spray (0.5%)	Six gauze pads (4 × 4 in.) attached on the back and six attached to the chest of each worker	Modified respirator with prefilters Blood (pre- and postshift and 12 hr postshift) Urine (pre- and during the shift; 12 hr post shift) Pads for surface contamination	Das et al., 1983

*For dermal studies with metals, PCBs, TCDD, amines, and pesticides, see the Appendixes.

Contaminant	Activity	Dermal Methods	Other Monitoring	Reference
Dichlorovos	Application with hand sprayer to interiors of residences for insect control	Pads (10.2 × 10.2 cm) of 8-ply gauze over Whatman chromatography paper (0.16 mm) with glassine paper backing placed inside and outside of polyester jumpsuits at forearms, lower legs, chest, and back, and head (on top and under hard hat) Hand rinse in 200 mL ethanol:water (50:50)	Personal breathing zone air samples Blood Urine	Gold and Holcslaw,1985
Dieldrin (1.1%, 0.55%)	Hand spraying of houses for disease vector control	Pads (10 × 10 cm) of filter paper (0.08 cm thick) attached to clothing on one side of the body and skin at matching sites on other (shoulder, back of wrist, and side of ankle) and also to skin of stomach and cheek (5 × 5 cm)		Fletcher, Press, and Wilson, 1959
Dieldrin (1.1%, 0.55%)	Hand spraying of houses for disease vector control	Filter paper pads (10 × 10 cm) (0.08 cm thick) impregnated with lanolin attached to clothing on one side of the body and skin at matching sites on other (shoulder, back of wrist, and side of ankle), and also to skin of stomach and cheek (5 × 5 cm)		Fletcher, Press, and Wilson, 1959
Diethyl phthalate Dibutyl phthalate Dioctyl adipate	Office where workers were experiencing headaches, eye and skin irritation while handling carbonless copy paper	Cotton gloves	Area air samples for total dust, formaldehyde organics	NIOSH, May 1982 (HETA 81-275-1122)

Contaminant	*Activity*	*Dermal Methods*	*Other Monitoring*	*Reference*
Fiberglass	Office building with computer facilities	Transparent adhesive tape applied to skin surface of the elbow or wrist of one arm used to collect fibers; if skin lesions were present, tape was applied to lesion	General area air samples Surface samples in offices and computer room Settled dust samples	NIOSH, April 1984 (HETA 83-409-1450)
Mancozeb ETU	Home garden mixing and applying with compressed air sprayer	Gauze pads (10.16 × 10.16 cm) stapled to clothing outside and underneath clothing at chest, back, forearms, ankles, and thighs Cotton gloves	Modified respirator with collecting pads (7.01 cm) Urine (pre- and postapplication)	Mumma, Brandes, and Gordon, 1985
PAHs (as pyrene)	Wood preserving plant where railroad crossties are impregnated with creosote oil in a pressurized vessel	Polypropylene pads (60 mm diam) pasted to the workers' skin at the jaw, right shoulder, right upper arm, right wrist, groin and right ankle. On one day workers wore Tyvek suits under their normal work clothing and on the second day they did not.	Personal air samples Urine	Van Rooij et al., 1993
Pentachlorophenol Tetrachlorophenol	Montana residents in treated log homes	Wet wipe samples from the palms of the hands of residents using Whatman smear tabs	Area air samples Bulk samples of treating chemicals Surface wipes Urine	NIOSH, April 1986 (HETA 84-53, 425-1680)
Pesticides	Residences	Bottle rinse of children's hands with 2-propanol (70 mL)	Area air sampling Soil Surface samples from floors and carpets	Lewis et al., 1991

REFERENCES

Beusterien, K. M., R. A. Etzel, M. M. Agocs, G. M. Egeland, E. M. Socie, M. A. Rouse, and B. K. Mortensen. 1991. Indoor air mercury concentrations following application of interior latex paint. *Arch. Env. Contam. Toxicol.* **21**:62–64.

Birkner, L. R., A. K. Nagayama, J. M. Bachman, G. R. Rosenblum, and X. J. Padilla. 1991. *Asbestos Abatement Related Contamination of a High Rise Office Building—Recognition, Evaluation and Control.* Salt Lake City, UT: American Industrial Hygiene Conference Abstract.

Budd, W. T., J. W. Roberts, and M. G. Ruby. 1990. *Field Evaluation of a High Volume Surface Sampler for Pesticides in Floor Dust.* Washington, DC: EPA, EPA/600/3-90/030.

Center for Disease Control (CDC). 1990. Mercury exposure from interior latex paint—Michigan. *Mortality and Morbidity Weekly* **39**:125–126.

Currie, K. L., E. C. McDonald, L. T. K. Chung, and A. R. Higgs. 1990. Concentrations of Diazinon, Chlorpyrifos and Bendiocarb after application in offices. *AIHA J.* **51**(1):23–27.

Das, Y. T., P. K. Taskar, H. D. Brown, and S. K. Chattopadhyay. 1983. Exposure of professional pest control operator to dichlorvos (DDVP) and residue on house structures. *Toxicol. Letters* **17**:95–99.

Decker, J. 1982. Case studies: The case of the dirty neighbor. *Appl. Occup. Env. Hyg.* **7**:292–293.

Diemel, J. A. L., B. Brunekreef, J. S. M. Boleij, K. Biersteker, and S. J. Veenstra. 1981. The Arhnem lead study. II. Indoor pollution and indoor/outdoor relationships. *Env. Res.* **25**:449–456.

EPA. May 1984. *Techniques for the Assessment of the Carcinogenic Risk to the U.S. Population Due to Exposure from Selected Volatile Organic Compounds from Drinking Water.* Washington, DC: Office of Drinking Water, EPA, PB21394-1.

EPA. 1985. *Guide for Decontaminating Building, Structures and Equipment at Superfund Sites.* Washington, DC: EPA, EPA600/2-85-028.

EPA. 1988. *Development of a High Volume Surface Sampler for Pesticides in Floor Dust.* Washington, DC: EPA, EPA/600/4-88/036.

EPA. 1989. *Exposure Factors Handbook.* Washington, DC: EPA, EPA600/8-89-043.

EPA. 1990. *Nonoccupational Pesticide Exposure Study (NOPES).* Research Triangle Park, NC: U.S. EPA, EPA 600/3-90/003.

EPA. 1992. *Dermal Exposure Assessment: Principles and Applications.* Washington, DC: EPA, EPA600/8-91-011B.

Fenske, R. A., K. G. Black, K. P. Elkner, C. Lee, M. M. Methner, and R. Soto. 1990. Potential exposure and health risks of infants following indoor residential pesticide applications. *Am. J. Pub. Health* **80**(6):689–693.

Fenske, R. A., P. B. Curry, F. Wandelmaier, and L. Ritter. 1991. Development of dermal and respiratory sampling procedures for human exposure to pesticides in indoor environments. *J. Exposure Anal. Env. Epidemiology* **1**:11–30.

Fergusson, J. E., and N. D. Kim. 1991. Trace elements in street and housedusts: Sources and speciation. *Sci. Total Env.* **100**:125–150.

Fletcher, T. E., J. M. Press, and D. B. Wilson. 1959. Exposure of spraymen to dieldrin in residual spraying. *Bull. WHO* **20**:15–25.

Gold, R. E., and T. Holcslaw. 1985. Dermal and respiratory exposure of applicators and residents to dichlorvos-treated residences. In Honeycutt, R. C., G. Zweig, and N. N. Ragsdale (eds.), *Dermal Exposure Related to Pesticide Use.* Washington, DC: American Chemical Society, pp. 253–264.

Hawley, J. K. 1985. Assessment of health risk from exposure to contaminated soil. *Risk Anal.* **5**:289–301.

Hirai, Y. I., and K. Tomokuni. 1993. Levels of chlordane, oxychlordane and nonachlor on human skin and in human blood. *Bull. Env. Contam. Toxicol.* **50**:316–324.

Kazen, C., A. Bloomer, R. Welch, A. Oudbier, and H. Price. 1974. Persistence of pesticides on the hands of some occupationally exposed people. *Arch. Env. Health* **29**:315–318.

Kurtz, D. A., and W. M. Bode. 1985. Application exposure to the home gardener. In R. C. Honeycutt, G. Zweig, and N. N. Ragsdale (eds.), *Dermal Exposure Related to Pesticide Use.* Washington, DC: American Chemical Society, pp. 137–161.

Lewis, R. G., A. E. Bond, R. C. Fortmann, L. S. Sheldon, and D. E. Camann. 1991. *Determination of Routes of Exposure of Infants and Toddlers to Household Pesticides: A Pilot Study.* Washington, DC: EPA, EPA/600/D-91/077.

Lewis, R. G., R. C. Fortman, and D. E. Camann. 1994. Evaluation of methods for monitoring the potential exposure of small children to pesticides in the residential environment. *Arch. Env. Contam. Toxicol.* **26**:37–46.

Lu, C., and R. A. Fenske. 1991. *Indoor Air and Surface Chlorpyrifos Residues Following Broadcast and Total Release Aerosol.* Salt Lake City, UT: American Industrial Hygiene Conference Abstract.

McKone, T. E., and D. W. Layton. 1986. Screening the potential risks of toxic substances using a multimedia compartment model: Estimation of human exposure. *Regul. Toxicol. Pharmacol.* **6**:359–380.

Matte, T. D., J. P. Figueroa, S. Ostrowski, G. Burr, L. Jackson-Hunt, and E. L. Baker. 1991. Lead exposure from conventional and cottage lead smelting in Jamaica. *Arch. Env. Contam. Toxicol.* **21**:65–71.

Morse, D. L., R. McLellan, and C. Christophersen. 1982. Potential pesticide exposure of migrant farmworkers living within spray areas. *J. Env. Health*, **44**(May/June):301–304.

Mumma, R. O., G. A. Brandes, and C. F. Gordon.

1985. Exposure of applicators and mixer-loaders during the application of mancozeb by airplanes, airblast sprayers, and compressed-air backpack sprayers. In R. C. Honeycutt, G. Zweig, and N. N. Ragsdale (eds.), *Dermal Exposure Related to Pesticide Use*. Washington, DC: American Chemical Society, pp. 201–219.

Nigg, H. H., R. C. Beier, O. Carter, C. Chaisson, C. Franklin, T. Lavy, R. G. Lewis, P. Lombardo, J. F. McCarthy, K. T. Maddy, M. Moses, D. Norris, C. Peck, K. Skinner, and R. G. Tardiff. 1990. Exposure to pesticides. In S. R. Baker and C. S. Wilkinson (eds.), *The Effect of Pesticides on Human Health*. Advances in Modern Environmental Toxicology, vol. 17. New York: Princeton Scientific, pp. 35–130.

NIOSH, Hazard Evaluation and Technical Assistance Report. March 1978. *Louisana State Univ., School of Dentistry, New Orleans, LA*. TA 78-9. Cincinnati, OH: NIOSH.

NIOSH, Hazard Evaluation and Technical Assistance Report. February 1979. *Louisana State Univ., School of Dentistry, New Orleans, LA*. TA 78-62. Cincinnati, OH: NIOSH.

NIOSH, Hazard Evaluation and Technical Assistance Report. July 1979. *Lincoln Hall, Lincolndale, NY*. TA 79-12. Cincinnati, OH: NIOSH.

NIOSH, Technical Assistance Report. 1980*a*. *Greif Brothers Corporation, Niagara Falls, NY*. TA 80-87-771. Cincinnati, OH: NIOSH.

NIOSH, Technical Assistance Report. 1980*b*. *Niagara Steel Finishing Company, Niagara Falls, NY*. TA 80-107-772. Cincinnati, OH: NIOSH.

NIOSH, Health Hazard Evaluation Report. May 1981. *Greif Brothers Corporation, Niagara Falls, NY*. HETA 81-213-886. Cincinnati, OH: NIOSH.

NIOSH, Health Hazard Evaluation Report. May 1981. *Cyanotype printing in an artist's workshop, Bucyrus, OH*. HETA 81-171-880. Cincinnati, OH: NIOSH.

NIOSH, Health Hazard Evaluation Report. July 1981. *Dept. of Transportation, August, ME*. HHE 80-118-928. Cincinnati, OH: NIOSH.

NIOSH, Health Hazard Evaluation Report. August 1981*a*. *U.S. Air Force Recruiting Station, Bridgeport, CT*. HETA 81-309-936. Cincinnati, OH: NIOSH.

NIOSH, Health Hazard Evaluation Report. August 1981*b*. *National Center for Health Statistics, Hyattsville, MD*. HETA 81-333-935. Cincinnati, OH: NIOSH.

NIOSH, Health Hazard Evaluation Report. September 1981. *New England Telephone Co., Manchester, NH*. HHE 80-176-955. Cincinnati, OH: NIOSH.

NIOSH, Health Hazard Evaluation Report. December 1981. *DHHS, Washington, DC*. HETA 81-125-1029; and IBM, Lexington, KY, and Gaithersburg, MD. HETA 81-352-1029. Cincinnati, OH: NIOSH.

NIOSH, Health Hazard Evaluation Report. January 1982. *Blue Cross of Northeastern New York, Inc., Slingerlands, NY*. HETA 81-58-1037. Cincinnati, OH: NIOSH.

NIOSH, Health Hazard Evaluation Report. May 1982. *General Telephone Company, York, PA*. HETA 81-275-1122. Cincinnati, OH: NIOSH.

NIOSH, Health Hazard Evaluation Report. July 1983. *Fort Stanwix National Monument, Rome, NY*. HETA 83-90-1326. Cincinnati, OH: NIOSH.

NIOSH, Health Hazard Evaluation Report. September 1983. *George H. Fallon, Federal Office Building, Baltimore, MD*. HETA 83-358-1362. Cincinnati, OH: NIOSH.

NIOSH, Health Hazard Evaluation Report. January 1984*a*. *Wappingers Central School District, Wappingers Falls, NY*. HETA 83-172-1409. Cincinnati, OH: NIOSH.

NIOSH, Health Hazard Evaluation Report. January 1984*b*. *Ozark National Scenic Riverways, Van Buren, MO*. HETA 83-424-1403. Cincinnati, OH: NIOSH.

NIOSH, Health Hazard Evaluation Report. February 1984. *West Virginia Air National Guard, 167th Tactical Airlift Group, Martinsburg, WV*. HETA 83-214-1424. Cincinnati, OH: NIOSH.

NIOSH, Health Hazard Evaluation Report. March 1984. *Rutgers University, Newark, NJ*. HETA 81-314-1435. Cincinnati, OH: NIOSH.

NIOSH, Health Hazard Evaluation Report. April 1984. *King Kwit Minit Market, Inc., Cincinnati, OH*. HETA 83-409-1450. Cincinnati, OH: NIOSH.

NIOSH, Health Hazard Evaluation Report. July 1984*a*. *Progress Federal Savings & Loan, Bridgeport, PA*. HETA 83-363-1480. Cincinnati, OH: NIOSH.

NIOSH, Health Hazard Evaluation Report. July 1984*b*. *Georgetown University, Washington, DC*. HETA 83-444-1481. Cincinnati, OH: NIOSH.

NIOSH, Health Hazard Evaluation Report. April 1986. *Montana Log Home Residents, Kalispell, MT*. HETA 84-53, 425-1680. Cincinnati, OH: NIOSH.

NIOSH, Health Hazard Evaluation Report. September 1987. *Federal Office Building, Evansville, IN*. HETA 86-434-1833. Cincinnati, OH: NIOSH.

NIOSH, Health Hazard Evaluation Report. January 1988. *Planned Parenthood of South Central Indiana, Bloomington, IN*. HETA 83-258-1859. Cincinnati, OH: NIOSH.

NIOSH, Health Hazard Evaluation Report. March 1989. *Barbados Ministry of Health, Bridgetown, Barbados*. HETA 88-372-1953. Cincinnati, OH: NIOSH.

NIOSH, Health Hazard Evaluation Report. 1991*a*. *Andrew Jackson Jr. High School, Crosslands, WV*. HETA 89-183-2101. Cincinnati, OH: NIOSH.

NIOSH, Health Hazard Evaluation Report. 1991*b*. *Exxon Valdez Alaska Oil Spill*. HETA 89-200-2111. Cincinnati, OH: NIOSH.

NIOSH, Health Hazard Evaluation Report. September 1991. *Western Primary School, Russiaville, IN*. HETA 91-143-2136. Cincinnati, OH: NIOSH.

Que Hee, S., B. Peace, C. S. Clark, J. R. Boyle, R. L. Bornschein, and P. B. Hammond. 1985. Evolution of efficient methods to sample lead sources, such as house dust and hand dust, in the homes of children. *Env. Res.* **38:**77–95.

Rinehart, R. D., and Y. Yanagisawa. 1993. Paraoccupational exposures to lead and tin carried by electrical cable splicers. *AIHA J.* **54:**593–599.

Roels, H. A., J. P. Buchet, R. R. Lauwerys, P. Bruaus, F. Claeys-Thoreau, A. Lafontaine, and G. Verduyn. 1980. Exposure to lead by the oral and the pulmonary routes of children living in the vicinity of a primary lead smelter. *Env. Res.* **22:**81–94.

Ross, J., H. R. Fong, T. Thongsinthusak, S. Margetich, and R. Krieger. 1991. Measuring potential dermal transfer of surface pesticide residue generated from indoor fogger use: Using the CDFA roller method. Interim report II. *Chemosphere* **22**(9/10):975–984.

Schneider, T., O. Nielsen, P. Bredsdorff, and P. Linde. 1990. Dust in buildings with man-made mineral fiber ceiling boards. *Scand J. Work Env. Health* **16:**434–439.

Shu, H., P. Teitelbaum, A. S. Webb, L. Marple, B. Brunck, D. Dei Rossi, F. J. Murray, and D. Paustenbach. 1988. Bioavailability of soil-bound TCDD: Dermal bioavailability in the rat. *Fund. Appl. Toxicol.* **10:**335–343.

Skowronski, G. A., R. M. Turkall, and M. S. Abdel-Rahman. 1988. Effects of soil on percutaneous absorption of toluene in male rats. *J. Toxicol. Env. Health* **26:**373–384.

Starr, H. G., F. D. Aldrich, W. D. McDougall, and L. M. Mounce. 1974. Contribution of household dust to the human exposure to pesticides. *Pest. Monitoring J.* **8**(3):209–212.

Van Rooij, J. G. M., E. M. A. Van Lieshout, M. M. Bodelier-Bade, and F. J. Jongeneelen. 1993. Effect of the reduction of skin contamination on the internal dose of creosote workers exposed to polycyclic aromatic hydrocarbons. *Scand. J. Work Env. Health* **19:**200–207.

Veckman, M. G. 1991. *Pesticide Contamination and Subsequent Decontamination of a Residential Subslab Ventilation System*. Salt Lake City, UT: American Industrial Hygiene Conference Abstract.

Wester, R. C., and H. I. Maibach. 1989. Skin contamination and absorption of chemicals from drinking water while bathing or swimming. In R. L. Bronaugh and H. I. Maibach (eds.), *Percutaneous Absorption: Mechanisms, Methodology, Drug Delivery*. 2nd ed. New York: Marcel Dekker, pp. 191–196.

Wright, C. G., and M. D. Jackson. 1974. A comparison of residues produced by spraying and fogging of diazinon in buildings. *Bull. Env. Contam. Toxicol.* **12**(2):177–181.

Wright, C. G., R. B. Leidy, and H. E. Dupree. 1984. Chlorpyrifos and diazinon detection on surfaces in dormitory rooms. *Bull. Env. Contam. Toxicol.* **32:**259–264.

Yankel, A. J., I. H. von Lindern, and S. D. Walter. 1977. The Silver Valley lead study: The relationship between childhood blood lead levels and environmental exposure. *J. Air Pollut. Control Assoc.* **27:**763–767.

PART III

Surface Monitoring

CHAPTER 6

Introduction to Surface Monitoring

In 1961 it was noted by H. J. Dunster that surface contamination monitoring had not become a tool of occupational hygiene in general, partly because of the difficulty of monitoring for non-radioactive materials on surfaces (Dunster, 1961). However, it was deemed a good practice to avoid the indiscriminate distribution of toxic materials through the working environment, and if the techniques of measurement were easier, it was likely that the occupational hygienist would find the monitoring of surface contamination to be as useful as it is to the radiological profession. Due to its high toxicity, many sampling programs in the 1950s and 1960s treated beryllium in the same manner as radiation when it came to surface contamination.

No one can argue the importance of a safe workplace or living environment. Surface monitoring is one means through which safety can be achieved. Health hazards from chemicals, microorganisms, and radiation can be assessed by collecting and testing samples from various surfaces, or by using direct reading instruments to measure volatile releases from surfaces and items such as clothing. Environments determined to be unsafe can then undergo decontamination (see Chapter 10). Decontamination is the process of removing or neutralizing contaminants that have accumulated on personnel and equipment. Decontamination protects end users from hazardous substances that may contaminate and eventually permeate the protective clothing, respiratory equipment, tools, vehicles, and other equipment used in the vicinity of the chemical hazard; it protects all plant or site personnel by minimizing the transfer of harmful materials into clean areas; it helps prevent mixing incompatible chemicals together; and it protects the community by preventing uncontrolled migration of contamination from the site. Surface sampling is often the key to identifying building and equipment contamination and verifying that a decontamination method is effective.

In some cases, air sampling will not find overexposures to a contaminant such as fibrous glass even though employees are complaining of the irritant effects of this dust and are experiencing eye, nose, and throat problems as well as skin rashes. Measurements of airborne fibrous glass dust may not exceed recommended standards but surface monitoring can confirm the presence of fibers. This situation can exist because the amount of dermatitis related to fibrous glass exposure does not necessarily correlate with the airborne concentration of fibrous glass fibers. The dermatitis is more due to skin contact with fibers that have settled on work surfaces rather than to contact with airborne fibers. The surface levels that can cause skin irritation are often much lower than airborne exposure limits designed to protect against inhalation exposures. The number of persons affected with dermatitis would depend on housekeeping practices, which allow surface levels to build up especially when the source is intermittent or when the airborne concentration is minimal.

TARGETED HAZARDS

Chemicals

Chemicals that can penetrate or injure the skin or that are highly toxic if ingested orally, or dusts that pose a significant inhalation or migration hazard if resuspended are the primary types of compounds for which surface contamination is a concern. The variety of chemicals for which surface sampling can be conducted is large, although the most common groups are amines, metals and other toxic dusts, polychlorobiphenyls (PCBs) and tetrachlorobenzodioxin (TCDD), and pesticides. Other chemicals that have been sampled are described in Chapter 4.

Amines

Because many amines are carcinogenic, permeate the skin, and have low vapor pressures allowing them to remain on surfaces, they are good candidates for surface sampling studies. 3,3'-Dichlorobenzidine used in the manufacture of polyethylene and polyvinylchloride resins and 4,4'-methylene bis chloroaniline (MOCA), a catalyst for urethane resins, are examples. Airborne concentrations of 3,3'-dichlorobenzidine were found in both the clean and dirty changing rooms of a resin manufacturing facility (NIOSH, May 1986). Wipe sampling confirmed surface contamination in both of these rooms. An air vent was found between the rooms and neither room was under positive pressure, which allowed the amine to leak in from the production areas. In many cases OSHA has issued substance specific standards for carcinogenic amines. Appendix A describes specific studies that have been performed to measure amine contamination.

Toxic Dusts

Surface accumulations of toxic dusts such as lead, arsenic, and beryllium can become resuspended in air, and thus may contribute to airborne exposures. Dusts can migrate to other areas including personal vehicles of workers and their homes by being carried on their personal clothing and hair. Appendix B contains descriptions of surface sampling situations involving these and other metals as well as some specific sampling methods used for collection.

One situation where surface sampling is necessary is in asbestos abatement work where residual materials on areas such as windowsills, pipes, and floor cracks is a concern. Another is a determination to see if residual dust, such as lead, is present on the worker's clothing, and therefore could be contributing to the worker's exposure. These accumulations are also referred to as residual dust, especially when collected from structural members or the ventilation system in a plant. Dustfall methods collect dust as it settles out and provides a record of the amount deposited in the time elapsed since the last cleaning of the sampling container.

A good example of the mechanisms through which dust can migrate and contaminate the interior of a building can be described using asbestos. Friable sprayed asbestos surfaces have low impact resistance and are easily damaged. Even minor physical contact, whether it be intentional and unavoidable during maintenance activities, accidental during routine activity, or deliberate through vandalism, can produce fiber release. Asbestos fiber contamination of a building interior occurs by three general modes: fallout, contact or impact, and reentrainment. Fiber fallout is primarily a consequence of the characteristics and condition of the ceiling material itself, while contact (impact) and reentrainment (secondary dispersal) result from activity within the structure. Each of the three modes has a characteristic rate of fiber dispersal.

Continuous, low level and long lived fiber fallout may occur without actual physical disruption of the fiber-bearing material as the adhesive in the sprayed-on material degrades, producing concentrations ranging from nearly zero for cementitious mixes in good repair to roughly 100 ηg/M^3 for deteriorating dry mix applications. Variations in the fallout rate are due to structure vibration, humidity, air movement from heating and ventilating equipment, and air turbulence and vibration caused by human activity.

PCBs and TCDDs

The widespread use of PCBs as a dielectric fluid in transformers, capacitors, and fluorescent lamp ballasts occurred before there was good data on their toxicity and potential carcinogenicity. Due to their stability and low vapor pressures, PCBs can remain on and in surfaces unchanged for years. When exposed to high heat, TCDDs and tetrachlorodibenzofurans (TCDFs) are formed. Many opportunities for leaks, spills, and fires have produced significant contamination of several office buildings and schools. These resulted in the first systematic use of wipe samples to determine levels of contamination as well as whether cleanups were effective. As a result, PCBs have provided the basis for many cleanup standards. PCB sampling studies and standards are discussed in Appendix C.

Pesticides

Although pesticides are best known for dermal studies performed during application and reentry, surface contamination as a result of improper application in offices, restaurants, residences, and schools is also a concern. In a study of remote living facilities where applicators of 2,4-D in forests were residing, contamination was suspected when urine results for 2,4-D were high in nonspray periods (Frank, Campbell, and Sirons, 1985). It was found that the urine results were the result of surface contamination in the living quarters. The available water for washing in the field living quarters was found to be limited. The following year, levels of surface contamination were much lower due to improved water supplies provided for washing. In this case biological monitoring led to the investigation of contamination as a source of continuing exposure outside of the workplace. Surface studies on pesticides are described in Chapter 5 and Appendix D.

Aerosol Fallout

Aerosol fallout occurs due to the difficulties in preventing the spread of mists, sprays, and granules (most commonly, pesticides) during application and from process upsets. It is difficult to predict the length of time required for surface contamination from these applications to dissipate to nonhazardous levels. Therefore three different measurements are commonly made: (1) the amount of total surface deposition produced as a result of the application or release, (2) the amount of residual contamination remaining over time, which often involves taking samples immediately after application and at increasing time intervals following, and (3) the amount of the residue that would most likely be removed by human contact. If samples represent only the portion that can be dislodged by worker contact, they are termed *dislodgeable residues* (in the case of field workers exposed to pesticides). Total deposition samples provide a baseline measurement of contaminant actually applied to a surface to which all results can be compared. Dislodgeable or removeable residues predict the amount available for human exposure. Several different collectors have been developed that are specific for spray deposition. One is to take 1 ft^2, on-target aluminum foils, mounted on corrugated cardboard, and place them randomly in a horizontal position in different areas where the spray is expected to reach (Ware et al., 1973). Other methods involve the use of mylar sheets or glass plates.

Volatile Chemicals

For example, one of the most common formaldehyde-containing resins is used to give fabric wrinkle-resistant properties. Occupational dermatitis has been associated with airborne formaldehyde levels as low as 0.08 ppm, and with bulk fabric samples having latent formaldehyde concentrations, as low as 200 ppm (by weight) (NIOSH, July 1984c).

The National Institute of Occupational Safety and Health (NIOSH) evaluated a textile operation because of reports of skin and eye irritation and loss of fingernails among employees working with textiles that contained formaldehyde (NIOSH, 1977). Work area air samples were analyzed for vaporous formaldehyde and fabric samples were analyzed for latent formaldehyde content in a laboratory. The medical evaluation included a medical questionnaire and skin examination of symptomatic production employees. The airborne formaldehyde concentrations ranged from 0.13 ppm to 0.57 ppm and all were below the NIOSH recommended ceiling of 1.0 ppm. The latent formaldehyde levels in four fabrics tested ranged from 580 ppm to 938 ppm suggesting that it was the source of the problems (Table 6-1). Three weeks after the initial determination, the latent formaldehyde content of these fabrics decreased by 86–91%. These data indicate that as storage time increases, the amount of available formaldehyde, and, hence, potential worker exposure decrease.

Mercury from a clinical thermometer plant was unintentionally carried on the clothing of workers to their homes (Zirschky and Witherell, 1987). Elevated airborne mercury vapor levels were found in some of the workers' homes and elevated urine mercury levels were found in some of the children of the workers.

Microorganisms

Surface sampling for microorganisms originated from concerns of the spread of infections from multiple-use eating utensils (restaurants, hospitals) and attempts to identify reservoirs of epidemic causing microorganisms in health care institutions. Current applications include the manufacture of spacecraft, submarines, laminar flow hood in clean rooms, and indoor air illness outbreaks including *Legionella*. Surface sampling for microorganisms is most commonly done to determine the potential for inhalation exposure either as a result of a heating, ventilating, and air conditioning (HVAC) system or resuspension into the air after being disturbed on a surface.

Similar to dusts, microorganisms can become airborne by being released from people or stirred up after they have settled on surfaces. A particular concern is bacteria tracked into buildings on

TABLE 6-1. Comparison of NIOSH Studies in Textile Mills: Symptoms and Formaldehyde Levels

Study No.	*Number of Employees (%) Reporting Symptoms*	*Air Levels (Avg.) in ppm*	*Bulk Sample Offgassing*
1	26/210 (12.4%) all symptoms 15/210 (7.15) skin irritation	0.13–0.57 (0.27)	580–938
2	44/56 (78.65) eye irritation 18/56 (32.1%) skin irritation	0.08–0.44 (0.26)	329–339
3	107/120 (89%) eye irritation 70/120 (58%) skin irritation	0.12–0.53 (0.36) 0.11–0.27 TWA	200–500
4	44/64 (69%) eye irritation 15/64 (23%) skin irritation	0.34–0.53 (0.47)	200
5	13/102 (13%) all symptoms 13/102 (13%) skin irritation	0.15–0.23 (0.18) 0.15–0.18 TWA	260–450
6		0.07–0.34	
7		0.15–0.30	

Source: From *NIOSH Health Hazard Evaluation Report*. July 1984. Lion Uniform Co., Beattyville, KY. HETA 83-301-1478. Cincinnati, OH: NIOSH.

the soles of shoes from the outside where they are in dust and soil, and for indoor dust, also containing bacteria, to be tracked further through a building. The activity of people and equipment within enclosed spaces is considered the principal factor leading to the buildup and spread of airborne microbial contamination. In one study of the contamination built up on floors and walls in operating rooms during three surgeries (Table 6-2), it appeared that an increase in airborne microbial contamination was followed by an increase in surface contamination as well (Goddard, 1965). However, unlike chemicals, the quantity of microbial contamination on surfaces reaches a plateau and then does not increase since microorganisms die away due to desiccation and other hazards.

If workers have cuts or abrasions on their skin, microbes can enter. Poultry workers have had a high prevalence of warts on their hands and it was suspected that the wart-causing virus often entered through breaks in the skin, which were common because the workers perform intense manual work with their hands that are also frequently moist (Cohen, 1974).

Offices and other buildings can be targets for buildups of microorganisms, especially if they have ventilation systems that recirculate all or a portion of the air. These HVAC systems are susceptible to moisture buildup, and once contaminated, can allow microbial buildup and subsequent spread throughout the building. Other sources of microbes in buildings include organic materials, humidifiers and vaporizers, and HVAC equipment such as cooling towers. Typical evidence of microbial contamination inside an HVAC system includes a muddy sediment, patchy white and brown areas on the insulation, dripping water lines, and white powdery substances on the surface. Porous insulation, moisture, and a carbon source, such as organic dust from outside air, are good conditions for the proliferation of microbes.

The role of carpeting as a reservoir for microorganisms is also important. In addition to surface sampling, bulk samples are often collected from carpets, ceiling tiles, and HVAC system filters for microbial culturing. The types of organisms found in surface and bulk samples are often identical to those obtained with air sampling and these samples are a useful screening tool prior to performing air sampling. In areas where carpeting is not essential for noise reduction, and where it is likely to be chronically exposed

TABLE 6-2. Levels of Surface and Airborne Microbial Contamination in an Operating Room

		Average Surface Microbial Contamination (colonies/ft²)	
Operation	*Average Airborne Microbial Contamination (colonies/ft³)*	*Floor*	*Walls and Ceiling*
No. 1: 8:00–9:50 First day	8.5	254	82
After mopping	—	156	—
No. 2: 13:00–14:40	14.1	403	165
After mopping	—	91	—
No. 3: 7:40–9:20 Second day	16.8	649	222

Source: From Goddard, K. R. 1967. Effect of ventilation on distribution of airborne microbial contamination—field studies. In B. R. Fish (ed.). *Surface Contamination.* London: Pergamon Press, pp. 313–323.

to stagnant water, it should be removed. Damp carpet fibers can be colonized by molds and bacteria, which can then become aerosolized as people walk across the carpet or when it is vacuumed. It follows that diseases are often associated with water leaks. Water damaged materials often support microbial growth long after they appear dry, and dead materials (antigens, spores, toxins, and irritants) may remain in such materials for years. Carpet cleaning is rarely effective in removing microbial contamination and overuse of disinfectants can cause additional problems for building occupants.

Submarines and other environments where the same air is recirculated for long periods of time are prone to microorganism buildups. A typical program for this type of environment could include measuring the microbial burden of the air, potable water, and internal surfaces of the vehicle at intervals during patrols; examining the changes in human flora and determining the carrier rates of infection indicators such as *Staphylococcus aureus* in nasal and skin swabs; examining the blood of crew members for increasing antibodies to agents such as *Mycoplasma pneumoniae*; and analyzing the sick bay attendance rates for illness that could be attributed to infectious agents (Morris, 1975). A frequently reported and difficult organism to deal with is *Pseudomonas aeruginosa*, since it has a significant resistance to many bacteriocides.

Hospitals are regularly monitored for microorganisms not only because of patient illnesses but also because of the frequent contact of body fluids and aerosols with structure surfaces and health care equipment. Burn units must be monitored extra carefully since burn patients have a high susceptibility to disease. Surgical suction equipment has been found to be contaminated due to foaming of bodily fluids allowing contamination with portions of the unit that were supposed to be sealed off (Hodgson and Ruis-Frutos, 1991).

Restaurants and other foodservice facilities may have outbreaks due to contamination from microorganisms such as *Salmonella*. Tests of surfaces in food preparation facilities as well as cooking and eating utensils can be useful in determining the source of an outbreak.

Certain agricultural environments and wood processing facilities also need to be evaluated. Plywood mills can have large populations of mold and fungal spores. In factories such as printing works and textile mills, where high humidity is required to maintain efficient production and the processes undertaken may produce organic dusts, an additional problem arises as organic materials can provide nutrition and encourage the growth of microorganisms (Ager and Tickner, 1983). Large outbreaks of dermatitis of microbial origin have been reported in celery workers (Birmingham, Key, and Tubich, 1961).

Construction projects in general have been shown to introduce high concentrations of spores through production of dust and dirt. If there are office buildings nearby, the dust will collect on the filters of the HVAC systems. During periods of high humidity, such as the summer, enough moisture can be present to allow the spores to multiply on the filter and spread.

Radiation

One of the first instances producing an awareness of the hazard of skin and oral contact with low level radiation resulted from the painting of watch and clock dials with a luminous paint containing a radioactive substance, which began in the United States in 1915 (Castle, Drinker, and Drinker, 1925; Bloomfield and Knowles, 1933; Schwartz et al., 1933). In 1925 it was determined that workers employed in applying a luminous paint containing radium often suffered from necrosis of the jaw, a chronic, progressive rotting away of the jawbone.

A very small amount (1–2 g) of powdered radium paint was poured into a porcelain crucible or ink well, a few drops of oil-based or water-based adhesive and distilled water were added, and the mixture was stirred with a glass rod until a desired consistency was obtained. The clock or watch dial was placed in the center of a small, circular holder; the crucible was held with the left hand and tilted until the liquid was at the very brim so that contact with the surface of the paint might be clearly visible. To keep the desired consistency, the paint was stirred frequently. The paint, a luminous zinc sulfide containing minute traces of copper combined with small amounts of radium bromide, was applied with fine brushes. It was the universal practice of the dial painters to point their brushes in their mouths. The jaw was the target rather than the mouth because radium binds to the bone much more readily than soft tissue, and once bound, continues to release radiation, producing more damage.

The exposures were more widespread, however. Dust collected in the workroom from various locations, such as tables, chandeliers, and wall beams, were luminous in the dark room. The hair, faces, hands, arms, necks, dresses, and underclothes, including the corsets of the female dial painters, were luminous in the dark following exposure to light. One worker noticed that her nasal discharges were luminous in her handkerchief. Dust from the machine shop below the painting room was luminous as well as the skin of the office workers and others in the plant not employed in the paint room. This finding suggested that the powdered base was being spread throughout the plant by the dial painters' clothing and skin.

In some plants daily sweeping was conducted with each worker taking care of her own workstation, causing the dust to spread even further. Since the powder used by the painters was extremely light, if a person breathed on it, it would blow about; to prevent this scattering, it should have been kept wet. Therefore, there were several routes of exposure: inhalation of the powder, absorption through the skin, and oral ingestion.

METHODS FOR IDENTIFYING HAZARDS

The time to identify surface contamination should be before air monitoring levels increase or personnel in nearby nonproduction areas start to complain. A number of methods for assessing surface and personal contamination have been developed, including wet and dry smears, adhesive tape sampling, and settled dust and spray deposition techniques. For surface samples, it must be remembered that quantitation is related to the specific area that was sampled and the contamination in other areas is a matter of professional judgment.

Wipe Sampling

Wipe sampling is useful for compounds that rapidly absorb through the skin as long as their physical characteristics are appropriate for this collection method. Surfaces that may be contacted by food or other materials ingested or placed in the mouth (chewing tobacco, gum, cigarettes) may be wipe sampled (including hands and fingers) to show contamination (OSHA, 1991). Wipe sampling methods have come under scrutiny recently with the result that the methodologies are producing more consistent results and, in at least one instance, the Lioy-Weisel-Wainman Sampler may provide reliable quantitative results.

Some unusual techniques may prove useful for investigations where the contaminants are unknown. A variation on wipe sampling for specific chemicals involves performing an AMES test on filter content where mutagens are suspected but the specific compounds are unknown. Filter wipes have also been cultured for microbes. Environmental surfaces have also been wiped with the same media used by dermatologists for patch testing and then used to perform this test on subjects when allergies are suspected to be due to this surface dust.

Chemicals for which wipe sampling is ineffective even though they can penetrate the skin include volatile solvents such as n-butyl alcohol, because their evaporation from surfaces can be rapid and sampling will not provide adequate quantitation. Most gases such as bromine and boron trifluoride do not redeposit on surfaces, so sampling for them is ineffective; however, some gases such as arsine and stibine may revert to their metallic forms after contact with surfaces and remain. Due to their volatile nature, most organic solvents are not suitable for wipes.

When accompanied by close observation of the operation in question, wipe sampling can help identify sources of contamination and poor work practices. Surface contamination may be readily apparent for colored compounds such as lead and cadmium pigments, but it may not be evident for surface deposition from lead fumes in a radiator shop or bumper (chromium) plating facility, or on dark and colored surfaces. In addition, the effectiveness of chemical protective clothing (CPC) such as gloves, aprons and respirators in these situations can be evaluated by wipe sampling the inner surfaces of the protective gear (and protected skin).

It can be difficult to determine whether equipment or instruments are effectively decontaminated after they have been used in a contaminated area, such as on a hazardous waste site or for sampling of concentrated materials. Wipe and or sniff sampling can be useful in determining whether these procedures are effective.

Aerosol Deposition and Dislodgeable Residues

There are several methods used to measure aerosol deposition: foam strips, tape, and surface vacuuming for dust or spray that has already settled. Tape samples are used primarily for surface asbestos contamination, but can be used for other dusts as well. It has been suggested that adhesive tape may be more efficient in taking samples from rough surfaces than filter paper (Chavalitnikul and Levin, 1984). Vacuum methodologies have improved and, when used with prescribed methodologies, several devices can produce quantitative results. A standardized method for carpet samples has been developed by the American Society for Testing and Materials. Occasionally a case can be made for collecting a bulk sample rather than wiping or vacuuming a surface, for example, when a mechanical or manual device is used to regularly vacuum or sweep surfaces and the dust is derived from a floor or carpet. Dust has also been collected from carpet sweepers and used to represent surface contamination. Dislodgeable residues are collected using several methods, including the PUF roller, Dow Drag Sled, CFDA Roller, and, for foliage, coupons and leaf punches.

Volatile Surface Contamination

Surface deposits of the volatile type generally cannot be determined through conventional surface sampling methods and other investigatory methods are thus necessary. In many cases, a field evaluation will depend on whether there is an instrument capable of detecting the contaminant of interest.

For those types of surface contamination that do not respond well to manual collection (such as wipe testing), direct reading instruments, for example, a mercury monitor, can be used. Other examples are general survey instruments, such as a photoionization analyzer for organic vapor contamination. In this case, it is important to remember that unless the instrument is calibrated with the contaminant in question, the results are all relative to the response of the instrument.

STANDARDS FOR SURFACE SAMPLING

There are few standards related to surface contamination; generally situations must be handled on a case-by-case basis. The health effects caused, the contribution of skin absorption or ingestion to the total dose, and air sample results must be considered when evaluating the results of wipe samples. For example, detection of lead on the surfaces of an office associated with a radiator shop or lead battery shop means that other individuals besides production workers are potentially exposed. Exposure could include younger people such as teenagers working after school, office workers, and customers.

Where samples collected over different areas are to be compared, results should be converted to the same units, such as $\mu g/ft^2$. There is always the possibility that false negative results, that is, nondetection of existing contamination, will occur because surface contamination is not removed by a wipe sample. It can be due to the selection of the wrong solvent or permeation of the contamination into a porous material. Dirt and grease on surfaces will adhere to wipes, obscuring sample results and making analyses impossible or difficult. In many instances it is also difficult to estimate how closely the amount of material removed from a surface by a method represents what would actually be removed by human skin contact.

There are two ways of presenting surface test

results: concentration (μg/g) of a contaminant in the dust and the amount of contaminant removed from a surface (surface loading). The first criteria is considered by many to provide a more accurate representation of the hazard. Concentration rather than loading is generally preferred when surface measurements are used to estimate dermal exposure. For example, lead concentration on a surface measures how much lead is in the dust, while lead loading measures how much lead is on a surface. Lead loading equals the amount of lead in the dust (concentration) times the amount of dust in a given area ($\mu g/g \times g/ft^2$). Lead loading levels are a better indication of the amount of lead available for human exposure. Contaminant concentration is not directly affected by cleaning or physical variation of the total dust levels because it is standardized to one weight, usually 1 g for dust, regardless of the amount of dust on the surface.

For wipe samples, it must be remembered that quantitation is related to the specific sampling area. It is generally impossible to wipe all areas of a surface, and other portions could have higher levels of contamination. This effect can be minimized by taking a sufficient number of samples or by compositing. Higher levels on one area of a work surface or desk versus another (left versus right) may be due to the workers using their hand of preference. Contamination of the interiors of vehicles and living quarters can account for continuing exposures to seasonal workers (Frank, Campbell, and Sirons, 1985).

In addition to the amount of concentration on a surface, an estimate should be made of the frequency of contact. A control switch for an overhead crane used several times an hour could result in a greater daily exposure (at a lower concentration) than a highly contaminated light switch that is touched twice a shift.

In general, for Occupational Safety and Health Administration (OSHA) compliance, wipe sampling is necessary to establish the presence of a toxic material posing a potential absorption or ingestion hazard. A citation for an ingestion hazard can be issued when there is a reasonable probability that a toxic material may be ingested and subsequently absorbed in areas where employees consume food or beverages (including drinking fountains). A citation for exposure to materials that can be absorbed through the skin or can cause a skin problem such as dermatitis shall be issued where appropriate CPC is necessary but not worn. Neither of these citations require any air sampling in addition to wipe sampling.

There are two primary considerations when issuing a citation for an ingestion or absorption hazard, such as a citation for lack of protective clothing. The first consideration is whether a health risk exists as demonstrated by a potential for an illness, such as dermatitis, and/or the presence of a toxic material that can be ingested or absorbed through the skin or in some other manner. The second consideration is whether there is a potential that the toxic material can be ingested or absorbed, meaning if it is present on the skin of the employee, which can be established by evaluating the conditions of use and determining if a health hazard exists.

The toxic substance must be of such a nature and exist in such quantities as to pose a serious hazard. The substance must be present on surfaces that have hand contact, such as lunch tables and cigarettes, or on other surfaces that present the potential for ingestion or absorption if contaminated, for example, a bottled water dispenser. The CPC or other abatement means must be effective in eliminating or significantly reducing exposure.

Standards for Wipe Samples

The simplest method for setting up a wipe sample standard is to qualitatively compare areas for relative contamination or use a zero acceptable criterion for areas that are supposed to be clean such as eating areas and personal vehicles. Guidelines or standards have been developed for some chemicals. California and OSHA have set a surface sampling standard MBOCA. Some companies have developed in-house standards. The Department of Housing and Urban Development (HUD) has developed a standard for lead abatement wipe samples and criteria have also been developed for asbestos.

Reentry levels for pesticides on foliage may be

appropriate for determining other pesticide surface contamination such as on equipment and vehicles associated with manufacturing or ancillary work to the application of the material. Reentry levels are often expressed as waiting intervals (days) to allow sufficient time for dislodgeable pesticide residues to dissipate to lower and thus safer concentrations. However, these can also be expressed as toxic dislodgeable (insecticide) residues (concentrations in $\mu g/cm^2$) or concentrations on foliage (Knaak and Iwata, 1982). Some examples are included in Table 6-3.

The British have established limits for surface contamination of beryllium. The method for deriving these limits is described as follows (Brooks, 1959): When a room has been decontaminated, it is normal to take smear samples, using filter papers, from the floor and walls over an area of 1 M^2. The height of the room is taken into account to convert this measurement to cubic meters, and it is assumed that all beryllium detected is dispersed uniformly within this volume and similarly throughout the room. The room is derestricted with a series of such samples giving results below 2 $\mu g/M^3$.

Fittings and apparatus are checked in a similar way, but it is often impossible to take a smear sample over 1 M^2 of surface, and the sample is taken over as large an area as is practicable. In such cases where the total amount of beryllium contamination is likely to be slight due to a small surface area, a figure of up to 25 μg is tolerated. Sometimes a variety of quantitative standards can exist for a single chemical, especially if individual facilities voluntarily set their own standards. Table 6-4 lists acceptable levels of beryllium surface concentrations which have been developed.

Background Levels and Detection Limits

In some cases, background levels have been used for surface cleanup standards (Oatman and Roy, 1986). In a study of emissions of TCDDs and TCDFs from a polyvinyl chloride (PVC) fire in a wooden warehouse, background samples were collected from the outside of a house in the main windward direction, which was unlikely to have been contaminated by the fire (Marklund et al., 1989). Sampling studies have also found that inherent concentrations of TCDFs and TCDDs may be in many office buildings representing background contamination (Kominsky, 1989).

Cleanup Criteria

How clean is clean after a decontamination effort? Several approaches have been used to set "safe" levels and are essentially similar to those used for surface sampling standards. The simplest is the use of expert opinions or applying standards used for other purposes. If a consensus among several experts is used, it is safer than if only one professional's judgment is considered. Another approach is to use background levels after sampling in several representative noncontaminated situations. Yet another approach is to use laboratory or instrument detection limits, which can also be considered the most conservative approach. For example, in a decontamination program for aromatic amines chemical spot tests were used to detect residual contamination (Weeks and Dean, 1978). These tests were capable of detecting the cancer-suspect agents at levels of 10 $\eta g/cm^2$ on stainless steel, 150 $\eta g/cm^2$ on painted surfaces, and 2–5 $\eta g/cm^2$ on concrete. When a test revealed no contaminant, the surface was considered clean.

An approach gaining in popularity is to perform a risk assessment using toxicity data, exposure assumptions, and safety factors. An examination of two methods used to establish decontamination guidelines following PCB-containing transformer fires is useful in understanding the difficulties in using risk assessments to set clean up levels. One method assumes that the major hazard to human health represented by PCBs is carcinogenesis, and a calculation is performed to obtain an estimate of the risk to humans by extrapolating animal testing data. This procedure calculates a dose that corresponds to an estimated lifetime cancer risk. The second approach is to calculate a safe human intake using no observed effect levels (NOELs) determined from animal experiments.

TABLE 6-3. Guidelines and Standards for Surface Sample Results

Compound	*Limit*	*Criteria*	*Source*[a]
Asbestos	≥ 1%	Abatement	Beaulieu, 1991
Asbestos	≥ 0.1%	Abatement	State of California
Azinphos-Methyl	3.1 μg/cm²	Field reentry	Knaak, 1980
Beryllium	25 μg/12 in²	MAC	Bolton, 1985
Beryllium	10^{-2} μg/cm²	Inactive and low activity areas	Saxby and Hole, 1965
Beryllium	5×10^{-1} μg/cm²	Control areas	Saxby and Hole, 1965
Beryllium	$<5 \times 10^{-2}$ μg/cm²	Contact surfaces	Saxby and Hole, 1965
Chlordane	50 μg/ft², walls		NIOSH, January 1988 (HHE 83-258-1859)
Dialifor	0.8 μg/cm²	Field reentry	Knaak, 1980
3,3′-Dichlorobenzidine	10 μg/100 cm²		NIOSH, May 1986 (HETA 84-58-1700)
Dimethoate	53 μg/cm²	Field reentry	Knaak, 1980
Dioxin	55 μg/M²		Bromley, Wilson, and Smith, 1988
Lead	200 μg/ft², floor 500 μg/ft², windowsills 800 μg/ft², window wells 200 μg/ft² exterior porch	Clearance for lead paint abatement; lead in settled dust in residences	HUD, Sept. 1990
MBOCA	100 μg/100 cm²		CAL/OSHA
Mercury	1 μg/M³	Detection limit of monitoring instrument	Zirschky and Witherell, 1987
Methidathion	0.6 μg/cm²	Field reentry	Knaak, 1980
Nor-nitrogen mustard hydrochloride	0.5 μg/dm²	Internal company standard	Thulin, 1993
Paraoxon	0.02 μg/cm²	Field reentry	Knaak, 1980
Parathion	0.09 μg/cm²	Field reentry	Knaak, 1980
PCBs	100 ηg/cm²		Perdek et al., 1991
PCBs	0.5 μg/100 cm²	Office building cleanup standard	NIOSH, 1986*b* (HETA 85-289-1738)
PCBs	1 mg/M²	Decontamination standard for worker reentry into transformer vault	EPA, 1985
PCBs	100 μg/M²	Decontamination standard for offices in same building	EPA, 1985
PCBs	10 μg/100 cm²	EPA standard for low-contact indoor impervious surfaces	EPA, 1987

[a]Source citations appear in the reference list at the end of this chapter.

TABLE 6-3. *(continued)*

Compound	*Limit*	*Criteria*	*Source*[a]
PCBs	10 µg/100 cm^2	EPA standard for high-contact solid surfaces indoors	EPA, 1987
PCBs	10 µg/100 cm^2 or 100 µg/100 cm^2 plus encapsulation	EPA standard for low-contact indoor nonimpervious surfaces	EPA, 1987
PCBs	100 µg/100 cm^2	Low-contact outdoor surfaces (both impervious and nonimpervious)	EPA, 1987
PCBs	10 µg/100 cm^2	Indoor solid surfaces and high-contact outdoor solid surfaces and indoor electrical vault areas	EPA, 1987
PCBs	10 µg/100 cm^2	Low-contact outdoor impervious solid surfaces	EPA, 1987
PCBs	10 µg/100 cm^2 or 100 µg/100 cm^2 plus encapsulation	Low-contact outdoor nonimpervious solid surfaces	EPA, 1987
PCBs	100 µg/M^2	NIOSH standard for surfaces that routinely contact workers' unprotected skin	NIOSH, June 1991 (HETA 91-27-2117)
TCDFs	50 ηg/M^2		Marklund et al., 1989
Phosalone	7 µg/cm^2	Field reentry	Knaak, 1980
Polychlorinated dibenzofurans (TCDFs)	3 ηg/M^2		State of California. In Schecter and Tiernan, 1985
Polychlorinated dioxins (PCDDs)	3 ηg/M^2		State of California. In Schecter and Tiernan, 1985
Sodium fluoroacetate	0.2 mg/100 cm^2	Protection for workers	LaGoy, Bohrer, and Halvorsen, 1992
TCDD	$\leq$ 0.75 µg/M^2, exterior building surfaces $\leq$ 0.01 µg/M^2, interior building surfaces	Decontamination of homes and schools after Seveso incident	Di Domenico et al., 1980
2,3,7,8-TCDD	10 ρg/M^2		Sherman et al., 1987
2,3,7,8-TCDD	1 ρg/cm^2		Wagoner, 1989
2,3,7,8-TCDD	5 µg/M^2		Fortunati, 1985
2,3,7,8-TCDD equivalents	1 ηg/M^2		NIOSH, September 1987 (HETA 86-434-1833)
2,3,7,8-TCDD equivalents	10 ηg/M^2		Kim and Hawley, 1985

TABLE 6-3. *(continued)*

Compound	*Limit*	*Criteria*	*Source*[a]
2,3,7,8-TCDD equivalents	25 ηg/M²		Kim and Hawley, 1985; National Research Council, 1988
TCDD equivalents	1 ηg/M²	Office building cleanup standard	NIOSH, 1986*b* (HETA 85-289-1738)
TCDD-PCDF (Total)	24 ηg/M²	Decontamination standard for worker reentry into transformer vault	EPA, 1985
TCDD-PCDF (Total)	3 ηg/M²	Decontamination standard for offices in same building	EPA, 1985

[a]Source citations appear in the reference list at the end of the chapter.

TABLE 6-4. Acceptable Levels of Beryllium Surface Concentrations (μg/cm²)

Surface	*Facility No. 1 1956*	*Facility No. 2 1958*	*British (Harwell) 1959*	*Facility No. 3 1961*	*LRL 1959*	*LRL 1960–1963*	*LRL 1967*
Floors and walls	0.02	0.08	0.0025	0.005	0.01 (LOD)	0.02 or with air monitoring up to 1.0	0.05 or with air monitoring up to 2.0
Room equipment	0.005	0.08	0.0025	0.005	0.01 (LOD)	0.01 or with air monitoring up to 0.5	0.05 or with air monitoring up to 2.0
Surplus equipment (for removal to non-Be areas)	0.001	0.02–0.006	—	—	0.01 (LOD)	0.001	0.01

Source: From Cohen, J. J., and R. N. Kusian. 1967. The significance of beryllium surface contamination to health. In B. R. Fish (ed.), *Surface Contamination*. London: Pergamon Press, pp. 297–301.
Note: LOD = limit of detection.
Wipe Methods:
Facility No. 1: Wipe 1.0 ft² with dry filter paper.
Facility No. 2: Wipe 12 in² with alcohol-wetted filter paper.
Facility No. 3: Wipe 100 cm² with dry filter paper.
Harwell: Wipe 1.0 M² with dry filter paper.
LRL: Wipe 100 cm² with dry filter paper.

Most of the risk assessments for TCDD have been based on the extrapolation of dose–response relationships for these compounds from animals to humans. The underlying assumptions can vary. Decontamination guidelines for the Binghamton transformer fire were based on the assumption that the major hazard of exposure to TCDFs and TCDDs, expressed as 2,3,7,8-TCDD equivalents, was the development of noncarcinogenic long-term health effects (Hryhorczuk et al., 1986). Decontamination guidelines for the San Francisco transformer fire were based on the assumption that the major hazard of exposure was carcinogenesis.

The Environmental Protection Agency (EPA) has not prescribed levels of contaminants that are acceptable to all Superfund sites; one reason is that potential synergistic effects of combinations of wastes cannot be adequately predicted (Anon., 1983). A formal, systematic approach needs to be developed for determining acceptable levels of contaminants in and on building and equipment surfaces. Related methods for determining acceptable levels of contaminants in soils at contaminated sites may be useful for developing such an approach. Examples of methods that should be evaluated include the multimedia environmental goals, the composite hazard index, the preliminary pollutant limit values, and the monitoring trigger levels (EPA, 1985).

Another approach used for developing cleanup standards is to categorize areas by the frequency of contact as well as the groups of people most likely to have contact. The following categories of surfaces were developed by the EPA (1987) for PCB spill cleanup:

High-contact residential/commercial surface: A surface in a residential/commercial area that is repeatedly touched, often for relatively long periods of time. Doors, wall areas below 6 ft high, uncovered flooring, windowsills, fencing, banisters, stairs, automobiles, and children's play areas, such as outdoor patios and sidewalks, are examples.

Low-contact residential/commercial surface: A surface that is rarely touched, such as interior ceilings, interior wall areas above 6 ft high, roofs, asphalt roadways, concrete roadways, wooden utility poles, unmanned machinery, concrete pads beneath electrical equipment, curbing, and exterior structural building components such as aluminum/vinyl siding, cinder block, asphalt tiles, and piping.

High-contact industrial surface: A surface in an industrial setting that is repeatedly touched, often for relatively long periods of time. Manned machinery and control panels are examples. High-contact industrial surfaces are generally of impervious solid material.

Low-contact industrial surface: A surface that is rarely touched, such as ceilings, walls, floors, roofs, roadways and sidewalks in the industrial area, utility poles, unmanned machinery, concrete pads beneath electrical equipment, curbing, exterior structural building components, indoor vaults, and piping.

Cleanup levels are often called action levels or reentry criteria. The EPA sets cleanup standards in site closure plans for hazardous waste cleanups (Perdek et al., 1991). The most perplexing question surrounding the setting of these levels, usually for decontamination activities, is how clean is clean? Decontamination target levels have been, and continue to be, established on a case-by-case basis by a variety of federal, state, and local agencies. Some examples of different cleanup levels that have been set for accidents involving PCB-containing transformers are in Appendix C.

Target levels for Superfund sites have been, and can be, set by a number of groups, including local and state health departments and federal agencies such as EPA, NIOSH, OSHA, NRC (National Research Council), Centers for Disease Control, and the surgeon general's office. Target levels for Army-unique materials such as explosives are proposed by the U.S. Army Toxic and Hazardous Materials Agency and approved by the Army surgeon general. Target levels are more stringent in cases where the site, buildings, or equipment is to be released for unrestricted/public use.

Sodium Fluoroacetate: A Case Study

One approach to develop cleanup standards for wipe samples was done in conjunction with a plant cleanup of sodium fluoroacetate (LaGoy, Bohrer, and Halvorsen, 1992). It was assumed that workers in contact with hard surfaces could get any material present on these surfaces on their hands and could subsequently ingest the material, or if the material was wet, it could be absorbed through the skin. To accurately calculate cleanup levels for sodium fluoroacetate on the wipe samples, the number of times a surface is likely to be contacted, the amount of surface dust that would be picked up on each contact event (this depends on several other factors including the amount of time the hand or arm is in contact with the surface, moisture on the hands, and the amount of the body area contacting the surface), and the amount of contacted material that would be ingested or absorbed must be known. Because it is extremely difficult to measure these factors, calculating cleanup levels for wipe samples is an inexact science.

The sodium fluoroacetate assessment assumed that all dust ingested came from surfaces in the facility. Therefore, the dust cleanup level could be applied that had already been developed using conventional risk assessment techniques, where a reference oral dose, body weight, duration of exposure, absorption factor, and ingestion rate are determined. The amount of dust on the surfaces was calculated using known deposition rates and air concentrations (Hawley, 1985). An air concentration of 1 mg/M^3 was assumed to produce approximately 2 g/100 cm^2 area over a 30-day period. By multiplying the soil/dust cleanup level of 100 mg/kg by the amount of dust on the 100-cm^2 surface used for a wipe sample, the cleanup level was determined to be 0.2 mg/100 cm^2 wipe sample.

Resuspension Factors

Pollutants in the soil can be resuspended as dust by wind erosion just as settled dusts in workplaces and residences can become airborne when disturbed by activities (Fig. 6-1). A particular fraction of these particles, that is, those less than or equal to 10 µm in diameter, may be inhaled by persons. The factors affecting dust resuspension include moisture content, presence of nonerodible surfaces (rocks and vegetation), surface crust stability, wind velocity, particle size, and soil roughness height. Moisture hinders the resuspension of dust by forming a cohesive matrix among the dust or soil particles, and when soil is saturated, resuspension will not occur. However, as the surface layer of moisture is removed by evaporation, resuspension occurs. Evaporation is influenced by wind speed, temperature, and dust characteristics.

Resuspension factors have been used to develop standards for surface contamination, primarily for radiation. The most likely mechanisms for contamination of air by particles redispersed from solid surfaces involve

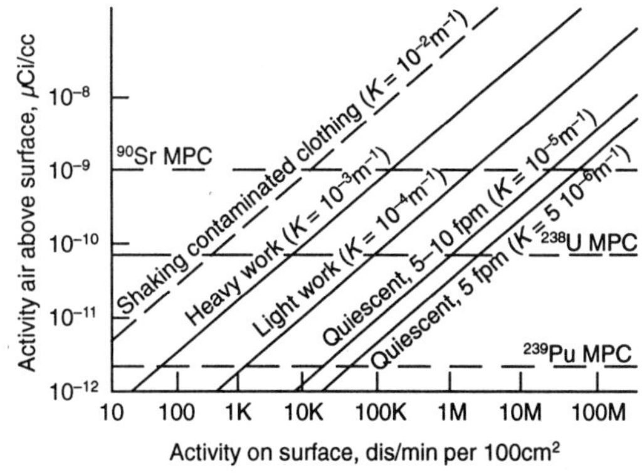

Figure 6-1. Air activity above a contaminated surface relative to contamination on the surface under different working conditions. (*K* = resuspension factor.)
Source: From R. B. Keely and T. K. Wenstrand. 1971. Impact of fuel reprocessing on the health physics professions. *Health Physics* **20:**144.

transfer of momentum from the activity of human beings, or from large surfaces in motion (Corn and Stein, 1965). After the particles are airborne, room air currents could theoretically keep unit density particles as large as 90 µm aloft. However, in reality very few particles as large as 5 µm are found. The reasons include the fact that although room air velocities approach 50 ft/min on average, air currents move down as well as up, and can deposit particles in addition to lifting them. The inertia of large particles in motion contributes to their rapid deposition by impaction on surfaces.

A resuspension factor is defined as the ratio of airborne contamination to surface contamination (Caplan, 1993). A *K* factor can be calculated to represent this ratio. The units vary, which is not a problem as long as the same ones are used for both the surface and airborne weights of the material as well as the surface area and air volumes.

$$K = \frac{\text{Air quantity per unit volume}}{\text{Surface quantity per unit area}} = \frac{\mu g/M^3}{\mu g/M^2} = \frac{\text{Air sampling}}{\text{Wipe sampling}}$$

where K is usually expressed as mg/ft^2 and mg/ft^3, or µg/M^2 and µg/M^3.

The usefulness of these factors has been demonstrated in radioactivity measurements but may not be appropriate in other situations. There are many variables involved in predicting how resuspension will affect a dust, including the physical properties of the dust; nature and condition of the surface; type, form, and amount of activity that disturbs the material; environmental factors (e.g., ventilation); and controls in place to minimize resuspension (e.g., wet methods). Tests usually involve performing air sampling during an activity and collecting wipe samples immediately following the activity.

A typical set of conditions that would be used to develop resuspension factors is as follows: undisturbed, that is, no movement during the tests; fans about 1 ft above floor level directed parallel to the floor surface for the entire test period; movement of a dolly or cart almost continuously along the length of the test area; and concurrent use of fans and movement of a dolly. Thus, the value of a resuspension factor will vary depending on the activities used to disturb the dust (Table 6-5). These are often referred to as K_1, K_2, and so on. The type of surface also affects the amount of a resuspension factor. In one study, unwaxed linoleum floors gave higher resuspension factors than the waxed polished linoleum surface (Jones and Pond, 1965). Tests are often done in isolated rooms (from the process) such as change rooms, because any airborne activity therein must arise from surface contamination of floors, walls, clothing, and shoes since no work is done with contaminants in this area.

The interpretation and application of resuspension factors must be done carefully as they may not always represent all possible conditions. In general, the lower the resuspension factor, the lower the concern that surface contamination will create a significant airborne hazard. It should be noted that this has nothing to do with the degree of oral hazard or the hazard from direct skin contact. However, it could reflect the degree of clothing contamination if the majority of the contamination were due to airborne material.

There are also sources of air contamination other than contaminated surfaces, such as building ventilation and work practices that deliberately disturb dusts (e.g., using pneumatic equipment, hammering or sweeping). It has been suggested that resuspension factors are likely to be proportional to the number of people in an area. In a study using air and wipe sampling, resuspension factors of 4.2×10^{-2} and 1.02×10^{-2} were calculated for beryllium (Mitchell and Eutsler, 1965).

TABLE 6-5. Variables Involved in the Resuspension of Dusts

Types of properties of the dust	Adhesive Cohesive Particle size distribution Particle density Chemical reactivity with normal air gases (oxygen, water, carbon dioxide)
Properties of the surface	Macrostructure Microstructure Adhesive properties with respect to the dust
Actions creating resuspension	Foot traffic Nonpowered wheel traffic Powered wheel traffic Vibration Air velocity

Source: After Caplan, K. 1993. The significance of wipe samples. *AIHA J.* **54**(2):70–75.

CORRELATIONS BETWEEN SURFACE LEVELS AND AIRBORNE LEVELS

The majority of the work that has been done to find correlations between surface and airborne levels has been done in the radiation field. Although K factors have attempted to provide a correlation between surface and likely airborne levels that would be created by resuspension of dusts, in general their application has not proved successful for chemical exposures. Table 6-6 provides an example. Therefore, if the concern is whether a significant airborne concentration might exist, then air sampling should be con-

TABLE 6-6. Air Lead Versus Surface Lead in Firing Ranges

Firing Range	*Number of Samples*	*Range (μg/M³)*	*Mean (μg/M³)*	*Number of Samples*	*Range (μg/100 cm²)*	*Mean (μg/100 cm²)*
A	4	30.9–477	158	3	794–12,000	4,457
B	5	168–746	337	5	55–67,000	16,200
C	4	71.0–114	90.3	6	10–4,350	983
D	1	84.7	84.7	0		
E	5	0.14–7.64	3.5	5	9–195	98

Source: Data from Caplan, K. 1993. The significance of wipe samples. *AIHA J.* **54**(2):70–75.

ducted. However, surface sampling can be useful in determining the source of airborne material.

In tests performed for contamination in a beryllium refinery, levels of surface contamination and corresponding general air concentrations were measured (Table 6-7). It was determined that for a wide range of surface contamination values there was a relatively narrow range of airborne dust concentrations, indicating that surface contamination had little influence on airborne concentrations at that facility. In general, higher air concentration ratios were associated with the higher surface concentrations, and it is more likely that this condition was due to activities occurring in the respective areas.

TABLE 6-7. Contamination in a Beryllium Refinery

Location	*Surface Smear (μg/cm²)*	*Air Concentration (μg/M³)*
Process areas	0.32–8.1	0.5–3.0
Auxiliary areas (maintenance, stockrooms)	0.02–0.8	0.5–1.5
Offices	0.01–0.3	0.1–0.5

Source: Data from Glauberman, H., W. R. Bootmann, and A. J. Breslin. 1967. Studies of the significance of surface contamination. In B. R. Fish (ed.), *Surface Contamination.* London: Pergamon Press, pp. 110–115.

SURFACE SAMPLING FOR SPECIFIC COMPOUNDS

Compound	*Media*	*Source*
Abate	37 mm 1.0 µm glass fiber filter, 100 cm^2 area	OSHA, 1988
Acetic acid	Whatman smear tab, wetted with deionized water, 100 cm^2 area	OSHA, 1991
2-Acetylaminofluorene	37 mm 1.0 µm glass fiber filter, 100 cm^2 area	OSHA, 1988
Acid black 128	37 mm 1.0 µm glass fiber filter, 100 cm^2 area	OSHA, 1988
Acid orange 74	37 mm 1.0 µm glass fiber filter, 100 cm^2 area	OSHA, 1988
Acid yellow 34	37 mm 1.0 µm glass fiber filter, 100 cm^2 area	OSHA, 1988
Acrylamide	37 mm 0.8 µm MCE filter moistened with water, 100 cm^2 area	Hills and Greife, 1988
Acrylamide	37 mm glass fiber filter premoistened with 0.3 mL of deionized or distilled water	Cummins et al., 1992
Aldicarb	37 mm 1.0 µm glass fiber filter, dry or wetted with isopropanol, 100 cm^2 area	OSHA, 1988
Aldicarb	Whatman smear tab, 100cm^2 area	NIOSH, January 1985 (HETA 78-4-1511)
Aldrin	37 mm 1.0 µm glass fiber filter, dry, 100 cm^2 area	OSHA, 1988
Allergins, house dust. *See* *Dermatophagoides pteronyssinus*		
Allethrin	37 mm 1.0 µm glass fiber filter, 100 cm^2 area	OSHA, 1991
Aluminum	Whatman 40 filter, dry or wetted with distilled water, 1 ft^2 area	NIOSH, September 1979 (HHE 79-9-615)
Aluminum trihydrate	37 mm 0.8 µm MCE filter, dry	NIOSH, June 1977 (HHE 77-39-400)
Amiben	37 mm 1.0 µm glass fiber filter, 100 cm^2 area	OSHA 1991
4-Aminodiphenyl	37 mm 1.0 µm glass fiber filter, 100 cm^2 area	OSHA, 1988
4-Aminodiphenyl	Whatman 41 filter, wetted with methanol, 100 cm^2 area, fluorescamine used for visualization	OSHA, 1991
4-Aminopyridine	37 mm 1.0 µm glass fiber filter, wetted with isopropanol, 100 cm^2 area	OSHA, 1991
Ammoniacal copper arsenate. *See* Arsenic; Copper		

Compound	*Media*	*Source*
Ammonium chloride	Whatman smear tab, wetted with deionized water, 100 cm^2 area	OSHA 1991
Ammonium nitrate	Whatman smear tab, wetted with deionized water, 100 cm^2 area	OSHA 1991
Aniline	Aromatic amine swipe test, 100 cm^2 area	CLI Colorimetric Laboratories, Inc.
Aniline and homologues	37 mm 1.0 μm glass fiber filter, 100 cm^2 area	OSHA, 1988
Anisidine (o, p)	37 mm 1.0 μm glass fiber filter, wetted with isopropanol, 100 cm^2 area	OSHA, 1991
Antimony	3 × 3 in. cotton gauze pad, wetted with deionized water, 100 cm^2 area	NIOSH, July 1992 (HETA 92-10-2234)
Antimony and compounds	Whatman smear tab, wetted with distilled water, 100 cm^2 area	OSHA, 1990 (ID-121)
Antimony and compounds	37 mm 0.8 μm MCE filter, wetted with distilled water, 100 cm^2 area	OSHA, 1990 (ID-121)
ANTU	37 mm 1.0 μm glass fiber filter, dry, 100 cm^2 area	OSHA, 1988
Arsenic	Whatman smear tab, wetted with distilled water, 100 cm^2 area	OSHA, 1990 (ID-105)
Arsenic	37 mm 0.8 μm MCE filter, wetted with distilled water, 100 cm^2 area	OSHA, 1990 (ID-105)
Arsenic	Whatman 50 filter, wetted with distilled water, 1 $in.^2$ area	NIOSH, 1983*a*
Arsenic	Whatman 41 filter, wetted with distilled water, 100 cm^2 area	OSHA, 1991
Arsenic	7 cm Whatman 42 filter, wetted with distilled or deionized water, 100 cm^2 area	Sheehy and Jones, 1993
Arsenic	Whatman 40 filter, dry, 0.5 ft^2 area	NIOSH, February 1976 (HHE 75-8-263)
Arsenic	Vacuuming using a personal air sampling pump and MCE filter in cassette	Polissar et al., 1990
Arsenic trichloride	Whatman 41 filter, dry, 100 cm^2 area	OSHA, 1991
Arsenic trifluoride	Whatman 41 filter, dry, 100 cm^2 area	OSHA, 1991
Asbestos	Cellophane tape, placed directly on microscope slide	Beaulieu, 1991
Asbestos	Vacuuming using a personal air sampling pump and MCE filter in cassette	NIOSH, September 1987 (HETA 86-434-1833)

Compound	*Media*	*Source*
Asbestos	Do not use Whatman or other paper filters, bulk preferred	OSHA, 1991
Asphalt fumes	37 mm 1.0 μm glass fiber filter, dry, 100 cm^2 area	OSHA, 1988
Atrazine	37 mm 1.0 μm glass fiber filter, 100 cm^2 area	OSHA, 1988
Atrazine	Whatman 41 filter, dry or moistened with solvent with which pesticide was formulated, 100 cm^2 area	NIOSH, December 1979*b* (HHE 77-126-646)
Auramine	37 mm 1.0 μm glass fiber filter, 100 cm^2 area	OSHA, 1988
Auramine hydrochloride	37 mm 1.0 μm glass fiber filter, 100 cm^2 area	OSHA, 1988
Azinphos-ethyl	37 mm 1.0 μm glass fiber filter, 100 cm^2 area	OSHA, 1988
Azinphos-methyl	37 mm 1.0 μm glass fiber filter, 100 cm^2 area	OSHA, 1988
Azodrin	Whatman 41 filter, dry or moistened with hexane or chloroform, 100 cm^2 area	NIOSH, December 1979*b* (HHE 77-126-646)
Bacteria	Sterile cotton Q-tip	
Bacteria, fastidious	Hycon® contact slide	Biotest Corp.
Bacteria, coliform	Hycon® contact slide	Biotest Corp.
Barium	Whatman smear tab, wetted with deionized water, 100 cm^2 area	OSHA, 1991
Barium, soluble compounds	37 mm 0.8 μm MCE filter, wetted with distilled water, 100 cm^2 area	OSHA, 1990
Baygon	37 mm 1.0 μm glass fiber filter, wetted with isopropanol, 100 cm^2 area	OSHA, 1988
Bendiocarb	Cotton gauze pad soaked in isopropanol	Currie et al., 1990
Benomyl	37 mm 1.0 μm glass fiber filter, 100 cm^2 area	OSHA, 1988
Benzidine	37 mm 1.0 μm glass fiber filter, 100 cm^2 area	OSHA, 1988
Benzidine	Whatman 41 filter, wetted with methanol, fluorescamine used for visualization, 100 cm^2 area	OSHA, 1991
Benzidine-based dyes	37 mm 1.0 μm glass fiber filter, 100 cm^2 area	OSHA, 1988
3,4-Benzpyrene	Whatman 1 filter	Ketcham and Norton, 1960
Beryllium	Whatman 1 filter, dry, 1 ft^2, 100 cm^2 or 1 M^2 area	Cohen and Kusian, 1965

Compound	*Media*	*Source*
Beryllium	Whatman 1 filter, wetted with alcohol, 12 in^2 area	Cohen and Kusian, 1965
Beryllium	Whatman smear tab, wetted with distilled water, 100 cm^2 area	NIOSH, 1984 (HETA 82-024-1428)
Beryllium	Adhesive tape	Routledge, 1968
Betasan	37 mm 1.0 µm glass fiber filter, 100 cm^2 area	OSHA, 1988
BHETA. *See* Bis-hydroxy ethyltallowamine		
Bidrin	Whatman 41 filter, dry or moistened with solvent with which pesticide was formulated, 100 cm^2 area	NIOSH, December 1979*b* (HHE 77-126-646)
Bis(2-dimethylamino) ethyl ether	Whatman 41 filter, 100cm^2 area	NIOSH, December 1978 (HHE 78-68-546)
Bis-hydroxy ethyltallowamine (BHETA)	3 × 3 in. cotton gauze pad, wetted with methanol, 100 cm^2 area	NIOSH, April 1987 (HETA 85-453-1787)
Bismuth	Whatman 40 filter, 0.5 ft^2 area	NIOSH, February 1976 (HHE 75-8-263)
Bismuth	3 × 3 in. cotton gauze pad, wetted with deionized water, 100 cm^2 area	NIOSH, July 1992 (HETA 92-10-2234)
Bladex	Whatman 41 filter, dry or moistened with solvent with which pesticide was formulated, 100 cm^2 area	NIOSH, December 1979*b* (HHE 77-126-646)
Borates, tetra; sodium salts, anhydrous	Whatman smear tab, wetted with deionized water, 100 cm^2 area	OSHA, 1991
Borates, tetra; sodium salts, decahydrate	Whatman smear tab, wetted with deionized water, 100 cm^2 area	OSHA, 1991
Borates, tetra; sodium salts, pentahydrate	Whatman smear tab, wetted with deionized water, 100 cm^2 area	OSHA, 1991
Boric acid	Whatman smear tab, wetted with deionized water, 100 cm^2 area	OSHA, 1991
Boron	Whatman smear tab, wetted with deionized water, 100 cm^2 area	OSHA, 1991
Boric oxide	Whatman smear tab, wetted with deionized water, 100 cm^2 area	OSHA, 1991
Botran	37 mm 1.0 µm glass fiber filter, 100 cm^2 area	OSHA, 1988
Bromine pentafluoride	Whatman smear tab, wetted with deionized water, 100 cm^2 area	OSHA, 1991
Cadmium	Whatman smear tab, moistened with distilled water, 100 cm^2 area	NIOSH, 1984 (HETA 82-024-1428)

Compound	*Media*	*Source*
Cadmium	37 mm 0.8 μm MCE filter, 100 cm² area	Tartre, 1992
Cadmium	3 × 3 in. cotton gauze pad, wetted with deionized water, 100 cm² area	NIOSH, July 1992 (HETA 92-10-2234)
Cadmium	Vacuuming using a personal air sampling pump and MCE filter in cassette, 0.25 M² area	Solomon and Hartford, 1976
Calcium hypochlorite	37 mm 1.0 μm glass fiber filter, wetted with 0.1% sulfamic acid, 100 cm² area	OSHA, 1991
Captafol	Whatman 41 filter, 100 cm² area	OSHA, 1988
Captan	37 mm 1.0 μm glass fiber filter, 100 cm² area	OSHA, 1988
Carbaryl	37 mm 1.0 μm glass fiber filter, 100 cm² area	OSHA, 1988
Carbofuran	Whatman 41 filter, 100 cm² area	OSHA, 1988
Carbon fibers	37 mm 0.8 μm MCE filter, 100 cm² area	NIOSH, August 1984 (HETA 82-289-1496)
Chlordane	Whatman smear tab, dry, 100 cm² area	NIOSH, January 1988 (HETA 83-258-1859)
Chlordane	Whatman smear tab, wetted with toluene, 4 in.² area	NIOSH, 1984 (HETA 83-444-1481)
Chlordane	2 × 2 in. cotton gauze pad, wetted with 8 mL hexane, 0.25 M² area	NIOSH, February 1991 (HETA 89-183-2101)
Chlorodiphenyl (42% and 54% chlorine). *See also* PCBs	3 × 3 in. cotton gauze pad, wetted with hexane, 100 cm² area	NIOSH, 1987*a* (HHE 85-414-1805)
Chlorpyrifos	37 mm 1.0 μm glass fiber filter, 100 cm² area	OSHA, 1988
Chlorpyrifos	Cotton ball, wetted with 10 mL 2-propanol	Wright, Leidy, and Dupree, 1984
Chlorpyrifos	Cotton gauze pad soaked with isopropanol	Currie et al., 1990
Chlorpyrifos	Surgical cotton gauze pad, wetted with distilled water	Fenske et al., 1990
Chlorpyrifos	2 × 2 in. cotton gauze pad, wetted with 8 mL hexane, 0.25 M² area	NIOSH, February 1991 (HETA 89-183-2101)
Chlorpyrifos	Whatman 41 filter, wetted with toluene, 100 cm² area	NIOSH, July 1984*a* (HETA 83-383-1480)
Chromated copper arsenate. *See* Arsenic; Chromium VI; Copper		
Chromates. *See* Chromium VI		
Chromic acid. *See* Chromium VI		

Compound	*Media*	*Source*
Chromium	Whatman smear tab, wetted with distilled water, 100 cm^2 area	OSHA, 1990 (ID-121)
Chromium	37 mm 0.8 μm MCE filter, wetted with distilled water, 100 cm^2 area	OSHA, 1990 (ID-121)
Chromium	3 × 3 in. cotton gauze pad, wetted with deionized water, 100 cm^2 area	NIOSH, July 1992 (HETA 92-10-2234)
Chromium	Whatman 40 filter, dry or wetted with distilled water, 1 ft^2 area	NIOSH, September 1979 (HHE 79-9-615)
Chromium	Vacuuming samples using personal air sampling pump and MCE filter in cassette	NIOSH, May 1981 (HETA 81-171-880)
Chromium VI	Spot test using 1 N sulfuric acid on a cotton Q-tip to wipe surface and drops of a 1% alcoholic solution of diphenyl carbazide for visualization	NIOSH, September 1975 (HHE 74-87-221)
Chromium VI	Whatman smear tab, wetted with distilled water used to wipe a 100 cm^2 area followed up with drops of 0.5 normal sulfuric acid and 1% alcoholic diphenylcarbazide solution for visualization	NIOSH, June 1981 (HETA 81-85-889)
Chromium VI	Low ash PVC filter, wetted with deionized water, 100 cm^2 area	OSHA, 1991
Ciodrin	Whatman filter, dry or moistened with solvent with which pesticide was formulated, 100 cm^2 area	NIOSH, December 1979*b* (HHE 77-126-646)
Cobalt	Whatman smear tab, wetted with distilled water, 100 cm^2 area	OSHA, 1990 (ID-121)
Cobalt	37 mm 0.8 μm MCE filter, moistened with distilled water, 100 cm^2 area	OSHA, 1990 (ID-121)
Coccidioides immitis	Cotton tipped swab soaked in sterile saline, 1 ft^2 area, which is then streaked directly onto Mycosel agar	NIOSH, November 1981 (HHE 80-183-991)
Copper	Whatman smear tab, moistened with distilled water, 100 cm^2 area	OSHA, 1990 (ID-121)
Copper	37 mm 0.8 μm MCE filter, wetted with distilled water, 100 cm^2 area	OSHA, 1990 (ID-121)
Copper	Whatman 40 filter, dry or wetted with distilled water, 1 ft^2 area	NIOSH, September 1979 (HHE 79-9-615)
Copper	Whatman 40 filter, 5 cm^2 area	NIOSH, August 1982 (HETA 81-212-1169)

Compound	*Media*	*Source*
CoRal	37 mm 1.0 μm glass fiber filter, 100 cm^2 area	OSHA, 1988
Cyanide	37 mm 0.8 μm silver membrane filter, 50 in^2 area	NIOSH, March 1987 (HETA 86-30-1785)
Cyanide	Whatman smear tab, wetted with deionized water, 100 cm^2	OSHA, 1991
2,4-D, Butyl ester	37 mm 1.0 μm glass fiber filter, 100 cm^2 area	OSHA, 1988
DDT	Whatman 41 filter, 100 cm^2 area	OSHA, 1988
DDVP	37 mm 1.0 μm glass fiber filter, 100 cm^2 area	OSHA, 1988
DEF	Whatman smear tab, wetted with distilled water, 100 cm^2 area	NIOSH, July 1984*b* (HETA 81-463-1477)
Demeton	37 mm 1.0 μm glass fiber filter, 100 cm^2 area	OSHA, 1988
Denatomium benzoate	37 mm 1.0 μm glass fiber filter, 100 cm^2 area	OSHA, 1991
Dermatophagoides pteronyssinus	Vacuum into polytetrafluoroethylene filters in cassettes	Swanson et al., 1989
o-Dianisidine	37 mm 1.0 μm glass fiber filter, 100 cm^2 area	OSHA, 1988
o-Dianisidine-based dyes	37 mm 1.0 μm glass fiber filter, 100 cm^2 area	OSHA, 1988
Diazinon	2 × 2 in. cotton gauze pad, wetted with 8 mL hexane, 0.25 M^2 area	NIOSH (HHE 89-183-2101)
Diazinon	Cotton ball, wetted with 10 mL 2-propanol	Wright, Leidy, and Dupree, 1984
Diazinon	3 × 3 in. cotton gauze pad, soaked with isopropanol	Currie et al., 1990
Diazinon	Whatman 41 filter, wetted with toluene, 100 cm^2 area	NIOSH, July 1984*a* (HETA 83-383-1480)
Dibrom	Whatman smear tab, 100 cm^2 area	NIOSH, January 1985 (HETA 78-4-1511)
o-Dichloroaniline	Aromatic amine swipe test, 100 cm^2 area	CLI Laboratories
3,3'-Dichlorobenzidine	37 mm 1.0 μm glass fiber filter, 100 cm^2 area	OSHA, 1988
3,3'-Dichlorobenzidine	37 mm 1.0 μm glass fiber filter, impregnated with sulfuric acid, 100 cm^2 area	OSHA, 1988 (Method 65)
3,3'-Dichlorobenzidine	11 cm Whatman 1 filter, moistened with methanol, 100 cm^2 area	NIOSH, June 1985 (HETA 84-128-1601)
3,3'-Dichlorobenzidine	Whatman smear tab, wetted with cyclohexane, 100 cm^2 area	NIOSH, November 1985 (HETA 80-035-1635)

Compound	*Media*	*Source*
3,3'-Dichlorobenzidine	Cotton gauze pad, moistened with isopropanol, 100 cm^2 area	NIOSH, May 1986 (HETA 84-58-1700)
Dichloroisocyanuric acid	37 mm 1.0 μm glass fiber filter, wetted with 0.1% sulfamic acid	OSHA, 1991
2,4-Dichlorophenoxyacetic acid	Cotton ball, wetted with 2 mL methanol, 0.1 m^2 area	Frank, Campbell, and Sirons, 1985
3,4-Dichloropropionanilide	37 mm 1.0 μm glass fiber filter, 100 cm^2 area	OSHA, 1988
3,4-Dichloropropionanilide	Whatman 41 filter, 100 cm^2 area	OSHA, 1991
Dicofol	Whatman 41 filter, 100 cm^2 area	OSHA, 1988
Dicrotophos	37 mm 1.0 μm glass fiber filter, 100 cm^2 area	OSHA, 1988
Diethylaminoethanol (DEAE)	Whatman smear tab, 100 cm^2 area	NIOSH, December 1989 (HETA 89-057-2003)
DEAE	Whatman 41 filter, 100 cm^2 area	NIOSH, September 1981 (HETA 81-247-958)
Dimethoate	37 mm 1.0 μm glass fiber filter, 100 cm^2 area	OSHA, 1988
4-Dimethylaminoazobenzene	37 mm 1.0 μm glass fiber filter, dry or wetted with methanol or isopropanol, 100 cm^2 area	OSHA, 1988
Dimethylaminopropionitrile	Whatman 41 filter, 100 cm^2 area	NIOSH, December 1978 (HHE 78-68-546)
Dimethyl 1,2-dibromo-2,2-dichloroethyl phosphate	37 mm 1.0 μm glass fiber filter, 100 cm^2 area	OSHA, 1988
1,1-Dimethylhydrazine	Fluorescamine, 0.35 mg/mL in 1,4-dioxane, drops on Whatman 42 filter paper wipes and observe for yellow fluorescence in black box	Weeks, Yasuda, and Dean, 1976
Dimethylpolysiloxane	Whatman smear tab, dry, 100 cm^2 area	NIOSH, May 1982*b* (HETA 81-396-1118)
Dinitrochlorobenzene (DNCB)	Whatman smear tab, wetted with cyclohexane, 100 cm^2 area	NIOSH, November 1985 (HETA 80-035-1635)
Dinitrotoluene (DNT)	Wooden Q-tip, wetted with acetone, 0.24 M^2 area	EPA, 1985
DNT	Cotton gauze pad, wetted with 97% isopropanol	Levine et al., 1985
Dipropylene glycol monomethyl ether	Whatman 41 filter paper, dry, 100 cm^2 area	NIOSH, August 1983 (HETA 81-304-1361)
Direct black 38	37 mm 1.0 μm glass fiber filter, 100 cm^2 area	OSHA, 1988
Direct blue 2	37 mm 1.0 μm glass fiber filter, 100 cm^2 area	OSHA, 1988
Direct blue 6	37 mm 1.0 μm glass fiber filter, 100 cm^2 area	OSHA, 1988

Compound	*Media*	*Source*
Direct blue 98	37 mm 1.0 μm glass fiber filter, 100 cm^2 area	OSHA, 1988
Direct brown 31	37 mm 1.0 μm glass fiber filter, 100 cm^2 area	OSHA, 1988
Direct brown 95	37 mm 1.0 μm glass fiber filter, 100 cm^2 area	OSHA, 1988
Disperse yellow 3	37 mm 1.0 μm glass fiber filter, 100 cm^2 area	OSHA, 1988
Disulfiram	37 mm 1.0 μm glass fiber filter, 100 cm^2 area	OSHA, 1988
Disulfoton	37 mm 1.0 μm glass fiber filter, 100 cm^2 area	OSHA, 1991
Disyston	37 mm 1.0 μm glass fiber filter, 100 cm^2 area	OSHA, 1988
2,4-Di-tert-butylphenol	Cotton swab, wetted with ethanol	O'Malley et al., 1988
Dyfonate	37 mm 1.0 μm glass fiber filter, 100 cm^2 area	OSHA, 1988
Elements (Al, As, Ba, Be, Ca, Cd, Co, Cr, Cu, Fe, Li, Mg, Mn, Mo, Ni, Pb, P, Pt, Se, Ag, Na, Sn, Te, Ti, W, V, Yt, Zn, Zr). *See also* Metals	Whatman smear tab, wetted with distilled water (ICP), 100 cm^2 area	NIOSH, 1991*a* (HETA 91-073-2165)
EPN	37 mm 1.0 μm glass fiber filter, 100 cm^2 area	OSHA, 1988
Escherichia coli	Calcium alginate swab moistened with buffer	Felix, Parrow, and Parrow, 1990
β-Estradiol	Cotton gauze pad, wetted with ispropanol-water, 1/25 M^2 area	NIOSH, March 1984 (HETA 81-314-1435)
Estradiol benzoate	Cotton gauze pad, wetted with ispropanol-water, 1/25 M^2 area	NIOSH, March 1984 (HETA 81-314-1435)
Estrone	Cotton gauze pad, wetted with ispropanol-water, 1/25 M^2 area	NIOSH, March 1984 (HETA 81-314-1435)
Ethacure 100	Aromatic amine swipe test, 100 cm^2 area	CLI Laboratories
Ethacure 300	Aromatic amine swipe test, 100 cm^2 area	CLI Laboratories
Ethion	37 mm 1.0 μm glass fiber filter, 100 cm^2 area	OSHA, 1988
Ethylene dibromide	Whatman 41 filter, 36 $in.^2$ area	NIOSH, November 1983 (HETA 83-408-1389)
Ethylene thiourea (ETU)	Whatman smear tab, dry	NIOSH, 1978 (HHE 77-67-499)
Fensulfothion	37 mm 1.0 μm glass fiber filter, 100 cm^2 area	OSHA, 1988
Fenthion	37 mm 1.0 μm glass fiber filter, 100 cm^2 area	OSHA, 1988

Compound	*Media*	*Source*
Fiberglass	Transparent tape, placed directly on glass slide	NIOSH, April 1984*a* (HETA 83-409-1450)
Fiberglass	37 mm 0.8 μm MCE filter, dry, 4 ft^2 area	NIOSH, April 1984*a* (HETA 83-409-1450)
Fiberglass	Vacuuming using a personal air sampling pump and MCE filter in cassette	NIOSH, September 1991 (HETA 91-143-2136)
Fluorides	Whatman smear tab, wetted with deionized water, 100 cm^2 area	OSHA, 1991
Fonofos	37 mm 1.0 μm glass fiber filter, 100 cm^2 area	OSHA, 1988
Formaldehyde. *See* Paraformaldehyde		
Formic acid	Whatman smear tab, wetted with deionized water, 100 cm^2 area	OSHA, 1991
Fungi	Hycon® contact slide	Biotest Corp.
Haloxon	Whatman 41 filter, 100 cm^2 area	OSHA, 1988
Heptachlor	37 mm 1.0 μm glass fiber filter, wetted with trimethylpentane, 100 cm^2 area	NIOSH, July 1978 (TA 77-66)
Hexachlorocyclopentadiene	Whatman filter, moistened with deionized water, 100 cm^2 area	NIOSH, August 1978 (TA 77-39)
Hydrazine	Whatman 42 filter, wetted with fluorescamine (0.35 mg/mL in 1,4-dioxane) drops, observed for yellow fluorescence under UV light	Weeks, Yasuda, and Dean, 1976
Hydrazine	Whatman 42 filter, wetted with o-phthalaldeyde (1 mg/mL in acetic acid) drops, observed for blue fluorescence under UV light	Weeks, Yasuda, and Dean, 1976
Hydrazine	Whatman 42 filter, wetted with m-phthalaldehyde (1 mg/mL in acetic acid) drops, observed for brown fluorescence under UV light	Weeks, Yasuda, and Dean, 1976
Hydrazine	Whatman 42 filter, wetted with p-phthalaldehyde (1 mg/mL in acetic acid) drops, observed for blue fluorescence under UV light	Weeks, Yasuda, and Dean, 1976
Hydrogen chloride (for liquid solutions)	Whatman smear tab, wetted with deionized water, 100 cm^2 area	OSHA, 1991
Hydrogen peroxide	Quant TM ether peroxide test that involves wiping a strip of treated litmus paper across the surface and comparing the reacted section of the paper to a colorimetric ppm scale	NIOSH, May 1980 (HHE 79-105-687)

Compound	*Media*	*Source*
Hypochlorites (as available chlorine)	37 mm 1.0 μm glass fiber filter, wetted with 0.1% sulfamic acid, 100 cm^2 area	OSHA, 1991
Iodine	Whatman smear tab, wetted with deionized water, 100 cm^2 area	OSHA, 1991
Indium	3 × 3 in. cotton gauze pad, moistened with deionized water, 100 cm^2 area	NIOSH, January 1992 (HETA 92-10-2234)
Isodecane	Cotton gauze pad, alcohol saturated, 100 cm^2 area	NIOSH, January 1980 (HHE 78-77-659)
Isofenphos	Gauze wetted with distilled water	Veckman, 1991
Lead	Whatman 40 filter, 0.5 ft^2 area	NIOSH, February 1976 (HHE 75-8-263)
Lead	Whatman 41 filter, wetted with distilled water, 100 cm^2 area	OSHA, 1990 (ID-121)
Lead	Whatman smear tab, wetted with distilled water, 100 cm^2 area	NIOSH, 1984 (HETA 82-042-1428)
Lead	Whatman filter, dry or wetted with distilled water, 1 ft^2 area	NIOSH, September 1979 (HHE 79-9-615)
Lead	Lead check swab as a spot test	SKC, 1993
Lead	Whatman 40 filter, moistened with acetic acid, drops of sodium sulfide for visualization	Askin and Alvarez, 1993
Lead	Spot test using 1% sodium sulfide, color change to form dark-brown or gray to black	Lerner and Hogan, 1985
Lead	37 mm 0.8 μm MCE filter, wetted with isopropyl alcohol, 100 cm^2 area	NIOSH, 1991*b* (HETA 91-290-2131)
Lead	Premoistened commercial baby wipe, 929 cm^2 area	NIOSH, May 1992 (HETA 90-84-2219)
Lead	Premoistened commercial hand towelette	NIOSH, August 1992 (HETA 91-209-2249)
Lead	Premoistened commercial wipe (with nonalcohol wetting agent), 1 ft^2 area	HUD, Sept. 1990
Lead	Direct reading X-ray fluorescence detection	HUD, Sept. 1990
Lead	3 × 3 in. cotton gauze, moistened with deionized water, 100 cm^2 area	NIOSH, July 1992 (HETA 92-10-2234)
Lead	Vacuuming using a personal air sampling pump and MCE filter in cassette, 0.25 M^2 area	Solomon and Hartford, 1976
Legionella pneumophilia	Sterile dacron swab, placed directly into buffered yeast extract	Cordes et al., 1981

Compound	*Media*	*Source*
Legionella pneumophilia	Sterile cotton swab placed in a sterile plastic container with 15–25 mL aliquot of water obtained from same source	Cordes et al., 1981
Lindane	37 mm 1.0 μm glass fiber filter, wetted with trimethylpentane, 100 cm^2 area	NIOSH, July 1978 (TA 77-66)
Lindane	Vacuuming with a personal air sampling pump and MCE filter cassette	NIOSH, 1980*a* (HETA 80-087-771)
Linuron	37 mm 1.0 μm glass fiber filter, 100 cm^2 area	OSHA, 1988
Lorsban	Whatman smear tab, wetted with distilled water, 100 cm^2 area	NIOSH, July 1984*b* (HETA 81-463-1477)
Magnesium	Whatman smear tab, wetted with distilled water, 100 cm^2 area	OSHA, 1990 (ID-121)
Magnesium	37 mm 0.8 μm MCE filter, distilled water, 100 cm^2 area	OSHA, 1990 (ID-121)
Malathion	37 mm 1.0 μm glass fiber filter, 100 cm^2 area	OSHA, 1988
Malathion	Cotton gauze pad, wetted with hexane	NIOSH, June 1986 (HETA 85-527-1704)
Maneb	37 mm 1.0 μm glass fiber filter, 100 cm^2 area	OSHA, 1988
Manganese	Whatman smear tab, wetted with distilled water, 100 cm^2 area	OSHA, 1990 (ID-121)
Manganese	37 mm 0.8 μm MCE filter, wetted distilled water, 100 cm^2 area	OSHA, 1990 (ID-121)
Man-made mineral fibers (MMMF)	Gelatinous foil	Schneider et al., 1990
MCPA	Cotton ball, wetted with ethanol	Hattula, Wasenius, and Arstila, 1979
MDI (can convert to MDA on surfaces in the presence of moisture, including skin)	Aromatic isocyanate swype test, 100 cm^2 area	CLI Laboratories
Mercury (aryl and inorganic compounds)	Jerome Model 411 Gold Film Mercury analyzer	Zirschky and Witherell, 1987
Mercury	Bachrach MV2 (UV) Mercury Sniffer	NIOSH, 1985 (HETA 84-90-1533)
Mercury	Whatman 40 filter, 0.5 ft^2 area	NIOSH, February 1976 (HHE 75-8-263)
Mercury	Cheesecloth, wetted with 1% nitric acid	van Netten and Teschke, 1988
Mercury	Mercury check swab as a spot test	SKC Inc., 1992
Mercury vapor	Jerome Model 411 Gold Film Mercury analyzer	Zirschky and Witherell, 1987

Compound	*Media*	*Source*
Mestranol	37 mm 1.0 μm glass fiber filter	Harrington et al., 1978
Metals	3 × 3 in. cotton gauze pad, soaked in isooctane, 2,500 cm^2 area	Perdek et al., 1991
Metals (30 different)	37 mm 0.8 μm MCE filter, dry or wetted with deionized water, 100 cm^2 area	Eller, 1992 (NIOSH Method No. 7300)
Metals (30 different)	3 × 3 in. cotton gauze pad, wetted with deionized water, 100 cm^2 area	NIOSH, March 1992 (HETA 88-207-2195)
Metals (29 different)	Whatman smear tab, dry or wetted with distilled water, 100 cm^2 area	NIOSH, 1991*a* (HETA 91-073-2165)
Methomyl	37 mm 1.0 μm glass fiber filter, 100 cm^2 area	OSHA, 1988
5-Methyl o-anisidine	37 mm 1.0 μm glass fiber filter, 100 cm^2 area	OSHA, 1988
4,4'-Methylene bis (2-chloro-aniline)	Aromatic amine swype test, 100 cm^2 area	CLI Laboratories
4,4'-Methylene bis (2-chloro-aniline)	Whatman smear tabs	Clapp et al., 1991
4,4'-Methylene bis (2-chloro-aniline)	37 mm 1.0 μm glass fiber filter, 100 cm^2 area	OSHA, 1988
4,4'-Methylene dianiline (MDA)	37 mm 1.0 μm glass fiber filter, 100 cm^2 area	OSHA, 1988
MDA	Aromatic amine swype test, 100 cm^2 area	CLI Laboratories
Methyl parathion	37 mm 1.0 μm glass fiber filter, 100 cm^2 area	OSHA, 1988
MICP	Whatman 41 filter, wetted with acetonitrile, 100 cm^2 area	OSHA, 1991
Microbials, total	Hycon® contact slide	Biotest Corp.
Mirex	Vacuuming with a personal air sampling pump and MCE filter cassette	NIOSH, 1980*a* (HETA 80-087-771)
MMMF. *See* Man-made mineral fibers		
MOCA. *See* 4,4'-Methylene bis (2-chloroaniline)		
Molybdenum	Whatman smear tab, wetted with distilled water, 100 cm^2 area	OSHA, 1990 (ID-121)
Molybdenum	37 mm 0.8 μm MCE filter, wetted with distilled water, 100 cm^2 area	OSHA, 1990 (ID-121)
α-Naphthylamine	Whatman 41 filter, wetted with methanol, 100 cm^2 area, fluorescamine used for visualization	OSHA, 1988

Compound	*Media*	*Source*
β-Naphthylamine	Whatman 41 filter, wetted with methanol, 100 cm^2 area, fluorescamine used for visualization	OSHA, 1988
Naphthylene diamine	Aromatic amine swype test, 100 cm^2 area	CLI Laboratories
NDI	Aromatic isocyanate swype test, 100 cm^2 area	CLI Laboratories
Nickel	Whatman smear tab, wetted with distilled water, 100 cm^2 area	OSHA, 1990 (ID-121)
Nickel	37 mm 0.8 μm MCE filter, wetted with distilled water, 100 cm^2 area	OSHA, 1990 (ID-121)
Nickel	3 × 3 in. cotton gauze pad, wetted with deionized water, 100 cm^2 area	NIOSH, July 1992 (HETA 92-10-2234)
Nickel	Whatman 40 filter, 5 cm^2 area	NIOSH, August 1982 (HETA 81-212-1169)
Nicotine	Cotton cloth, wetted with water	Gehlbach, Williams, and Freeman, 1979
Nitric acid (liquids)	Whatman smear tab, wetted with deionized water, 100 cm^2 area	OSHA, 1991
p-Nitroaniline	37 mm 1.0 μm glass fiber filter, 100 cm^2 area	OSHA, 1988
4-Nitrobiphenyl	37 mm 1.0 μm glass fiber filter, 100 cm^2 area	OSHA, 1988
Nitrocellulose	Wooden Q-tip, wetted with acetone, 0.24 M^2 area	EPA, 1985
Nitroglycerin	Wooden Q-tip, wetted with acetone, 0.24 M^2 area	EPA, 1985
p-Nitrophenol	Whatman 41 filter, 100 cm^2 area	OSHA, 1988
Nor-nitrogen mustard chloride	10 × 10 cm Chifonet (rayon) cloth, wetted with 2 mL toluene	Thulin, 1993
Norethindrone	37 mm 1.0 μm glass fiber filter	Harrington et al., 1978
Nudrin	Whatman 41 filter, dry or moistened with MIBK or hexane	NIOSH, December 1979*b* (HHE 77-126-646)
Octachlorocyclopentene	Whatman filter, wetted with deionized water, 100 cm^2 area	NIOSH, August 1978 (TA 77-39)
Oil		Zsigmond, 1985
Organic vapors (aliphatic and aromatic hydrocarbons)	Whatman smear tab, wetted with distilled water, 100 cm^2 area	NIOSH, April 1984*b* (HETA 82-284-1456)
Oxalic acid	Whatman smear tab, wetted with deionized water, 100 cm^2 area	OSHA, 1991
Oxydemeton methyl	37 mm 1.0 μm glass fiber filter, 100 cm^2 area	OSHA, 1988

Compound	*Media*	*Source*
Paraformaldehyde	Filter soaked in 1% sodium bisulfite used to wipe a 100 cm^2 area, placed into 20 mL of bisulfite solution immediately following	NIOSH, January 1984*a* (HETA 83-312-1400)
Parathion	37 mm 1.0 μm glass fiber filter, 100 cm^2 area	OSHA, 1988
Particulates	Personal air sampling pump and filter in cassette used to vacuum sample	Que Hee et al., 1985
PCBs. *See also* Chlorodiphenyl	Whatman smear tab, saturated with reagent grade methanol	Lees, Corn, and Breysse, 1987
PCBs	Whatman smear tab, saturated with toluene, 100 cm^2 area	NIOSH, April 1984*b* (HETA 82-284-1456)
PCBs	Whatman smear tab, saturated with cyclohexane	Orris et al., 1986
PCBs	Whatman smear tab, wetted with distilled water, 75–100 cm^2 area	NIOSH, June 1984 (HETA 80-212-1474)
PCBs	Whatman filter, saturated with hexane, 1 ft^2 area	Hryhorczuk et al., 1986
PCBs	Cotton ball, wetted with petroleum ether and acetone (4:1)	Maroni et al., 1981
PCBs	Whatman smear tab, moistened with pesticide quality cyclo-hexane, 100 cm^2 area	NIOSH, May 1982*a* (HETA 82-068-1111)
PCBs	Whatman 40 filter, dry or wetted with xylene, 100 cm^2 area	NIOSH, October 1984 (HETA 80-7-1520)
PCBs	3 × 3 in. cotton gauze pad, wetted with 8 mL hexane, 0.25 m^2 area	NIOSH, 1986*b* (HETA 85-289-1738)
PCBs	2 × 2 in. cotton gauze pad, wetted with 4 mL hexane, 0.01 m^2 area	NIOSH, 1986*b* (HETA 85-289-1738)
PCBs	3 × 3 in. cotton gauze pad, soaked in isooctane, 2,500 cm^2 area	Perdek et al., 1991
PCBs	37 mm 0.8 μm MCE filter or backup pad, dry, 100 cm^2 area	NIOSH, May 1978 (HHE 77-7A-7B-486)
PCBs	Vacuuming with a personal air sampling pump and MCE filter cassette	NIOSH, 1980*a* (HETA 80-087-771)
PCDD/PCDF	Glass wool fiber, soaked in hexane, 1 ft^2 area	Hryhorczuk et al., 1986
PCDD/PCDF	3 × 3 in. cotton gauze pad, wetted with 8-ml hexane, 0.25 m^2 area	NIOSH, 1986*b* (HETA 85-289-1738)
PCDD/PCDF	2 × 2 in. cotton gauze pad, wetted with 4-ml hexane, 0.01 m^2 area	NIOSH, 1986*b* (HETA 85-289-1738)

Compound	*Media*	*Source*
Pentaborane	Whatman smear tab, wetted with deionized water, 100 cm^2 area	OSHA, 1991
Pentachlorophenol	37 mm 1.0 μm glass fiber filter, 100 cm^2 area	OSHA, 1988
Pentachlorophenol	Whatman smear tab, wetted with distilled water, 100 cm^2 area	NIOSH, 1986*a* (HETA 84-053-1680)
Pentaerythritol	Wooden Q-tip, wetted with acetone, 0.24 M^2 area	EPA, 1985
Phenylene diamine	37 mm 1.0 μm glass fiber filter, 100 cm^2 area	OSHA, 1988
Phenylene diamine	Aromatic amine swype test, 100 cm^2 area	CLI Laboratories
Phenylhydrazine	Whatman 42 filter, fluorescamine (0.35 mg/ml in 1,4-dioxane) drops, observed for yellow fluorescence in UV light	Weeks, Yasuda, and Dean, 1976
Phenylhydrazine	Whatman 42 filter, o-phthalaldehyde (1 mg/ml in acetic acid) drops, observed for blue fluorescence in UV light	Weeks, Yasuda, and Dean, 1976
Phenylhydrazine	Whatman 42 filter, m-phthalaldehyde (1 mg/ml in acetic acid) drops, observed for brown fluorescence in UV light	Weeks, Yasuda, and Dean, 1976
Phenylhydrazine	Whatman 42 filter, p-phthalaldehyde (1 mg/ml in acetic acid) drops, observed for blue fluorescence in UV light	Weeks, Yasuda, and Dean, 1976
N-phenyl-2-naphthylamine	37 mm 1.0 μm glass fiber filter, 100 cm^2 area	OSHA, 1988
Phorate	37 mm 1.0 μm glass fiber filter, 100 cm^2 area	OSHA, 1988
Phosdrin	37 mm 1.0 μm glass fiber filter, 100 cm^2 area	OSHA, 1988
Phosdrin	Whatman smear tab, 100 cm^2 area	NIOSH, January 1985 (HETA 78-4-1511)
Phosphoric acid	Whatman smear tab, wetted with deionized water, 100 cm^2 area	OSHA, 1991
Phosphorus pentasulfide	Whatman smear tab, wetted with deionized water, 100 cm^2 area	OSHA, 1991
Phosphorus pentaoxide	Whatman smear tab, wetted with deionized water, 100 cm^2 area	OSHA, 1991
Phosvel	37 mm 1.0 μm glass fiber filter, 100 cm^2 area	OSHA, 1988
Polyamines	Cotton gauze, alcohol saturated, 100 cm^2 area	NIOSH, January 1980 (HHE 78-77-659)
Polymethacrylates	Cotton gauze, alcohol saturated, 100 cm^2 area	NIOSH, January 1980 (HHE 78-77-659)

Compound	*Media*	*Source*
Potassium dichromate. *See* Chromium VI		
Potassium hydroxide	Whatman smear tab, wetted with deionized water, 100 cm^2 area	OSHA, 1991
Progesterone	Cotton gauze, wetted with ispropanol-water, 1/25 M^2 area	NIOSH, March 1984 (HETA 81-314-1435)
Propoxur	37 mm 1.0 μm glass fiber filter, 100 cm^2 area	OSHA, 1991
1-(2-Pyridyl)piperazine	37 mm 1.0 μm glass fiber filter, 100 cm^2 area	OSHA, 1988
Pydrin	Whatman smear tab, wetted with distilled water, 100 cm^2 area	NIOSH, July 1984*b* (HETA 81-463-1477)
Pydrin	37 mm 1.0 μm glass fiber filter, 100 cm^2 area	OSHA, 1991
1-(2-Pyridyl) piperazine	37 mm 1.0 μm glass fiber filter, 100 cm^2 area	OSHA, 1991
Rabon	37 mm 1.0 μm glass fiber filter, 100 cm^2 area	OSHA, 1988
Radium	2.4 cm filter paper	EPA, 1985
RDX	Wooden Q-tip, wetted with acetone, 0.24 M^2 area	EPA, 1985
Refractory ceramic fibers. *See* Man-made mineral fibers		
Resmethrin	Whatman 41 filter, 100 cm^2 area	OSHA, 1991
Ronnel	37 mm 1.0 μm glass fiber filter, 100 cm^2 area	OSHA, 1988
Rozol		NIOSH, 1980*b* (HETA 80-092-769)
Sarin	37 mm 1.0 μm glass fiber filter, 100 cm^2 area	OSHA, 1988
Silver	Whatman smear tab, wetted with distilled water, 100 cm^2 area	OSHA, 1990 (ID-121)
Silver	37 mm 0.8 μm MCE filter, wetted with distilled water, 100 cm^2 area	OSHA, 1990 (ID-121)
Silvex	37 mm 1.0 μm glass fiber filter, 100 cm^2 area	OSHA, 1988
Sodium bisulfite	Whatman smear tab, wetted with deionized water, 100 cm^2 area	OSHA, 1991
Sodium chloro-compounds	37 mm 1.0 μm glass fiber filter, wetted with 0.1% sulfamic acid, 100 cm^2 area	OSHA, 1991
Sodium dichloroisocyanurate	37 mm 1.0 μm glass fiber filter, wetted with 0.1% sulfamic acid, 100 cm^2 area	OSHA, 1991
Sodium hydroxide	Whatman smear tab, wetted with deionized water, 100 cm^2 area	OSHA, 1991

Compound	*Media*	*Source*
Sodium metabisulfite	Whatman smear tab, wetted with deionized water, 100 cm^2 area	OSHA, 1991
Stainless steel fibers	37 mm 0.8 μm MCE filter, 100 cm^2 area	NIOSH, August 1984 (HETA 82-289-1496)
Staphylococcus aureus	Calcium alginate swab moistened with buffer	Felix, Parrow, and Parrow, 1990
Steroids	37 mm 1.0 μm glass fiber filter	Harrington et al., 1978
Streptococcus fecalis	Calcium alginate swab moistened with buffer	Felix, Parrow, and Parrow, 1990
Sudan I	37 mm 1.0 μm glass fiber filter, 100 cm^2 area	OSHA, 1988
Sudan III	37 mm 1.0 μm glass fiber filter, 100 cm^2 area	OSHA, 1988
Sulfamethazine	Whatman 41 filter, 100 cm^2 area	OSHA, 1988
Sulfotep	37 mm 1.0 μm glass fiber filter, 100 cm^2 area	OSHA, 1991
Sulfuric acid	Whatman smear tab, wetted with deionized water, 100 cm^2 area	OSHA, 1991
2,4,5-T	Whatman 42 filter, 100 cm^2 area	OSHA, 1988
Tantalum	Whatman smear tab, wetted with deionized water, 100 cm^2 area	OSHA, 1991
2,3,7,8-TCDD. *See* also PCDD/ PCDF	3 × 3 in. cotton gauze pad, soaked in isooctane, 2,500 cm^2 area	Perdek et al., 1991
2,3,7,8-TCDD	Vacuuming with a personal air sampling pump and MCE filter cassette	NIOSH, 1980*a* (HETA 80-087-771)
TDA	Aromatic amine swype test, 100 cm^2 area	CLI Laboratories
TDI (Can convert to Toluene diamine on surfaces in the presence of moisture)	Aromatic isocyanate swype test, 100 cm^2 area	CLI Laboratories
Tellurium	Whatman smear tab, wetted with distilled water, 100 cm^2 area	OSHA, 1990 (ID-121)
Tellurium	37 mm 0.8 μm MCE filter, wetted with distilled water, 100 cm^2 area	OSHA, 1990 (ID-121)
TEDP	37 mm 1.0 μm glass fiber filter, 100 cm^2 area	OSHA, 1988
Temephos	37 mm 1.0 μm glass fiber filter, 100 cm^2 area	OSHA, 1991
TEPP	37 mm 1.0 μm glass fiber filter, 100 cm^2 area	OSHA, 1988
Terbufos	37 mm 1.0 μm glass fiber filter, 100 cm^2 area	OSHA, 1988
Terbufos	Whatman smear tab, 100 cm^2 area	NIOSH, 1983c (HETA 81-465-1323)

Compound	*Media*	*Source*
p-Tert-butylphenol	Cotton swab, wetted in ethanol	O'Malley et al., 1988
Testosterone	Cotton gauze pad, wetted in ispropanol-water, 1/25 M^2 area	NIOSH, March 1984 (HETA 81-314-1435)
Testosterone proprionate	Cotton gauze pad, wetted in ispropanol-water, 1/25 M^2 area	NIOSH, March 1984 (HETA 81-314-1435)
Tetrachlorophenol (in water)	Surgical cotton gauze pad (12-ply), 6 in^2 area	Fenske, Horstman, and Bentley, 1987
Tetrachlorophenol	Whatman smear tab, wetted with distilled water, 100 cm^2 area	NIOSH, 1986*a* (HETA 84-053-1680)
Tetramethrin	37 mm 1.0 μm glass fiber filter, 100 cm^2 area	OSHA, 1991
Tetrasodium pyrophosphate	Whatman smear tab, wetted with deionized water, 100 cm^2 area	OSHA, 1991
Tetryl	Wooden Q-tip, wetted with acetone, 0.24 M^2 area	EPA, 1985
Thallium	Whatman smear tab, wetted with distilled water, 100 cm^2 area	OSHA, 1990 (ID-121)
Thallium	37 mm 0.8 μm MCE filter, wetted with distilled water, 100 cm^2 area	OSHA, 1990 (ID-121)
Thiophanate	37 mm 1.0 μm glass fiber filter, 100 cm^2 area	OSHA, 1988
Tin, inorganic	Whatman smear tab, wetted with distilled water, 100 cm^2 area	OSHA, 1990 (ID-121)
Tin, inorganic	37 mm 0.8 μm MCE filter, wetted with distilled water, 100 cm^2 area	OSHA, 1990 (ID-121)
Tin	3 × 3 in. cotton gauze pad, wetted with deionized water, 100 cm^2 area	NIOSH, July 1992 (HETA 92-10-2234)
TNF. *See* 2,4,7-Trinitro-fluorene-9-one)		
o-Tolidine	37 mm 1.0 μm glass fiber filter, 100 cm^2 area	OSHA, 1988
o-Tolidine	Aromatic amine swype test, 100 cm^2 area	CLI Laboratories
o-Tolidine-based dyes	37 mm 1.0 μm glass fiber filter, 100 cm^2 area	OSHA, 1988
Toluene diamine	Aromatic amine swype test, 100 cm^2 area	CLI Laboratories
Torak	37 mm 1.0 μm glass fiber filter, 100 cm^2 area	OSHA, 1988
Trace metals. *See* Elements; Metals		
Trichloroisocyanuric acid (as available chlorine)	37 mm 1.0 μm glass fiber filter, wetted with 0.1% sulfamic acid, 100 cm^2 area	OSHA, 1991

Compound	*Media*	*Source*
Trimethyl phosphite	Whatman 41 filter, dry or moistened with solvent with which pesticide was formulated, 100 cm^2 area	NIOSH, December 1979*b* (HHE 77-126-646)
2,4,7-Trinitro-fluorene-9-one (TNF)	Whatman 41 filter, dry, 100 cm^2 area	NIOSH, December 1981 (HETA 81-352-1029)
2,4,6-Trinitrotoluene	Wooden Q-tips, wetted with acetone, 0.24 M^2 area	EPA, 1985
Tris 2,3-dibromopropyl phosphate	37 mm 0.8 μm MCE filter, dry, 100 cm^2 area	NIOSH, June 1977 (HHE 77-39-400)
Tungsten	Whatman 40 filter, 5 cm^2 area	NIOSH, August 1982 (HETA 81-212-1169)
Uranium	2.4 cm cellulose filter paper	EPA, 1985
Vanadium	Whatman smear tab, wetted with water, 100 cm^2 area	NIOSH, 1991*a* (HETA 91-073-2165)
Vapona	Whatman smear tab, 100 cm^2 area	NIOSH, January 1985 (HETA 78-4-1511)
Vapona	Whatman 41 filter, dry or moistened with solvent with which pesticide was formulated, 100 cm^2 area	NIOSH, December 1979*b* (HHE 77-126-646)
Yeasts and molds	Hycon® contact slide	Biotest Corp.
Zectran	37 mm 1.0 μm glass fiber filter, 100 cm^2 area	OSHA, 1988
Zeranol	Cotton gauze, wetted with isopropanol, 100 cm^2 area	NIOSH, March 1985 (HETA 82-257-1571)
Zinc	Whatman 40 filter, dry or wetted with distilled water, 1 ft^2 area	NIOSH, September 1979 (HHE 79-9-615)
Zinc	Whatman 40 filter, 5 cm^2 area	NIOSH, August 1982 (HETA 81-212-1169)
Zinc bromide	Whatman smear tab, wetted with deionized water, 100 cm^2 area	OSHA, 1991
Zirconium	Whatman smear tab, wetted with distilled water, 100 cm^2 area	OSHA, 1990 (ID-121)
Zirconium	37 mm 0.8 μm MCE filter, wetted with distilled water, 100 cm^2 area	OSHA, 1990 (ID-121)

REFERENCES

Ager, B. R., and J. A. Tickner. 1983. The control of microbiological hazards associated with air-conditioning and ventilation systems. *Ann. Occup. Hyg.* **27**(4):341–358.

Anonymous. 1983. Act II—How clean is clean? *Hazardous Waste Report* **5**(9):13.

Askin, D., and B. Alvarez. 1993. Sodium sulfide instantly reveals lead on surfaces. *Occup. Health and Safety*, January, p. 34.

Beaulieu, H. 1991. Asbestos contamination of abatement equipment surfaces. *Appl. Occup. Env. Hyg.* **6**(7):583–587.

Birmingham, D. J., M. M. Key, and G. E. Tubich. 1961. Phototoxic bullae among celery harvesters. *Arch. Dermatol.* **83:**73–87.

Bloomfield, J. J., and F. L. Knowles. 1933. Health aspects of radium dial painting. II. Occupational environment. *J. Ind. Hyg.* **15**(5):368–382.

Bolton, N. E. 1985. *Industrial Hygiene*, quarterly report, 1st quarter, April, 1962. Department of Energy, Oak Ridge National Laboratories.

Bromley, J., D. C. Wilson, and E. T. Smith. 1988. Remedial measures following accidental release of dioxin. *Chemosphere* **6:**687–703.

Brooks, R. O. 1959. *The Control of Beryllium Handling at A. E. R. E. Harwell, Medical Division, Atomic Energy Research Establishment*. Report No. 3000. British Atomic Energy Research Establishment.

CAL/OSHA. 1980. General Industry Safety Orders, Title, 8, GISO-5215, Title 8, 4,4'-Methylenebis (2-chloroaniline), *Register* 80, No. 38-9-20-80, pp. 442.6–442.16. State of California, Occupational Safety and Health Administration Sacramento, CA

Caplan, K. 1993. The significance of wipe samples. *AIHA J.* **54**(2):70–75.

Castle, W. B., K. R. Drinker, and C. K. Drinker. 1925. Necrosis of the jaw in workers employed in applying a luminous paint containing radium. *J. Ind. Hyg.* **7**(8):371–382.

Chavalitnikul, C., and L. Levin. 1984. A laboratory evaluation of wipe testing based on lead oxide surface contamination. *AIHA J.* **45**:418–426.

Cohen, R. C. 1974. Desensitization of hospital staff to streptomycin. *Tubercule* **35**:142.

Clapp, D. E., G. M. Piacitelli, D. D. Zaebst, and E. Ward. 1991. Assessing exposure to 4,4'-methylene bis(2-chloroaniline) (MBOCA) in the workplace. *Appl. Occup. Env. Hyg.* **6**(2):125–130.

Cohen, J. J., and R. N. Kusian. 1965. The significance of beryllium surface contamination to health. In G. W. Royster and B. R. Fish (eds.), *Surface Contamination*. New York: Pergamon Press.

Cordes, L. G., A. M. Wiesenthal, G. W. Gorman, J. P. Phair, H. M. Sommers, A. Brown, V. L. Yu, M. H. Magnussen, R. D. Meyer, J. S. Wolf, K. N. Shands, and D. W. Fraser. 1981. Isolation of *Legionella pneumophila* from hospital shower heads. *Ann. Int. Med.* **94**:195–197.

Corn, M., and F. Stein. 1967. Mechanisms of dust redispersion. In B. R. Fish (ed.), *Surface Contamination*. London: Pergamon Press, pp. 45–54.

Cummins, K., D. Morton, D. Lee, E. Cook, and R. Curtis. 1992. Exposure to acrylamide in chemical sewer grouting operations. *Appl. Occup. Env. Hyg.* **7**(6):385–391.

Currie, K. I., E. C. McDonald, L. T. K. Chung, and A. R. Higgs. 1990. Concentrations of diazinon, chlorpyrifos, and bendiocarb after applications in offices. *AIHA J.* **51**(1):23–27.

Di Domenico, A., et al. 1980. Accidental release of 2,3,7,8-tetrachlorodibenzo-p-dioxin (TCDD) at Seveso, Italy: III. Monitoring of residual TCDD levels in reclaimed buildings. *Ecotoxicol. and Env. Safety* **4**:321–326.

Dunster, H. J. 1961. The monitoring of surface contamination and its place in radiological protection. *Ann. Occup. Hyg.* **4**:148–151.

Eller, P. (ed). 1992. *NIOSH Manual of Hazard Evaluation*, 3d ed. Vols. 1 and 2 with 1985, 1987, and 1987 supplements. Cincinnati, OH. NIOSH.

EPA. 1985. *Guide for Decontamination of Building Structures and Equipment at Superfund Sites*. Washington, DC: EPA, EPA 600/2-85-028.

EPA. 1987. *Polychlorinated Biphenyls Spill Cleanup Policy: Final Rule*. 40 CFR Pt.761. FR52:10,688–10,710.

Felix, C. W., C. Parrow, and T. Parrow. 1990. Utensil sanitation. *J. Env. Health* **53**(2):13–15.

Fenske, R. A., S. W. Horstman, and R. K. Bentley. 1987. Assessment of dermal exposure to chlorophenols in timber mills. *Appl. Ind. Hyg.* **2:**143–147.

Fenske, R. A., K. G. Black, K. P. Elkner, C. Lee, M. M. Methner, and R. Soto. 1990. Potential exposure and health risks of infants following indoor residential pesticide applications. *Am. J. Pub. Health* **80**(6):689–693.

Fortunati, G. U. 1985. The Seveso accident. *Chemosphere* **14**(6/7):729–737.

Frank, R., R. A. Campbell, and G. J. Sirons. 1985. Forestry workers involved in aerial application of 2,4-dichlorophenoxyacetic acid (2,4-D): Exposure and urinary excretion. *Arch. Env. Contam. Toxicol.* **14**:427–435.

Gehlbach, S. H., W. A. Williams, and J. I. Freeman. 1979. Protective clothing as a means of reducing nicotine absorption in tobacco harvesters. *Arch. Env. Health* **34**:111–114.

Goddard, K. R. 1965. Effect of ventilation on distribution of airborne microbial contamination—field studies. In G. W. Royster and B. R. Fish (eds.), *Surface Contamination*. New York: Pergamon Press, pp. 88–94.

Harrington, J. M., G. F. Stein, R. O. Rivera, and A. V. deMorales. 1978. The occupational hazards of formulating oral contraceptives—A survey of plant employees. *Arch. Env. Health* **33**: 12–15.

Hattula, M. L., V. Wasenius, and A. U. Arstila. 1979. The exposure to MCPA in the use of clearing saw. *Chemosphere* **7**:473–476.

Hawley, J. K. 1985. Assessment of health risk from exposure to contaminated soil. *Risk Anal.* **5**:289–302.

Hills, B. W., and A. L. Greife. 1988. Evaluation of acrylamide exposures. *Appl. Ind. Hyg.* **1**(3):148–152.

Hodgson, E. S. and C. Ruis-Frutos. 1991. A case report of contaminated operating theatre multipurpose equipment: A potential hazard for health care workers. *Ann. Occup. Hyg.* **35**(3):341–346.

Hryhorczuk, D. D., P. Orris, J. R. Kominsky, J. Melius, W. Burton, and D. L. Kinkamp. 1986. PCB, PCDF and PCDD exposure following a transformer fire: Chicago. *Chemosphere* **15**(9/12):1297–1303.

HUD. Sept. 1990. *Lead-Based Paint: Interim Guidelines for Hazard Identification and Abatement in Public and Indian Housing*. Washington, DC: Office of Public and Indian Housing, Dept. of Housing and Urban Development.

Jones, I. S., and S. F. Pond. 1967. Some experiments to determine the resuspension factor of Plutonium from various surfaces. In B. R. Fish (ed.), *Surface Contamination*. London: Pergamon Press, pp. 83–92.

Ketcham, N. H., and R. W. Norton. 1960. The hazards to health in the hydrogenation of coal. III. The industrial hygiene studies. *Arch. Env. Health* **1**:30/194–41/207.

Kim, N. K., and J. Hawley. 1985. *Reentry Guidelines*. Binghamton State Office Building, Document 0549, Bureau of Toxic Substances Assessment, Division of Environmental Health Assessment. Albany, NY: NY State Dept. of Health.

Knaak, J. B. 1980. Safe levels of foliar residues. *Res. Rev.* **75**:81–96.

Knaak, J. B., and Y. Iwata. 1982. The safe level concept and the rapid field method: A new approach to solving the reentry problem. In *Pesticide Residues and Exposure*. Washington, DC: American Chemical Society, pp. 23–39.

Kominsky, J. R. 1989. Background concentrations of polychlorinated dibenzofurans (PCDFs) and polychlorinated dibenzo-p-dioxins in office buildings in Boston, MA. *Chemosphere* **18**(1/6):599–608.

LaGoy, P. K., R. L. Bohrer, and F. H. Halvorsen. 1992. The development of cleanup criteria for an acutely toxic pesticide at a contaminated industrial facility. *AIHA J.* **53**:298–302.

Lees, S. J., M. Corn, and P. N. Breysse. 1987. Evidence for dermal absorption as the major route of body entry during exposure of transformer maintenance and repairmen to PCBs. *AIHA J.* **48**(3):257–264.

Lerner, S. I., and D. J. Hogan. 1985. Detection of inorganic lead contamination with sodium sulfide. *JOM* **27**:293–294.

Levine, R. J., M. J. Turner, Y. S. Crume, M. E. Dale, T. B. Starr, and D. E. Rickert. 1985. Assessing exposure to dinitrotoluene using a biological monitor. *JOM* **27**(9):627–638.

Marklund, S., R. Andersson, M. Tysklind, and C. Rappe. 1989. Emissions of PCDDs and PCDFs from a PVC-fire in Holmsund, Sweden. *Chemosphere* **18**(1/6):1031–1038.

Maroni, M., A. Colombi, S. Cantoni, E. Ferioli, and V. Foa. 1981. Occupational exposure to polychlorinated biphenyls in electrical workers. I. Environmental and blood polychlorinated biphenyls concentrations. *Brit. J. Ind. Med.* **38**:49–54.

Mitchell, R. N., and B. C. Eutsler. 1967. A study of beryllium surface contamination and resuspension. In B. R. Fish (ed.), *Surface Contamination*. London: Pergamon Press, pp. 349–353.

Morris, J. E. W. 1975. Microbial pollution in submersibles. *Ann. Occup. Hyg.* **17**:245–246.

National Research Council. 1988. *Acceptable Levels of Dioxin Contamination in an Office Building Following a Transformer Fire*. Washington, DC: National Academy Press.

NIOSH, Health Hazard Evaluation Report. September 1975. *Industrial Platers, Inc., Columbus, OH*. HHE 74-87-221. Cincinnati, OH: NIOSH.

NIOSH, Health Hazard Evaluation Report. February 1976. *Hedstom Union Co., Bedford, PA*. HHE 75-8-263. Cincinnati, OH: NIOSH.

NIOSH, Health Hazard Evaluation Report. 1977. *Ottenheimer and Sons, Inc., Dawson Springs, KY*. HHE 77-74-720. Cincinnati, OH: NIOSH.

NIOSH, Health Hazard Evaluation Report. June 1977. *Fisher Body No. 2 Plant, Grand Rapids, MI*. HHE 77-39-400. Cincinnati, OH: NIOSH.

NIOSH, Health Hazard Evaluation Report. 1978. *St. Clair Rubber Co., Marysville, MI*. HHE 77-67-499. Cincinnati, OH: NIOSH.

NIOSH, Health Hazard Evaluation Report. May 1978. *Union Electric Co., St. Louis, MO*. HHE 77-7A-7B-486. Cincinnati, OH: NIOSH.

NIOSH, Health Hazard Evaluation and Technical Assistance Report. July 1978. *Platte Chemical Co., Fremont, NE*. TA 77-66. Cincinnati, OH: NIOSH.

NIOSH, Health Hazard Evaluation and Technical Assistance Report. August 1978. *Morris Forman Wastewater Treatment Plant, Metropolitan Sewer District, Louisville, KY*. TA 77-39. Cincinnati, OH: NIOSH.

NIOSH, Health Hazard Evaluation Report. December 1978. *Lear Siegler, Inc., Marblehead, MA*. HHE 78-68-546. Cincinnati, OH: NIOSH.

NIOSH, Health Hazard Evaluation Report. September 1979. *Arapahoe Aluminum and Brass Foundry, Inc., Englewood,* CO. HHE 79-9-615. Cincinnati, OH: NIOSH.

NIOSH, Health Hazard Evaluation Report. December 1979*a*. *St. Charles Furniture Corp., Wright City,* MO. HHE 79-103-640. Cincinnati, OH: NIOSH.

NIOSH, Health Hazard Evaluation Report. December 1979*b*. *Shell Chemical Co., Rocky Mountain Arsenal, Denver,* CO. HHE 77-126-646. Cincinnati, OH: NIOSH.

NIOSH, Technical Assistance Report. 1980*a*. *Grief Brothers Corp., Niagara Falls, NY.* TA 80-087-771. Cincinnati, OH: NIOSH.

NIOSH, Hazard Evaluation and Technical Assistance Report. 1980*b*. *Rutgers University, Newark, NJ.* HETA 80-092-769. Cincinnati, OH: NIOSH.

NIOSH, Health Hazard Evaluation Report. January 1980. *R. L. Polk Co., Cincinnati, OH.* HHE 78-77-659. Cincinnati, OH: NIOSH.

NIOSH, Health Hazard Evaluation Report. May 1980. *RCA Corp., Marion, IN.* HHE 79-105-687. Cincinnati, OH: NIOSH.

NIOSH, Health Hazard Evaluation Report. May 1981. *Cyanotype Printing in an Artist's Workshop, Bucyrus, OH.* HETA 81-171-880. Cincinnati, OH: NIOSH.

NIOSH, Health Hazard Evaluation Report. June 1981. *Valley Chrome Platers, Bay City, MI.* HETA 81-85-889. Cincinnati, OH: NIOSH.

NIOSH, Health Hazard Evaluation Report. September 1981. *Boehringer Ingelheim, Ltd., Ridgefield, CT.* HETA 81-247-958. Cincinnati, OH: NIOSH.

NIOSH, Health Hazard Evaluation Report. November 1981. *Naval Biosciences Laboratory, Oakland,* CA. HHE 80-183-991. Cincinnati, OH: NIOSH.

NIOSH, Health Hazard Evaluation Report. December 1981. *DHHS, Washington, DC.* HETA 81-125-1029. Cincinnati, OH: NIOSH.

NIOSH, Health Hazard Evaluation Report. March 1982. *City of Norwood, Norwood, OH.* HETA 82-17-1067. Cincinnati, OH: NIOSH.

NIOSH, Health Hazard Evaluation Report. March 1982*a*. *Miamitown Grade School, Cincinnati, OH.* HETA 82-068-1111. Cincinnati, OH: NIOSH.

NIOSH, Health Hazard Evaluation Report. March 1982*b*. *Keebler Co., Cincinnati, OH.* HETA 81-396-1118. Cincinnati, OH: NIOSH.

NIOSH, Health Hazard Evaluation Report. August 1982. *N.P.C. Systems, Inc., Milford, NH.* HETA 81-212-1169. Cincinnati, OH: NIOSH.

NIOSH. 1983*a*. *Industrial Hygiene Surveys of Occupational Exposure to Wood Preservative Chemicals.* Cincinnati, OH: NIOSH.

NIOSH, Health Hazard Evaluation Report. 1983*b*. *Harley Davidson Motor Co., Milwaukee, WI.* HETA 81-317-1202. Cincinnati, OH: NIOSH.

NIOSH, Health Hazard Evaluation Report. 1983*c*. *Hopkins Agricultural Chemical Company, Atlanta, IL.* HETA 81-465-1323. Cincinnati, OH: NIOSH.

NIOSH, Health Hazard Evaluation Report. August 1983. *Robertson Paper Box Company, Monteville, CT.* HETA 81-304-1361. Cincinnati, OH: NIOSH.

NIOSH, Health Hazard Evaluation Report. November 1983. *U.S. Forest Service, Dillon District, Frisco,* CO. HETA 83-408-1389. Cincinnati, OH: NIOSH.

NIOSH, Health Hazard Evaluation Report. 1984. *Chemetco, Inc., Alton, IL.* HETA 82-024-1428. Cincinnati, OH: NIOSH.

NIOSH, Health Hazard Evaluation Report. January 1984*a*. *Champion Technology Center, Hamilton, OH.* HETA 83-312-1400. Cincinnati, OH: NIOSH.

NIOSH, Health Hazard Evaluation Report. January 1984*b*. *Wappingers Central School District, Wappingers Falls, NY.* HETA 83-172-1409. Cincinnati, OH: NIOSH.

NIOSH, Health Hazard Evaluation Report. March 1984. *Rutgers University, Newark, NJ.* HETA 81-314-1435. Cincinnati, OH: NIOSH.

NIOSH, Health Hazard Evaluation Report. April 1984*a*. *King Kwit Minit Market, Inc., Cincinnati, OH.* HETA 83-409-1450. Cincinnati, OH: NIOSH.

NIOSH, Health Hazard Evaluation Report. April 1984*b*. *Port Authority of New York and New Jersey, Elizabeth Industrial Park Site, Elizabeth, NJ.* HETA 82-284-1456. Cincinnati, OH: NIOSH.

NIOSH, Health Hazard Evaluation Report. June 1984. *Pacific Gas and Electric Company, San Francisco,* CA. HETA 80-212-1474. Cincinnati, OH: NIOSH.

NIOSH, Health Hazard Evaluation Report. July 1984*a*. *Progress Federal Savings & Loan, Bridgeport,* PA. HETA 83-383-1480. Cincinnati, OH: NIOSH.

NIOSH, Health Hazard Evaluation Report. July 1984*b*. *Colorado River Indian Reservation, Parker,* AZ. HETA 81-463-1477. Cincinnati, OH: NIOSH.

NIOSH, Health Hazard Evaluation Report. July 1984*c*. *Lion Uniform Co., Beattyville, KY.* HETA 83-301-1478. Cincinnati, OH: NIOSH.

NIOSH, Health Hazard Evaluation Report. July 1984*d*. *Georgetown University, Washington, D.C.* HETA 83-444-1481. Cincinnati, OH: NIOSH.

NIOSH, Health Hazard Evaluation Report. August 1984. *Schlegel Corp., Rochester, NY.* HETA 82-289-1496. Cincinnati, OH: NIOSH.

NIOSH, Health Hazard Evaluation Report. October 1984. *GSA Switchgear Shop, Washington, DC.* HETA 80-7-1520. Cincinnati, OH: NIOSH.

NIOSH, Health Hazard Evaluation Report. 1985. *J. Butler, D.D.S., Wellston, OH.* HETA 84-90-1533. Cincinnati, OH: NIOSH.

NIOSH, Health Hazard Evaluation Report. January 1985. *Shell Chemical Co., Axis, AL.* HETA 78-4-1511. Cincinnati, OH: NIOSH.

NIOSH, Health Hazard Evaluation Report. March

1985. *Manufacturing Chemists, Inc., Indianapolis, IN*. HETA 82-257-1571. Cincinnati, OH: NIOSH.

NIOSH, Health Hazard Evaluation Report. June 1985. *Harshaw/Filtrol, Louisville, KY*. HETA 84-128-1601. Cincinnati, OH: NIOSH.

NIOSH, Health Hazard Evaluation Report. November 1985. *Bofors-Nobel/Lakeway Corporation, Muskegon, MI*. HETA 80-035-1635. Cincinnati, OH: NIOSH.

NIOSH, Health Hazard Evaluation Report. 1986*a*. *Montana Log Home Residents, Kalispell, MT*. HETA 84-053-1680. Cincinnati, OH: NIOSH.

NIOSH, Health Hazard Evaluation Report. 1986*b*. *Page Belcher Federal Building, Tulsa, OK*. HETA 85-289-1738. Cincinnati, OH: NIOSH.

NIOSH, Health Hazard Evaluation Report. 1986c. *Inland Steel, East Chicago, IN*. HHE 82-309-1630. Cincinnati, OH: NIOSH.

NIOSH, Health Hazard Evaluation Report. May 1986. *Hilton-Davis Chemical Co., Cincinnati, OH*. HETA 84-58-1700. Cincinnati, OH: NIOSH.

NIOSH, Health Hazard Evaluation Report. June 1986. *Canyon de Chelly National Monument, Chinle, AZ*. HETA 85-527-1704. Cincinnati, OH: NIOSH.

NIOSH, Health Hazard Evaluation Report. 1987*a*. *New Mexico State Highway Department General Office Building*. HETA 85-414-1805. Cincinnati, OH: NIOSH.

NIOSH, Health Hazard Evaluation Report. 1987*b*. *Commercial Office Building, Boston, MA*. HETA 86-472-1832. Cincinnati, OH: NIOSH.

NIOSH, Health Hazard Evaluation Report. March 1987. *Vimar Corp., Boulder, CO*. HETA 86-30-1785. Cincinnati, OH: NIOSH.

NIOSH, Health Hazard Evaluation Report. April 1987. *Sperry Rand Corp., Great Neck, NY*. HETA 85-453-1787. Cincinnati, OH: NIOSH.

NIOSH, Health Hazard Evaluation Report. September 1987. *Federal Office Building, Evansville, IN*. HETA 86-434-1833. Cincinnati, OH: NIOSH.

NIOSH, Health Hazard Evaluation Report. January 1988. *Planned Parenthood of South Central Indiana, Bloomington, IN*. HETA 83-258-1859. Cincinnati, OH: NIOSH.

NIOSH, Health Hazard Evaluation Report. December 1989. *Cincinnati Electronics Corp., Cincinnati, OH*. HETA 89-057-2003. Cincinnati, OH: NIOSH.

NIOSH, Health Hazard Evaluation Report. 1991*a*. *Carbonnaire Co., Palmerton, PA*. HETA 91-073-2165. Cincinnati, OH: NIOSH.

NIOSH, Health Hazard Evaluation and Technical Assistance Report. 1991*b*. *New England Lead Burning Co., (NELCO), Eaton Metals, Salt Lake City, UT*. HETA 91-290-2131. Cincinnati, OH: NIOSH.

NIOSH, Health Hazard Evaluation Report. February 1991. *Andrew Jackson Junior High School, Cross Lanes, WV*. HETA 89-183-2101. Cincinnati, OH: NIOSH.

NIOSH, Health Hazard Evaluation Report. June 1991. *LTV Steel, East Chicago, IN*. HETA 91-27-2117. Cincinnati, OH: NIOSH.

NIOSH, Health Hazard Evaluation Report. September 1991. *Western Primary School, Russiaville, IN*. HETA 91-143-2136. Cincinnati, OH: NIOSH.

NIOSH, Health Hazard Evaluation Report. March 1992. *Northwest Incinerator, Philadelphia, PA*. HETA 88-207-2195. Cincinnati, OH: NIOSH.

NIOSH, Health Hazard Evaluation Report. May 1992. *Kansas City, KS, Police Department, Kansas City, KS*. HETA 90-84-2219. Cincinnati, OH: NIOSH.

NIOSH, Health Hazard Evaluation Report. July 1992. *Kreisler Industrial Corp., Elmwood Park, NJ*. HETA 92-10-2234. Cincinnati, OH: NIOSH.

NIOSH, Health Hazard Evaluation Report. August 1992. *Seaway Painting, Inc., Annapolis, MD*. HETA 91-209-2249. Cincinnati, OH: NIOSH.

Oatman, L., and R. Roy. 1986. Surface and indoor air levels of polychlorinated biphenyls in public buildings. *Bull. Env. Contam. Toxicol.* **37**:461–466.

O'Malley, M. A., C. G. T. Mathias, M. Priddy, D. Molina, A. A. Grote, and W. E. Halperin. 1988. Occupational vitiligo due to unsuspected presence of phenolic antioxidant byproducts in commercial bulk rubber. *JOM* **30**(6):512–516.

Orris, P., J. R. Kominsky, D. Hryhorczuk, and J. Melius. 1986. Exposure to polychlorinated biphenyls from an overheated transformer. *Chemosphere* **15**(9/12):1305–1311.

OSHA. 1988. *Chemical Information Manual*. Washington, DC: Dept. of Labor.

OSHA. 1990. *Analytical Methods Manual for Organic Compounds*. Salt Lake City, UT: Salt Lake City Technical Center, OSHA.

OSHA. 1991. *OSHA Technical Manual*, 2d ed. Washington, DC: Dept. of Labor.

Perdek, J. M., F. J. Freestone, D. Sandifer, and A. Sherman. 1991. Closure of a dioxin incineration facility. *Chemosphere* **23**(8/10):1295–1305.

Polissar, L., K. Lowry-Coble, D. A. Kalman, J. P. Hughes, G. van Belle, D. S. Covert, T. M. Burbacher, D. Bolgiano, and N. K. Mottet. 1990. Pathways of human exposure to arsenic in a community surrounding a copper smelter. *Env. Res.* **53**:29–47.

Que Hee, S. S., B. Peace, C. S. Clark, J. R. Boyle, R. L. Bornschein, and P. B. Hammond. 1985. Evolution of efficient methods to sample lead sources, such as house dust and hand dust, in the homes of children. *Env. Res.* **38**:77–95.

Rappe, C., S. Marklund, L. Kjeller, P. Bergqvist, and M. Hansson. 1985. Strategies and techniques for sample collection and analysis: Experience from the Swedish PCB accidents. *Env. Health Perspect.* **60**:279–292.

Ross, J., T. Thongsinthusak, H. R. Fong, S. Margetich, and R. Krieger. 1990. Measuring potential dermal transfer of surface pesticide residue generated from indoor fogger use. An interim report. *Chemosphere* **20**(3/4):349–360.

Routledge, R. 1968. Possible health risk from beryllium oxide ceramic rectifiers of 1000 H.P. rail motor coaches. *Ann. Occup. Hyg.* **11**:17–21.

Saxby, W. N., and J. A. Hole. 1965. Practical aspects of surface contamination control at A.W.R.E. In G. W. Royster and B. R. Fish (eds.), *Surface Contamination*. New York: Pergamon Press.

Schecter, A., and T. Tiernan. 1985. Occupational exposure to polychlorinated dioxins, polychlorinated furans, polychlorinated biphenyls, and biphenylenes after an electrical panel and transformer accident in an office building in Binghamton, NY. *Env. Health Perspec.* **60**:305–313.

Schneider, T., O. Nielsen, P. Bredsdorff, and P. Linde. 1990. Dust in buildings with man-made mineral fiber ceiling boards. *Scand. J. Work Env. Health* **16**:434–439.

Schwartz, L., F. L. Knowles, R. H. Britten, and L. R. Thompson. 1933. Health aspects of radium dial painting. I. Scope and findings. *J. Ind. Hyg.* **15**(5):362–367.

Sheehy, J. W., and J. H. Jones. 1993. Assessment of arsenic exposures and controls in gallium arsenide production. *AIHA J.* **54**(2):61–69.

Sherman, A., et al. 1987. Final permit application, USEPA mobile incineration system at the James Denney Farm site, McDowell, MS. USEPA, Hazardous Waste Engineering Research Laboratory, Releases Control Branch, Edison, NJ, SKC, Inc. 1992. *SKC Comprehensive catalog and air sampling guide*. Eighty Four, PA: SKC, Inc.

Solomon, R. L., and J. W. Hartford. 1976. Lead and cadmium in dusts and soils in a small urban community. *Env. Science and Tech.* **10**:773–777.

Spicer, R. C. and S. R. White. 1991. *Asbestos Dust Contamination of Documents: Airborne Exposure and Decontamination*. Salt Lake City, UT: American Industrial Hygiene Conference Abstract.

Swanson, M. C., A. R. Campbell, M. J. Klauck, and C. E. Reed. 1989. Correlations between levels of mite and cat allergens in settled and airborne dust. *J. Allergy Clin. Immunol.* **83**:776–783.

Tartre, A. 1992. Investigation of surface contamination in a cadmium pigment facility. *Appl. Occup. Env. Hyg.* **7**(5):318–322.

Thulin, H. 1993. Determination of nor-nitrogen mustard hydrochloride in air and on surfaces by using filter or wipe sampling and a derivatization-gas chromatographic procedure. *AIHA J.* **54**(2):76–81.

van Netten, C., and K. E. Teschke. 1988. Assessment of mercury presence and exposure in a lighthouse with a mercury drive system. *Env. Res.* **43**:48–57.

Veckman, M. G. 1991. *Pesticide Contamination and Subsequent Decontamination of a Residential Subslab Ventilation System*. Salt Lake City, UT: American Industrial Hygiene Conference, Abstract.

Wagoner, D. A. 1989. Closure plan for the Denney Farm site, EPA ID No. MOT300010980, USEPA Region VII, Kansas City, KS, January 31.

Waldron, A. C. 1985. The potential for applicator-worker exposure to pesticides in greenhouse operations. In R. C. Honeycutt, G. Zweig, and N. N. Ragsdale (eds.), *Dermal Exposure Related to Pesticide Use*. Washington, DC: American Chemical Society, pp. 311–321.

Ware, G. W., D. P. Morgan, B. J. Estesen, W. P. Cahill, and D. M. Whitacre. 1973. Establishment of reentry intervals for organophosphate-treated cotton fields based on human data: I. Ethyl and methyl parathion. *Arch. Env. Contam. Toxicol.* **1**:48–59.

Weeks, R. W., and B. J. Dean. 1978. Decontamination of aromatic amine cancer-suspect agents on concrete, metal, or painted surfaces. *AIHA J.* **39**:758–762.

Weeks, R. W., S. K. Yasuda, and B. J. Dean. 1976. Fluorescent detection of hydrazines via fluorescamine and isomeric phthalaldehydes. *Anal. Chem.* **48**:159–161.

Wright, C. G., R. B. Leidy, and H. E. Dupree. 1984. Chlorpyrifos and diazinon detection on surfaces in dormitory rooms. *Bull. Env. Contam. Toxicol.* **32**:259–264.

Zirschky, J., and L. Witherell. 1987. Cleanup of mercury contamination of thermometer workers' homes. *AIHA J.* **48**(1):81–84.

CHAPTER 7

Surface Sampling for Chemicals

COLLECTION METHODS: OVERVIEW

Techniques

Surface sampling methods range from the use of hand pressure to move a filter against a surface, vacuuming, coupons, and mechanical devices designed to slide or roll for nonvolatile compounds to the use of direct reading instruments to measure volatile surface contamination.

The most common surface sampling method used for chemicals is wipe sampling. For simplicity the term *wipe* will be reserved for those methods using hand pressure to move media across a surface. Wipe sampling has also been termed swipe, smear, and smair sampling. All are terms used to describe similar techniques used for assessing surface contamination. It has been said that the word *swipe* originates from the idea that a long single stroke with a paper filter that covered an area of 100 cm^2 could be made (Cohen and Kusian, 1965). However, the long single stroke is rarely used now; instead the most common techniques use the "Z" or "S" motion. A *smear* sampler that has an abrasive mechanism in which a piece of filter paper is mechanically wiped over a fixed area surface while maintaining a constant contact pressure has been used (Fish et al., 1965). Samples are sometimes termed *smair* samples if they are obtained by filter paper collection of particles made airborne by the action of air jets impinging on the contaminated surface.

Another method is the use of paper, cloth, tape, or microscope slides coated with an adhesive to press against the test surface to collect a sample of particles. Other collection media/methods include gauze, commercially available wet wipes, and vacuum cleaners. Some methods are designed to determine how much fallout occurs to a surface from a process such as fogging or spraying, while others are used to measure dislodgeable residues. In the first case measurements are made during the application while in the second measurements are made following the application. These methods have not been validated against each other and comparisons are difficult. Results are not easily duplicated for many of the methods. For this reason, research continues to develop and refine surface sampling techniques so these problems are overcome.

Surface Characteristics

Surface characteristics such as porosity or impermeability, smoothness or roughness, and the presence or absence of moisture have a marked effect on the potential for resuspension or release on contact of contaminants. For example, it has been found nearly impossible to get any beryllium resuspension from a wet surface (Cohen and Kusian, 1965). The physical nature of the contaminated surface (porous versus nonporous or smooth) is important since particles will be deposited in surface cracks and crevices where they are not removed by the wiping. On the other hand, because smooth surfaces are more easily cleanable they are likely to be cleaner while rough surfaces may have higher loadings. Nonporous or impervious solid surfaces for Environmental Protection Agency (EPA) purposes include metals, aluminum siding, and enameled or laminated surfaces. Porous surfaces, also called nonimpervious surfaces for EPA purposes, include wood (Table 7-1), concrete, asphalt, and plasterboard, and can allow contamination to permeate to a considerable depth. In these situations a core sample may be more appropriate than a wipe.

Even the smoothest, most highly polished surface contains microscopic cracks and fissures from which it is difficult to dislodge all of the contamination. Rough and porous surfaces have much lower removal efficiencies when being wiped than smooth surfaces such as Formica (Chavalitnitikul and Levin, 1984). Adhesive tapes have been found to provide a better removal efficiency in taking samples from rough surfaces than wiping with filter papers. Waxes and polishes on surfaces can absorb contaminants and can be more difficult to decontaminate or to use for surface sample retrieval. In the case of a surface from which it is difficult to dislodge material, such as a carpet, vacuuming methods are better than wiping. Depending on the types of surfaces, the percent of surface contamination removed by, or remaining after, wiping (and subsequent decontamination) will vary.

TABLE 7-1 Results of Sampling for Beryllium on Wood

Sample	*Result* (*μg Be/ft*^{2})
First wipe (5 in. by 8 in.) Whatman No. 41	79
Second wipe (5 in. by 8 in.) Whatman No. 41	67
Third wipe (5 in. by 8 in.) Whatman No. 41	75
Cheesecloth and water	150
Wood from floor	1,860

Source: From Mitchell, R. N., and B. C. Eutsler. 1965. A study of beryllium surface contamination and resuspension. In G. W. Royster and B. R. Fish (eds.), *Surface Contamination*. New York: Pergamon Press, pp. 349–353.

Sampling Media

Filters

Laboratory-grade filters are the most common media used. Generally there are two types of filters recommended by the Occupational Safety and Health Administration (OSHA) for collecting wipe samples (OSHA, 1991). Glass fiber (GF) filters (37 mm, 1.0 μm) are used for materials analyzed by high-performance liquid chromatography (HPLC) and often for substances analyzed for gas chromatography (GC). Mixed cellulose ester (MCE) air sampling filters or cellulose filtration type filters are generally used for metals, and may be used for anything not analyzed by HPLC. Since MCE filters are very hygroscopic, they cannot be successfully tared for field use.

Filters are fragile, and when using solvents extreme care must be used or they will be damaged. In some studies round filters have been trimmed to a square size, for example, Whatman filter paper number 42 cut to 10 cm by 10 cm (Chavalitnitikul et al., 1984). Chromatographic paper has been used. Although 37 mm is a common size for MCE and GF filters, the size of surface media often varies depending on the method. Larger filters have been found to give better removal efficiencies when 10 cm by 10 cm square filters were compared with 7 cm round filters (Chavalitnitikul and Levin, 1984). The expected concentration may also affect the choice. The smear tab is a specialized shape of filter that is convenient as it has a small handle

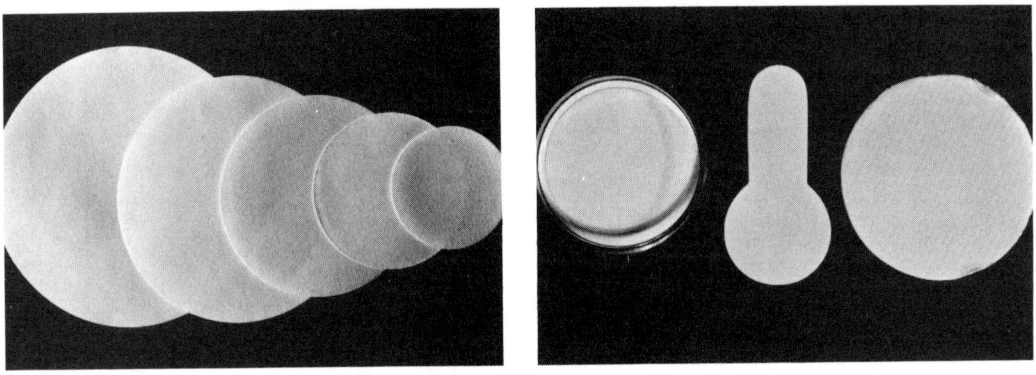

Figure 7-1. Various filter sizes and a smear tab.
Source: Photos by Ed Wesly.

that can be gripped while wiping. When preloading a set of vials with smear tabs, they should be inserted with the tab end out. Figure 7-1 shows some of the types of filter media available for wipe sampling.

Filter papers vary in their ability to absorb materials. In a test using oil as the transfer medium a greater mass of oil was transferred to Whatman 50 paper than to Whatman 3 paper, indicating the composition of filter is equally as important as contact time and pressure (McArthur and Lees, 1992). In a second study comparing GF filters, Whatman 50, Whatman 3, cotton cloth, paper towels, and aluminum, the greatest mass was transferred to the GF filters followed by Whatman 50. Therefore, not only is filter selection important but overall media (McArthur, 1993). Table 7-2 lists characteristics of Whatman filters used for surface sampling.

Other Materials

A wide variety of commercially available materials have also been used for wipe sampling. Cotton surgical gauze is sometimes used rather than filter papers, especially for polychlorinated biphenyl (PCB) sampling, and will hold up better on rough surfaces than many types of filters. Cotton balls have also been used to sample for 2,4-D using methanol as the solvent. Cotton-tipped swabs with wooden stems work best for wipe tests requiring toxic solvents to be used. Prepackaged baby wipes are currently used to collect lead samples (NIOSH, 1991*b*). Scott Paper Company "Wash-a-bye Baby" wipes were tested by the National Institute of Occupational Safety and Health (NIOSH) and were found to contain very low levels of background lead contamination. NIOSH now recommends commercial hand towelettes for lead surface sampling instead of the baby wipes (NIOSH, 1992*b*).

Commercial premoistened media such as baby and hand wipes do not have uniform wetness. In boxes the liquid tends to settle so it is increased in the bottom wipes. One way to minimize this condition is to rotate the container to uniformly distribute the liquid. Individually packaged wipes can dry out over time as well. Premoistened commercial materials contain a variety of chemicals including alcohols. Some of these chemicals may be interferents in either the sampling or analytical procedures. For this reason, the Department of Housing and Urban development (HUD) specifies that commercial wipes used for lead must not contain alcoholic wetting agents. Chifonet (rayon) cloths (Johnson & Johnson) have been used to sample for an amine compound (Thulin, 1993). Facial tissues have been used to dry wipe for soot suspected of containing dioxins (Rappe et al., 1985). Medical quality adhesive cloth, labels, and cellophane tape have been used for surface sample for dusts.

TABLE 7-2. Characteristics of Whatman Filters Used for Surface Sampling

Filter No.	*Wgt. (g/M^2)*	*Thickness*	*Surface Hardness*	*Ash (%)*	*Retention 98% Efficient at (μ)*	*Wet Strength*	*Sizes (cm)*	*Description*
1	87	0.18	SM	0.06	11	L	4.25, 5.5, 7, 9, 11, 12.5, 15, 18.5, 24, 27, 32, 40	Universal paper for general lab filtrations and qualitative analysis with a retention rating of 11 μm. Widely used for clarifying liquids in routine lab applications and for air pollution monitoring.
40	95	0.2	GR	0.01	8	L	4.25–40	Medium retention and filtering with retention rating of 8 μm. General purpose gravimetric paper recommended for silica in steel, calcium oxalate, and well-digested barium sulfate.
41	91	0.19	GR	0.01	20–25	L	4.25–32	Very open textured rapid filtering paper with retention rating of 20–25 μm for coarse and gelatinous precipitates such as iron and aluminum hydroxide. Also used for quantitative air pollution analysis as paper tape for impregnation when determining gaseous compounds at high flow rates.
42	100	0.2	GR	0.01	2.5	FC	4.25–40	Very retentive and slow filtering for extremely fine particulates such as barium sulfate or metastannic acid. Retention rating of 2.5 μm.
43	95	0.22	GR	0.01	16	FC	4.25–40	Intermediate in retention between 40 and 41 and twice as fast as 40. Typical applications include foodstuffs analysis, soil analysis, and particulate collection in air pollution monitoring.
44	80	0.18	GR	0.01	3	FC	4.25–40	Very retentive slow filtering with a rating of 3 μm. Similar in filtration quality to No. 42 but lighter in weight and thinner with lower residual ash.
50	94	0.12	SG	0.025	2.7	FC	4.25–40	Most retentive with a rating of 3 μm. Slowest filtering of low ash hardened grades. Retains finest crystalline precipitates. Finish helps keep paper free from loose surface fibers.

Source: Data from *Scientific Products Catalogue*. 1992. Chicago, IL: Scientific Products Co.
Notes: SM = smooth normal hardness. SG = smooth hard glazed surface. GR = slightly grained surface. L = suitable for gravity or low suction filtration, but care must be taken to prevent rupture of the paper. FC = filtering capacity.

If substituting media in an analytical method, do a pretest comparing new media to old because adjustments may be required. For example, some commercial premoistened wipes (including baby wipes) have many irregularities in their structure that may require longer digestion periods. Larger size materials (such as baby wipes) may also require special handling to get good extraction when prepared and analyzed using traditional filter methods. Other considerations in the selection of wipe media include ease of use in the field, robustness, and the ability to minimize cross-contamination between wipes.

Preparation of Media

Preweighing allows for determining concentration (μg/g) on media. However, tared wipe media can change characteristics in the field if not handled carefully. Moisture can be picked up or lost, and skin oils can contaminate media or add to the weight.

Media have been used with and without preextraction for many compounds including lead and pesticides. A blank must be analyzed for background contamination prior to selecting the media, however, and along with the samples after collection. Media designed to be used as bandages are often very clean anyway. While there have been some concerns about contamination in commercial media, these are considered to be minimal as long as the media are pretested for the contaminant to be sampled the first time they are used, and for each survey blanks of the media are included for analysis with the samples.

Where very low detection levels are needed or where an interferent is discovered, preextraction is necessary. Soxhlet extraction is a method for extracting nonvolatile and semivolatile organic compounds from solids. The Soxhlet extraction process ensures intimate contact of the sample matrix with the extraction solvent. Examples of extraction solvents (all pesticide quality or equivalent) are toluene/methanol (10:1), acetone/hexane (1:1), and methylene chloride. Exchange solvents include hexane, 2-propanol, cyclohexane, and acetonitrile. If contamination from skin oils or other potential interferents are suspected in the samples, the extract can be cleaned up using a florisil column. Soxhlet preextraction can also be used to remove sizing and other additions from media prior to extraction.

Whether or not to use a solvent is often a question. Solvents are not required, but they can enhance collection if appropriate for the contaminant under investigation. On the other hand, if a surface is already moist, solvents may dilute the sample. It has been stated that dry wipe samples are not as representative of real contact exposure as moistened wipe samples because the skin surface is most likely going to be moist from perspiration (NIOSH, 1979). One method effective in improving recovery of contaminant from porous surfaces is to first wet the surface with a solvent and then wipe with an absorbent type of material such as gauze or an absorbent pad (Klingner, 1992).

There is much debate over solvent selection. Solvents that increase the recovery of material from surfaces may not accurately mimic skin moisture. In this regard, a saline solution or water are considered the most appropriate solvents. Purity of solvents is important. Although they need not be spectroscopic grade, they should be of sufficient purity not to contaminate the sample. An example is PCBs, which are most commonly sampled using pesticide grade hexane. Distilled or deionized water should be used rather than tap water. Another concern with solvents is contaminating the surface with an additional chemical, or in the case of porous surfaces, increasing the permeation of the contaminant into it. OSHA (1991) directs its compliance officers to use only distilled water as the solvent for wiping surfaces that contact food or tobacco products.

It is important that the same amount of solvent be used for each sample (as long as the areas are consistent), which may be accomplished by premeasuring the solvent onto the media (e.g., 2 mL for each filter), or by dipping the medium into the solvent and squeezing hard (gauze, cotton puffs). Sometimes methods are combined, such as doing a dry wipe on a very dusty surface, followed by a wet wipe to remove residual contamination. Table 7-3 lists common

TABLE 7-3. Common Solvents Used in Wipe Sampling

Compound	*Solvent*
PCBs	Hexane
Aromatic amines	Methanol
4-Aminodiphenyl Azinphos methyl Toxaphene DDVP Diazinon Dieldrin Dinitrotoluenes Lindane Malathion Parathion	Ethylene glycol
4-Aminopyridine Aniline Anisidine Benzidine Heptachlor Nitroglycerin Pentachloronaphthalene TEDP Tetrachloronaphthalene Trinitrotoluene (TNT)	Isopropanol
Metals and salts Low-chain hydrocarbons	Distilled water
Bases Amines Hydrazines	Dilute acids
Acids Phenols Thiols (mercaptans)	Dilute bases
Nonpolar hydrocarbons	Organic solvents

solvents used in wipe sampling. For those who do not care to assemble materials individually, wipe sampling kits are available (Fig. 7-2).

Sampling Strategy

The first step in developing a sampling strategy in which wipe sampling will be performed is to identify as closely as possible the type and expected concentration of contaminant(s). In any one survey it is best to be consistent and use the same size and shape media. For comparing results from different surveys this is best as well. The decision to use wipe sampling as the collection in a survey should be made after evaluating its advantages and limitations. Wipe samples are inexpensive, fast, and simple to perform. They are useful as a screening tool, especially for trace elements. However, as a quantitative measurement they have several drawbacks, including operator bias and poor reproducibility. They are limited largely to trace elements and other inorganic analysis, and are sufficient for surface loading data (g/cm^2) but not for the concentration (μg/g) of the analyte in the dust. Wipes are not suited for sampling carpets or other absorbent materials, and the results may not reflect actual skin pickup. The amount of material recovered from a wipe is dependent both on technique (number of traverses across a surface, surface size to media size) as well as strategy (sequential or composite). The differences in wrist position (and therefore pressure) during vertical and horizontal wiping motions can also produce a significant amount of sample-to-sample variability.

When one of the components to be tested for is very expensive and difficult to analyze, such as TCDD, attempts have been made to use a less expensive contaminant that is also present in the mixture to be sampled. In a study on surface contamination following a PCB-containing transformer fire, a larger number of PCB surface samples was collected to demonstrate the range of cleanliness of surfaces throughout the building in order to support the use of a smaller number of TCDF/TCDD samples as being representative (NIOSH, 1986*b*). The TCDF/TCDD samples were collected side-by-side with the PCB samples to determine if a statistical relationship existed. The existence of a statistical relationship between PCB and TCDF/TCDD would permit the use of a PCB concentration to predict the corresponding TCDF/TCDD concentration.

Area

In a single survey it is best to use the same size sampling area for all samples unless the surface or object to be sampled makes doing so impossible. If different surveys are to be compared, it is

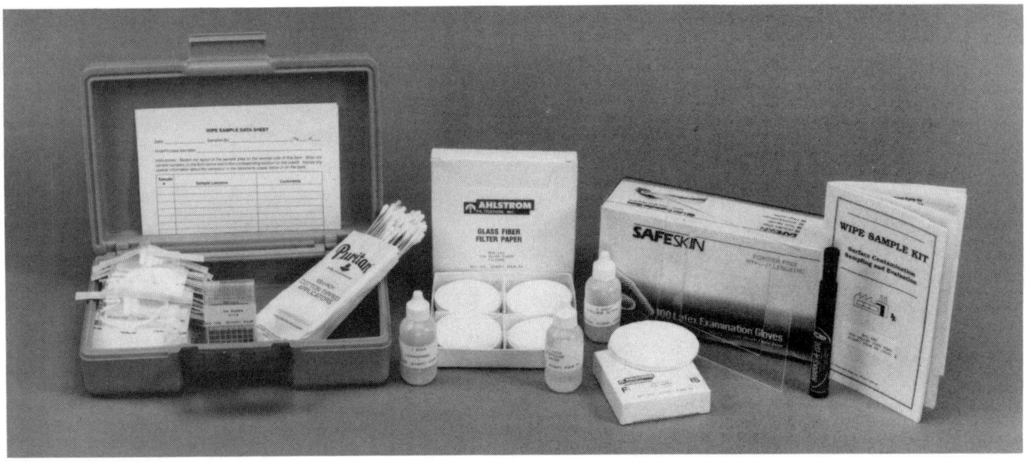

Figure 7-2. Wipe sampling kit.
Courtesy SKC Inc.

best once again to use the same sampling size for all chemicals. OSHA methods use a 100 cm^2 sampling area, which is the most common, but any dimension can be used. HUD specifies a 1 ft^2 area for lead abatement sampling.

In situations where handles, knobs, latches, and other small surfaces are being sampled along with larger areas a correction factor can be applied to give comparable areas (Frank, Campbell, and Sirons, 1985). Where different size areas must be wiped, the size should be documented. Even though all the results should be converted to the same units, for example, in^2, cm^2, or ft^2, it is still a good idea to document in the table of the results what size area was actually wiped. Typical areas are 100 cm^2, 300 cm^2, 1,000 cm^2, and 1 ft^2. If low levels are anticipated, one way to meet analytical detection limits is to double the size of the surface area sampled.

Use of Templates

Templates are commonly used to assure consistency in the size of area sampled. Both disposable and reusable templates can be used. If reusable, they must be decontaminated in between samples, which is one reason they are often constructed of galvanized or stainless steel rather than absorbent materials such as plastic. Another option is to cover them with a material such as aluminum foil and replace the foil each time. One way to speed up the use of templates is to cut holes in aluminum pie plates and then dispose of them after each sample. Templates have also been cut from 8.5 × 11 inch overhead transparency material.

One way of using a template is to place it on the surface to be sampled and then outline the area lightly with a soft pencil. When templates are used on smooth surfaces they are often taped down to free the sampler's hands for performing the collection. The tape can then be left down to indicate the area sampled to avoid resampling during a survey.

Figure 7-3 *(left)* shows the size of the template used by OSHA and Figure 7-3 *(right)* shows a template being used to take a sample inside of a tank. Another strategy in situations involving curved surfaces is to use a metal tape measure to size the area and draw on the surface with a pencil or other suitable marker.

An alternative to using templates is to cut filter paper to the desired size of the sample, for example, 10 cm by 10 cm, and place the paper over the exact surface to be sampled. The paper is then pressed evenly over the entire surface with a gloved hand (Chavalitnitikul, Levin, and Chen, 1984). If several or all fingers are used, then equal pressure should be applied by all. Another practice is to use a single finger to maintain a firm, steady pressure on the center of the paper. This

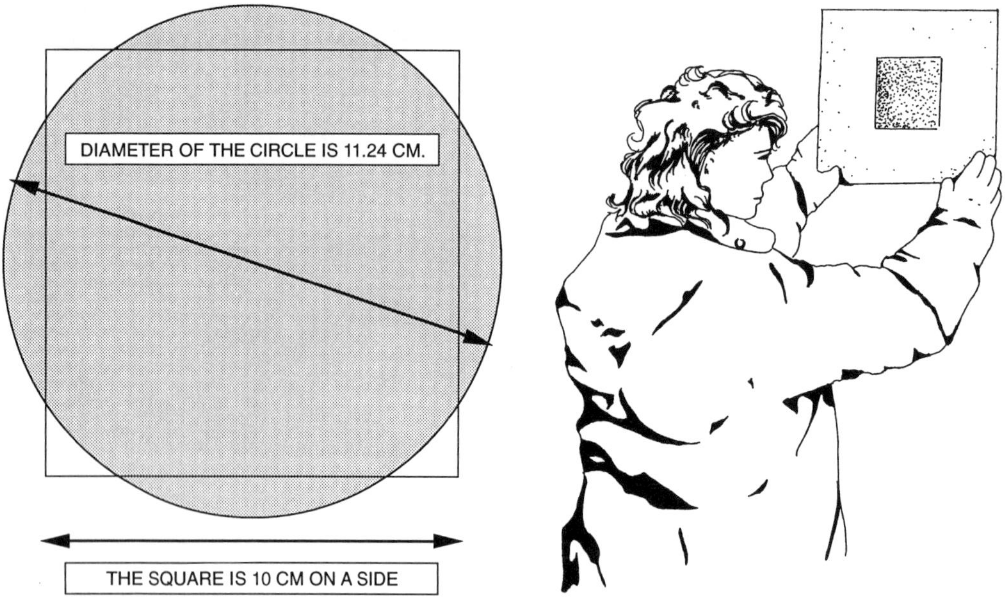

Figure 7-3. A template for OSHA sampling (*left*) and the template in use (*right*).
Source: Template from *OSHA Technical Manual*, 2d ed., Washington, DC, 1991. Drawing by Renea Joslin.

practice is best for wipes using smaller pieces of media such as a 5-cm diameter Whatman number 1 filter. To minimize variations, one person should perform all the tests using a predetermined pressure, often the maximum that can be exerted without harming the medium.

Avoiding Contamination

Samples can become contaminated from the hands of the samplers or, worse yet, sampling professionals might expose themselves to the contaminant. Therefore, where possible media can be held with a clamp that is decontaminated between samples, or the sampling professional can wear gloves. Always wear clean latex, polyethylene, or nitrile gloves when handling filters. Gloves should be disposable and should not be powdered. Due to problems with plasticizers being released, gloves that contain them should not be used. A new set of gloves should be used with each individual sample to avoid contamination of the filter by hand and the subsequent possibility of false positives, and to prevent contact with the substance. When several samples need to be collected, multiple pairs of thin gloves can be donned to save time. Some industrial hygienists have reported successfully donning as many as five pairs at a time. After each sample the outermost pair is removed and discarded.

Timing and Frequency

Most often surface samples are collected on a one time only basis in order to make a recommendation to improve a program (e.g., better housekeeping or local exhaust to minimize airborne contamination); however, regular repeat surveys to determine the effectiveness of cleaning programs or engineering controls will provide better assurance that they are effective. The sampling survey interval and frequency (number of samples collected per unit area of the surfaces to be sampled at the site) are determined by the likelihood of the processes producing contamination, and in well-established plants this may be further modified as the result of previous history. Some facilities using highly toxic materials such as beryllium have used a periodic (e.g., quarterly) monitoring program.

Areas that are supposed to be clean, such as changing rooms and lunchrooms, are important to sample regularly. In addition, a number of obvious contamination buildup points should be visited and checked regularly: frequently used doorways, finger plates around essential controls, changing room surfaces on the plant side of the changing facilities, and operatives monitoring equipment in the plants. In order to minimize the effects of day-to-day variation, five daily work surface wipes can be obtained whenever possible during a period of several consecutive workdays. A control location is also good to select such as a medical department. If there are several workers' stations, wipes can be taken at each station for comparison.

Locations

If multiple samples are to be taken at a work site, prepare a rough sketch of the area(s) or room(s) to be wipe sampled along with the locations of key surfaces (e.g., Fig. 7-4). Often air sampling locations are also included on the same diagram. In a study of the location illustrated by Figure 7-4, high levels of lead had been found in soil samples collected at a scrap metal reclaiming operation and there was concern about employees exposure (NIOSH, 1988). Wipe and air samples were collected in representative areas throughout the facility to identify the presence of airborne and surface contamination.

Where there are high concentrations of highly stable materials (e.g., heavy metals) that pose a significant oral toxicity concern, surface sampling should be done in both production and nonproduction areas. Another strategy is to target the areas where the concentration is sus-

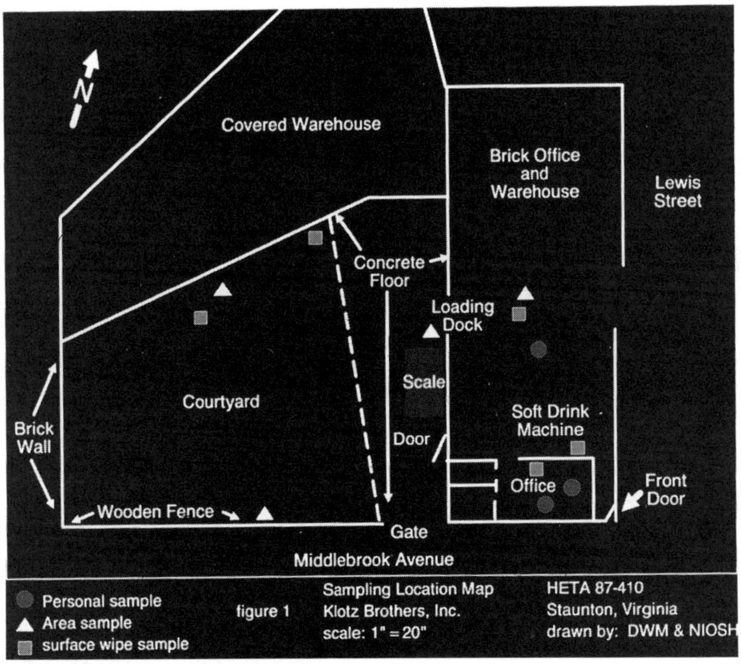

Figure 7-4. Air and wipe sampling locations at a scrap metal facility with high levels of lead in the soil.

pected to be heaviest such as floors. Sometimes reference areas that are known not to have any contamination could be in a different room or building on a site or in a hotel room or other building off site.

Weighted Random Sampling

The strategy for weighted random sampling of surfaces incorporates a scheme for random sampling of locations, weighted by likely frequency of human skin contact. Different work spaces are first divided into three broad categories by occupancy or frequency of use. As an example, an office building would be divided into (1) office space, (2) hallways and reception areas, and (3) storage areas. The work surfaces are then divided into seven categories by likelihood of skin contact: (1) floors; (2) ceilings; (3) high-contact work surfaces such as computer keyboards and desk tops; (4) low-contact work surfaces such as bookshelves and file cabinets; (5) high-use wall areas such as door knobs and light switches, as well as the areas around them; (6) high-contact wall areas (between 3 ft and 6 ft above the floor) including room dividers; and (7) low contact wall areas (below 3 ft and above 6 ft from the floor). A system of weighting factors (Table 7-4) is needed to characterize the contact an occupant might have with each surface. The probability of selection for any given surface for the random sampling is weighted by a factor according to the frequency of contact with the surface by the worker. This approach is similar to that used by the EPA for setting cleanup levels according to the usage of an area and type of surface.

TABLE 7-4. Weighting Factors

Surface	*Office*	*Hallway*	*Storage*
Floors	0.15	0.05	0.10
Ceilings	0.05	0.05	0.05
High contact Work	1.0	NA	NA
Low contact work	0.5	0.1	0.5
High use wall	0.5	0.3	0.5
High contact wall	0.4	0.2	0.3
Low contact wall	0.15	0.1	0.15

Source: From NIOSH, Health Hazard Evaluation Report. February 1988. 50 *Staniford St., Office Building, Boston*, MA. Cincinnati, OH: NIOSH.
Note: NA = Not applicable.

To accomplish the weighted random sampling of surfaces, an inventory of the existing surfaces and structural configuration in the building must be completed. Each room is assigned a designation and all of the surfaces in each room are listed on a statistical data input form. The information from the statistical data input form is entered into a computer database and converted to weighted surfaces. A computer program reads the database and produces a new database of surfaces, including their areas (square feet), and then weighs the areas according to the weighting factors. This new database of weighted areas is then randomly sampled by a computer program using a uniform random number generator to select the sampling locations.

The Grid System

Another sampling approach is to set up a grid system and collect a specific number of samples inside each grid box. Since this strategy is commonly used in buildings suspected of contamination, it is described further in Chapter 10.

Sample Compositing

Whether to take a single surface sample or several samples and have them analyzed is a point of discussion. There can be a significant amount of variability on a single surface or within a single dwelling. If the intent is to characterize and estimate the exposure over a large surface such as a work bench or several similar surfaces such as the tables in a lunchroom, collecting many individual samples for separate analysis and calculating the average of all the samples may provide a more useful estimate of the potential exposure. Or, after several samples are collected they can be composited for a single analysis. Compositing can make it easier to compare the sampling results of several dwellings.

Compositing is done for two different purposes. In situations where the detection level for a contaminant is very low, several wipes may be collected, composited, and treated as a single sample. Samples for dioxins and dibenzofurans are often collected in this manner. In one study the dioxin wipe sample consisted of a composite of four 0.25 m^2 wipe samples for a total area of 1.0 m^2 (NIOSH, 1986*b*). The second situation is when an average surface contamination result is desired, several samples taken in a pattern over a surface such as a floor or wall can be analyzed together. This will average out the effects of hot spots and zero values.

In some instances where a large area must be sampled, compositing can be done to represent an entire surface such as a ceiling or each wall in a room. In one study (Clarke, 1991), a composite sample contained up to 14 individual samples taken to represent a floor, wall, or ceiling in a given room of a manufacturing building. In the composited samples, floors were not mixed with ceilings or walls, and so on, in a given room. A composite confirmation sample was one in which a replicate sample was taken adjacent to each sample that was used in the composite. These replicate samples were kept discrete (not composited) and analyzed independently to show that no hot spots were diluted by the compositing process.

In this study the frequency of sampling, expressed as one sample per ft^2, for composite samples was 1,000 (minimum: one composite per room composed of a minimum of two individual samples; maximum: 14 individual samples per composite). For composite confirmation samples, the frequency was 10% of composited samples.

Another compositing strategy takes into account the activities of the subjects whose exposure is being evaluated. This approach is most often taken for studies of children's exposures in their homes. After the locations where the child spends time are identified, an estimate of the percent of time spent actively in each location is made. A compositing strategy is developed by adjusting the area (and thus the number of samples) to be proportional to the time spent in each area. For example, assume that a composite is to consist of five individual areas with each sample over an area of one square foot. An evaluation of one household finds that a child spends 20% of its awake time in the bedroom, 40 percent in the family room and another 40% in the kitchen. The exposure-weighted composite sample would be distributed as shown in Table 7-5.

TABLE 7-5. Exposure Weighting Strategy for Composited Samples

Room	*Time Spent (%)*	*Area to Be Sampled*	*Number of Samples*
Family	40	2 ft^2	2
Bedroom	20	1 ft^2	1
Kitchen	40	2 ft^2	2
Total samples/ composite			5

It is easier to collect composite samples by using vacuum methods than by using wipe sampling methods, however vacuum methods are best suited to sampling carpets and are therefore limited. Each location is vacuumed into one collection container and no decontamination of the vacuum is required in between samples. (A detailed discussion of vacuum methods appears later in this chapter.) Composite wipes are generally placed in a single container for analysis as a single sample. If the composite is significantly larger than the normal sample volume, an analytical method may need to be redesigned to address changes in procedures, thus increasing the time and cost of analysis.

WIPE SAMPLING

Various strategies for wiping exist (Table 7-6): wiping across the surface in either an "S" or a "Z" motion; wiping across horizontally or up and down; using a series of progressively decreasing circles or squares to fill up a circle or a square. To some degree the shape of the template will dictate the motion: a circular template would be done with a circular motion, and a square with either a square, horizontal, or vertical motion.

TABLE 7-6. Wipe Sampling Methods

Method	*Surface Type*	*Wipe Media*	*Area*	*Sampling Procedure*	*Shipping Container*	*Units*	*Reference*
Proposed ASTM Standard	Hard (floors, windows)		Template (12 × 12 in.) or measured area	Wipe with "S" motion L → R, F → B. Fold wipe. Repeat "S" motion L → R, F → B.	Centrifuge tube (50 mL)	μg/ft^2	ASTM, 1993
Georgia Tech	Hard	Little Ones baby wash cloths	Measured area	Wipe with "S" motion F → B, L → R. Fold wipe. Repeat "S" motion F → B, L → R.	Centrifuge tube (50 mL)	μg/ft^2	Georgia Technical Research Institute, 1993
Farfel	Hard	Nonalcohol wipes	Template (12 × 12 in.) or measured area	Wipe with "S" motion F → B, L → R. Fold wipe inside. Repeat "S" motion.	Ziploc™ bags	μg/ft^2	Farfel and Chisolm, 1990
HUD	hard	Commercial nonalcohol premoistened wipes	Template (12 × 12 in.) or meas. area	Wipe with "S" motion F → B, L → R. Fold wipe inside. Repeat "S" motion 90° to first wipe.	Polypropylene tube (50 mL)	μg/ft^2	HUD, 1990
Rabinowitz			Preweighed filter paper, Whatman 541	930 cm^2	Resealable polyethylene bags	μg/wipe	Rabinowitz et al., 1985
LWW	Hard	Three preweighed polyethylene filters (3.8 × 6.35 cm)	Template (27.3 × 4 cm)	Wipe within template with filter no. 1 (moistened with Type I water). Wipe within template with filter no. 2 (moistened with Type I water). Wipe within template with filter no. 3 (dry).	Plastic bag	μg/ft^2 μg/g	Lioy, Wainman, and Weisel, 1993

NIOSH	Hard	Gauze (2 × 2 in.) wetted with 1–2 mL distilled water Wash 'n Dri wipes (individually packaged)	Disposable template (10 × 10 cm)	Wipe with "S" motion three or four vertical strokes. Fold wipe inside. Wipe with "S" motion three or four horizontal strokes. Fold wipe inside. Wipe with "S" motion three or four vertical strokes.	Ziploc™ bag	μg/ft²	NIOSH, 1992
Stark		Preweighed cotton gauze				μg/g	Stark et al., 1982
State of MA	Hard	Individually wrapped alcohol medical wipes	Template (1 ft²)	Wipe area once L → R.	Plastic tube	μg/ft²	Timperi, 1992
State of NC	Hard	Johnson & Johnson Baby Wipes	Template (1 ft²) or measured area	Wipe with "S" motion. Rewipe with "S" motion 90° to first pass.	Ziploc™ bag	μg/ft²	Hayes, J., 1992
Vostal	Hard (uncarpeted)	Disposable paper towel (14 × 20 cm) moistened with 20% denatured alcohol or 1:150 benzalkonium chloride	Template (1 ft²)			μg/ft²	Vostal et al., 1974

Source: From EPA. 1994. The National Human Exposure Assessment Survey (NHEXSUS) Workshop. Research Triangle Park, NC: U.S. Environmental Protection Agency.
Notes: L → R = left to right and F → B = front to back.

Care should be taken not to rewipe any sections that have been wiped previously.

Repeat wipes may be useful. For surveys where quantitative results are important, such as those for which a surface standard exists, repeat wipes should be performed. Generally it has been found that after three wipes the majority of surface contamination is collected. Studies have found that most repeat wipe values are lower in concentration than the value for the first wipe, but this technique is useful for determining how much total contaminant is present. In one study, a repeat wipe over the same area detected an average of 55% of the initial wipe concentration, although there was a wide variation in actual results (Lichtenwalner, 1992). Certain types of surfaces may require additional samples in order to be certain that the majority of the contamination has been removed. For the smear check to be realistic, at least 50% of any removable surface dust must be retained on the filter paper for estimation (Brooks, 1959). These results can also be useful for planning decontamination strategies. It is best to use a fixed template in these instances since pencil or other markings might be removed. The template stays in place until all samples are collected. The results of sampling for each area are then added together.

The inability of a wipe medium to effectively hold onto sampled contaminant may result in adherence of sampled material to the sample container, thus possibly leading to lower recoveries. Therefore, wipe samples are best shipped in bottles rather than bags because a rigid container, plastic or glass, is easier to rinse out than a plastic bag, to make sure that none of the material collected on the wipe is lost.

After the analytical results are received the samples are tabulated as shown in Table 7-7, which gives the results for a survey in an office building where there was a concern that the toner in the photocopy machine contained trinitrofluorene (TNF), a possible carcinogen.

Wipe Sampling for OSHA Concerns

1. Preload a group of vials with appropriate filters. Make sure the vials have labels.
2. Always wear clean impervious gloves when doing wipes. Disposable gloves are preferable, and can prevent contamination of future samples as well as to oneself. A clean set of gloves should be used with each sample. The selection of gloves will depend on the contaminants being sampled and the types of solvents used.

TABLE 7-7. Swipe Sample Results, IBM, Gaithersburg, MD, May 19, 1981

Location	*TNF Detected (ηg)*	*Swipe Area (in.²)*	*Removable TNF (ηg/in.²)*
3800 Printing subsystem			
Near vacuum	ND	16	—
Near toner transfer	ND	16	—
Back of door enclosing drum	233	16	15
Next to cyclone bag (relay box)	37	16	2
Vacuum box (top)	57	16	4
Copier II			
Inside exit pocket	ND		—
At operator position	ND	5	—
Right caster well	ND	8	—
Bottom frame near drum	471	13	36

Source: From NIOSH, Health Hazard Evaluation Report. December 1981. *Washington, DC*. HETA 81-125-1029, *DHHS*. Cincinnati, OH: NIOSH.
Notes: Limit of detection was 30 ηg per sample. The limit of quantitation was 120 ηg per sample.
ND = Not detected.

3. Prepare a diagram of the area or rooms to be wipe sampled along with the locations of key surfaces.
4. Label the sample vial with the place where the sample is being collected and a unique number. Withdraw the filter or other medium from the vial. If a damp wipe sample is needed, moisten the filter with a specific amount of distilled water or other solvent as recommended for the contaminant being sampled.
5. Wipe approximately 100 cm^2 of the surface to be sampled using a template with an opening exactly 100 cm^2. The purpose is to have consistent areas to compare. Even if standards are not available, samples should be comparable for determining which areas are the most contaminated. For surfaces smaller than 100 cm^2, use a template of the largest size possible. Be sure to document the size of the area wiped. For curved surfaces, the wiped area should be estimated as accurately as possible and then documented.
6. Maximum pressure should be applied when wiping. To assure that all portions of the partitioned area are wiped, start at the outside edge and progress toward the center making concentric squares of decreasing size.
7. If the filter dries out during the wiping procedure, discard the filter, reduce the area to be wiped by one-half, and repeat the wiping procedure with a new filter.
8. Without allowing the filter to contact any other surface, fold the filter with exposed sides against each other and then fold it over again (Fig. 7-5). Put the filter in its sample vial, cap the vial, and place a corresponding number at the sample location on the diagram. Some substances, such as benzidine, must have solvent added to the vial as soon as the wipe is placed inside.
9. Include notes with the sketch giving any further description (lunch table in shop area next to quality control lab; painted wood) that may prove useful when evaluating sample results, for example, employee's names who work in the area.
10. At least one blank filter should be folded and put into a vial. Put on clean gloves and remember that no contact with surfaces is important. Also provide a sample of the solvent used as a blank in case it is needed.
11. Samples that can evaporate must be contained within airtight bottles or samples will be lost.

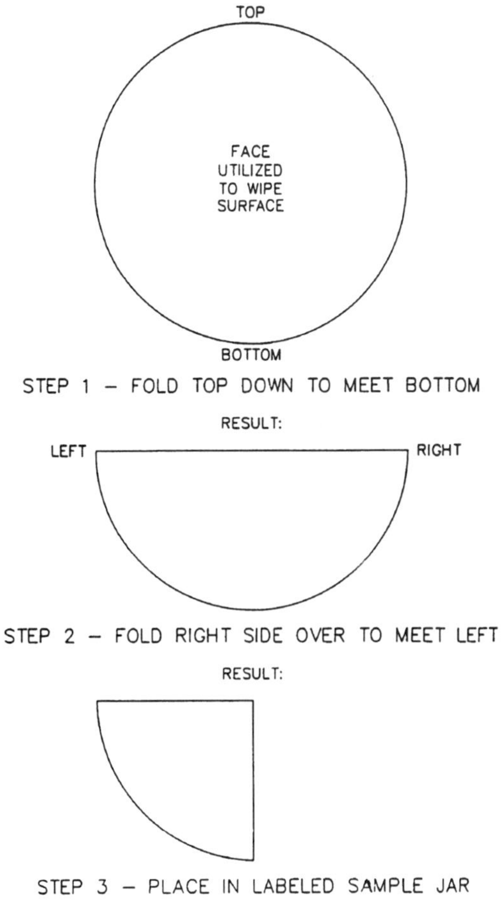

Figure 7-5. Folding procedure for wipes.

Variation on OSHA Sampling Procedure

1. Assemble preweighed MCE filters in 37 mm plastic two-stage cassettes and a 100 cm^2 circular open template.
2. Don a clean pair of latex gloves for each sample.
3. Open the cassette by taking the first stage off and lift the filter out of the cassette with

pointed tweezers. Wipe the surface in a circular motion while applying uniform pressure.
4. Replace filter in the original plastic cassette.

Dry Filter Method

Dry wipes can be used for liquid residues. OSHA recommends dry wiping for skin, chemical protective clothing (CPC), or surfaces that contact food or tobacco products if distilled water is not used.

1. Using the tip of the thumb, wipe a 2.4-cm-diameter filter paper disk in a "Z" of "S" pattern over a representative portion of the surface to be sampled. The length of the wipe should be 50 cm. The pressure-bearing portion of the filter paper disk will be about 2 cm wide; therefore, the area of the surface that is sampled will be approximately 100 cm^2.
2. Avoid contacting excess dirt when wiping an area.

Wipe Sampling for HUD Concerns

Commercial premoistened hand wipes are used for lead abatement sampling. Since HUD regulations require that a 1 foot by 1 foot area be wiped, it is helpful to create a variety of plastic templates in different shapes that meet this criterion. One for floors might be square; another should be rectangular to fit a typical windowsill. Since this method is specific for lead paint abatement situations, it is described in Appendix B. NIOSH has also developed a method that has been evaluated for its efficiency in collecting lead dust (see the section on commercial premoistened wipes).

Whatman Smear Tab Method

Surface wipe samples have been collected by applying moderate pressure to the backs of pesticide-quality cyclohexane-moistened Whatman No. 50 smear tabs and wiping a unit area of approximately 100 cm^2 (Orris et al., 1986). A fresh, disposable, polyvinyl chloride glove was worn for each wipe sample to prevent cross-contamination of the samples. After wiping the surface, the smear tab was folded face-inward, then folded inward once more, and sealed in a 20-mL glass vial with a Teflon-lined screw cap.

In a study for metals contamination, Whatman smear tabs were moistened with water, and donning disposable vinyl gloves, a 15 cm by 15 cm area was wiped with a series of horizontal left-to-right strokes (NIOSH, 1991*a*). The gloves were changed after each sample to prevent cross-contamination. Care was taken to use the same method and wiping pressure for each sample. The samples were placed in glass scintillation vials for transportation to the laboratory. In this instance, laboratory analysis was performed for elements using inductively coupled plasma (ICP).

Method for Commercial Premoistened Wipes

Surface wipe samples were collected using commercial premoistened baby wipes as follows (NIOSH, 1992): An area measuring 30.5 cm by 30.5 cm was marked on a flat surface. Disposable gloves were put on, the first wipe from the package was discarded, the second wipe was handled for an imaginary (approximate) sampling time and placed in a clean labeled Zip-Loc™ bag (this is a sample blank), and the third wipe was folded in half and placed on the surface to be sampled. The wipe was rubbed in an "S" pattern over the entire measured area, then refolded with the dust side in, rubbed in an "S" pattern again, at a 90-degree angle to the first "S" pattern, refolded, and rubber over the surface a third time, in the same direction as the first. The wipe was then folded and placed in a clean labeled Zip-Loc™ bag. To reduce possible cross-contamination, the disposable gloves were discarded after each sample.

The HUD procedure has also been modified for use in industrial situations (NIOSH, 1991*b*). One modification is as follows: A flat surface of about 1 ft^2 was measured and disposable gloves were donned. Taking a baby wipe from its container and folding the wipe in half, the entire area was wiped using a series of horizontal strokes in an "S" pattern without lifting the wipe. Refolding the wipe with the dust side in, the area was rewiped in an "S" pattern a second time at a 90-degree angle to the first pattern. Folding the wipe again, the area was wiped yet a third time in an "S" pattern at a 90-degree angle to the previous pattern. The folded baby wipe was then placed in a sealed plastic bag. Care was taken to use the same technique and wiping pressure for each sample to reduce variation in collection efficiency. As usual, a fresh disposable glove was used for each surface.

Lioy-Weisel-Wainman Quantitative Surface Sampler

A flat surface wipe sampler has been developed to quantitatively measure the concentration (μg/g) and surface loading (μg/cm^2) of dust on flat surfaces (Lioy, Wainman, and Weisel, 1993). The Lioy-Weisel-Wainman (LWW) sampler has been tested under conditions that controlled particle deposition in a chamber for two types of particles—road dust and potting soil—and for three different types of surfaces—painted shelving, formica, and wood paneling. The results for replicate analyses demonstrated that the sampler had greater than 90% efficiency for the capture of deposited dust. The LWW wipe sampler consists of two sections, a template and movable plate-filter retainer. It uses a template to map a specific area for the quantitative collection of dust and to control the movement of a collection plate. The moveable plate traces the rectangular opening within the template. The filter media used to sample a surface is a ragged polyethylene drain disc material that is cut into rectangles of 3.8 cm × 6.35 cm. Self-closing forceps are used when handling the filters.

Procedure

1. Select a flat nonporous area to be sampled and place the precleaned template with the silicon padding facing down on the surface.
2. Place a clean, uncontaminated work surface, such as aluminum foil, near the sampling location.
3. Place the filter retainer frame and block on the work surface. The notches in the frame should face down.
4. Select the filter set to be used to collect the sample.
5. Carefully unfold the aluminum foil that contains the filter set. If any foil tears off, be sure to collect the pieces and wrap them in the foil with the filters after collecting the sample.
6. Using the forceps, remove the filters from the aluminum foil and place them along with the foil on the work surface.
7. Pick up one of the filters by its edge.
8. Place the filter into the frame so the filter edges are touching the sides of the frame and the fold is facing down.
9. Continue to hold the filter edge with the forceps.
10. With your other hand, attach the red handle to the filter retainer block using the Velcro and match the lines on the block to the lines on the frame.
11. Gently press the block down on top of the filter and into the frame until it is flush with the work surface. The edges of the filter should be clamped between the block and the frame.
12. Release the filter from the forceps.
13. Remove the handle from the block.
14. Pick up the unit and gently press down onto the block until it snaps into the frame.
15. Wet the filter with type 1 reagent water by either dipping it into a petri dish filled with water or by applying the water with a wash bottle.
16. Shake the unit gently several times to remove excess water.
17. Place the filter wet side down on the surface at one end of the template. The sides of the block covered by the filter should be aligned along the length of the template.
18. With little or no vertical pressure applied to the block, slide the filter unit across the length of the template, stopping approximately 1 inch from the opposite end.

19. Lift the filter unit a few millimeters off of the surface and place it down at the edge of the template opposite from the starting position. (Sliding the filter unit completely to the end may push dust to the extreme edge of the template, making it difficult to recover.)
20. Slide the filter unit back across the length of the template, stopping approximately 1 inch from starting position.
21. Lift the filter unit a few millimeters off of the surface and place it down at the edge of the template, returning it to the starting position.
22. Repeat steps 17 through 20 twice so that the filter is passed back and forth over the sampling area a total of three times.
23. Turn the filter unit upside down and hold it over the aluminum foil that the filters were wrapped in.
24. Using thumb and index finger, grab the exposed edges of the block and slide the block and filter out of the frame.
25. Remove the filter from the block using the forceps and place it on the aluminum foil wrapping.
26. Repeat steps 7 through 24 for the remaining two filters.
27. Carefully fold the filters in half and wrap them in the aluminum foil. Prior to weighing and analyzing, the samples must be stored in a refrigerator.
28. Place the sample in a plastic bag for transport with the first filter dust side up and subsequent filters with the dust side toward the previously used filters.

Gauze and Cotton Ball Methods

Gauze has been used to sample for PCBs, TCDDs, chlorophenols, and pesticides. In a study by Oatman and Roy (1986), double-layered gauze strips (2 in. by 4 in.) were cut from individually wrapped gauze pads. The strips underwent solvent extraction to remove existing contaminants and were then put into hexane-rinsed, disposable test tubes (16 mm by 100 mm). The tubes were identified by numbers and capped with aluminum foil.

A template (10 cm by 10 cm) was used to outline the surface area to be sampled. A fresh, disposable latex glove was placed on one hand of the sampler. The treated gauze was removed from the test tube with hexane-rinsed forceps, wrapped into a wad around the forceps tips with the gloved hand, and moistened with hexane. The sample was taken by wiping the complete area within the template with a horizontal motion and then with a vertical motion. The completed sample was returned to the test tube and sealed with aluminum foil. Field blanks were obtained by following the above procedure with the exception that the hexane-moistened gauze wad was held on the forceps tips for 10 seconds before being replaced in the test tube. All surface wipe samples were collected by the same individual and stored in a refrigerator until analyzed. Prior to analysis, the gauze wipes were warmed to room temperature.

Cotton balls are generally used for smooth surfaces such as stainless steel and Formica. A pair of clean disposable plastic gloves is used for the collection of each sample. An example procedure would be to use a pipette to wet cotton balls with up to 2 mL of solvent and then swabbing the surfaces in two directions. The areas are then swabbed a second time using dry cotton balls, and both swabs are placed in vials, sealed, and retained for analysis.

Alternatively, the balls can be dipped in the solvent or placed inside a vial and allowed to become saturated with the solvent. After saturation, the cotton balls are removed from the solvent with sterile forceps, placed against the top of the vial, and squeezed with the forceps to remove a portion of the excess solvent. If excess solvent is deliberately retained, care must be used to squeeze it out during wiping. After sampling, the balls are placed in vials.

Swab Methods

This method is similar to that used for leak testing radiation sources. Analysis of these samples is qualitative, but will reflect the general degree of surface contamination. Cotton swabs with wooden stems work best. This technique has been used to collect explosives such as dinitrotoluene (DNT), trinitrotoluene (TNT), and RDX (EPA, 1985). An advantage of this technique is that solvents can be used since the swab is a small surface area and the hands do not touch the surface. This should not be confused with another method called swabbing, which is skin washing with gauze pads (see Chapter 12).

Procedure (Roxbury, 1985)

1. Use nanograde quality solvents. For pesticides, acetone with pesticide grade hexane in a 1:4 acetone/hexane ratio has been used. Acetone has been used for explosives. Place the solvent in a glass stoppered glass jar for transport to the site. At the site, put a small amount of the solvent into a scintillation vial. Assemble 10-mL test tubes with Teflon-lined screw caps.
2. Using a cotton swab with a wooden stem, wipe off a square area of approximately 0.24 M^2 on the surface to be sampled. If sampling an area of known contamination, select an area of 4 $in.^2$ in the center of the contamination. A grid is useful as a guide. Mark the spots that were sampled.
3. While holding a swab by the wooden tip, saturate it in 20–30 mL of the solvent from the large bottle. With the swab, continue wiping the sampling area back and forth in a vertical direction applying moderate pressure. Wipe several times. Turn over the swab and wipe back and forth in a horizontal direction.
4. Wrap each swab in aluminum foil and place the wrapped swab in a clean, labeled test tube with a Teflon-lined lid, and screw the cap down.
5. When all circles have been swabbed, dip a swab into the solvent, wrap it in foil, and put it into a jar labeled "blank."
6. Preserve the collected samples and blank at 4°C in a refrigerated box.

Procedure for Q-Tips

1. Alternatively, mark five 2-in. (5-cm)-diameter circles distributed at the four corners and center of a 1-M^2 area for building surfaces, or one 2-in. (5-cm)-diameter circle for vents and other surfaces.
2. Dip a Q-tip in the small scintillation vial of solvent and swab one circle at a time, dipping the Q-tip in the solvent before and after each circle.
3. When all circles have been swabbed, tightly seal the small vial with a Teflon-lined cap and discard the used swab. This bottle is the sample.
4. Preserve the collected samples and blank at 4°C in a refrigerated box.

Static Surface Sampling Pressure Method

Static or touch sampling works well for wet surfaces, especially when surfaces are rough or the sampling media are delicate and may tear during wiping (Fenske, Horstman, and Bentley, 1987). One method is to use Whatman No. 1 cellulose filter disks (42.5 mm) and place them on a surface for 1 minute under a 300-gram weight. When used to sample wet pentachlorophenol-treated lumber, the filter disks were placed into 15-mL screw cap culture tubes containing 10 mL of 0.1 N NaOH to leach the contaminant from the filter. Another method is to place the filter in contact with the wet surface, pick it up, and place it in contact with another part of the surface until the same area is covered from which a wipe sample would collect, such as 100 cm^2.

Hand Press Methods

Cotton Gloves

Hand press methods are an attempt to make a surface sampling method that replicates the degree of exposure to the human hand. Natural cotton jersey gloves, preextracted with hexane, are used in the hand press test to screen for contaminants in house dust (Roberts and Camann, 1989). The surface area of the hands of the sampling technician is determined prior to the test. The gloves, worn over a clean pair of powderless surgeon's gloves, were pressed 100 times into a dust-spiked piece of carpet. Each hand press consisted of simultaneously placing both hands on the surface and leaning from the shoulders over the hands for approximately 2 sec. Gloves should be included as blanks. It was determined that for the detection limits required for the various pesticides for which analysis was conducted, the cotton gloves press test would be able to screen for moderate pesticide levels in dust down to about 1 ppm. A high volume pump and filter cassette or similar sampling system would be required for greater sensitivity or to collect a larger sample for multiple tests or bioassays.

Bare Hand Press

A variation of the cotton glove method is the use of a bare hand to collect a sample from a surface. This method is only applicable for contaminants that are of low toxicity or are poor skin penetrants. Bare hand presses have been used to identify surface contamination from house dusts contaminated with pesticides (Lewis, Fortmann, and Camann, 1991). A template can be used to identify the sampling area. One person is often used to perform all hand presses in a single survey. Careful precleaning of the hand with soap and water is essential. It must dry for several minutes. Then it is pressed palm down repeatedly for sample collection progressing from one end of the template to the other. The number of presses used to sample a surface has varied from 10 to 100 times for each sample in different studies. It can be useful to have the sampling person practice applying a uniform pressure by pressing on a scale covered with aluminum foil to achieve a uniform pressure each time (such as 12 lb).

After pressings over the sampling surface, the hand is carefully rinsed into a clean sample bottle with 70 mL of 2-propanol or other solvent. (For more information on skin washing methods see Chapter 12.) The number of hand presses that can be performed in a day is limited because removal of the oils from the hand by the solvent is a concern. The selection of the bare hand press as a method must be done with care. It is best used in situations where the nature of the contaminant and its concentration are well known. Collection of material from the hand must be done promptly (within 2 to 3 minutes) to avoid absorption (and loss) of some sampled contaminants through the skin. A comparison of the bare hand press (followed by an isopropanol/water rinse) with wipe sampling and the polyurethane foam (PUF) roller technique found that the hand method removes less pesticide residue from carpets than either the PUF roller or wipe sampling (Fenske and Lu, 1992). The PUF roller method is described in a section later in this chapter.

Shipping and Analysis of Samples

Shipping surface samples containing solvents may be a problem and may delay receipt at the laboratory from normal air times. For example, hexane, which is used to sample PCBs, is highly flammable and cannot be shipped by air. If shipped in uncontaminated vials that are the proper size, wipes can be extracted in the same vial.

ADHESIVE SAMPLING

Cloth tape, labels, and cellophane tape with adhesive backings have all been used for sample collection. There has also been some discussion that adhesive cloths might be useful as pads or other collectors. Adhesive collectors were found to be more efficient for collecting surface samples from plywood than filter paper wipes (Chavalitnitikul, Levin, and Chen, 1984). Cellophane tape works well for fibers and has been used for both fiberglass and asbestos.

Adhesive Labels

Adhesive labels have been used to sample surfaces for dust containing lead in houses (Lepow, 1975). Preweighed self-adhesive labels (Avery #5615, 1⁄16 in. by 3.5 in., 21.5 cm^2) were equilibrated for 24 hours before sampling and following sampling before the total weight was recorded. A label was usually pressed once on a single area, although it was often necessary to press several times on a given area to obtain a single sample.

Pebbles and paint chips were avoided or removed. The sample was placed in a wax bag, stored away from the sun to prevent dehydration, and delivered to the laboratory within two to three days. Information was kept as to the exact location of the samples. The labels were ashed digested with acid and filtered prior to analyses on an atomic absorption spectrometer.

Collection of Tape Samples

The primary use of tape methods is to assess surface contamination of dusts, primarily in the asbestos industry, although the methodology was developed to collect dust for environmental and forensic purposes (Nichols, 1985). Vinyl-coated paper tape has been used to collect metals on surfaces (NIOSH, October 1990). These samples are then wet-ashed and diluted with nitric and perchloric acids, filtered, and analyzed by the same NIOSH method as air samples. The advantage of cellophane tape when used for residual asbestos dust is that the tape can be mounted directly on a slide and inspected under a phase contrast microscope.

Prior to the implementation of this technology, the primary means for determining if surface contamination was present was a visual inspection of surfaces and equipment. Sticky tape sampling has also been used to collect beryllium dusts from surfaces (Routledge, 1968).

Between 1987 and 1989, 244 samples were collected from the equipment of 13 different work crews (Beaulieu, 1991). Typical equipment sampled included respirators and related equipment such as belts, boots, hoses (air and water), and quick disconnect fittings (Fig. 7-6). Sampling was also performed on the decontamination units, air movers, flexible ducting, vacu-

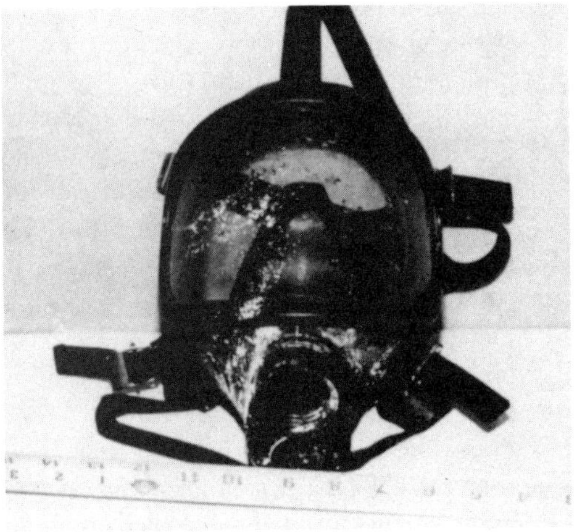

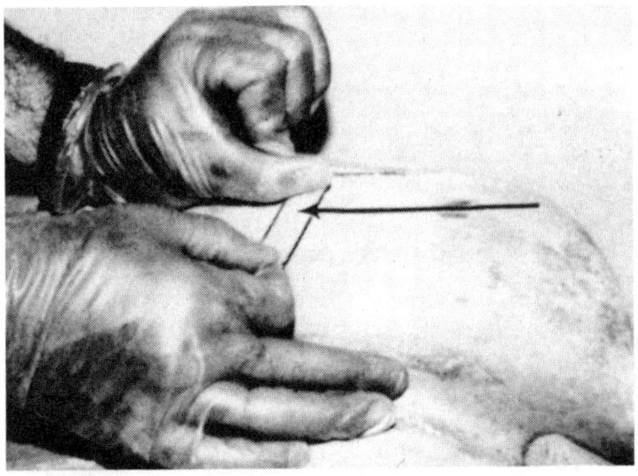

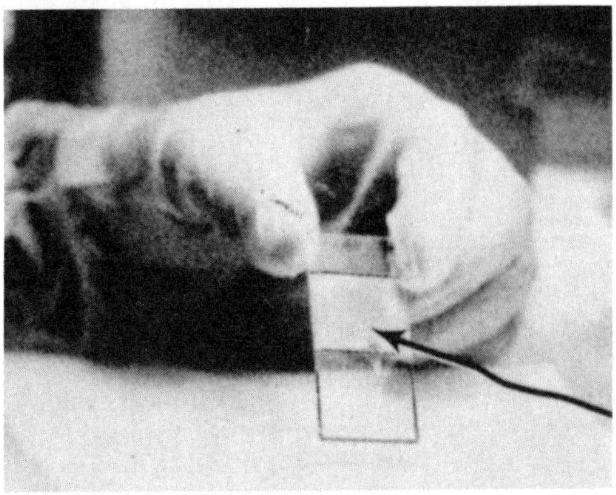

Figure 7-6. *Above:* Front view of a full face respirator with readily visible, heavy, friable asbestos surface contamination (white spots). *Top right:* Collection of a strip tape sample on the surface of a scoop shovel. *Right:* A portion of the cellophane tape sample mounted in oil on the surface of a second microscope slide. This sample is ready for optical microscopic analysis.
Source: All three illustrations from H. J. Beaulieu. 1992. Asbestos contamination of abatement equipment surfaces. *Appl. Occup. Env. Hyg.* 6(7):583–587.

ums, shovels, ladders, scaffolding, and even air sampling pumps. Analysis of the tape for asbestos was performed via polarized light microscopy. Results were expressed as a type and percentage of asbestos fibers of the total surface contamination (e.g., 30% amosite). The analytical procedure involves placing refractive index oil with one layer of oil underneath the tape and one layer on top of the tape.

Procedure

1. Prepare strip tape slides in a noncontaminated area by placing a clean strip of cellophane tape (2 cm by 8 cm), sticky side down, onto a clean slide. A tab is made on the end of the tape to allow for labeling and handling (to pull the tape away from the slide for sampling).
2. Before sampling, place a sample number of the tab of the tape on the slide. Don single-use, surgical latex gloves.
3. Select a sampling site and remove the piece of tape from the slide and touch the sampling surface with the sticky side down several times. A 10-cm square surface area has been shown to be effective.
4. After each surface sample, the tape is then pressed back onto the slide, sticky side down, in preparation for analysis. The tape is then replaced on the surface of its slide. The completed sample slide should be placed into a clean, zip lock bag for transport to the laboratory.
5. A sampling data sheet must be completed, logging the sampling location, date, and other pertinent information.

Surface Sampling Strips

Surface sampling strips, such as those available from RJ Lee (Fig. 7-7A), are an example of a commercially prepared kit used to collect particulate from most surfaces such as floors, walls, duct work, furniture, and other surfaces typically sampled using conventional techniques. The strips are then sent back to the manufacturer where they are analyzed using specially developed techniques. Each sampling strip consists of a single-sided adhesive sampling surface and a tab portion with a label. The sampling surface is on the labeled tab side. The tab portion is to be used for handling purposes only and is not part of the sampling medium. A kit comes with applicators and ampoules containing activator solutions, practice strips, plastic bags, sample boxes, and a set of directions.

Procedure

1. Remove the applicator and activator ampoule from the plastic bag. Snip or cut the tip of the activator ampoule and apply the solution across the surface of the applicator (Fig. 7-7*B*).
2. Carefully remove the sampling strip from the box, close the box, and place the strip (label side up) on the top of the closed box so that the lid surface can be used for the activation process.
3. While grasping the tabbed end of the sampling strip with one hand, place the applicator lightly on the strip and quickly pull the sampling strip past the applicator to activate the specially formulated adhesive surface. Do not press the applicator too hard (Fig. 7-7C). The objective is to make the adhesive tacky, not wet.
4. Quickly place the tacky surface face down on the area to be sampled. This should be done within 5–10 sec of activation.
5. Press down firmly, running your finger over the entire adhesive area for about 3–5 sec while keeping hold of the tabbed end.
6. Remove the sampling strip with an upward motion similar to removing a Band-Aid. Return the strip to the original box with the tacky side up and the tabbed end protruding from one side of the box (Fig. 7-7*D*). Place the box in the plastic bag provided.
7. Discard the applicator and empty ampoule.
8. Return the plastic bags with media strips enclosed to the manufacturer.

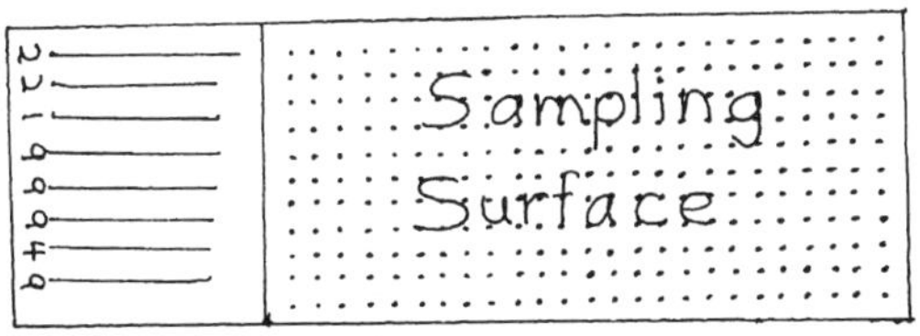

Figure 7-7A. RJ Lee Group surface sampling strip consisting of a single-sided adhesive sampling surface and a tab portion with a label.

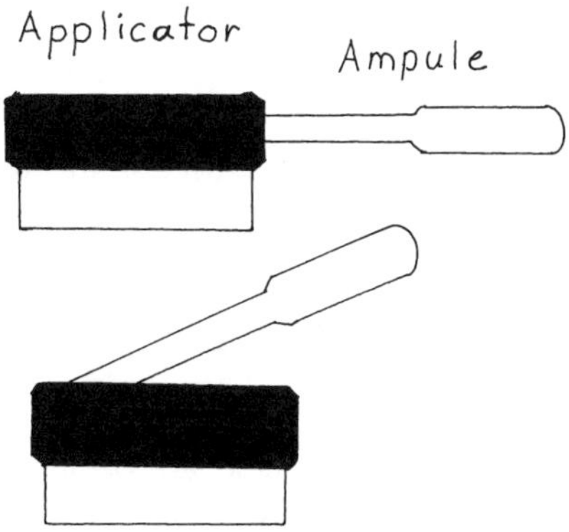

Figure 7-7B. Applicator and ampule from the RJ Lee Group surface sampling strip kit.

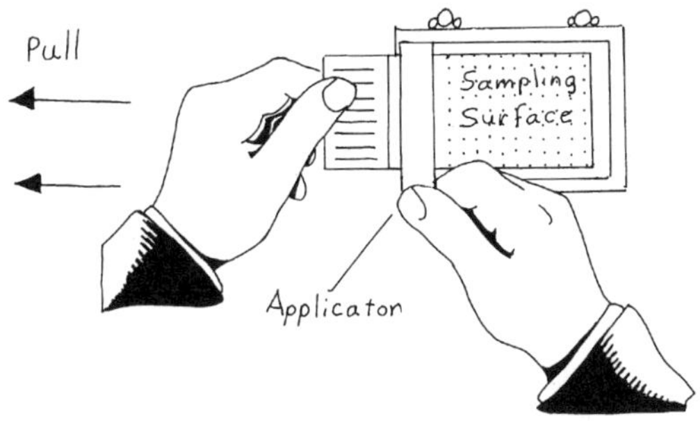

Figure 7-7C. Activating the adhesive surface of the RJ Lee Group surface sampling strip.

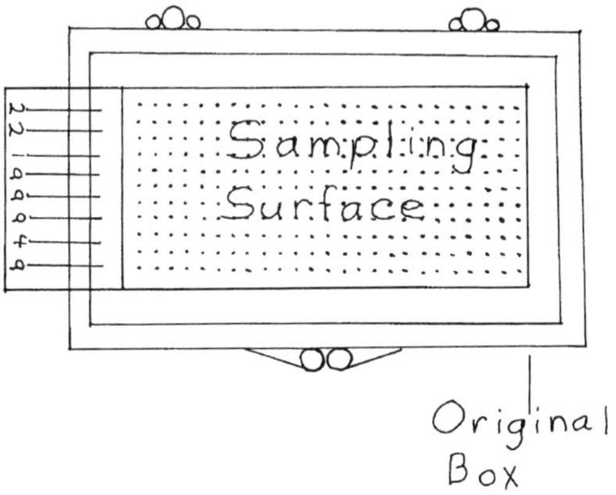

Figure 7-7D. Storing a used RJ Lee Group surface sampling strip in its original box.

Other Sticky Surfaces

Dusts settled on horizontal surfaces can be sampled with sticky gelatinous foils (Schneider et al., 1990). Double sided tape has also been affixed to surfaces in residences (Weschler, 1978). After several days of exposure to estimate the settling rate of the dust, the tapes were transferred to specimen mounts and examined under a scanning electron microscope. Another variation uses 30 cm by 40 cm glass plates that have been greased by pouring a mixture of paraffin and petroleum ether 40/60 on them and allowing the petroleum ether to evaporate (Diemel et al., 1981). The plates were placed in the living rooms of the houses, at a height of approximately 2 M, usually on cupboards. Three continuous samples of 28 days were taken. After sampling, the paraffin plus collected dust was removed by rinsing the plates with petroleum ether 40/60. The suspensions were centrifuged at 4,000 rpm for 5–10 min. After decanting the paraffin/petroleum ether mixture, the dust was resuspended in petroleum ether and collected on a preweighed cellulose filter. The centrifugation-resuspension step was necessary to avoid irreversible paraffin uptake by the cellulose filters.

LEACHING METHODS

Rough surfaces may be sampled using the leaching method. The compound of interest is leached from the surface with solvent impregnated filter paper (Weeks, Dean, and Yasuda, 1976). For aromatic amines, a filter paper is placed on the surface and five drops of methanol (or other appropriate solvent) are applied to the paper's center. The paper is kept in intimate contact with the surface until it dries. It is then removed and a visualization reagent is applied (to the surface of paper facing down) by streaking from one edge of the filter paper to the other edge. After a suitable reaction period, the paper is examined for color formation.

VACUUMING METHODS

Vacuum methodologies have become an important aspect of surface sampling especially for collecting residential samples, and, therefore, the methodologies have been refined at least as much as those for wipe sampling, if not more. Vacuum methods include the HVS3, an elaborate aparatus developed under an EPA contract; the Sirchee-Spittler variation of the Dustbuster; the "blue nozzle," a specialized collecting head attached to a vacuum pump; and the Cincinnati DVM portable air sampling pump and cassette. For all of these methods, accurate characterizations of particle size and cut point are important.

Some vacuum methods have been used to sample smooth, hard surfaces, such as wooden floors and paving; however, vacuum methods are more effective for sampling carpets than filter wiping methods. Vacuum sampling is sometimes called "surface sweeps." In some cases, a bulk sample of dust from a household vacuum is collected. The amount of information that can be gained from this type of sample is very limited because there is no information on the period in which the dust collected, the area in which it was collected, or the size of the sampled area. Therefore these samples are useful for screening purposes only.

The advantages of vacuum methods include the collection of adequately sized samples providing enough material for detailed analyses; larger sample volumes allowing for more repetitions during sampling, providing better sample area coverage; the direct comparison of indoor dust concentrations to those in outdoor soil; and the ability to obtain dust loading, analyte surface loading, and concentration data. Disadvantages can include the collection of dust that is inaccessible (and, therefore, nonrepresentative) for exposure; variable sampling efficiency between devices and for different surfaces; the requirement of sampling apparatus that is more costly than typical wipe media; and the need for more sampling time (including time to clean and decontaminate the devices in between samples). Table 7-8 describes different vacuum methods.

All vacuum setups need to be checked carefully for leaks at connections. Vacuum samplers must be cleaned between samples, which is time consuming. Elbows on larger units can be difficult to clean, although tongue depressors can help. The larger diameter on the sampling tube of the vacuum samplers reduces plugging, but it also increases sampling time. Also, although larger inlets are easier to use, they cannot get into corners on window wells and other cramped areas. The length of time required to collect a sample can increase significantly if a house is clean. In one instance it took almost 1.5 hours to collect a 2 g sample in a house (EPA, 1990).

When vacuum methods are used to collect samples from carpets, a fresh collector is usually used for each room or sample. Although some units have been configured with filter cassettes, a tared Teflon bottle is preferable as a collection container. However, taring entire cassettes or bottles creates the problem of avoiding deposition of skin oils during handling, and therefore clean fresh gloves are required during field handling. The bottles can build up a static charge if shaken a lot during shipment.

Samples are often screened through a 1 mm sieve to remove objects such as twigs, glass frag-

TABLE 7-8. Vacuum Sampling Methods

Method	*Surface Type*	*Type of Vacuum*	*Flow Rate/ Collection Time*	*Sampling Procedure*	*Sampling Collector*	*Particle Sizes*	*Reference*
DVM (Univ. of Cincinnati)	Carpeted or bare floor	Personal air sampling pump and tubing (3 mm)	2 L/min	Three passes over a 22 × 22 cm area	Preweighed 37 mm MCE filter in cassette with a 45° nozzle in front		Que Hee et al., 1985
DVM (three-city study)	Hard	Personal air sampling pump and tubing (1.3 cm)	2.5 L/min/1.5–2 sec/stroke	Pass 1: L → R covering entire 25 × 25 cm area. Pass 2: F → B. Pass 3: L → R.	Preweighed polycellulose acetate (0.8 μm) with a 45° nozzle in front		EPA, 1993
ASTM 5438.93	Carpeted	HVS3 upright vacuum cleaner with a nozzle, cyclone cm), butterfly valve, pump, collection bottle and filter bag	20 ft^3/min. (16 ft^3/min with PUF plug)/10 min	Template/area: 0.5 m to 1.5 m in length, 13 cm wide. Make four double passes at 0.5 m/sec over each area until sufficient sample is collected	Cyclone with a 200 g capacity with or without PUF plug	0.5 μm and >	ASTM, 1993
Modified HVS3	Carpeted or bare floor	Canister vacuum cleaner with 16 in. nozzle with a flared, serrated end and a 14.5 in. cyclone	2 min.	Pass 1: L → R covering entire 1 ft^2 area with 50% overlap. Pass 2: F → B.	Preweighed Teflon liners (100 mL)	0.5 μm and >	EPA, 1992*a*
MRI Cyclone	Hard or soft	Canister vacuum cleaner with a 1 in. PVC pipe nozzle and cyclone	1 ft^2/2 min	Overlapping passes of 1 ft^2 area rotating nozzle 180° during procedure.	37 mm cassette or collection bottle	1–2,000 μm	EPA, 1992*b*

Source: From EPA. 1994. The National Human Exposure Assessment Survey (NHEXSUS) Workshop. Research Triangle Park, NC: U.S. Environmental Protection Agency.
Notes: L → R = left to right and F → B = front to back.

ments, insects, and paper, and then through a 150 μm sieve prior to analysis. The higher flow rates on the larger vacuums bias the samples for smaller particles while the lower flow rate of the personal air sampling pump induces a bias toward collection of larger size particles. Samples using different types of vacuum methods may be difficult to compare because of differences in flow rates and the presence or absence of agitators.

Personal Sampling Pump Method

The personal air sampling pump and filter cassette method has been standardized and is often referred to as the University of Cincinnati (DVM) method. The sampling pump is attached with Tygon tubing (3 mm internal diameter) to a 37 mm diameter three-stage cassette with a 0.8 μm MCE or other filter inside. A crimped stainless steel tube or clean plastic nozzle is attached to the inlet side of the filter cassette with Tygon tubing. A 25 × 25 cm area is sampled using three passes over the surface both horizontally and vertically taking 2 seconds for each. Flow rates range from 2 Lpm to 3 Lpm. In general, this method is limited to the collection of stable pesticides and metals.

The small size of the opening to the filter cassette can plug up frequently during sampling. Therefore the use of a clear plastic nozzle allows the sampler to see when the nozzle is plugged with dust or other material. If the nozzle plugs, the material is pushed into the sample cassette with a small pointed object and sampling continues. Plastic nozzles can generally be disposed of while stainless steel nozzles are expensive and therefore need to be decontaminated so they can be reused.

A more general method has a piece of Tygon tubing attached to the front of the cassette. A 45-degree angle is the best for the end of the tubing because it has been found to provide the best collection efficiency. (The flexibility of Tygon is an advantage over other tubing such as polypropylene and Teflon because it allows inaccessible surfaces such as windowsills, corners, and ledges to be sampled as well as floors and other large flat surfaces.) The thumb should be kept on the spine of the tubing and the tube should always be moved in one direction, usually across the widest portion from left to right (if right-handed). A variation involves placing a plastic disposable syringe tip in front of the cassette as a vacuum nozzle rather than a piece of Tygon tubing. The syringe tip is changed each time a sample is collected.

The portable air sampling pump method can also be prone to inlet losses. The shape and angle of the inlet affect sampling efficiency. It is difficult to get good reproducibility in area coverage from sample to sample. Tared cassettes require special handling in the field. There is no reliable spiking method available to use for cassettes for field use. Problems have also occurred from cross-sample contamination due to inadequate cleaning of the inlet and tubing between samples. Because of the low sampling flow rate and static electricity forces, dust tends to cling to the side of the cassette. This condition makes it difficult to accurately reweigh the filter and often requires that cassettes be washed prior to analyses.

The type of surface also has a significant impact on sampling efficiency for this vacuuming method. Surfaces ranging from wood to textured linoleum to different types of carpet have been tested. Smooth surfaces can be sampled with a stainless steel sampling tube because its sampling geometry and the surface are relatively constant. If a surface has cracks, steep depressions, or corrugations, such as some windowsills, then Tygon tubing should be used due to its flexibility. Just as for wipes, repeating the motion of the vacuum over the same surface can increase efficiency.

A comparison of the personal air sampling pump filter cassette method and the wipe test was performed on floors of residences with lead dust contamination. The wipe method yielded higher results on floors. However, the vacuum method was considered suitable for use on carpets and upholstered furniture (Menrath, Clark, and Bornschein, 1992).

General Procedure

1. Calibrate a personal air sampling pump at 2 Lpm. Attach a tube and a filter in a 37 mm cassette. Depending on the analysis, the type

of filter will vary. Another short length of tubing is attached to the inlet of the cassette.

2. Start the pump and use the exposed end of the second piece of tubing like a vacuum cleaner.
3. Move the sample collector through the work area, stopping at 10 sites or more that represent the most likely places where dust might collect. Each sampled spot should be marked with an "X" on a diagram, and the specific area should be described on a list, such as windowsill, left sleeve, cuff, top of pipe.
4. The amount of time spent sampling each site will be determined by filter loading. If the dust is readily visible, the filter will rapidly become loaded.

High Volume Vacuum

The HVS3 is a high volume surface sampler designed to collect samples of surface dust (Fig. 7-8). It was developed to measure pesticides in house dust. It is a high-powered vacuum cleaner equipped with a nozzle that can be adjusted to a specific static pressure and air flow rate. The dust goes to a cyclone that removes particles greater than 5 μm from the air stream for collection in a bottle. Use of this sampler is limited to floors or other large flat surfaces because it cannot reach small or uneven areas such as windows and upholstery.

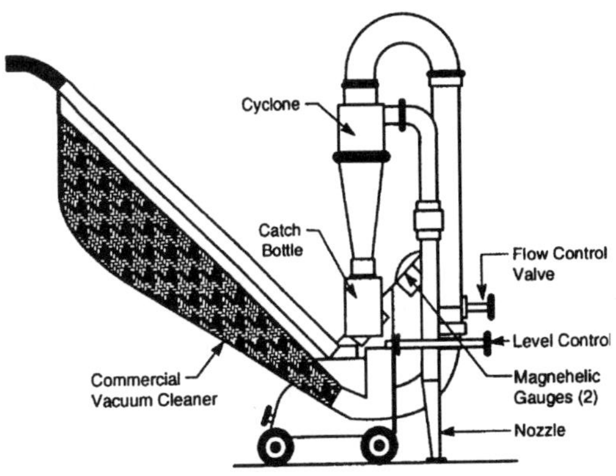

Figure 7-8. The HVS3 carpet dust sampler. *Source:* R. G. Lewis, R. C. Fortmann, and D. E. Camann. 1994. Evaluation of methods for monitoring the potential exposure of small children to pesticides in the residential environment. *Arch. Env. Contam. Toxicol.* **26**:37–46.

This vacuum method has had problems with inlet losses of sample. There is no specified pressure drop that needs to be developed across filter sampling surfaces. Flow rates are not calibrated. Tared vessels must be handled carefully to avoid contamination in the field. It is difficult to obtain good reproducible area coverage between samples. There is no reliable spiking method for field spikes. The type of sampling surface has a significant impact on sampling efficiency.

The sampling procedure calls for laying out eight 46 cm by 137 cm (18 in. by 54 in.) folding frame rectangles, securing them with masking tape, setting the HVS3 flow rate and nozzle pressure drop, sampling four of these rectangles, and continuing the sampling for the other four if less than 2 grams of material have been collected. Because the HVS3 overhangs the sampling area and some maneuvering room is required behind the sampled area, occasionally the marked sampling areas do not have sufficient clearance. Sometimes the masking tape is difficult to remove. In these instances, furniture has to be moved. Between runs, the HVS3 must be cleaned using brushes and a mixed solvent (acetone: hexane, 50:50) rinse over the entire sampling train between the nozzle and the PUF plug holder.

The blue nozzle dust collector has been piloted in certain HUD studies and consists of three major units: the (blue) nozzle, a vacuum pump, and a filter cassette to collect the dust. The specially designed angle-cut blue Teflon nozzle fits over the cassette with "O" rings to seal it. The sampling rate is 16 Lpm. Tubing interconnects these components and a vacuum gauge is connected to the pump to provide a means to monitor the vacuum. The large nozzle (4" × 12") allows samples to be collected faster than with the personal air sampling pump. This device is still under study.

ASTM Method for Collecting Dust from Carpeted Floors

The American Society for Testing and Materials (ASTM) method for the collection of carpet-embedded dust is applicable to a variety of carpeted surfaces, such as home carpets, and has been tested for level loop and plush pile carpets specifically (ASTM, 1993). The sampling apparatus is essentially the HVS3 vacuum, which was developed for the EPA. While there have been some variations on this device, the ASTM method specifically limits the specifications for a proper vacuum. The dimensions of the nozzle size, cyclone diameter, cyclone inlet diameter, and so forth must be such that the vacuum can produce a flow rate that will provide a cut diameter of 5 μm at the same velocity that will provide a horizontal velocity of 40 cm/sec at 10 mm from the nozzle in carpet material. While this requirement allows for some variation in design, the edges and corners of the sampling nozzle must be rounded to prevent catching the carpet material, and gaskets in joints must be made of material that will not absorb sampled materials. Cyclones must be made of aluminum or stainless steel and the catch bottle must be made of clear glass or fluorinated ethylene propylene. The suction source can be any commercial vacuum as long as it is capable of drawing 12 Lps through the system with all components connected.

One method for assuring a defined sampling area is to use measuring tapes placed parallel to each other on the carpet. The measuring tapes should be between 0.5 m and 1.5 m apart and extended as far as practical. Masking tape is used to hold them in place.

The wheels and nozzle tip should be cleaned with laboratory tissue immediately prior to sampling. The nozzle is moved between the two measuring tapes starting at the end. It should be moved at approximately 0.5 m/sec back and forth four times for each strip. The nozzle is then angled over to the second strip on the next pass and four more double passes are performed. After a 0.5 M^2 area is sampled the bottle is checked to see how much dust has been collected. The ASTM estimates that a dust level of 6 mm in a 55 mm diameter catch bottle corresponds to approximately 6–8 g of sampled material. Hair, carpet fibers, and other large objects should be excluded from the sample when estimating the quantity collected.

Methanol is recommended as the decontamination agent for the vacuum in between samples.

DIRECT READING SURFACE SAMPLING METHODS

Spot Tests

Chemical spot tests have been used to identify surface contamination, usually after first stage decontamination has taken place (Weeks and Dean, 1978). These tests involve a color change if a positive reaction occurs and are usually specific for certain chemical groups or substances such as metals and aromatic amines. These tests have been particularly successful with porous surfaces, which cannot be efficiently sampled with wipe samples. The level of difficulty ranges from rubbing a cartridge that is squeezed beforehand to mix chemicals to adding drops of various reagents in sequence in the field.

Reagents can be dropped directly onto a surface or the surface can be wiped with a filter and the test performed on the filter. Both methods have advantages and drawbacks. A permanent discoloration on a floor in a production area may not be a problem, but in an office it is likely to be undesirable. Many reagents used for spot testing are toxic and their use on eating surfaces may pose a problem requiring decontamination after testing. Filters may not remove all surface contamination and the contaminant may be diluted if a solvent is used. Also solvents other than water must be compatible with the spot testing reagents.

During surveys it is a good idea to photograph surfaces on which spot testing is performed, including the results. Metals such as lead and chromium VI can be sampled using these tests. For information, see Appendix B.

Colorimetric Surface Swypes

Surface "swypes" are sold by CLI Colorimetric Laboratories. They are absorbent pads impregnated with colorimetric reagent indicators to provide a visual determination of contamination on work surfaces and skin. A color indication within 2–3 minutes of placing the wipe in solvent is a positive determination. The solvent is drawn up through the pad via capillary

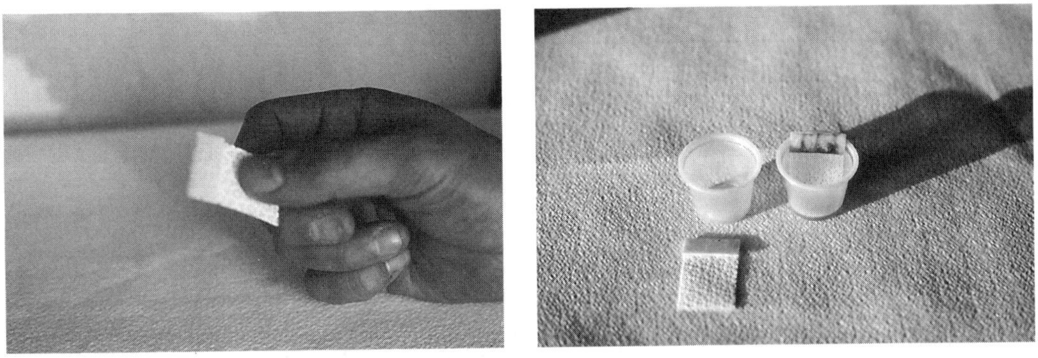

Figure 7-9. Amine CLI swipe: held in hand ready to sample (*left*) and development of sample (*right*).
Source: Both illustrations from CLI Colorimetric Labs.

action concentrating the contamination in the colorimetric detection zone. A clear, plastic backing on the pad allows for the attachment of a handle and prevents the solution from contacting the user's skin. Also, when the front surface of the pad is obscured by dirt from the sampling environment, the color indication can be viewed from the back of the pad. One medium is utilized, which changes to a different color depending on what amine has been detected. Swype kits are available for aromatic amines (Fig. 7-9) and aromatic isocyanates such as methylene bisphenyl isocyanate (MDI) and toluene diisocyanate (TDI).

pH Paper

Acids and bases (or alkalis) can be detected by their reaction with pH paper. For example, ammonia and amines are very basic and can be detected by a high pH; however, pH paper should not be used in lieu of some of the amine specific methods described in Appendix A. This method can also be used as a first identification if an unknown spill is detected. Acids turn litmus paper blue, and bases turn it pink.

Fluorescence

For compounds that have natural fluorescence, ultraviolet (UV) light has been used to detect their contamination on surfaces. Polycyclic aromatic hydrocarbons (PAHs) are the most common and can be found in coal derived and petroleum derived oils. A handheld black light in a darkened room will indicate whether contamination is present but not how much. When surfaces are illuminated with broad spectrum UV lamps, any compounds that fluoresce will be detected; therefore, potentially harmless fluorescent materials are identified whereas nonfluorescing carcinogens are not. Another method is to use an instrument developed to detect and quantitate fluorescence. At least two have been developed and they are based on the use of a UV producing lamp, often mercury, coupled with a fluorescence detector. While there are some problems with interferents, these can be minimized. A detailed discussion on the operation of these types of instruments is included in Chapter 13.

Dislodgeable Residue Methods

Dislodgeable residue methods measure that portion of surface contamination likely to be removed by human contact. They are frequently used to sample carpets in residential studies. These studies often combine aerosol deposition measurements if the concern is the percent of overall residue that can be removed. Table 7-9 describes the most common methods and Figure 7-10 shows the PUF and Dow drag sled samplers.

Rolling methods may represent human expo-

TABLE 7-9. Dislodgeable Residue Methods

Method	*Surface Type*	*Wipe Media*	*Area*	*Sampling Procedure*	*Shipping Container*	*Reference*
Dow Drag Sled	Carpet	Denim pad or moist towelette	10 cm × length sampled	Weighted sled pulled across area in two directions.	Glass jar stored at dry ice temperature	Vaccaro and Cranston, 1990
CDFA	Carpet	17 × 17 in. percale sheet	17 × 17 in.	Weighted roller rolled over covered area 10 times.	Glass jar stored at dry ice temperature	Ross et al., 1991
PUF Roller	Carpet, bare floors, turf	Polyurethane	7.6 cm × length sampled	PUF roller pulled over area in two passes.	Glass jar stored at dry ice temperature	Hsu, Camann, and Schattenburg, 1990

Source: From EPA. 1994. The National Human Exposure Assessment Survey (NHEXSUS) Workshop. Research Triangle Park, NC: U.S. Environmental Protection Agency.

sure better than flat dragging and wiping methods. Carpet samples can be affected by RH in the room (EPA, 1994). Rooms with higher RH have produced higher recoveries from carpets sampled for pesticide residue. This condition may be due to retention of the moisture in the pesticide formulation that was applied, which would decrease binding.

PUF Roller

The PUF roller consists of a weighted roller fitted with a PUF cover that simulates the pressure applied to a surface by a crawling child weighing 9 kg/(20 lb). It was specifically developed as a dislodgeable residue sampler to estimate dermal exposure from surface contact. The precleaned dry or moistened PUF ring is secured on the 3 inch by 1.75 inch (OD) aluminum roller. The sampling areas of 800 cm^2 (8 cm by 100 cm) are outlined with a template that exposes the surface to be sampled. The PUF is dipped in distilled water and compressed to remove the excess water immediately prior to loading onto the roller. Two passes in each area should be made.

The matrix of polyurethane is more similar to skin than the media used with other devices for dislodgeable residues. The sampler can be used dry or wet or alternatively on a moist surface, and works well on both smooth and uneven surfaces including turf. When used to sample a moist surface, the transfer of material was increased, however the variability between samples also increased (EPA, 1994). Its constant pressure can simulate that of a child or adult, and samples have shown good reproducibility. The PUF hardware is expensive and must be special ordered. Dust loadings or analyte concentration in the dust cannot be determined. It cannot sample for most organic compounds. When compared to the hand press, the PUF roller technique produced similar results (Hsu, Camann, and Schattennburg, 1990).

California Department of Food and Agriculture Roller

The California Department of Food and Agriculture (CDFA) roller technique was developed to examine dermal transfer of pesticides from carpets treated with an indoor fogger. For example, a 12 kg foam-covered rolling cylinder was rolled over a percale cotton/polyester fabric (1,840 cm^2) that was placed over the area of carpet to be sampled and a plastic sheet was placed over the cloth sheet (Ross et al., 1991). The roller was rolled over the plastic/cloth/carpet sandwich 10 times. One forward push and one backward pull constituted one roll. Care was taken not to press down on the roller, which would have added extra weight. After rolling, the plastic was discarded and the cloth was care-

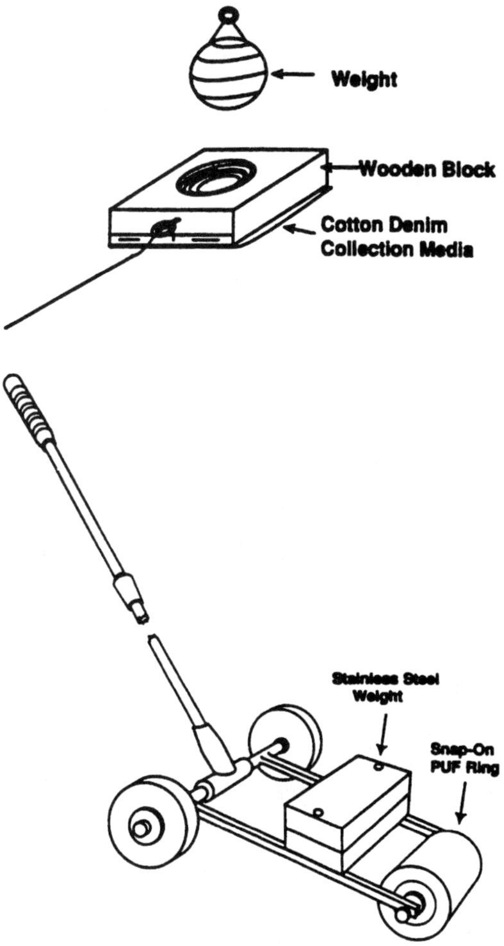

Figure 7-10. *Top:* Dow drag sled. *Bottom:* PUF roller sampling instrument.
Source: Both illustrations from D. E. Camann, H. J. Harding, S. R. Agrawal, and R. G. Lewis. 1993. Comparison of transfer of surface chlorpyrifos residues from carpet by three dislodgeable residue methods. In *Proceedings of the 1993 EPA/Air and Waste Management Association International Symposium*. Pittsburgh, PA: Air and Waste Management Association.

fully removed from the carpet and placed into a wide-mouthed quart jar. The jar was sealed with aluminum foil, capped, and placed on dry ice.

The CDFA roller samples a larger area than other dislodgeable residue samplers. The roller can be difficult to maneuver and suffers from operator bias. It is heavy and therefore difficult to transport. It is difficult to get reproducible samples due to its heavy weight. The cotton bedsheet sampling media is bulky and unlike skin. Like many other samplers, it cannot be used to determine dust loadings or analyte concentration in the dust.

When gauze pad residues were compared to the CDFA roller method, it was determined that the roller transferred approximately 1–3% of the floor residue. After comparing the carpet roller results with that of dosimeter clothing worn by subjects performing exercise on the carpets, it was indicated that the carpet roller method was a good surrogate for human exposure studies to chlorpyrifos and d-trans allethrim when applied in pesticide foggers indoors.

Dow Drag Sled

Dow Chemical designed a device called the "Dow Drag Sled" for indoor dislodgeable residue measurements. It consists of a block of plywood (3 inches by 3 inches by ¾ inch) weighted with a lead ball that exerts the approximate pressure of a 10-kg (22.5 lb) child standing or crawling. A removable denim pad is attached across the entire bottom of the block. The roller consists of a 2 foot by 4 inch diameter sewer pipe, filled with 25 lb of lead shot ballast and wrapped in a sheet of high density PUF. The path to be wiped is taped. A common size is 48 inches. When multipled by the 3-inch width of the sampler, 1 ft^2 sampling area is achieved. The sled is dragged at a rate of 6–8 cm/sec to do a single pass; twenty passes are used for each sample. The denim pad is removed and replaced after each "drag" and placed inside a container on dry ice for shipment. The Drag Sled has also been used to sample turf.

The sled is inexpensive to use, simple to operate and has shown good reproducibility. The roller is simple in design and can be assembled from materials available in most hardware stores. Its use is limited to smooth, flat surfaces. The cotton denim sampling matrix is unlike skin and it cannot be used to determine dust loading. The sampling cloth tends to bind and shift from the original position, the plastic cover can stick to the roller due to static electricity buildup, and transfer on carpet is affected by roll orientation relative to the lay of the carpet fibers (Camann et al., 1993).

SPECIAL SITUATIONS

Scraping

Occasionally situations occur where a material is released and sticks to a surface, forming a crust. In such cases, sampling the top layer (1–2 mm) of a square 0.25 M^2 area using steel hand scrapers can be useful. Steel hand scrapers are similar to the spatulas used for mortar in bricklaying. Building surfaces (except where walls are painted) respond well to this technique. It is good to collect 100–500 g of coarse dust and store the dust in clean, dark glass jars. Analysis can be done by extracting the scraping with a suitable solvent and shaking vigorously. Examples of situations where scraping is more effective than wiping include tanks with lead impregnated in their metal interiors and soot. Painted surface should be avoided.

Sampling Whole Articles

Articles such as dishware, small tools, or sample bottles on which surface contamination is suspected can be sampled using immersion and rinsing techniques. A pesticide (Paraquat) dispenser nozzle was checked for contamination by removing the container cap or cover and by inverting the container, placing the nozzle end into a glass jar containing 250 mL of distilled water (Staiff et al., 1975). The edge of the jar was sealed to the dispenser container with masking tape to prevent leakage, and the jar and container were then shaken vigorously for one minute in order to rinse contamination from the nozzle. The rinse samples were analyzed for paraquat content to determine the amount of nozzle contamination available for oral exposure.

Articles from houses such as kitchen plates have been selected for rinsing to determine if contamination from spraying or fogging of an insecticide was present (Wright and Jackson, 1974). Plates were placed in a plastic bag at varying intervals (0.2, 1, and 4 days) after treatment of the homes and were immediately sent to the laboratory for analysis. Another method used when articles have been exposed to sprays is to wipe the article with a cotton ball soaked with a solvent such as ethanol (Hattula, Wasenius, and Arstila, 1979).

Settled Dust

All processes that generate dusts or fumes and are open to the air will release some particulates that will settle on surfaces. Although settled dust samples may also be classified as a type of bulk sample, they can be useful in estimating the types of airborne exposures or for developing air sampling strategies. This type of sample can only be considered representative of surface contamination if collected from surfaces such as rafters, windowsills, and the tops of bookcases and refrigerators where their presence is not due to a spill but to the "settling out" of airborne dust and particles. Settled dust has been collected from the top of electrical switch gear boxes after a fire for TCDD analysis (NIOSH, 1986*b*).

Sampling sites often bear visual signs of dustiness. One strategy is to monitor areas not cleaned for several months; another is to collect samples from relatively inaccessible locations. It is good to observe the variations in surface dust throughout the process.

A concern with settled dust is the potential for resuspension, therefore producing inhalation dust exposures and clothing contamination. Sometimes the respirable fraction is separated out prior to analysis; however, in theory the bulk of settled dust is already less than 10 μm. Settled dust samples collected on sites such as main rafter supports are likely to reflect the composition of airborne dust accumulated since the facility was constructed. Other samples collected from unobstructed surfaces within a facility may be indicative of more recent deposition of airborne dust. Surface dust can also reflect contamination brought from the outside or other areas of a plant. The floor is common to sample in this instance. The following are typical surfaces sampled for settled dust:

Catwalks
Overhead pipelines

Ledges
Top of equipment (grinding hoods, gas generators, presses)
Door frames
Floors
Conveyor belts
Rafters
Top of circuit breaker box
Bookshelves
Tops of room dividers
Louvers of air supply vents

Dustfall is one of the oldest methods used to measure the amount of suspended dust that has settled. After sitting out for a period, such as one month, the collected dust can be weighed and a dust fall rate can be calculated. If a specific contaminant (stable, generally inorganic) such as lead is of interest, additional analyses can be performed and a lead fall rate can be calculated. Dustfall methods only look at what is transferred to the site via the air and do not capture larger particles.

A typical dustfall method uses a polyethylene bucket with a 491 cm^2 opening placed on the floor (Polissar et al., 1990). Dust has been collected for up to three calendar quarters from the bottom of the bucket by using a personal air sampling pump to vacuum it up into a filter cassette for transport to the lab. In one instance it was used to sample for arsenic contamination in homes near a copper smelter.

Another method for collecting settled dust is to use a porcelain funnel placed in a metal ring for support with a porcelain beaker placed underneath to collect the dust. This technique has been used in steel mills to collect fumes in the rolling mill plant, the coke oven, and the blast and electric furnace areas for benzo(a)pyrene analysis (Tanimura, 1968). An additional method is to remove the top of a three-stage air sampling filter cassette and allow it to stand open for a period of time. The following chemicals are frequently analyzed in settled dust:

Asbestos
Beryllium
Cadmium
Coal
Cobalt
Coke dust
Fiberglass
Fly ash
Lead
Limestone
Metals, trace
Mineral wool
Nickel
Pesticides (lindane, mirex)
Silica
Silver
Talc
Vegetable dusts

A soft paintbrush can be used to brush settled dust from smooth surfaces into glassine or zip lock envelopes. No. 5 artists' brushes previously rinsed in distilled water, ethanol, and 1,1,2-trichloro-1,2,2,-trifluoroethane were used for house dust in one study (Weschler, 1978). A different brush should be used for each sample to avoid cross-contamination.

Aerosol Deposition

Another term frequently used for samplers to collect aerosol deposition, regardless of the type of media they are composed of, is *coupons*. These methods are used primarily to verify the effectiveness (%) of (follow-up) sampling measurements for dislodgeable residues. The coupon approach is the standard approach used for setting worker reentry levels based on dislodgeable residues remaining on pesticide-treated foliage. Coupons simulating the treated surface (carpet, wood, etc.) are placed on or near the treated areas before pesticide application and collected at appropriate time intervals after application, placed in a container, and shaken in a solution of wetting agent to remove the dislodgeable residues. Filters, gauze and foam pads, mylar sheets, aluminum foil and plates, glass dishes and plates, and carpet swatches are examples of media that have been used. Gauze is considered a good estimate of the behavior of a contaminant on an absorbing surface, whereas the harder, shiny materials, such as aluminum foil and mylar, represent the behavior of a contaminant on a nonabsorbing surface (Ross et al., 1990).

If aerosol deposition is desired, total residues can also be extracted from these collectors using appropriate solvents. For dislodgeable residues, wipes of surfaces are often performed. Coupons placed prior to application allow quantitation of deposition to provide a good baseline to compare subsequent wipe samples to and determine sampling efficiency. Large differences commonly result when deposition samples are compared to wipes. Sequential surface samples are often collected at different time intervals after aerosol deposition in order to measure the dissipation of chemicals over time. Dissipation occurs with virtually all chemicals and is one reason measurements of aerosol deposition are unlikely to reflect exposures at times after the actual deposition.

Filter Paper

Filter paper has been used to collect aerosol deposition. In one study, two No. 44 Whatman filter papers, 24 cm in diameter, were placed on a raft and two filter papers were placed on a dock where there was concern about drift of mosquito insecticide into estuary waters when it was applied aerially (Wang, Lenahan, and Tucker, 1987). Filter papers were spaced 3 M apart at the north and south ends of the test dock.

Filter paper was also used in a study at a pilot coal conversion plant when it was noticed that workers had speckles on their faces (Ketcham and Norton, 1960). In order to ascertain the source of these speckles, large rounds of Whatman filter paper were placed on music stands at various points around the facility and the results were compared to what was found on the workers.

Pads

Pads similar to those used for dermal dosimetry have been placed on surfaces in residences during pesticide spray application to measure surface residue. The pads are constructed in the same way as for dermal monitoring and frequently consist of three layers: a glassine paper backing (10.2 cm by 10.2 cm) with an equal size sheet of filter paper (Whatman chromatography Paper, 0.16 mm thickness) used as a second layer, and the top layer of 8-ply gauze pad (Steri-Pad). The layers are fastened together with strips of masking tape, leaving a 6.4 cm by 6.4 cm area exposed. Pads were placed on top of the refrigerator, stove, kitchen table, and kitchen floor (center) prior to insecticide (DDVP) application and were collected 2 hours posttreatment. Pads from all locations (within each house) were combined and analyzed as a single sample using the procedures for dermal pads.

Gauze pads (Fig. 7-11) can be placed on an elevated stand if drift from spraying is of interest. Platforms are placed at an angle with respect to the wind direction.

Mylar Sheets

Mylar sheets have been used to collect sprays. One method is to tape the sheets to pressed hardboard (Wilson et al., 1980). To measure the width of a helicopter's spray pattern and to obtain information on drift (with the helicopter at an 80 ft height applying 2,4,5-T with a microfoil boom), mylar sheets (9 in. by 9 in.) were placed on the ground at intervals at 80 ft, 160 ft, 320 ft, 640 ft, and 960 ft on each side of the spray path (Lavy, Shepard, and Bouchard, 1980). A total of three replications were attached to 9 in. by 9 in. floor tile to keep them from being moved by the wind or the helicopter. Immediately after the spraying was completed, the mylar strips were removed from the tile and placed in jars of methanol in a manner similar to that used with gauze pads. They have also been folded and stored in wide mouth glass jars after sampling and extracted in the laboratory.

Aluminum

Aluminum sheets (400 cm^2, food grade foil) have been used to measure fallout from pesticide foggers used inside homes. The sheets were placed in room corners 1 M from each corner

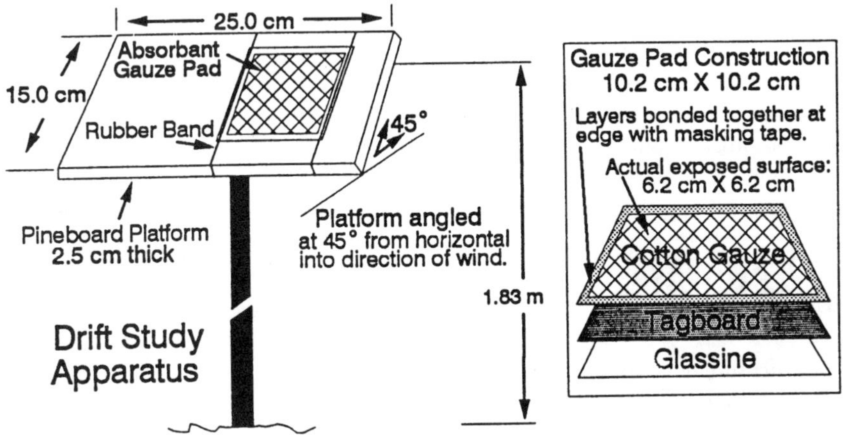

Figure 7-11. Insecticide drift monitoring apparatus and gauze monitoring pad construction.
Source: From M. E. Byers, S. T. Kamble, and J. F. Witkowski. 1993. Drift during center-pivot chemigation of chlorpyrifos with and without crop oil. *Bull. Env. Contam. Toxicol.* **51**:61; copyright © 1993 by Springer-Verlag New York Inc.

(Ross et al., 1990). Swabbing with a solvent-soaked gauze pad was then used to remove material from the foil.

Aluminum plates have also been placed on tables prior to insecticide application indoors (Wright, Leidy, and Dupree, 1984). For analysis the plates were rinsed with hexane and the rinse was analyzed for the insecticide. In a study to compare residues produced by spraying and fogging of Diazinon, aluminum pie plates (22.9 cm diam.) were placed on a shelf inside an open wall cabinet, on the countertop, and on the floor in the center of the kitchen (Wright and Jackson, 1974). In the bedroom they were suspended 168 cm from the floor in the center of the room, on the floor in the center of the room, and 15 cm from the center of the outside wall. Three plates were positioned side by side, but not touching, at each site.

Glass Plates and Dishes

Glass plates have been used to measure surface fallout during spraying in greenhouses (Waldron, 1985). The most common application for this technique is to estimate residue likely to land on foliage, which is often preferred over foliage analysis because of the ease in conducting several experiments over a period of time by replacing the plates rather than waiting for the pesticide to completely dissipate from the treated foliage. Also, measurement of residue from the upper and under surfaces of the glass plate provides a means of determining the plant coverage from different application methods. Glass slides coated with magnesium oxide provide a means of determining pesticide droplet deposition from low volume pesticide application, but are not considered practical for use with high volume applications because the spray may wash the magnesium coating from the slides. Other variations have included glass saucers and culture dishes (Wright and Jackson, 1971; Haverty et al., 1983).

Carpet Swatches

Carpet swatches (7.6 cm by 15.2 cm by 1.3 cm) were placed on the floor of residences 24 hours prior to insecticide application and taken up immediately before treatment (Wright and Leidy, 1982). A second sample was placed in the same floor site immediately upon completion of termite treatment and removed 24 hours later. The carpet swatches were analyzed to detect the presence of any chlordane or heptachlor. Three circles (2.4 cm in diameter) were punched from the midline of each swatch and were tared in a Soxhlet thimble. They were extracted for 4 hours with 200 mL of chloroform:methanol (1:1) and the liquid was analyzed.

VOLATILE SURFACE CONTAMINATION

When does a measurement for a volatile compound fall into the surface category rather than air sampling? Although this is a gray area, when a measurement is 1 in. to 12 in. from a surface it can be assumed that the source is the surface—unless there is a process that is actively generating the contaminant nearby. If a measurement is in the breathing zone or in the middle of a room (general area) away from surfaces likely to be contaminated, it can be categorized as air sampling rather than surface sampling. As is the case with other contaminants, surface sampling for volatile materials is usually done to determine if skin or clothing exposures are a concern. This type of sampling is useful for many compounds for which wipe sampling is not effective, such as

Acetone
Acetylene tetrabromide
Acrylonitrile
Allyl alcohol
Allyl glycidyl ether
Aluminum oxide
Ammonia
Ammonium sulfamate
sec-Amyl acetate
Amyl nitrate
Benzene
(OSHA, 1991)

Ionization Detectors

For many volatile contaminants, a general survey monitor with a photoionization detector (PID) or a flame ionization detector (FID) can be used (Fig. 7-12). The probe is moved around the article to see if there are any increases in levels existing on equipment, instruments, tools, and other objects over background. In some instances screening for the presence of volatile materials on a surface can be useful to determine if further testing or decontamination is necessary. Another application is the determination of residual dry cleaning solvent in clothing, which can be present if the clothing is immediately placed in protective plastic and does not get a sufficient offgassing period. In this case the most popular instruments for organic vapors are the PID and FID. Recently a combination PID/FID has also become available. As with other general survey instruments, both PID- and FID-based instruments will have different responses for organic vapors relative to the gas to which it is calibrated. A brief description of the operating principles of these instruments follows. For more detailed information, other resources on air monitoring instruments are available (Ness, 1991).

PID

There are two basic PID designs. In one, the lamp is contained within the instrument housing and one set of electronics applies to all lamps. In the other design, the lamp is incorporated into a probe and there is a separate set of electronics for each probe/lamp. The result is a difference in the cost as well as the frequency of lamp replacement, the former being less expensive. The all-in-one design can be held in one hand. The limit of detection for most contaminants is approximately 1 ppm. The PID has a large linear range and is a good general detector for aliphatic and aromatic hydrocarbons, halohydrocarbons, alcohols, ketones, aldehydes, ethylene oxide, arsine phosphine, total reduced sulfur components including hydrogen sulfide, and glycol ethers.

A strategy that is sometimes used is adjusting the response of an instrument calibrated with one gas to the sensitivity needed for another gas. This can be done using response factors to multiply the reading or utilizing the span adjustment instead. In the first case, the sampling professional can consult charts that give the re-

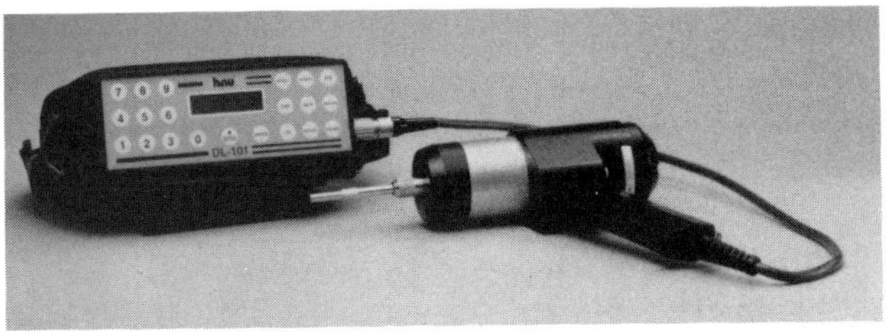

Figure 7-12. *Left:* HNU DL-101 PID. *Below:* The Foxboro TVA-1000 vapor analyzer, an FID/PID combination.
Courtesy of HNU Systems Inc. and The Foxboro Company.

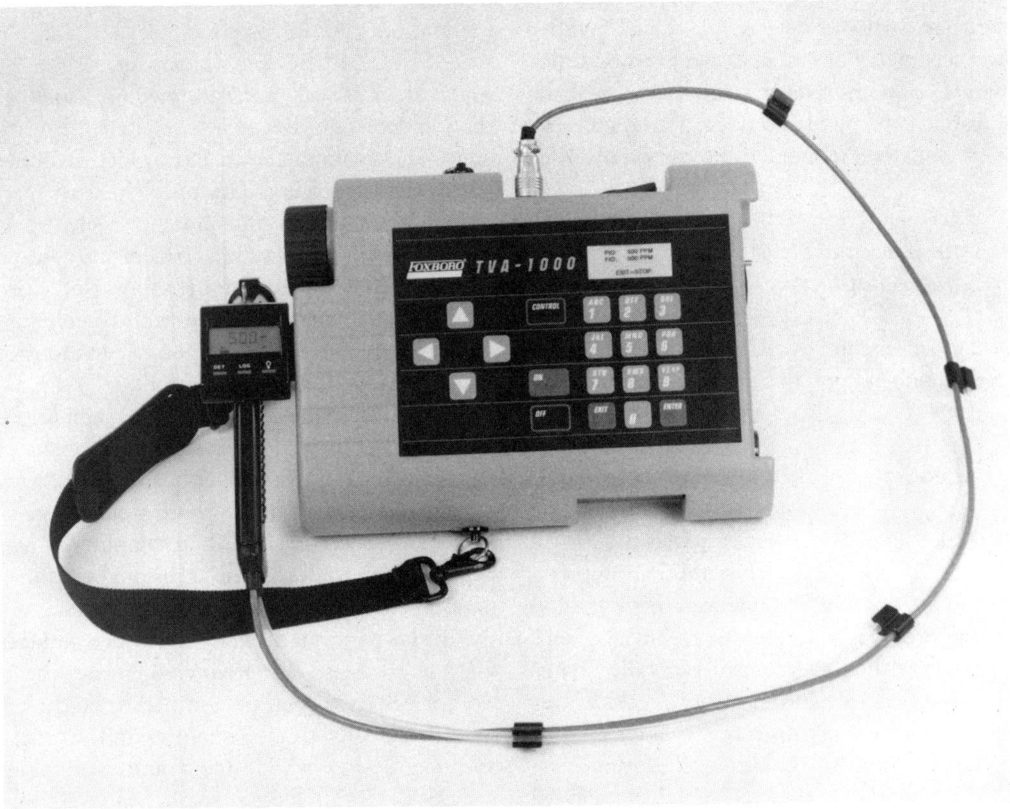

sponse factor for a different compound than that used for calibration and multiply the measurements accordingly. In the second case, an instrument is calibrated using isobutylene, and the span is adjusted to respond as if this gas were benzene (55 ppm of benzene is equivalent to approximately 100 ppm of isobutylene, if using a 10.2 eV lamp). The use of a span adjustment provides more accuracy than multiplying measurements. This method is often chosen rather than calibrating directly with a concentration of the contaminant of interest because the calibration gas may not be readily available or may be very toxic.

FID

Another detection method utilized for low-level hydrocarbon contamination is FID. General survey FIDs respond to almost all organic compounds, but the response is greater to aliphatic hydrocarbons. While FIDs do not respond to atoms other than carbon, other atoms can alter an instrument's sensitivity to carbon by altering the environment around the carbon atom. For example, compounds containing oxygen, such as alcohols, ethers, aldehydes and esters, and nitrogen-containing compounds, such as amides, amines, and nitriles, have a lower response than that observed for hydrocarbons. Halogenated hydrocarbons will be detected, although with a lower sensitivity compared to most combustibles. The FID is insensitive to water, inert gases, and inorganic compounds and has a negligible response to carbon monoxide and carbon dioxide.

General Use of a PID/FID for Large Equipment

All measurements should be made from the same distance in order to be comparable.

Procedure

1. Make sure prior to field use that the instrument is fully charged. During charging of an instrument where the lamp is contained in the probe, it is important to have a probe attached or the unit will not fully charge and will not show the battery check. With a full charge most instruments should last 8 hours, although colder temperatures can decrease this time. If needed, lead acid gel packs are available that will extend battery life up to 36 hours.
2. When changing lamps, depending on the energy (eV) of the lamp, the span may have to be changed.
3. Adjust the zero of the instrument. If the span setting is changed after the zero is set, rezero the instrument.
4. Position the end of the intake probe in close proximity to the area or item to be sampled because of the low flow rate associated with most instruments. Set the instrument to the highest operating range and then switch to the more sensitive (lower) ranges if nothing is detected.
5. Use slow sweeping movements to avoid bypassing problem areas.

Frequently Encountered Compounds

Mercury

Mercury vapor can be released from surface contamination over long periods of time and absorbed through the skin (Hursh et al., 1989). Many devices still contain mercury, such as thermometers, sphygmomanometers, barometers, and manometers. Many older switches also contain mercury. The problem with mercury contamination is that mercury easily vaporizes at room temperature, where it can be breathed or absorbed through the skin. Contamination can occur on shoes, cart wheels, and other mobile items. It is also possible to monitor smaller articles for contamination.

If droplets of mercury are visible, sampling is not required. Instead these spills or droplets of mercury should be immediately cleaned up with a vacuum system equipped with a mercury-absorbent exhaust filter and then sampling should be performed to determine if residual contamination exists. All operations involving mercury should be performed over impervious surfaces free of crevices. Elevated concentrations in workplaces have been determined to be the result of residual mercury remaining in the cracks and recesses of wood floors and worktables (NIOSH, 1982). Floors, some walls, exhaust hoods, and other surfaces in mercury work areas should be painted or coated with hard, low-porosity materials.

Mercury testing was used to determine the effectiveness of decontamination of thermometer workers' homes that were contaminated as a result of mercury brought home on their clothing (Zirschky and Witherell, 1987). During the decontamination of homes, every exposed surface of the home was washed or dusted. In addition, all dishes, pottery, appliances, and similar personal effects were cleaned. To minimize the intrusion on the family, personal items within drawers (except kitchen items) and closets were not cleaned. After most of the home had been decontaminated, an interim monitoring showed that personal effects, such as clothing, were still contaminated. All such items were laundered or allowed to air. HgX was placed in the machine during the wash cycle. The wash and rinse waters then were collected and treated as a hazardous waste. A few washing machines were too contaminated to be cleaned either in this manner or by taking the machine apart and cleaning all parts by hand, and therefore were replaced.

In the gold film technique for mercury detection a thin gold film that is part of a piezoelectric sensor undergoes an increase in electrical resistance proportional to the mass of mercury in the sample. The Jerome 411 mercury monitor has an internal pump that draws a precise volume of air over the sensor at a flow rate of 750 mL/min. Mercury in the sample is adsorbed and integrated by the sensor, registering it as a proportional change in electrical resistance. It can collect samples in two modes: a 3 sec period for screening and a 12 sec period for better quantitation. The measurements are displayed on a digital readout. Its sensitivity is reported as 0.0003 mg/M^3.

Calibration of these instruments with an atmosphere of mercury is difficult outside a laboratory with a very specialized mercury vapor generator setup. Therefore, for most users, it is best to send the unit back to the factory for calibration. Prior to each use, the sampling professional should check an instrument's general response to mercury and the condition of the charcoal in the zero filter.

Mercury Contamination on Small Objects

Procedure Number 1

The following is an example of how a sniff test can be used to identify mercury contamination (Arizona Instrument Co.). The same procedure is applicable for organic vapor identification with a PID or FID.

1. Enclose the suspect material in a polyethylene bag or close-fitting airtight container for 8 hours at room temperature (76°–80°F, 24°–30°C), or place the bag in an oven set at 125°F ± 5°F (52°C ± 2°C) for 1 hour.
2. Make a small slit in the bag or lift the lid of the container high enough to insert the probe of a mercury vapor analyzer.
3. If the mercury vapor concentration is greater than 0.01 mg/M^3, the material is contaminated.

Procedure Number 2

Another technique used for mercury contamination is to wipe a surface with a filter and then sniff the filter with a direct reading instrument. This may be useful for surfaces that are hard to reach (e.g., under sinks) and for heavy objects such as refrigerators. If the same size area is wiped each time, it may provide a better averaging than the traditional method of spot sampling. This test eliminates variation due to distance when measurements are performed, since using a ruler to verify that all measurements are being taken at the same distance from a surface is tedious and is rarely done; instead the distance is usually estimated and measurements are generally within a window of 6–12 in. away.

Mercury Contamination in Dental Offices

One method for large areas, such as floors, where volatile contaminants are suspected is to perform a mapping survey. A direct reading instrument is used to make a series of samples, each of which is the same distance from the previous sample. A map of the floor is gradually developed indicating where areas of high concentration are located. This is especially useful for dental offices (Fig. 7-13) and labs where mercury contamination is a concern. Typical surfaces sampled in dental offices include carpeting, baseboards, sink drain traps, patient chairs, amalgam mixing counters, walls, and linoleum.

Formaldehyde

Skin rashes have been associated with exposure to free formaldehyde from resin systems used in

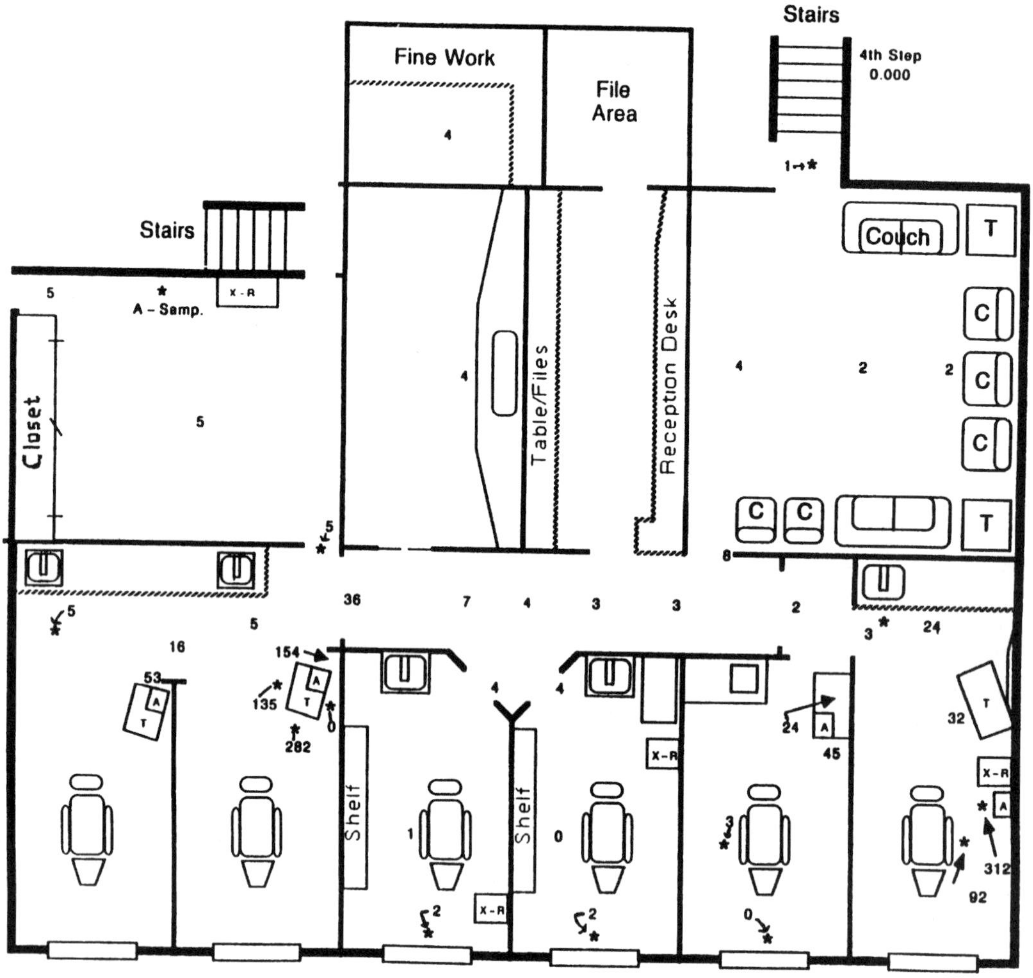

Figure 7-13. Dental office layout showing sampling sites.
Source: From NIOSH, Health Hazard Evaluation Report. April 21, 1987. Rothan & Rothan, DDS, NEED LOCATION PER OTHER NIOSH ITEMS. HETA 87-147. Cincinnati, OH: NIOSH.

the preparation of permanent press clothing. There is a definite correlation between the age of a resin treated fabric and the latent formaldehyde content. Among textile workers, symptoms are more commonly associated with postcured fabrics, which have a higher level of free formaldehyde; however, if the fabric has been stored in an open ventilated area, levels should have decreased significantly over what was originally present.

One control that can be used is to air fabrics in a ventilated chamber while adding heat to drive the formaldehyde out of the cloth, possibly by unrolling bolts of cloth at one end and rolling them back up at the other end. Proper temperature, humidity, and airing time would need to be determined beforehand.

Only a few real time instruments can be used to monitor for formaldehyde: infrared (IR), and voltametric and colorimetric detection systems. The IR is generally not used, since the levels of concern for formaldehyde, 1 ppm and less, are below the reliable detection limits of most instruments. The CEA TGM 555 is a portable wet chemical analyzer that is capable of continuously monitoring for a number of compounds utilizing colorimetry. Sample air is continuously drawn through an absorbing reagent that removes the compound of interest from the airstream and transfers it into a liquid reagent system that undergoes a color change. The intensity of the color is read at a specific visible wavelength. The unit can monitor for other compounds besides formaldehyde, mostly inorganic, but this requires a separate set of reagents for each type of contaminant.

Testing Fabrics and Garments

Screening Methods

One method used to test clothing is to take an unopened box of the material and make a hole large enough to withdraw an air sample. The sample is collected onto whatever media or with whatever instrument is needed. Bulk samples of fabric can also be analyzed in the laboratory. One method for textiles is to suspend samples of textile material on a wire above distilled water in a sealed container heated to approximately 49°C in a drying oven. Aliquots of the distilled water from each container are then analyzed for formaldehyde using visible spectroscopy according to NIOSH Method 9001 (NIOSH, 1989).

Sorbent Methods

There are two basic methods for collecting integrated samples of gases and vapors. The first involves active collection wherein a battery powered pump pulls air through an appropriate medium that collects the contaminant(s) of interest. The second method, passive collection, involves exposing the sampler to the contaminated air and allowing the compounds of interest to simply diffuse or permeate it. Collection media for gases and vapors either adsorb contaminants onto a sorbent, allowing them to be easily separated in the laboratory, or absorb them in a reagent as a result of a contaminant's solubility or a reaction that takes place to form another compound. Of the sorbents, the most common is charcoal, and it can be used for a wide variety of organic vapors. Another sorbent that can be used for organic vapors and can also be thermally desorbed is tenax. Passive media, such as organic vapor badges or others that measure formaldehyde or mercury, are the easiest to use whereas pumps and tubes require calibration and more equipment but can sample a wider range of concentrations. For more information on the basics of these air sampling methods, other resources are available (Ness, 1991).

A method used to test garments for volatile contaminants for which there is no direct reading instrument available, but the contaminant can be analyzed on a passive monitoring dosimeter, is as follows: The garment is sealed in plastic (Redmond and Schappert, 1987). A small slit is made in the sealed garment package and an organic vapor monitor is inserted and placed between folds of the garment. The bag is immediately sealed with tape and intermittently massaged during the next one to two days. The samples are analyzed by gas chromatography. One application for this technique is for residual dry cleaning fluid: perchloroethylene.

Worker clothing has also been sampled after it was worn using this technique (NIOSH, 1992). In one situation a worker became ill after using a spray adhesive. The clothing he was wearing at the time of the incident was placed in a sealed plastic bag and an organic vapor dosimeter was placed in the bag for approximately seven hours. A PID was also used to screen the clothing while inside the bag. The organic vapor badge was then analyzed for the components in the adhesive.

REFERENCES

ASTM. 1993. Proposed Standard Practice for the Field Collection of Dust Samples Using Wipe Sampling Methods for Lead Determination by Atomic Spectrometry Techniques. Philadelphia, PA: American Society for Testing and Materials.

Beaulieu, H. J. 1991. Asbestos contamination of abatement equipment surfaces. *Appl. Occup. Environ.* **6**(7):583–587.

Brady, E. U., and Y. H. Atallah. 1986. Effectiveness of

candidate barrier sprays for managing residues of chlordane on plywood. *Bull. Env. Contam. Toxicol.* **37**:467–474.

Brady, E. U., R. Tippins, J. Perry, J. R. Young, and R. D. Wauchope. 1991. Chlorpyrifos exposure of workers entering sweet corn after chemigation. *Bull. Env. Contam. Toxicol.* **46**:343–350.

Camann, D. E., H. J. Harding, S. R. Agrawal, and R. G. Lewis. 1993. Comparison of transfer of surface chlorpyrifos residues from carpet by three dislodgeable residue methods. In *Proceedings of the 1993 EPA/Air and Waste Management Association International Symposium*. Pittsburgh, PA: Air and Waste Management Association.

Chavalitnitikul, C., and L. Levin. 1984. A laboratory evaluation of wipe testing based on lead oxide surface contamination. *AIHA J.* **45**(6):418–426.

Chavalitnitikul, C., L. Levin, and L. Chen. 1984. Study and models of total lead exposures of battery workers. *AIHA J.* **45**(12):802–808.

Clarke, A. N. 1991. Results of an investigation of an old manufacturing facility for levels of polychlorinated dibenzofurans and polychlorinated dibenzodioxins. *Chemosphere* **23**(8/10):1001–1008.

Cohen, J. J., and R. N. Kusian. 1965. The significance of beryllium surface contamination to health. In C. W. Royster and B. R. Fish (eds.), *Surface Contamination*. New York: Pergamon Press, pp. 345–348.

Currie, K. L., E. C. McDonald, L. T. K. Chung, and A. R. Higgs. 1990. Concentrations of diazinon, chlorpyrifos, and bendiocarb after application in offices. *AIHA J.* **51**(1):23–27.

Diemel, J. A. L., B. Brunekreef, J. S. M. Boleij, K. Biersteker, and S. J. Veenstra. 1981. The Arnhem lead study. II. Indoor pollution and indoor/outdoor relationships. *Env. Res.* **25**:449–456.

EPA. 1985. *Guide for Decontaminating Building, Structures and Equipment at Superfund Sites*. Washington, DC: EPA, EPA 600/2-85-028.

EPA. 1988. *Field Evaluation of a High Volume Surface Sampler for Pesticides in Floor Dust*. Washington, DC: EPA, EPA/600/3-90/030.

EPA. 1990. *Non-occupational Pesticide Exposure Study. (NOPES)*. EPA 600/3-90-003. Research Triangle Park, NC: Atmospheric Research and Exposure Assessment Laboratory.

EPA. 1992*a*. *Engineering Study to Explore Improvements in Vacuum Dust Collection, Final Report*. Office of Pollution Prevention and Toxics. Washington, DC: U.S. Environmental Protection Agency.

EPA. 1992*b*. *Quality Assurance Project Plan for the Comprehensive Abatement Performance Study*. Office of Pollution Prevention and Toxics. Washington, DC: U.S. Environmental Protection Agency.

EPA. 1993. *Urban Soil Lead Abatement Demonstration Project*. EPA 600/AS-93-001. Office of Health and Environmental Assessment. Research Triangle Park, NC: U.S. Environmental Protection Agency.

EPA. 1994. The National Human Exposure Assessment Survey (NHEXSUS) Workshop. Research Triangle Park, NC: U.S. Environmental Protection Agency.

Farfel, M. R., and J. J. Chisolm. 1990. Health and environmental outcomes of traditional and modified practices for abatement of lead-based paint. *Am. J. Pub. Health* **80**:1240.

Fenske, R. A., and C. Lu. 1992. *Dermal Exposure to Pesticide-Contaminated Surfaces*. Boston: American Industrial Hygiene Conference, Abstract.

Fenske, R. A., S. W. Horstman, and R. K. Bentley. 1987. Assessment of dermal exposure to chlorophenols in timber mills. *Appl. Ind. Hyg.* **2**:143–147.

Fish, B. R., R. L. Walker, G. W. Royster, and J. L. Thompson. 1965. Redispersion of settled particulates. In G. W. Royster and B. R. Fish (eds.), *Surface Contamination*. New York: Pergamon Press, pp. 111–129.

Frank, R., R. A. Campbell, and G. J. Sirons. 1985. Forestry workers involved in aerial application of 2,4-dichlorophenoxyacetic acid (2,4-D): Exposure and urinary excretion. *Arch. Env. Contam. Toxicol.* **14**:427–435.

Georgia Technical Research Institute. 1993. *Wipe Sampling Procedures: Inspecting for Lead Hazards and Lead-based Paint Risk Assessment*. Athens, GA: Georgia Technical Research Institute.

Gold, R. E., and T. Holcslaw. 1985. Dermal and respiratory exposure of applicators and residents to dichlorovos-treated residences. In R. C. Honeycutt, G. Zweig, and N. N. Ragsdale (eds.), *Dermal Exposure Related to Pesticide Use*. Washington, DC: American Chemical Society, pp. 253–264.

Hattula, M. J., V. Wasenius, and A. Arstila. 1979. The exposure to MCPA in the use of clearing saw. *Chemosphere* **7**:473–476.

Haverty, M. I., M. Page, P. J. Shea, J. B. Hoy, and R. W. Hall. 1983. Drift and worker exposure resulting from two methods of applying insecticides to pine bark. *Bull. Env. Contam. Toxicol.* **30**:223–228.

Hayes, J. 1992. Dust sampling protocol, State of North Carolina.

Hsu, J. P., D. P. Camann, and H. Schattennburg. 1990. New dermal exposure sampling technique. In *Proceedings of the EPA/AWMA International Symposium: Measurement of Toxic and Related Pollutants*. Pittsburgh, PA: Air and Waste Management Association, pp. 489–497.

HUD. 1990. *Lead-based Paint: Interim Guidelines for Hazard Identification and Abatement in Public and Indian Housing*. Department of Housing and Urban Development, Washington, DC: U.S. Government Printing Office.

Hursh, J. B., T. W. Clarkson, E. F. Miles, and L. A. Goldsmith. 1989. Percutaneous absorption of mercury vapor by man. *Arch. Environ. Health* **44**(2):120–127.

Ketcham, N. H., and R. W. Norton. 1960. The hazards to health in the hydrogenation of coal. II. The industrial hygiene studies. *Arch. Env. Health* **1**:30/194–41/207.

Klemmer, H. W., E. Leitis, and K. Pfenninger. 1975. Arsenic content of house dusts in Hawaii. *Bull. Env. Contam. Toxicol.* **14**:449–452.

Klingner, T. 1992. New developments in surface contamination monitoring for aromatic amines. In *Proceedings of the Conference for Advanced Composites*. Cincinnati, OH: ACGIH, pp. 43–46.

Lavy, T. L., J. S. Shepard, and D. C. Bouchard. 1980. Field worker exposure and helicopter spray pattern of 2,3,5,-T. *Bull. Env. Contam. Toxicol.* **24**:90–96.

Lee, I. N., et al. 1987. Additivity of detector responses of a portable direct-reading 10.2 eV photoionization detector and a flame ionization gas chromatograph for atmospheres of multicomponent organics: Use of PID/FID ratios. *AIHA J.* **48**(5):437–441.

Lepow, M. L., L. Bruckman, M. Gillette, S. Markowitz, R. Rubino, and J. Kapish. 1975. Investigations into sources of lead in the environment of urban children. *Env. Res.* **10**:415–426.

Lewis, R. G., R. C. Fortmann, and D. E. Camann. 1994. Evaluation of methods for monitoring potential exposure of small children to pesticides in the residential environment. *Arch. Env. Contam. Toxicol.* **26**:37.

Lewis, R. G., A. E. Bond, R. C. Fortmann, L. S. Sheldon, and D. E. Camann. 1991. *Determination of Routes of Exposure of Infants and Toddlers to Household Pesticides: A Pilot Study*. Washington, DC: EPA, EPA/600/D-91/077.

Lioy, P. J., T. Wainman, and C. Weisel. 1993. A wipe sampler for the quantitative measurement of dust on smooth surfaces: Laboratory performance studies. *J. Exp. Anal. Env. Epidemiol.* **3**:315.

Lichtenwalner, C. P. 1992. Evaluation of wipe sampling procedures and elemental surface contamination. *AIHA J.* **53**:657–659.

McArthur, B. 1993. *The Transfer of Oil from a Contaminated Surface to Selected Surface Sample Media*. New Orleans, LA: American Industrial Hygiene Conference, Abstract.

McArthur, B. R., and P. S. J. Lees. 1992. *The Effect of Contact Time and Contact Pressure on the Transfer of Oil to Wipe Sample Media*. Boston, MA: American Industrial Hygiene Conference, Abstract.

Maroni, M., A. Colombi, S. Cantoni, E. Ferioli, and V. Foa. 1981. Occupational exposure to polychlorinated biphenyls in electrical workers. I. Environmental and blood polychlorinated biphenyls concentrations. *Brit. J. Ind. Med.* **38**:49–54.

Mathews, T. G. 1982. Evaluation of modified CEA Instruments, Inc. Model 555 Analyzer for the monitoring of formaldehyde vapor in domestic environments. *AIHA J.* **43**(8):547–552.

Menrath, W. G., C. S. Clark, and R. L. Bornschein. 1992. *A Comparison of Two Methods for Determining the Risk of Exposure to Lead-Contaminated Dust*. Boston, MA: American Industrial Hygiene Conference, Abstract.

Mitchell, R. N. and B. C. Eutsler. 1965. A study of beryllium surface contamination and resuspension. In G. W. Royster and B. R. Fish (eds.), *Surface Contamination*. New York: Pergamon Press, pp. 349–353.

Ness, S. A. 1991. *Air Monitoring for Toxic Exposures*. New York: Van Nostrand Reinhold.

Nichols, G. 1985. Scotch Magic Tape—An air to the microscopist for dust examination. *Microscope* **33**:247–254.

NIOSH, Health Hazard Evaluation Report. September 1979. *Arapahoe Aluminum and Brass Foundry, Inc., Englewood, CO*. HHE 79-9-615. Cincinnati, OH: NIOSH.

NIOSH, Technical Assistance Report. 1980. *Greif Brothers Corp., Niagara Falls, NY*. TA 80-087-771. Cincinnatti, OH: NIOSH.

NIOSH, Health Hazard Evaluation Determination Report. December 1982. *Ohio Thermometer Co., Springfield, OH*. HETA 82-364-1243. Cincinnati, OH: NIOSH.

NIOSH, Health Hazard Evaluation Report. 1986*a*. *Hilton-Davis Chemical Company, Cincinnati, OH*. HETA 84-058-1700. Cincinnati, OH: NIOSH.

NIOSH, Health Hazard Evaluation Report. 1986*b*. *Page Belcher Federal Bldg., Tulsa, OK*. HETA 85-289-1738. Cincinnati, OH: NIOSH.

NIOSH, Health Hazard Evaluation Report. February 1988. *Klotz Brothers, Inc., Stanton, VA*. HETA 87-410-1868. Cincinnati, OH: NIOSH.

NIOSH, Health Hazard Evaluation Determination Report. October 1989. *Meyersdale Manufacturing Co., Meyersdale, PA*. MHETA 88-269-1993. Cincinnati, OH: NIOSH.

NIOSH, Health Hazard Evaluation Report. October 1990. *Thomson Consumer Electronics, Inc., Circleville, OH*. HETA 89-244-2068. Cincinnati, OH: NIOSH.

NIOSH, Health Hazard Evaluation Report. 1991*a*. *Carbonnaire Co., Palmerton, PA*. HETA 91-073-2165. Cincinnati, OH: NIOSH.

NIOSH, Health Hazard Evaluation Report. 1991*b*. *M&J Painting Company, Covington, KY*. HETA 91-006-2193. Cincinnati, OH: NIOSH.

NIOSH, Health Hazard Evaluation Report. 1991*c*. *New England Lead Burning Co., (NELCO), Eaton Metals, Salt Lake City, UT*. HETA 91-290-2131. Cincinnati, OH: NIOSH.

NIOSH. 1992. Lead in surface wipe samples, draft method 0700. In *NIOSH Manual of Analytical Methods*. Cincinnati, OH: NIOSH.

NIOSH, Health Hazard Evaluation Determination Report. March 1992. *IMC Corp., Sterlington, LA*. HETA 91-338-2187. Cincinnati, OH: NIOSH.

NIOSH, Health Hazard Evaluation Report. August 1992. *Independence Police Department, Indoor Range, Independence, MO*. HETA 90-168-2248. Cincinnati, OH: NIOSH.

NIOSH. March 2, 1992. *Lead in Surface Wipe Samples, Method (Draft) 0700*. Issued as addendum to the NIOSH manual of analytical methods, 3d ed., vols. 1 and 2, with 1985, 1987 and 1989 supplements. P. Eller, ed. Cincinnati, OH: U.S. Dept. of Health and Human Services, Public Health Service, Centers for Disease Control, National Institute for Occupational Safety and Health.

Oatman, L., and R. Roy. 1986. Surface and indoor air levels of polychlorinated biphenyls in public buildings. *Bull. Env. Contam. Toxicol.* **37:**461–466.

Orris, P., J. R. Kominsky, D. Hryhorczuk, and J. Melius. 1986. Exposure to polychlorinated biphenyls from an overheated transformer. *Chemosphere* **15**(9/12):1305–1311.

OSHA. 1991. *OSHA Technical Manual*, 2nd ed. Washington, DC: OSHA.

Polissar, L., K. Lowry-Coble, D. A. Kalman, J. P. Hugher, G. van Belle, D. S. Covert, T. M. Burbacher, D. Bolgiano, and N. K. Mottet. 1990. Pathways of human exposure to arsenic in a community surrounding a copper smelter. *Env. Res.* **53:**29–47.

Que Hee, S. S., B. Peace, C. S. Clark, J. R. Boyle, R. L. Bornschein, and P. B. Hammond. 1985. Evolution of efficient methods to sample lead sources, such as house dust and hand dust, in the homes of children. *Env. Res.* **38:**77–95.

Rabinowitz, M., A. Leviton, H. Needleman, D. Bellinger, and C. Waternaux. 1985. Environmental correlates of infant blood lead levels in Boston. *Env. Res.* **38:**96.

Rappe, C., S. Marklund, L. Keller, P. Bergqvist, and M. Hansson. 1985. Strategies and techniques for sample collection and analysis: Experience from the Swedish PCB accidents. *Env. Health Perspec.* **60:**279–292.

Redmond, S. F., and K. R. Schappert. 1987. Occupational dermatitis associated with garments. *JOM* **29**(3):243–244.

Roberts, J. W., and D. E. Camann. 1989. Pilot study of a cotton glove press test for assessing exposure to pesticides in house dust. *Bull. Env. Contam. Toxicol.* **43:**717–724.

Roberts, J. W., W. T. Budd, M. G. Ruby, V. R. Stamper, D. E. Camann, R. C. Fortmann, L. S. Sheldon, and R. G. Lewis. 1991. A small high volume surface sampler (HVS3) for lead, pesticides and other toxics substances in house dust. Paper No. 91-150.2. In *Proceedings of the 84th Annual Meeting of Air & Waste Management Association*. Vancouver, British Columbia.

Ross, J., T. Thongsinthusak, H. R. Fong, S. Margetich, and R. Krieger. 1990. Measuring potential dermal transfer of surface pesticide residue generated from indoor fogger use: An interim report. *Chemosphere* **20**(3/4):349–360.

Ross, J., H. R. Fong, T. Thongsinthusak, S. Margetich, and R. Krieger. 1991. Measuring potential dermal transfer of surface pesticide residue generated from indoor fogger use: Using the CDFA roller method. Interim report II. *Chemosphere* **22**(9/10):975–984.

Routledge, R. 1968. Possible health risk from beryllium oxide ceramic rectifiers of 1,000 H.P. rail motor coaches. *Ann. Occup. Hyg.* **11:**17–21.

Royster, G. W., and B. R. Fish. 1967. Techniques for assessing "removeable" surface contamination. In G. W. Royster and B. R. Fish (eds.), *Surface Contamination*. New York: Pergamon Press, pp. 201–207.

Roxbury, K. D. (1985). *Handbook: Dust Control at Hazardous Waste Sites*. Washington, DC: EPA, EPA-540/2-85/003.

Schneider, T., O. Nielsen, P. Bredsdorff, and P. Linde. 1990. Dust in buildings with man-made mineral fiber ceiling boards. *Scand. J. Work Env. Health* **16:**434–439.

Schuresko, D. D. 1980. Portable fluorometric monitor for detection of surface contamination by polynuclear aromatic compounds. *Anal. Chem.* **52:**371–373.

Staiff, D. C., S. W. Comer, J. F. Armstrong, and H. R. Wolfe. 1975. Exposure to the herbicide, paraquat. *Bull. Env. Contam. Toxicol.* **14**(3):334–340.

Stark, A. D., R. F. Quah, J. W. Meigs, and E. R. DeLouise. 1982. The relationship of environmental lead to blood-lead levels in children. *Env. Res.* **27:**372.

Tanimura, H. 1968. Benzo(a)pyrene in an iron and steel works. *Arch. Env. Health* **17:**172–177.

Thulin, H. 1993. Determination of nor-nitrogen mustard hydrochloride in air and on surfaces by using filter or wipe sampling and a derivatization-gas chromatographic procedure. *AIHA J.* **54**(2):76–81.

Timperi, R. 1992. Dust collection protocol, State of Massachusetts.

Vaccaro, J. R., and R. J. Cranston. 1990. Evaluation of Dislodgeable Residues and Absorbed doses of Chlorpyrifos Following Indoor Broadcast Application of Chlorpyrifos-based Emulsifiable Concentrate. Internal report. Midland, MI: Dow Chemical Co.

Vostal, J. J., E. Taves, J. W. Sayre, and E. Chamey. 1974. Lead analysis of house dust: A method for the detection of another source of lead exposure in inner city children. *Env. Health Perspec.* **7:**91.

Waldron, A. C. 1985. The potential for applicator-worker exposure to pesticides in greenhouse operations. In *Dermal Exposure Related to Pesticide Use*, Washington, DC: American Chemical Society.

Wang, T. C., R. A. Lenahan, and J. W. Tucker. 1987. Deposition and persistence of aerially-applied Fenthion in a Florida estuary. *Bull. Env. Contam. Toxicol.* **38:**226–231.

Weeks, R. W., and B. J. Dean. 1978. Decontamination of aromatic amine cancer-suspect agents on concrete, metal, or painted surfaces. *AIHA J.* **39**:758–762.

Weeks, R. W., Jr., B. J. Dean, and S. K. Yasuda. 1976. Detection limits of chemical spot tests toward certain carcinogens on metal, painted, and concrete surfaces. *Anal. Chem.* **48**(14):2227–2233.

Weschler, C. J. 1978. Characterization techniques applied to indoor dust. *Env. Sci. and Tech.* **12**:923–926.

Wilson, B. W., C. M. Cisson, W. R. Randall, J. E. Woodrow, J. N. Seiber, and J. B. Knaak. 1980. Organophosphate risk assessment: Field testing of DEF with the scaleless chicken. *Bull. Env. Contam. Toxicol.* **24**:921–928.

Wood, G. W., and D. K. R. Stewart. 1976. Fenitrothion residues in blueberry fields after aerial forest spraying. *Bull. Env. Contam. Toxicol.* **15**(5):623–629.

Wright, C. G., and M. D. Jackson. 1971. Propoxur, Chlordane, and Diazinon on porcelain china saucers after kitchen cabinet spraying. *J. Econ. Entomol.* **64**(2):457–459.

Wright, C. G., and M. D. Jackson. 1974. A comparison of residues produced by spraying and fogging of Diazinon in buildings. *Bull. Env. Contam. Toxicol.* **12**(2):177–181.

Wright, C. G., and R. B. Leidy. 1982. Chlordane and heptachlor in the ambient air of houses treated for termites. *Bull. Env. Contam. Toxicol.* **28**:617–623.

Wright, C. G., R. B. Leidy, and H. E. Dupree. 1984. Chlorpyrifos and Diazinon detection on surfaces in dormitory rooms. *Bull. Env. Contam. Toxicol.* **32**:259–264.

Zirschky, J., and L. Witherell. 1987. Cleanup of mercury contamination of thermometer workers' homes. *AIHA J.* **48**(1):81–84.

CHAPTER 8

Surface Sampling for Microorganisms

Many microbials can exist in both viable (living) and nonviable states. Viable microorganisms such as bacteria, fungi, yeasts, and molds originate from sprays or splashes of media, from the agitation of dusts, and from sneezes and coughs of which only the small particles (<10 μm) remain in the air long enough to travel any distance. The ability to divide and multiply is what enables collected samples of microbials to be detected with a high degree of sensitivity. A single cell collected on a moist solid surface containing sufficient nutrients will divide repeatedly to form a mass of cells visible to the human eye. Examples of nonviable agents that are occasionally sampled include pollens and insect parts. Grains, clusters of cells, and skin scales are much larger-size particles (10–50 μm) than bacteria (Macher and First, 1984). Spores, which can be formed by fungi and certain bacteria, can be both viable and nonviable and are capable of causing disease in both forms. Surface sampling is most appropriate for nonviable forms; however there are methods that can sample for viable organisms.

Most bacteria are 1–5 mm in size and are classified through their nutritional and growth requirements, shape (round or rod), ability to utilize certain compounds, oxygen needs, metabolites produced, and the type of stain they take in the Gram stain test (positive or negative). There are four main factors that influence bacterial growth: temperature, nutrient supply, availability of stagnant water, and presence of particulate matter for binding. Temperature is the most important factor for many bacteria. While some thermophilic organisms can exist at elevated temperatures, most bacteria exist in a range of 20°–45°C. Nutrients can include nitrites; by-products of other microbials since the growth products of one organism may support another; certain chemical additives often used for water treatment; nonmetallic materials such as insulation, rubber parts, gaskets, and sealants; and atmospheric contamination by dusts and insects.

The fungi class includes yeasts, mold, mildew, and mushrooms. Soil is the most common habitat of the fungi, although many of the primitive fungal groups are aquatic. Fungi occur on the surface of decaying plant or animal materials in ponds and streams or grow on top of aqueous industrial fluids such as metalworking coolants. They are common in grain handling facilities, paper mills, plywood mills, fruit warehouses, and agricultural environments as well as indoor air environments. Fungal species commonly encountered include *Aspergillus*, which is ubiquitous in the soil and air, especially in agricultural products and in standing water, whose spores are known to cause a variety of pulmonary effects; and *Histoplasma* and *Cryptococcus*, found in bird droppings.

A unique stage of the fungus life cycle is the spore stage, consisting of a wide variety of shapes in a very broad size range (<2 mm to >100 mm; Burge, 1985). In this stage they form a durable coating over the exterior and become dormant. Spores can be classified by size, morphology, and color, and thus into different taxonomic groups. Since spores are relatively hardy structures, they can survive on surfaces in dry environments and become airborne when disturbed. Fungal spores are released into the air either by mechanical means, such as wind or other agitation, or biologically by specialized (active) spore discharge mechanisms usually occurring during periods of high relative humidity (Burge, 1985).

Systems in which water is used as a reservoir, particularly those with recirculation, may provide a suitable environment for a food chain of microorganisms (Ager and Tickner, 1983). The types of microorganisms that will develop in such circumstances will depend on the nutrient content of the water, its pH, and temperature. A wide range of microorganisms are capable of growth in water, and once an initial colony is established, its metabolic products may provide nutrients for the subsequent appearance of other species. The differing water, nutrient, pH, and temperature requirements between species make it unlikely that full growth potential of any one organism in these circumstances can continue for a prolonged period of time and instead the result is a succession of different microorganisms. Such a growth chain may consist of bacteria, fungi, algae, and amoebae. A humidifier water tank or reservoir colonized in this way is likely to form a surface slime on the sides, or if conditions are favorable, a crust layer, which may contain a range of viable and dead organisms together with cell wall components and spores.

Legionnaires' disease became a concern when it became apparent that aerosol from contaminated cooling towers could enter fresh air vents and spread this agent through the heating, ventilating, and air conditioning (HVAC) system in buildings. *Legionella pneumophila*, the agent in this case, is a rod-shaped, slow-growing, gram-negative bacterium. In water the bacteria multiply at 25°–42°C but are able to survive a much wider temperature range for long periods (they have been isolated from tap water stored at ambient temperatures for 14 months; Kurtz, 1988). The bacteria are ubiquitous in the environment. They can coexist with amoebae and can grow on blue-green algae. The vast majority of outbreaks have been associated with *Legionella* sero group 1, but other sero groups, if detected, are also of concern, and control measures should be initiated if they are detected.

Legionella sero group 1 has been isolated from a variety of surface and potable aquatic habitats, including water fountains in office buildings. It is viable in tap water for more than a year. Hot water tanks, and in particular their bottom sediments, are excellent media for its survival and proliferation. Sources of piped water such as recirculating water-cooling tower systems, whirlpool baths, and industrial cutting/grinding fluid have been associated with sudden large outbreaks. The route of infection is inhalation of aerosols; however, surface swab sampling of sections in the water systems, such as shower heads and sediment, along with bulk samples of water, are the primary means used to identify its presence.

Antigens such as animal dander are capable of stimulating the production of antibodies that produce allergic diseases. Sources of airborne antigens include bacteria, fungi, pollen, insect body parts and skin scales (dander), and saliva of mammals (ACGIH, 1989). Allergens that can exist in dusts in residences and offices have proven useful to sample. These include mites of the genus *Dermatophagoides* and species *Euroglyphus maynei*, which are sightless, eight-legged Acaridae. Only 0.3 M long, they feed on human skin flakes and thrive in 70% relative humidity at 21°C (Lundblad, 1991). They are commonly known as house dust mites. The most important sites for infestation are those associated with textiles: carpets, curtains, upholstered furniture.

SAMPLING STRATEGIES

Although microbials have certain characteristics that make them difficult to collect and analyze, the collection methods are very simple. The basic strategy is to collect the material and either through direct examination on a microscope or through growth in various culture media demonstrate the presence of microorganisms. While there are some standard methods used for sampling, their applicability depends on whether viable or nonviable organisms are being collected and on the sampling situation. There is no one agar medium on which all microorganisms will grow rapidly enough to be countable after a relatively short incubation period and no one assay procedure can completely characterize the microbial contamination on a surface.

The literature should be reviewed and a sampling method should be selected based on the specific situation under evaluation. Selection should take into account sampling location(s), type of agent, expected concentration, analytical methods, and organism characteristics. The principal factors that influence the selection of a particular technique are the type and chemical composition of the surfaces, expected levels and types of microorganisms, presence of bactericides, and objective of the sampling test (AIHA, 1986). Some tests are designed only to provide an index of sanitation whereas others are concerned with preuse quantitation of microorganisms on surfaces. There are five basic methods for enumerating microorganisms on surfaces: contact plates, swabbing, direct surface agar plating, rinsing, and vacuum sampling.

All sampling devices and media should be sterilized before each use. Most samplers can be adequately disinfected by swabbing with isopropanol or sodium hypochlorite (bleach). All media should be prepared within days of use or even the same day if possible in order to minimize the potential for contamination by normal microorganisms in the air. Malt extract agar is recommended for the general detection of fungi while agar containing casein peptone, soy peptone, and sodium chloride is used for bacteria (ACGIH, 1989). Trypticase soy agar has been used to collect and support the growth of fungi and bacteria (McJilton et al., 1990). In order to make a culture medium more specific, antibiotics and other compounds are often added to inhibit growth of certain microbes. As an example, inhibitory mold agar promotes fungal growth. Rose-Bengal-Streptomycin has also been recommended as a useful medium as it yields high colony counts and impedes colony spreading; however, it is sensitive to direct sunlight and must be shielded when sampling outdoors.

The simplest type of surface to sample is that which is visibly contaminated with microbial growth. The bacteria can be green to greenish-brown feltlike growth and can be present on a variety of surfaces such as books, papers, desks, chairs, cabinets, and plants in contaminated rooms. If the growth is heavy, it may be scraped and placed directly into sterile distilled water. A variation is to take the contaminated piece such as a ceiling tile and press it directly onto the sampling agar surface.

If sampling to determine if contamination or cleaning is effective, one technique used for hospital floors is to sample before cleaning, after cleaning, and at four additional intervals. Typical areas sampled in hospitals for surface contamination are:

Work rooms
Instrument washing areas
Sterile instrument storage
Sterile linen storage
Doctors' dressing rooms
Scrub rooms
Substerilizing rooms
Interior corridors
Operating rooms
Air handling system interiors

Sanitation in food handling and preparation facilities is important. To obtain quantitative measurements of microorganisms on kitchen equipment or utensils, defined areas must be sampled. Swabs of work and equipment surfaces can evaluate the effectiveness of cleaning procedures; however, swabbing eating utensils is seldom done because they are rarely associated with disease transmission (Bryan, 1974). Precision of results is affected by the area sampled, the number of times the same area is sampled, the number of samples taken, the methods of sampling, the tests used, and the phase of process or preparation at the time of sampling.

Swabbing the contact surfaces of equipment such as cutting boards, grinders, and slicing machines and testing the swabs for the presence of foodborne pathogens would indicate the potential for cross-contamination. However, if a foodborne outbreak is suspected, the food itself is usually sampled rather than equipment or workers.

COLLECTION TECHNIQUES

Contact Plates

Contact plate sampling involves pressing a solidified nutrient agar surface against a sample surface to be examine, removed, covered, and incubated before counting colonies on agar. Rodac agar plates are the best known type of agar contact plate and are the most widely used due to their commercial availability, simplicity, and portability. They are commercially available in presterilized disposable packages and are very easy to use. These plates are designed so that the bottom part of the plate can be filled with agar, resulting in a raised surface of culture medium for contact with the surface to be sampled. The top part of the plate fits over the bottom part without touching the agar surface.

Consistent results can be achieved if the sampling professional makes sure that the entire meniscus of the agar contacts the surface to be sampled without sliding over it. Since microorganisms are unevenly distributed on most surfaces, a specific sampling area should be marked off. A common size is a 100 in.^{2} area. Five Rodac plates are sufficient to sample this area. The total number of bacteria is estimated as follows:

$$\text{Total bacteria/100 in.}^2 = \frac{\text{Total bacteria/5 plates} \times 100\ \text{in.}^2}{3.9\ \text{in.}^2 \times 5}$$

Hycon® contact slides consist of a flexible culture-medium-coated film board. The culture medium is sealed into a transparent case that serves as a resealable shipping and incubation chamber for the exposed slide. These slides come in four varieties, each with a different type of agar: (1) total microbial count, (2) detection of fastidious bacteria, (3) selective detection of yeasts and molds, and (4) selective detection of coliform bacteria. Hycon® slides have a flexible carrier that allows good contact with curved as well as flat surfaces. They have a larger surface area than conventional Rodac plates (Fig. 8-1).

Coated slides can also be prepared in house and used in the same manner as Rodac plates, but they are especially useful for nonviable organisms. Properly prepared, they will allow the organisms to be preserved. A variation of using a coated surface is using a chunk of agar. A plunger and cylinder apparatus can be used,

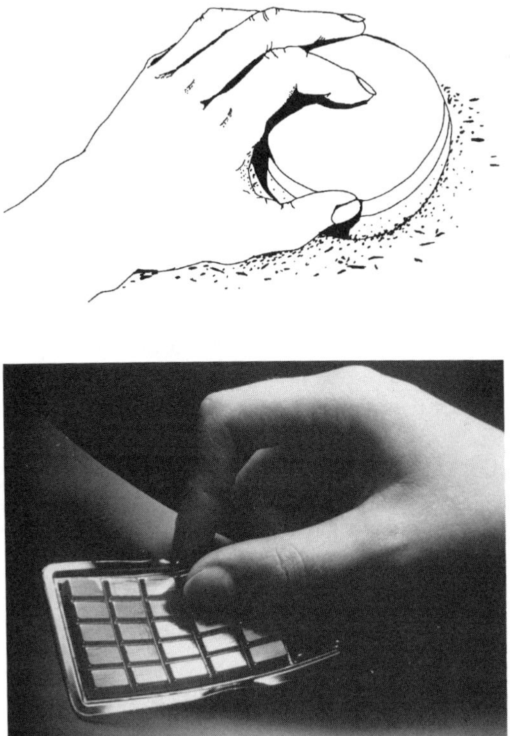

Figure 8-1. *Top:* Method of applying Rodac plate to surface. *Bottom:* Hycon® contact slide
Source: Drawing by Renea Joslin. Photo courtesy of Biotest Diagnostics Corporation.

such as a sterilized 20 mL or 50 mL syringe filled with sterile agar (MacCulloch and Cornere, 1973). The plunger pushes the agar out of the cylinder against the surface to be tested. The agar is sliced with a sterilized knife and placed in a petri dish for incubation. It can be difficult to make a smooth cut so that the next sampling surface contacts smoothly. Sausage casings have also been used rather than the cylinder and plunger (Walter, 1955).

Contact plates coated with trypticase soy agar with lecithin and polysorbate 80 have been used to sample the sides of immersion tanks in hospital burn units for bacteria (Turner, Higgins, and Craddock, 1974). A total of 15 plates, 5 from each side and 5 from the bottom of the tank, were used for each sample. Sampling was also repeated after scrubbing and rinsing.

Rodac plates have been used to sample clothing in a clean room before and after use (Kereluk, Meyer, and Pilgrim, 1965). Each item of clothing was separately packaged after cleaning and sealed in plastic bags. Both the clothing and the interior of the plastic bags were sampled. After being worn for 4 hours, the clothing was sampled again. Rodac plates with 110 agar have been used to sample a wooden pallet that lined the bottom of a metal, clean linen cart (Byrnes and Bland, 1980). A greater than 100 count growth of organisms identified the pallets as potential sources of recontamination for the hospital linen.

Contact plates are very portable and easy to use in the field. The plate is held in one hand, and using an equal pressure for each sample, the agar side is pressed against the surface to be sampled. For rough surfaces a slight rocking motion will provide better contact. Caution should be used so that the contact plate does not slip or slide on the surface. The time that contact plates are held next to the sample surface, often 5 seconds, should be consistent from sample to sample. Although rigid plastic contact plates are limited to flat surfaces, those of pliable plastic can be used on curved surfaces. In general, this method is limited to smooth surfaces. At least one study has found that fabric impinged bacteria do not imprint on Rodac plates with any degree of regularity (Wetzler, Quan, and Schatzle, 1971).

The primary disadvantage of direct contact methods is their inability to sample surfaces with high contamination and the interference of counts by confluence growth of mold or spreading colonies (Goulet et al., 1983). It is not possible to dilute samples collected on contact plates; therefore, this method is limited to situations where low levels of microorganisms are present. The presence of spreading colonies makes accurate counts difficult. A limitation of Rodac plates is that it is impossible to count colonies on the standard Rodac contact plate when bacterial contamination is very high. One way to get around this is to use a reflectance method (Jedlicka and Hill, 1975). First the reflectance of prepoured agar is measured and it is measured again after samples have been collected and incubated for 48 hours. With this method bacterial colonies will turn red, which lowers the reflectance of the medium. When compared with swab methods, the contact plate provided better recovery and repeatability for flat firm surfaces (Niskanen and Pohja, 1977).

Tape

Scotch tape imprints have been used to collect spores for qualitative identification of the presence of molds and other compounds. This technique has also been used for rapid identification of mold colonies growing on organic materials (Kozak and Gallup, 1985). After the tape is pressed against the surface, the exposed tape is stained and observed microscopically or placed in a small petri dish and covered with agar for culturing. Mylar tape has been used to sample the surfaces of red meat (Fung, Lee, and Kastner, 1980).

Velvet Pads

Sterile velvet pads of a standard size and shape can also be used to make an imprint on a surface and then imprinted onto agar. As an alternative they are rinsed in a sterile solution. The rinse method provided better recovery by a factor of up to 20 in one study and yielded consistent bacterial recoveries of 93% when rinsed in saline (Raahave, 1975).

Membrane Filters

The membrane filter technique uses a 5 μm membrane filter that is applied directly to a moist surface such as body tissue. Bacteria are absorbed into the filter and trapped in the membrane. The filter is then placed on a nutrient medium for culture and quantitation. In a study comparing this technique with Rodac plates and velvet pads, the filters recovered significantly more bacteria for contaminated surfaces (Craythorn et al., 1980).

Wipes and Swabs

Swabbing methods work in one of two ways. A cotton Q-tip or sterile pad or puff is used to wipe a surface and is then either wiped directly across an agar surface or immersed in a solution to remove the collected microorganisms. The solution is then plated with an appropriate culture medium. Most swabbing methods are best used to screen for gross contamination. It is a simple and easy-to-use field test. The most common swabs are cotton-tipped wooden swabs. Another version, sometimes called an "elephant" swab technique, consists of a sterile gauze sponge wrapped around the end of a sterile tongue depressor blade.

Sterile gauze pads by themselves can also be used to collect surface wipe samples for analysis of surface fungi. Calcium alginate swabs dissolve in Ringer's solution and sodium hexametaphosphate, thus freeing the microorganisms they collect. They have been found to produce higher counts than the cotton swab (Higgins, 1950). Calcium alginate swabs are limited, however, to collecting microorganisms that are not inhibited by either alginate or sodium hexametaphosphate. Membrane filters can be cultured after being used to filter calcium alginate swab solutions.

To use, an individually wrapped sterile calcium alginate swab is aseptically removed from its wrapper and inserted into a vial containing 4.5 mL of buffer. The swab is moistened and excess liquid is deposited against the inside of the vial. The swab is then moved across the testing surface, reversing direction between successive strokes while rotating the swab between the fingers. To sample glasses and cups with a swab, the outer rim as well as the inner rim surface is sampled. After sampling, the swab is placed in the vial and the stick of the swab is broken against the side of the vial below the point of handling.

Sterile swabs (Q-tips) of either cotton or Dacron are useful for sampling small inaccessible areas such as water spouts and drains. Cotton swabs can be used to collect air conditioning unit condensate as well as other suspect surface materials (McJilton et al., 1990). Showers and faucets have been swabbed for *Legionella* by using a Dacron swab to dislodge the sediment that has built up within the fixture (Stout et al., 1982). Cotton-tipped swabs soaked in sterile saline solution have been used to sample surface areas of up to 1 $ft.^2$ The swabs are then inoculated onto agar.

Depending on the situation, swabs can be used for identification or for routine testing if a source is known to be present. In one hospital where an outbreak of Legionnaires' disease occurred, the microorganism was found to be ubiquitous in the water system. The highest concentrations were found in the sediment of the various water sites, including faucets, showers, and hot water tanks. Sterile swabs should be used to wipe the surface of interest. If possible, a template should be used to delineate the area to be swabbed. The swabs are then stroked against the surface of a culture plate containing agar; plates are incubated and then examined. Swab method results may vary because different types of soils and dusts to which microorganisms adhere are removed at different rates depending on the chemical and physical properties of the surface; as with any wiping technique, the size of the area and the pressure applied will affect results.

Porous surfaces are best sampled using thorough rubbing with wet and/or dry swabs to get sufficient abrasion to dislodge microbes from the surface. Swabs were evaluated for their effectiveness in food service sanitation programs, and although the test itself was found to be useful, for periodic inspections it was not. In the event of a suspected salmonella epidemic, it is effective to test utensils such as plates, cups, glasses, silverware, and food preparation tools for contamination. Individually wrapped sterile calcium alginate swabs and sterile vials of neutralizing buffer solution are commonly used. A swab is aseptically removed from its wrapper and then inserted into a vial containing 4.5 mL of the buffer. The swab is moistened and excess liquid is deposited against the inside of the vial. For culturing, Q-tip type swabs can also be streaked directly on a petri dish with selective media in it.

Swabs have been used to collect spores of *Bacillus globigii* using cotton wool pledgets (Darlow, Simmons, and Roe, 1969). Sterile cotton wool pledgets were moistened in neutralizing buffer while being held with a forceps. Then 1.5 in. by 1 in. areas were swabbed with the cotton, still held with the forceps. The swabs were placed in 1.5 mL of the buffer, which also contained 0.5% lecithin, and were shaken for two minutes to remove the spores. For culturing, 0.25 mL aliquots were pipetted aseptically into each of four sterile petri dishes. Ten milliliters of molten plate count agar with 0.001% cycloheximide cooled to 45°C was poured into each dish and mixed by a standard technique. The dishes were allowed to stand on the bench for 1 hour before incubation at 37°C for 24 hours.

The duplicate swab technique uses two swabs for each sampling surface. The first swab is moistened in 9 mL of quarter strength Ringer's solution contained in a small screw cap bottom, rubbed over the surface, and is then broken off into the bottle of Ringer's. The second swab is used to remove excess moisture and any remaining microbes on the sampling surface, and is broken off into the same bottle of Ringer's.

One strategy for performing swabs on shower heads for *Legionella* is as follows: The internal and external surfaces are scraped with a sterile cotton swab and the swab is placed in a sterile plastic container along with a 15–25 mL aliquot of water obtained from the same shower after the head is reattached (Cordes et al., 1981). Swabs can also be used to sample sediment in water systems where microbial contamination such as *Legionella* is suspected. The sediment from disassembled parts, such as mixing valves and shower heads, is dislodged with a sterile Dacron swab, placed directly into buffered yeast extract broth with the dacron swab and cultured (Cordes et al., 1981).

Higher recoveries have been obtained when several similar sites are swabbed with a single swab rather than when one site is sampled with one swab. The result of sampling several sites with one swab is a composite sample that provides an average value of the surface contamination.

A modification of the swab method involves using a material such as sterilized velveteen mounted on a curved piece of metal, which is then moistened by rolling over a nutrient agar surface, and rolled once over the surface to be tested. Then the material is rolled over a nutrient culture agar, which is then incubated.

Another screening method for surface contaminants, including human pathogens such as *C. immitis*, uses moistened sterile cellulose sponges that are vigorously rubbed over the designated area, which can be as large as several square meters (NIOSH, 1981). The sponge is then introduced into a liquid medium and incubated. For *C. immitis* specifically, Saborouds dextrose broth with cycloheximide is used, and after incubation it is inoculated into rodents.

The disadvantages of the swab method are incomplete and inconsistent removal of surface bacteria. This problem is likely due to the many variables involved in swab sampling including pressure applied to the swab, moisture content of the swab, length of swabbing time, and fat content and texture of the surface. The swab method has been found to be appropriate for flexible and uneven surfaces and heavily contaminated surfaces (Goulet et al., 1983).

Scraping is an alternative to swabbing and has been used for food surfaces. On porous surfaces this method may be preferable to swabbing. One test found that the cotton swab method generally removed <10% of the microorganisms present when compared with scraping (Williams, 1967).

Direct Surface Agar Plate Method

The direct surface agar plate method involves pouring sterile melted agar into a tested surface and leaving it to solidify under a sterile cover. After incubation, the colonies at the agar interface are counted. Small items can be placed in a petri dish and covered with agar (Angelotti and Foter, 1958). The most common application is in laboratories, while field applications are limited because most surfaces are subject to disturbances in environments having significant temperature variations. This method cannot be used on surfaces containing chemicals that might be absorbed into the agar and inhibit the growth of the microorganisms. It is not useful for heavily contaminated surfaces since the growth will be so heavy that it will be hard to identify individual colonies. An advantage is that it measures microorganisms directly on the surface without the many variables associated with collecting devices.

Vacuuming

Vacuum cleaners have been used to collect dust for identification of hardy microorganisms such as house mites (Lundblad, 1991). A clean bag placed in a traditional vacuum can be used. Hand battery-powered vacuums have also been modified for sample collection (Haddock and San Nicolas, 1989). A short piece of plastic tubing is inserted in the suction nozzle and fixed in place with silicone plastic sealant, which is attached to a filter holder containing a membrane filter support pad in which the sample is collected. Dust was collected from carpet, a chair, and fabric-covered partitions in an office where there were concerns about the indoor air. Mattresses have also been vacuumed for dust mite excreta. Each sample should be collected in a separate bag in between which the vacuum is cleaned.

The vacuum probe sampler consists of a piece of Teflon tubing with a critical orifice connected to a conical aluminum chamber that houses a membrane filter. Under vacuum, surface particles impinge on the filter. The filter is removed, overlaid with a nutrient medium, incubated, and the colonies are counted. An evaluation provided 88% recoveries of surface contamination using this method (Peterson and Bond, 1969).

Another way of performing vacuuming is to have a canula connected by tygon tubing to either a slit sampler or an all-glass impinger. Viable microorganisms are impinged against an agar surface in the slit sampler or into a liquid medium in the impinger.

Some microorganisms cannot survive prolonged exposure to the airflow. When compared to the swab technique, the vac-probe recovered twice as many microorganisms. In general, this technique is suitable for sampling large surface areas where the level of microbial contamination is relatively low such as laminar low clean rooms (AIHA, 1986).

Rinse Method for Objects

Contaminated objects can either be immersed in a sterile fluid, or the fluid can be brought into contact with the surface being examined. Objects such as stainless steel, glass, or Lucite panels have had their surfaces sampled after being transferred to a sterile plastic bag containing 100 mL of distilled water with 0.5% peptone and 0.005% Tween 80 (Kereluk, Meyer, and Pilgrim, 1965). The bag was sealed and shaken vigorously for 2 minutes. Following this treatment, pour plates were made from the wash water to determine total numbers of bacteria.

This method is considered more accurate than swabbing because the entire surface is tested (Angelotti and Foter, 1958). Problems due to the variation in contamination on a surface are minimized. Surfaces such as food, which tend to retain bacteria, can produce low counts using this method.

Another variation that can be used for small objects is to take the object and make an impression with it directly onto an agar plate. This was used for oculars of microscopes (Paul et al., 1989). An impression of each ocular was performed directly onto a blood agar plate, following which each gall ocular was cultured with a premoistened sterile swab and then inoculated directly into the surface of a blood agar plate to determine if bacteria or fungi were present.

A spray gun technique has been developed that sprays a sterile rinse fluid against a specific area to remove microorganisms (Clark, 1965). The instrument recirculates the rinse fluid to a reservoir where it can be recovered and cultured. The disadvantages of the rinse method are the lack of friction to remove surface contaminants and its limitation to small objects.

Settling Plates

Setting out culture dishes to collect settling spores is similar to the methods used for settled dust and surface contamination from aerosols. Settling plate samples have been used to collect spores by exposing the bottom halves of empty, sterile, plastic petri dishes to the open air (Darlow, Simmons, and Roe, 1969). When the exposure time is complete, they are closed with a sterile lid. Molten plate count agar is added and mixed for analysis. Open petri dishes with nutrient agar are left out from 0, 1/2, and 1–4 hours and have been found to have a bias for collecting large particles (NIOSH, 1980*a*). Open settling surfaces that are uncoated can be used for hardy spores, can be left out for unlimited periods of time, and have the same bias toward large particles as coated petri dishes.

Plates can be placed in pairs in several different locations. They should not be placed directly underneath a ventilation system discharge vent. Different sampling times can be used for each one in the pair, especially if there are concerns about oversampling due to high concentrations being present.

The plates are covered and incubated and the total number of colonies growing on each plate is counted. A variation involves the use of stainless steel strips similar to the glass and mylar plates used to collect chemical aerosols. Sterile stainless steel strips are placed in the same environment as the surface of interest, and after a predetermined period of exposure the strips are transferred to bottles containing 1% sterile peptone water and subjected to ultrasonic energy or mechanical agitation (Favero et al., 1968). The rinse fluid is then cultured. This technique has been used primarily to measure surface contamination in spacecraft assembly areas and in laminar flow clean rooms used for the assembly and test of space hardware requiring dry heat sterilization (AIHA, 1986). This method may be inaccurate when the level of microbial contamination is low.

In a comparison of the use of Rodac agar plates (3.9 $in.^2$) and petri dishes (9.6 $in.^2$) as settling plates, no significant difference in the recovery of organisms from aerosol settling in either type of plate was noted (Kereluk, Meyer, and Pilgrim, 1965). The Rodac plates appeared to recover a slightly higher number of organisms. The slightly higher recovery was attributed to the lower sides of the Rodac plates. In comparing these plates it was noted that:

1. The organisms that collected on the petri plate concentrated around the center whereas those that collected on the Rodac plate were scattered over the entire plate.
2. The Rodac plate used less agar.
3. Rodac plates are smaller, thus requiring less incubator space.

Skin Samples

Skin cultures are occasionally done if there is a concern that the source of a dermatitis is a microbe found in the environment. Skin and nail scraping are often performed in conjunction with skin cultures. At this point a dermatologist should be involved. Skin cultures were collected from employees working in bio-pond waste treatment areas who were complaining of skin abscesses and other skin problems (NIOSH, 1983). Seven workers reported either skin abscess or folliculitis of the hands over the past one and one-half years. Bulk samples were collected from the various treatment ponds and cultured using the same media. Results were reviewed to see if there were any organisms in common known to be pathogens.

Tape has been used to remove microorganisms from human skin. This technique, often called tape stripping, is useful for identifying the distribution of bacteria on the skin. After the pressure sensitive tape is applied to the skin, it is removed and either covered with agar in a petri plate or placed on a prepoured plate. Each strip will remove a single layer of skin cells and the adhering bacteria (Ulrich, 1964). As many as 14 strippings have been performed. This technique is used to indicate the depth at which the organisms are found.

A variation involves the use of an adhesive film distributed evenly on a small plastic disc (Kooyman and Simons, 1965). This procedure allows for the rapid sampling of large groups of people for bacteria. It will provide information on the distribution and localization of the organisms on the skin surface if sufficient samples are collected.

Another method to sample depths of microorganism penetration in skin is scraping the skin with a scalpel. This procedure must be done under the direction of a physician. When scraping was compared with using adhesive tape, the tape was found to give satisfactory results (NIOSH, 1984).

Hands of workers can be rinsed with water or wiped with filters to collect microorganisms, but there is considerable variation and workers frequently have staphylococci and clostridia on their skin. If they handle raw meat or poultry, salmonella is usually present. Filters are used to identify reservoirs of epidemic causing bacteria and as a surveillance technique to evaluate general levels of cleanliness in food service establishments and health care facilities. The most common method for hands involves inserting the hands to the wrist in 1-quart size polyethylene freezer bags that have been sterilized with ethylene oxide and that contain a known volume of sterile sampling solution (AIHA, 1986). After inserting the hand, the subject holds the bag opening tightly around the wrist. The hand is then rubbed against the wall of the bag to agitate and dislodge the microorganisms. The fluid is then cultured. Skin washing and wiping techniques are further described in Chapter 11.

STORAGE AND SHIPMENT OF SAMPLES

Containers should be sterilized prior to use and shipping packages should insulate samples from environmental stresses, especially heat and freezing cold. Prompt shipment and proper sample storage following collection is critical for viable organisms. A rule of thumb is to get viable samples to a laboratory within 24 hours (ACGIH, 1989). During storage the sample temperature should be maintained as close as possible to that of the source (APHA, 1985). Samples taken on agar will begin to grow almost immediately following collection. Blanks should be included of sample (swab, coated slide, tape) and culture media.

ANALYSIS

Methods

Prior to sampling, an appropriate laboratory should be selected for analyses. Many clinical laboratories specialize in medical samples such as throat and other human cultures and do not have experience in analyzing environmental samples. Some laboratories specialize in mycology, the study of fungi, while antigen, endotoxin, and virus sampling often are still research techniques, and arrangements for analysis must be made with laboratories conducting research in a given area. *Legionnella* is one organism that was difficult to have cultured, but due to the wide interest many laboratories can now identify.

Analytical methods are direct, meaning the organism or its toxin is identified, or they are indirect, in that a skin bioassay or immunological assay on blood for an allergic reaction to that organism is performed and considered evidence that an individual has been exposed. Direct methods include microscopy that may be optical, electron microscopy, or epifluorescence (which requires that the sample be stained) and culturing followed by a variety of chemical tests for specific properties of microbes. Biochemical tests can be performed to identify metabolites, especially those considered toxic. Some direct reading tests for certain materials of this sort are available such as a test for house mite excreta.

A test kit is available that provides a semiquantitative determination of the level of mite infestation. For each sample, a measuring spoon of fine dust is mixed with the test fluid (potassium hydroxide and methanol). A colorimetric dip stick is placed in the mixture and the resulting color change when the guanine forms an azo dye of reproducible color intensity is compared to a scale to determine guanine content. The concentrations are classified as follows: light (0.06 mg/g), medium (0.25 mg/g), and strong (>1 mg/g).

Sampling professionals should be aware that not all microorganisms can be cultured, and some are extremely small and difficult to see in an optical microscope. In a situation where a food chain has occurred, the original microorganisms may no longer be present.

Interpretation of Results

It is not uncommon to find fungi such as fusarium, aspergillus, penicillium, and alternaria, which are ubiquitous in indoor and outdoor environments, in samples. Their presence alone does not constitute a health hazard (Howard, 1984). In the case of microorganisms such as *Staphylococcus epidermis*, which is commonly present on human skin, although these organisms are capable of causing disease in humans, the incidences are rare unless one's resistance is compromised by trauma, surgery, medication, or disease.

A standard of 100 colonies or less per utensil food contact surface was established in 1950 by the National Research Council (NRC, 1950). For example, the presence of predominantly *Bacillus* species on a sample suggests contamination is of nonhuman origin because these bacteria are found readily everywhere and in the spore stage can survive heat, cold, and drying (Robinton and Mood, 1968). On the other hand, finding primarily *Staphylococcus* or *Streptococcus* would suggest human contamination.

The most notable microorganisms are those not normally associated with areas of human habitation. Agents associated with hypersensitivity pneumonitis include *A. polyphaga*, *Aureobasidium* sp., and *Thermoactinomyces* sp. (NIOSH, 1983).

SURFACE MICROBIAL STUDIES

Contaminant	*Activity*	*Surface Methods*	*Other Sampling*	*Reference*
House dust mites	Indoor air quality investigation in an office building for allergy producers	Vacuum cleaner sampling of textile covered surfaces in office area (carpet, chair, partitions) and colorimetric test for mite excreta	Area air sampling for bacteria and fungi	Lundblad, 1991
Storage mites	Framing where house was suspected of being contaminated with mites from barn	Work clothing, cowhides, sofa and mattresses were sampled using vacuuming method	Barn floors vacuumed	Leskinen, Kalliokoski, and Heikkinen, 1991
Legionella pneumophila	Hospital	Dacron swab samples of showers and faucets at each of 13 nursing units and five offices or labs for identification Monthly samples at five showers and faucets		Stout et al., 1982
Legionella pneumophila	Water supply of hospital	Initial and routine swabs of showers and faucets in order to determine the source of endemic Legionnaires' disease		Stout et al., 1982
Legionella pneumophila	Hospital with concerns of the role of showers in sites where nosocomial Legionnaires' disease had occurred	Swab samples of shower heads with sterile cotton swab on internal and external surfaces	Bulk water samples from several sites on potable water system	Cordes et al., 1981
Legionella pneumophila	Hospital with concerns of the role of showers in sites where nosocomial Legionnaires' disease had occurred	Sediment from disassembled mixing valves and shower heads dislodged with a sterile Dacron swab and placed in culture media	Bulk water samples from several sites on potable water system	Cordes et al., 1981

Contaminant	*Activity*	*Surface Methods*	*Other Sampling*	*Reference*
Legionella pneumophila	Investigation of legionellosis outbreak at an inn	Swabs with cotton tipped applicators moistened with water from shower heads and a dehumidifier unit	Bulk sample of hair and organic debris from whirlpool pump strainer Water samples from water reservoir, kitchen skin faucet, outdoor swimming pool, indoor whirlpools, and dehumidifier sump	Witherell et al., 1983
Bacillus globigii	Animal lab involved in skin painting studies with carcinogens studied for the potential for spread of materials during typical activities (spores were substituted for carcinogens)	Swab samples collected on horizontal surfaces in treatment and animal housing room to determine spread of spores Settling plates also used to collect spores	Area air samples Bulk samples of animal bedding	Darlow, Simmons, and Roe, 1969
Bacteria	Disinfection of immersion tanks in a hospital burn unit	Contact plates with agar used to sample the surfaces of the tanks before and after scrubbing and rinsing, and after disinfection Swab samples of tank drain, overflow pipe, and turbines	Bulk sample of tank water after use	Turner, Higgins, and Craddock, 1974
Histoplasma capsulatum	Research and development laboratory with bird droppings inside ventilation system	Settled dust samples, including pigeon droppings, from inside the HVAC system for identification of *Histoplasma capsulatum* Wipe samples for *H. capsulatum* before and after fumigation of the HVAC system		NIOSH, 1983 (HETA 83-312-1400)

Contaminant	*Activity*	*Surface Methods*	*Other Sampling*	*Reference*
Bacteria: *Staphylococcus* sp. Baccillus	Clean room where electronic wafers were fabricated and 17 microscopes were shared over 3 shifts by 52 employees	An impression of each ocular was performed directly onto an agar plate and each glass ocular was swabbed with a premoistened sterile swab, which was then inoculated directly onto agar		Paul et al., 1989
Virus	Manufacturer of electronic components where employees in department using microscopes had high incidence of conjunctivitis	Sterile swabs of envelope surfaces placed in viral transport media	Conjunctival swabs for bacteria	Doyle et al., 1989
Bacteria	Sanitary landfill workers using heavy equipment (tractor) and spray irrigation	Contact plates from workers' hands and surface of rooms and control panel on landfill compactor	Personal breathing zone total dust and metals inside tractor cabin and outside for fungi and bacteria Area air sampling at fixed points downwind from spray irritation points	Rahkonen, Kttala, and Liokkanen, 1987
Bacteria	Insulation workers with skin problems	Cotton swab cultures of skin and scalp in the region of the headband of the hardhat to determine if irritation from refractory ceramic fibers (RCF) under hat allowed infection to develop due to fecal and oral contamination	Skin scrapings examined for RCF fibers	NIOSH, January 1981 (HHE 80-233-793)

Contaminant	*Activity*	*Surface Methods*	*Other Sampling*	*Reference*
Bacteria Fungi	Musical instrument repair shop where employees and management personnel had swollen lumps under their arms	Settling plates of blood and agar culture plates or petri dishes in bagging room, instrument repair, offices, and display areas Swabs inside air conditioning unit, supply ducts, dust collector in buffing room and on shag rug	Air samples for bacteria, fungi, sulfuric acid, chromic acid, respirable dust, and organic vapors Bulk dusts	NIOSH, August 1978 (HHE 78-65-514)
Molds Fungi	Facility manufacturing pressure switches and cockpit voice recorders where an outbreak of illness occurred	Petri dishes used as settling plates throughout work area	Air samples for organic vapors and metals	NIOSH, July 1980 (HHE 80-110-724)
Fungi	Newspaper printing facility where employees were concerned about contagious fungus in shower rooms and hand dermatitis	Surface samples in shower room and workers' skin	Skin scrapes Personal breathing zone air samples for solvents and vapors Bulk solvents of hand washing soaps, solvents, and inks	NIOSH, September 1976 (HHE 75-187-329)
Bacteria Fungi: *Aspergillus* *Penicillium* *Cladosporium*	School with widespread fungal contamination	Surface swabs for fungi on upper side false ceiling, air handling unit, diffuser, and duct	Bulk samples of filters from air handling units in HVAC system	NIOSH, January 1979*a* (TA 78-68)
Bacteria Yeast	Manufacture of small parts for the automotive industry (metalworking)	Swab samples on screw machines, broacher, and slotter for cultures	Personal breathing zone air samples for oil mist Bulk samples of cutting oils for bacterial growth and pH	NIOSH, February 1978 (HHE 77-77-464)

Contaminant	*Activity*	*Surface Methods*	*Other Sampling*	*Reference*
Bacteria: *Bacillus subtilis* Fungi	Printing factory where employees were suffering from an influenza-like illness	Sterile swabs from areas with accumulations of dust from beams, ventilator grids, and the floor Settling plates (2 min, 4 M in height) placed throughout the shop and at compressed air vents of machines	Area air sampling at three points in the continuous stationary dept.	Parrott and Blyth, 1980
Bacteria Fungi	Research lab where insects are reared and studied with high prevalence of occupational allergies among employees	Swab samples of surfaces Settling plates within the air handling system on each side of the air filter	Area air sampling for moth scales and fungi inside and outside the insectary Total dust and particle size air samples	NIOSH, May 1983 (HETA 82-2-1312)
Fungi: *Alternaria* sp. *Cladosporim* sp. *Epicoccum* sp. *Aspergillus* sp.	Office building with employee complaints of eye irritation, mucosal irritation, skin and respiratory irritation	Water stained and nonstained ceiling tiles pressed against sampling agar surface	Area air sampling for fungi on different floors of building, during changing of the HVAC filters, and in two surrounding office buildings as a control for ammonia, carbon dioxide, carbon monoxide, formaldehyde, nitrogen oxides, ozone, organic vapors, and total dust	NIOSH, November 1986 (HETA 86-410-1772)
Fungi	Office with employee complaints of poor air quality	Surface wipes with sterile gauze pads on return air grilles and supply diffuser	Area air sampling for carbon dioxide, bacteria, and fungi inside the building and for bacteria and fungi outside the building Bulk samples of insulation	NIOSH, March 1992 (HETA 91-257-2184)

Contaminant	*Activity*	*Surface Methods*	*Other Sampling*	*Reference*
Cocciodioides immitis	Lab performing research in human pathogens	Cotton tipped wooden swab samples (1 ft^2) of suspect and nonsuspect surfaces		NIOSH, November 1981 (HETA 80-183-991)
Bacteria Fungi	Office with poor air circulation and the presence of oppressive odors	Settling plates (open petri dishes) placed out in pairs (one for 15 min and 45 min) in three different locations—lunchroom, office area, and auditing area—and in a private residence as a control		NIOSH, April 1982 (HETA 81-469-1096)
Bacteria Fungi	Office building where employees had persistent flu-like illnesses	Settling plates (3 min) in the corridor and elsewhere in the building	Area air samples for fungi, bacteria, and pesticides High volume samples for respirable and total dust Blood Nasal swabs	NIOSH, April 1983 (GHETA 82-168-1302)
Molds: *Fusarium* *Aspergillus* *Penicillium* *Alternaria*	Middle school with indoor air quality concerns	Wipe samples for molds in the library based on identified growths on ceiling tiles and books		NIOSH, June 1987 (HETA 86-73-1804)
Bacteria Fungi	Office with indoor air problems	Smear samples of various surfaces of the furnace and HVAC system using throat swabs Petri dish settling plates with blood agar (1 hr)	Area air samples for organic vapors, nitrogen oxides, ozone, and carbon monoxide	NIOSH, January 1979*b* (HHE 78-69)
Allergens in dust: *Dermatophagoides pteronyssinus* *D. farinae*	Residences suspected of having mite and cat allergens in the house dust	Vacuum samples from bedroom mattresses and living room carpet collected on polytetrafluoroethylene filters	High volume air samples from living room and bedroom	Swanson et al., 1989

Contaminant	*Activity*	*Surface Methods*	*Other Sampling*	*Reference*
Bacteria: *Streptococci* *Klebsiella* *Proteus*	Cleaning procedures for machines used to slice meat in shops and cafes	Duplicate (30 cm^2) segments from the top and bottom surfaces of slicing blade, carving knives (1 cm^2, 4 cm^2), and can opener sampled using calcium alginate swabs after cleaning was performed	Bulk samples of used cleaning solution	Gilbert and Maurer, 1968
Bacteria: *Escherichia coli* *Staphylococcus aureus* *Streptococcus fecalis*	Comparison of disposable and reusable eating utensils used in food service operations at their point of use	Calcium alginate swabs moistened with buffer used to sample the food contact surface		Felix, Parrow, and Parrow, 1990
Bacteria: *Staphylococcus* *Bacillus* *Micrococcus* *Pseudomonas*	Investigation of contamination in hospital operating rooms, scrub areas, and dressing rooms and the effectiveness of disinfection procedures	Periodic samples collected with contact plates on operating lights, tables, anesthesia equipment, monitors and pillows, walls and floors		Suzuki et al., 1984
Bacteria: *Staphylococcus* *Bacillus* *Corneybacteria*	Study to determine the microbial contamination of cloth (continuous and individual) and paper towels placed in public restrooms	Rodac contact samples on towel surfaces		Robinton and Mood, 1968
Salmonella	Hospital (infant) nursery with *Salmonella* outbreak	Dust vacuumed into membrane support filter from rug placed at nursery entrance to determine if *Salmonella* was being carried in on staff's footwear		Haddock and San Nicolas, 1989
Bacteria: *Bacillus sp.* *Diptheroids*	Office where employees have developed red spots	Surface swabs in office	Area air samples for organic vapors and dusts Bulk humidifier water for fungi	NIOSH, February 1979 (TA 78-70)

REFERENCES

ACGIH Committee on Bioaerosols. 1989. *Guidelines for the Assessment of Bioaerosols in the Indoor Environment*. Cincinnati, OH: ACGIH.

Ager, B. P., and J. A. Tickner. 1983. The control of microbiological hazards associated with air-conditioning and ventilation systems. *Ann. Occup. Hyg.* **27**(4):341–358.

American Industrial Hygiene Association. 1986. *Biohazards Reference Manual*. Alexandria, VA: AIHA Biohazards Committee.

American Public Health Association. 1985. *Standard Methods for the Examination of Water and Waste Water*, 16th ed. New York: APHA.

Angelotti, R., and M. J. Foter. 1958. A direct surface agar plate laboratory method for quantitatively detecting bacterial contamination on nonporous surfaces. *Food Res.* **23**:170–174.

Birmingham, D. J., M. M. Key, and G. E. Tubich. 1961. Phototoxic bullae among celery harvesters. *Arch. Dermatol.* **83**:73–87.

Bryan, F. L. 1974. Identifying foodborne disease hazards in food service establishments. *J. Env. Health* **36**:537–540.

Bryan, F. L. 1978. Impact of foodborne diseases and methods of evaluating control programs. *J. Env. Health* **40**:315–323.

Byrnes, G. E. and L. A. Bland. 1980. Environmental health impact in the hospital laundry. *J. Env. Health* **42**(5):258–262.

Burge, H. A. 1985. Fungus allergens. *Clin. Rev. Allergy* **3**:319–329.

Clark, D. S. 1965. Method of estimating the bacterial population on surfaces. *Can. J. Microbiol.* **11**:407–413.

Cohen, S. R. 1974. Dermatologic hazards in the poultry industry. *JOM* **16**:94–97.

Cordes, L. G., A. M. Wiesenthal, G. W. Gorman, J. P. Phair, H. M. Sommers, A. Brown, W. V. Yu, M. H. Magnussen, R. D. Meyer, J. S. Wolf, K. N. Shands, and D. W. Fraser. 1981. Isolation of *Legionella pneumophilia* from hospital shower heads. *Ann. Internal Med.* **94**:195–197.

Craythorn, J. M., A. G. Barbour, J. M. Matsen, M. R. Britt, and R. A. Garibaldi. 1980. Membrane filter contact technique for bacteriological sampling of moist surfaces. *J. Clin. Microbiol.* **12**(2):250–255.

Darlow, H. M., D. J. C. Simmons, and F. J. C. Roe. 1969. Hazards from experimental skin painting of carcinogens. *Arch. Env. Health* **18**:883–893.

Doyle, L., K. Gallagher, B. S. Heath, and W. B. Patterson. 1989. An outbreak of infectious conjunctivitis spread by microscopes. *JOM* **31**(9):758–762.

Favero, M. S., J. J. McDade, J. A. Robertsen, R. K. Hoffman, and R. W. Edwards. 1968. Microbiological sampling of surfaces. *J. Appl. Bacteriol.* **31**:336–343.

Felix, C. W., C. Parrow, and T. Parrow. 1990. Utensil sanitation. *J. Env. Health* **53**(2):13–15.

Fung, D. Y. C., C. Y. Lee, and C. L. Kastner. 1980. Adhesive tape method for estimating microbial load on meat surfaces. *J. Food Protect.* **43**:295–297.

Gilbert, R. J., and I. M. Maurer. 1968. The hygiene of slicing machines, carving knives and can-openers. *J. Hyg. Camb.* **66**:439–449.

Goddard, K. R. 1967. Effect of ventilation on distribution of airborne microbial contamination—field studies. In G. W. Royster and B. R. Fish (eds.), *Surface Contamination*. New York: Pergamon Press, pp. 349–356.

Goulet, J., G. L'evesque, J. R. Morean, and L. A. Roth. 1983. A new simple method for microbiological sampling of meat surfaces. *Can. J. Microbiol.* **29**:631–636.

Haddock, R. L., and A. San Nicolas. 1989. Infant salmonellosis. *J. Env. Health* **52**:106–107.

Higgins, M. 1950. A comparison of the recovery rate of organisms from cotton, wool and calcium alginate wool swabs. *Pub. Health Lab. Ser. Bull.* **9**:50–51.

Hodgson, E. S., and C. Ruis-Frutos. 1991. A case report of contaminated operating theatre multipurpose equipment: A potential hazard for health care workers. *Ann. Occup. Hyg.* **35**(3):341–346.

Howard, W. A. 1984. Incidence and clinical characteristics of mold allergy. In Y. Al-Doory and J. Domson (eds.), *Mold Allergy*. Philadelphia, PA: Lea & Febinger.

Jedlicka, G. J., and W. M. Hill. 1975. A reflectance method for the enumeration of surface bacteria. *J. Food Sci.* **40**:647–648.

Kereluk, K., R. Meyer, and A. J. Pilgrim. 1967. A preliminary investigation of microbial surface contamination in various clean room environments. In G. W. Royster and B. R. Fish (eds.) *Surface Contamination*. New York: Pergamon Press, pp. 191–206.

Kooyman, J., and R. W. Simons. 1965. "Sticky disc" sampling of skin microflora. *Arch. Dermatol.* **92**:581–584.

Kozak, P. P., and J. Gallup. 1985. Endogenous mold exposure: Environmental risk to atopic and nonatopic patients. In H. B. Gammage and S. V. Kaye (eds.), *Indoor Air and Human Health*. Chelsea, MI: Lewis Pubs. Inc.

Kurtz, J. B. 1988. *Legionella pneumophilia*. *Ann. Occup. Hyg.* **32**(1):59–61.

Leskinen, L., P. Kalliokoski, and P. Heikkinen. 1991. *Storage Mites Are Carried into Farm Houses from the Farm Work Environment*. Salt Lake City, UT: American Industrial Hygiene Conference, Abstract.

Lundblad, F. P. 1991. House dust mite allergy in an office building. *App. Occup. Env. Hyg.* **6**(2):94–96.

MacCulloch, D., and B. M. Cornere. 1973. A method for bacteriological sampling of surfaces by direct application of culture media. *J. Clin. Pathol.* **26**(12):977–978.

Macher, J. M., and M. W. First. 1984. Personal air samplers for measuring occupational exposures to biological hazards. *AIHA J.* **45**(2):76–83.

McJilton, C. E., et al. 1990. Bacteria and indoor odor problems—three case studies. *AIHA J.* **51**(10):545–549.

Morris, J. E. W. 1975. Microbial pollution in submersibles. *Ann. Occup. Hyg.* **17**:245–246.

National Research Council. 1950. Minimum requirements for effective machine dishwashing. Committee on Sanitary Engineering and Environment, Division of Medical Sciences. *Hospitals* **24**:92.

Nichols, G. 1985. Scotch Magic Tape—An air to the microscopist for dust examination. *Microscope* **33**:247–254.

NIOSH, Health Hazard Evaluation Report. September 1976. *Cincinnati Enquirer, Cincinnati, OH.* HHE 75-187-329. Cincinnati, OH: NIOSH.

NIOSH, Health Hazard Evaluation Report. February 1978. *Buckeye Automatic Co., McArthur, OH.* HHE 77-77-464. Cincinnati, OH: NIOSH.

NIOSH, Health Hazard Evaluation Report. August 1978. *Carleton Stewart Music Co., Mason City, IA.* HHE 78-65-514. Cincinnati, OH: NIOSH.

NIOSH, Health Hazard Evaluation Report. January 1979*a*. *School of Veterinary Medicine, Tuskegee Institute, Tuskegee, AL.* TA 78-68. Cincinnati, OH: NIOSH.

NIOSH, Hazard Evaluation and Technical Report. January 1979*b*. *Social Security Administration, Richmond, IN.* TA 78-69. Cincinnati, OH: NIOSH.

NIOSH, Hazard Evaluation and Technical Report. February 1979. *Central Intelligence Agency. Washington, DC.* TA 78-70. Cincinnati, OH: NIOSH.

NIOSH, Health Hazard Evaluation Report. July 1980*a*. *Commonwealth of Massachusetts, Dept. of Labor and Industries, Div. Occupation Hygiene, Boyleston, MA.* TA 80-19. Cincinnati, OH: NIOSH.

NIOSH, Health Hazard Evaluation Report. July 1980*b*. *Fairchild Industrial Products, Commack, NY.* HHE 80-110-724. Cincinnati, OH: NIOSH.

NIOSH, Health Hazard Evaluation Report. January 1981. *Davis Bessie Nuclear Power Station, Toledo Edison Co., United Engineers and Contractors Co., Oak Harbor, OH.* HHE 80-233-793. Cincinnati, OH: NIOSH.

NIOSH, Health Hazard Evaluation Report. November 1981. *Naval Biosciences Laboratory, Oakland, CA.* HHE 80-183-991. Cincinnati, OH: NIOSH.

NIOSH, Health Hazard Evaluation Report. April 1982. *Cincinnati Income Tax Bureau, Cincinnati, OH.* HETA 81-469-1096. Cincinnati, OH: NIOSH.

NIOSH, Health Hazard Evaluation Report. April 1983. *Hubert H. Humphrey Bldg., Washington, DC.* GHETA 82-168-1302. Cincinnati, OH: NIOSH.

NIOSH, Health Hazard Evaluation Report. May 1983. *Metabolism and Radiation Research Laboratory (MRRL), Fargo, ND.* NETA 82-2-1312. Cincinnati, OH: NIOSH.

NIOSH, Health Hazard Evaluation Report. 1983. *E. I. Dupont de Nemours & Co., LaPorte, TX.* HETA 81-069-1390. Cincinnati, OH: NIOSH.

NIOSH, Health Hazard Evaluation Report. January 1984. *Champion Technology Center, Hamilton, OH.* HETA 83-312-1400. Cincinnati, OH: NIOSH.

NIOSH, Health Hazard Evaluation Report. April 1984. *King Kwit Minit Market, Inc.* HETA 83-409-1450. Cincinnati, OH: NIOSH.

NIOSH, Health Hazard Evaluation Report. November 1986. *HFCA–Meadows East Building, Baltimore, MD.* HETA 86-410-1772. Cincinnati, OH: NIOSH.

NIOSH, Health Hazard Evaluation Report. June 1987. *South Campbell County Middle School, Alexandria, KY.* HETA 86-73-1804. Cincinnati, OH: NIOSH.

NIOSH, Health Hazard Evaluation Report. March 1992. *Ohio Civil Rights Commission, 200 Goodall Complex, Cincinnati, OH.* HETA 91-257-2184. Cincinnati, OH: NIOSH.

Niskanen, A., and M. S. Pohja. 1977. Comparative studies on the sampling and investigation of microbial contamination of surfaces by the contact plate and swab methods. *J. Appl. Bacteriol.* **42**:53–63.

Parrot, W. F., and W. Blyth. 1980. Another causal factor in the production of humidifier fever. *J. Soc. Occup. Med.* **30**:63–68.

Paul, M., J. Himmelstein, S. Weinstein, G. Pransky, C. McDougal, B. Brogie, and S. Legendre. 1989. Ocular infections and the industrial use of microscopes. *JOM* **31**(9):763–766.

Peterson, N. J., and W. W. Bond. 1969. Microbiological evaluation of the vacuum probe surface sampler. *Appl. Microbiol.* **18**(6):1002–1006.

Raahave, D. 1975. Experimental evaluation of the velvet pad rinse technique as a microbiological sampling method. *Acta Pathol. Microbiol. Scand.* **83B**:416–424.

Rahkonen, P., M. Kttala, and I. Liokkanen. 1987. Working conditions and hygiene at sanitary landfills in Finland. *Ann. Occup. Hyg.* **31**(4A):505–513.

Robinton, E. D., and E. W. Mood. 1968. A study of bacterial contaminants of cloth and paper towels. *Am. J. Pub. Health* **58**:1452–1459.

Stout, J., V. L. Yu, R. M. Vickers, J. Zuravleff, M. Best, A. Brouwn, R. B. Yee, and R. Wadowsky. 1982. Ubiquitousness of *Legionella pneumophila* in the water supply of a hospital with endemic Legionnaires' disease. *New Eng. J. Med.* **306**:466–468.

Suzuki, A., Y. Namba, M. Matsuura, and A. Horisawa. 1984. Bacterial contamination of floors and other surfaces in operating rooms: A five-year survey. *J. Hyg. Camb.* **93**:559–566.

Swanson, M. C., A. R. Campbell, M. J. Klauck, and C. E. Reed. 1989. Correlations between levels of mite and cat allergens in settled and airborne dust. *J. Allergy Clin. Immunol.* **83:**776–783.

Turner, A. G., M. M. Higgins, and J. G. Craddock. 1974. Disinfection of immersion tanks (Hubbard) in a hospital burn unit. *Arch. Env. Health* **28:**101–104.

Ulrich, J. A. 1964. Techniques of skin sampling for microbial contaminants. *Health Lab. Sci.* **1:**133–136.

Van Assendelft, A., et al. 1979. Humidifier associated extrinsic allergic aleolitis. *Scand. J. Work Env. Health* **5:**35.

Walter, W. G. 1955. Symposium on methods for determining bacterial contamination on surfaces. *Bacteriol. Rev.* **19:**267–284.

Wetzler, T. F., T. J. Quan, and K. Schatzle. 1971. Critical analysis of the microflora of toweling. *Am. J. Pub. Health* **61**(2):376–393.

Williams, M. L. B. 1967. A new method for evaluating surface contamination of raw meat. *J. Appl. Bacteriol.* **30**(3):498–499.

Witherell, L. E., L. A. Orciari, K. C. Spitalny, R. A. Pelletier, W. B. Cherry, L. H. Orrison, L. F. Novick, K. M. Stone, and R. M. Vogt. 1983. Isolation of *Legionella pneumophila* from recreational whirlpool spas. *J. Env. Health* **46:**77–80.

CHAPTER 9

Surface Sampling for Low Level Radiation

Surface contamination from radioactive materials is a problem from two points of view. In the first place, the contamination can be a health hazard to the people working in the area due to inhalation or ingestion of the radioactive material. The second problem is that surface contamination may spread, causing contamination of equipment and other areas where it may not be suspected. Inhalation generally is the primary route of exposure for radioactive materials from contaminated surfaces. Airborne contamination produces surface radioactive contamination and, conversely, surface contamination produces radioactive airborne contamination.

Overexposures to radiation can occur as a result of inhalation, oral ingestion, surface skin exposure, and deep body skin penetrating exposures. Since radiation at the levels most commonly encountered in occupational situations does not have any warning signs to indicate an exposure is occurring, it is particularly important to perform surveys. Figure 9-1 shows the depth to which the various radioactive particles can penetrate.

Control programs for radioactive materials almost always include some monitoring for surface contaminants. Surface contamination monitoring can provide a general indicator of the degree of control being maintained over operations with radioactive material. Regular surface testing of radiation sources is often a state licensing requirement for the owner of the radiation source. Health department regulations often require leak testing (Table 9-1) of naturally occurring and accelerator-produced radioactive material (NARM) sealed sources. The Nuclear Regulatory Commission (NRC) and its member states require specific education and training for persons who perform leak testing.

The rate of release of radioactivity from surfaces is affected by particle size, density, humidity, temperature, air turbulence, surface composition and condition, and chemical state of the material (Spangles and Willis, 1965). Visual contamination is not a useful indicator of excessive surface contamination because deposits of UO_2, U_3O_8, and UF_4 are visible on work surfaces and clothing at levels greater than about 2,000 alpha dpm per 100 cm^2, while accumulations of uranyl fluoride or the oxides enriched in U^{235} may not be visible even at much higher activity levels (Schultz and Becher, 1963).

Radioactive surface contamination can be described as total residual, removable, loose, and fixed. Removable or free contamination is considered as the amount remaining on a dry filter

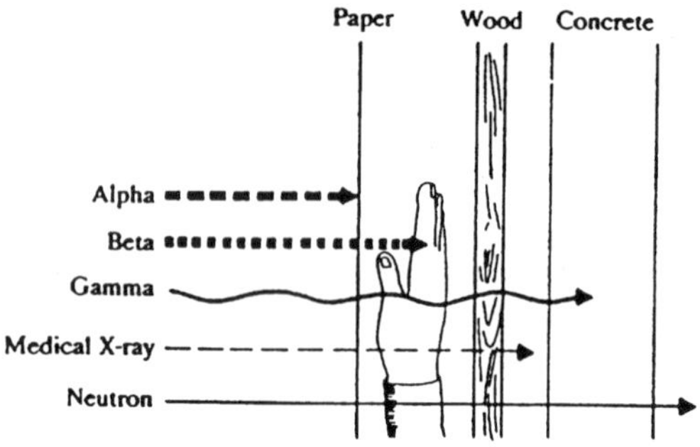

Figure 9-1. Sketch illustrating the ability of different forms of ionizing radiation to penetrate paper, the human body, wood, and concrete. *Source:* From NRC. n.d. *Working Safely with Nuclear Gauges*. NUREG/BR-0133. Washington, DC: U.S. Nuclear Regulatory Commission.

after it is used to wipe a 100 cm^2 area or, alternatively, it is material that can be easily removed by sucking dust into a vacuum. Loose contamination is that which cannot be removed without applying decontamination agents. Fixed contamination is not easily removed from a surface, and usually requires removal of some portions of the surface or dismantling of the contaminated parts. Total residual contamination is a combination of all three types.

Surface contamination can occur through direct contact with workers' hands or personal protective equipment, or through gravitational deposition of radiation. Once testing has determined that surface contamination exists, deeper testing of chips from surfaces may be required.

Routine contamination surveys should incorporate techniques to detect both removable and fixed contamination and should be conducted according to the following frequency recommendations (DOE, 1992):

1. Prior to transfer of equipment and material from one radiological buffer area to another.
2. Prior to transfer of equipment and material from highly contaminated areas within radiological buffer areas unless precautions such as bagging or wrapping are taken prior to transfer.
3. Daily, at contamination area control points, change areas, or protective clothing removal stations or per shift in high use situations.
4. Daily, in lunchrooms and office space located in radiological buffer areas.
5. Weekly, in routinely occupied radiological buffer areas.
6. Weekly, or upon entry if entries are less frequent, in areas where radioactive materials are handled or stored.
7. Weekly, or upon entry if entries are less frequent, where contamination boundaries or postings are located.

TABLE 9-1. Examples of Sources That Are Leak Tested

Source	*Radionuclide*	*Activity*
Level indicators	Cs^{137}	3.0 Ci, 100 mCi, 2 Ci, 1 Ci, 5 Ci, 500 mCi, 10 mCi, 25 mCi
	Am^{241}, neutron emitter	500 mCi
Electron capture detector in gas chromatograph	H^3	0.25 Ci
Sulfur analyzer	Am^{241}	550 mCi
Density meter	Cs^{137}	200 mCi
	Cd^{109}	5 mCi
	Fe^{55}	45 mCi
Metal analyzer	Fe^{55}	45 mCi
	Cd^{109}	5 mCi

8. During initial entry into a known or suspected contamination area, periodically during work, upon completion of a job, or as specified in a radiological work permit.
9. Areas identified as either contaminated with, or having the potential for being contaminated with, highly radioactive particles should be surveyed weekly. However, these areas must be surveyed daily during periods of work that may result in the generation of these particles.

Surface contamination that exceeds the standards, like airborne contamination, requires restriction of the area. Contaminated materials and equipment exceeding total or removable contamination levels are usually only conditionally released from a site for immediate placement in another radiation area. Controls must be in place during transit to prevent exposure and contamination of the transport vehicle and personnel. Whenever surface contamination is determined to be present, controls to prevent the inadvertent transfer of removable surface contamination to areas outside the identified radiation areas are necessary. These include posting, monitoring personnel and property at the exit, and using personal protective equipment. Types of controls include conspicuous visual and/or audible alarms, locked entries, and barricades.

Posting is used to identify areas of significant surface contamination. Different signs are used to identify areas with various radioactive levels. The classification categories for surface contamination are in Table 9-2. Signs with the standard radiation symbol and barriers are used. Ropes, tape, and chains have all been used to designate the boundaries of posted areas and are color coded similarly to the signs.

DETECTION EQUIPMENT

The type of radiation to be measured generally determines what instrument will be selected to perform measurements. The most common direct reading instruments used for radiation surveys are Geiger Meuller (GM) counters, ionization chambers, and portable scintillation detectors (Table 9-3).

Geiger-Mueller Detectors

The GM counter has been the most widely used detector. It has been popular because it is highly sensitive to even the smallest radiation; it can be used with many different types of radiation; it has a very high voltage pulse output; it is very portable and easy to use; and its cost is reason-

TABLE 9-2. Criteria for Posting Contamination and High Contamination Areas

Area	*Criteria*	*Posting*
Contamination	Levels (dpm/100 cm^2) > 1 time, but ≤ 100 times Table 9-7 values	"CAUTION, CONTAMINATION AREA" "RWP Required for Entry"
High contamination	Levels (dpm/100 cm^2) > 100 times Table 9-7 values	"DANGER, HIGH CONTAMINATION AREA" "RWP Required for Entry"
Fixed contamination	No removable contamination and total contamination levels exceed Table 9-7, column 3, values	"CAUTION, FIXED CONTAMINATION"

Source: Data from DOE. June 1992. *Radiological Control Manual.* DOE/EH-0256T. Washington, DC: U.S. Dept. of Energy, Assistant Secretary for Environment, Safety and Health.
Note: RWP = radiation work permit.

TABLE 9-3. Radiation Survey Instruments

Detector	*Radiation Measured*	*Full Scale Readings*	*Minimum Energy Measured*	*Directional Dependence*
Ionization chamber	β, X, γ	3 mR/hr to 500 R/hr	20 keV for X-rays; variable for betas	Low for X or γ
GM counter	β, X, γ	0.2 to 20 mR/hr to 800 to 80,000 cpm	20 keV for X-rays; 150 keV for betas	Low for X or γ
Scintillation counter	β, X, γ, neutrons	0.02 to 20 mR/hr	20 keV for X-rays; variable for betas	Low for X or γ
Alpha scintillation counter	α	100 to 10,000 α/min	Variable	High

able. It is not suitable if an accurate quantitation of exposure rate is necessary, but for screening purposes it is a good instrument to detect contamination.

The GM counter typically measures beta and gamma radiation. It has a metal or plastic detector probe, about 4 in. long, on a cable extending from the meter case, although some models do not have a probe. The basis of radiation detection in the GM counter is the production of ions by radiation as it passes through a gas, usually helium, argon, or neon. The gas is housed within the detector probe, which is actually the GM tube itself, that consists of positive and negative electrodes and the detector gas. The radiation creates negative electrons that move toward the positive electrode that, in turn, produce an electric current. The rate at which this current is produced depends on the intensity of the radiation to which the probe is exposed. The signal is expressed in units of milliRoentgens per hour (mR/hr). The lowest scale is the most sensitive and should be used to detect low level contamination.

A thin Mylar film, called a window, is located at the measuring end of the probe. This window has to be very thin to allow weakly penetrating radiations such as alpha and beta to enter. Great care must be taken not to puncture this window with sharp objects when using the detector probe. If the window is punctured, the GM probe must be replaced prior to further use. On many of these probes there is a sliding shield that can be opened or closed by twisting the end of the probe, or the end of the probe can be pulled out of an external shield cover. Generally, radiation surveys are performed with the probe in the open unshielded, exposed position so the probe can detect both beta and gamma radiation. When the shield is closed, beta radiation is blocked out, so the probe detects only gamma rays. When using the GM detector, the probe should be placed approximately 1 in. above the surface to be checked for possible contamination from liquid radiation or to locate other sources of radiation.

If a GM detector is used in a very high radiation field, it may read low or zero on the meter because the tube must be able to recover between detections. The GM counter cannot be used to detect low energy alphas and betas, including low energy beta from tritium and low concentrations of I^{125} or C^{14}. It can be used to detect radiation from Cs^{137}, P^{32}, Tc^{99m}, I^{131}, Ra^{226}, Co^{60}, Ir^{192}, and Au^{198}.

Ionization Chambers

In the portable ionization chamber, also called a "Cutie Pie," the radiation is allowed to penetrate a specifically known quantity of gas (usually helium or argon) within the sensitive volume of the detector. As the ion pairs are created within the sensitive volume, the charges migrate toward positive and negative electrodes within the chamber. This movement of electric charge constitutes what is known as an electric current. The amount of current produced depends on the number of ions created that, in turn, depends on the amount of radiation presented to the chamber. The amount of current produced per unit of time is measured as an exposure rate in units of Roentgens/hr (R/hr) or mR/hr. These instruments tend to be rather expensive, are relatively insensitive to low levels of radiation, and should not be used to detect areas of radioactive contamination. Proper zeroing is very important when using ionization detectors.

Comparison of Ionization Chambers and GM Counters

The ionization survey meter is similar to a GM counter in portability, but often has a large detection chamber as part of the instrument housing rather than in an external probe. The following comparisons apply: (1) An ionization instrument is not energy dependent, however the GM counter is; (2) ionization instruments generally require higher voltage (and more batteries); (3) ionization instruments often have higher scale ranges; and (4) ionization instruments are also used for X-ray measurements because of larger detector chambers, faster response times, and energy dependence.

Scintillation Detectors

The portable scintillation detector is more sensitive than the GM counter, especially in the detection of X- and gamma-ray emitting sources such as I^{125}, as well as medium and higher energy radiations, and therefore it is useful for locating lost or misplaced radiation sources. This type of detector looks and operates much the same as the GM counter with the exception of the detector probe. The probe for this detector is somewhat larger than that of the GM, but instead of a detector gas, a sodium iodide crystal is utilized. On interaction with X and gamma rays, small flashes of light, known as scintillations, are produced. Though too faint to be detected with the unaided eye, the flashes of light are detected by a light sensitive electronic device known as a photomultiplier tube, which converts these flashes of light to electrical pulses that, in turn, create the readout on the scale of the instrument. Like the GM, it usually has several scales of operation, commonly in units of mR/hr. Because of the crystal, special care must be taken to protect the probe from mechanical jarring or rapid changes or extremes in temperature. These conditions can produce crystal fractures that will cause the instrument to malfunction.

Scintillation detectors can also be used on some types of GM instruments instead of the usual probe. Scintillation probes typically consist of a thin wafer of sodium iodide crystal (activated with thallium) or a larger detector crystal. Compared to GM probes, these scintillation probes are much more efficient detectors of lower energy gamma radiation.

Neutron Detectors

Methods of detection for neutrons vary according to the neutron source's energy. Slow neutrons are detected by nuclear reactions with either B^{10} or with material that has a high cross-section for fission with low neutron energies. The boron chamber consists of a small cylinder containing boron fluoride gas or B^{10} in solid form. This detector functions as a proportional counter to detect the alpha particles released from the B^{10} to Li^7 reaction. Neutron instruments generally have a large (10 in. or more) round "Bonner" sphere as the detection chamber. Scintillation detectors are also used for neutron detection. The energy of the neutrons detected is a function of the scintillation crystal used. The crystal is impregnated with a material that gives off ionizing radiation when bombarded by neutrons. The crystal may be either solid or liquid in form. These instruments are very specific for neutrons and should never be used for general purposes. For this reason their operation is usually restricted to health physicists.

SAMPLING METHODS

Screening Surfaces for Total Contamination Using Instruments

Performance of radiation surveys should include dose rate measurements of the general area, dose rates at a distance of 30 cm from a source or surface of interest to evaluate potential whole body exposures, and dose rates on contact with potential sources of radiation where there is a possibility for hands-on work. Contamination surveys are frequently done after a grid has been developed for survey blocks (Fig. 9-2). Multiple test points are often measured within a group of related grid blocks to determine representative values. This approach allows for testing without biased scanning for hot spots to build a statistical distribution necessary for a representative assessment.

Monitoring should be performed only by trained and qualified personnel using properly calibrated instruments. Calibration procedures should be developed for each instrument type and should include frequency of calibration, precalibration requirements, primary calibration requirements, periodic performance test requirements, calibration record requirements, and maintenance requirements. Calibrations must use National Institute of Standards and Technology (NIST) traceable sources. For contamination monitoring the calibration is always done with reference to an area of 100 cm^2, regardless of the detector's window area. This standardization is necessary to ensure that the results obtained with different instruments are comparable. Instruments should bear a label or tag with the date of calibration and the date the next calibration is due. Never change a detection probe on an instrument unless it has been calibrated for use with that specific probe. Efficiencies of detector probes, even of the same model, may vary greatly from one probe to another. Changing a probe without having the

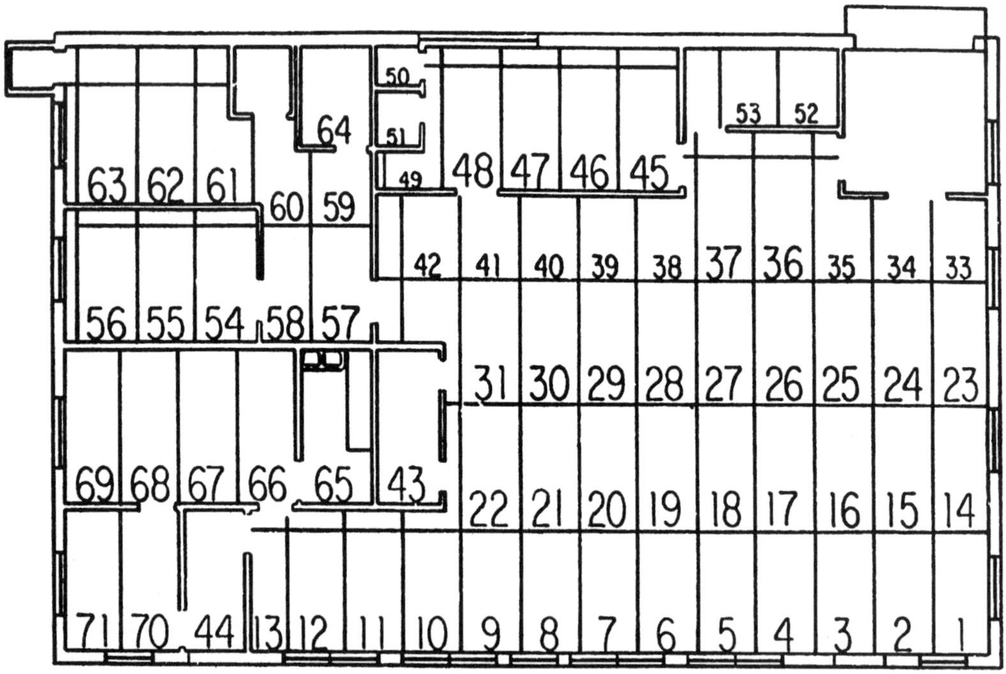

Figure 9-2. Floor/ceiling map grid (floor/ceiling areas are numbered the same).
Source: From EPA. 1985. *Guide for Decontaminating Buildings, Structures, and Equipment at Superfund Sites*. EPA 600/2-85-028. Washington, DC: Environmental Protection Agency.

calibration rechecked or adjusted could lead to serious errors in exposure readings. Radiation instrument response to interfering ionizing and nonionizing radiation and environmental conditions should be determined. The effects such interfering radiation have on an instrument should be known prior to use.

Instruments used to perform radiation surveys should also be response checked daily or prior to operation. Functional tests should be used to assess instrumentation designs that include alarms or that involve a process control. A functional test should be developed to test all components involved in an alarm or trip function and performed at least annually. When response checks are not within ±20% of the expected value, the instrument should be taken out of service. When response checks are not feasible, such as with instruments used to measure neutrons or tritium, compensatory actions should be established to ensure proper instrument performance. Usually certain areas are selected as control areas to compare measurements made where radiation contamination is suspected.

During any survey in which the quantity of radiation is unknown or it is suspected that it is high, the proper procedure is to stand at least 3 ft away from the radiation source with the probe or instrument face (in the case of an internal detector) facing the source to be measured. The instrument's batteries should always be checked using the battery check mode prior to operation. Batteries should be checked every 2–3 months even if an instrument is not being used. After turning an instrument on, do not change the scale ranges rapidly because many ionization instruments will not function properly if not given at least 4 sec waiting time before switching to the next range. Starting with the high scale ranges, slowly work toward the lower scale ranges, noting the deflection of the needle on the readout. If the needle starts to move in the higher scale ranges, the source contains a significant amount of radiation. As you move toward the source, increase the scale. Care should be taken not to change scales too quickly or the instrument's response may be delayed producing a false negative. A general rule is to select a scale that gives a good reading above 30% of the scale range. The higher the exposure rate, the closer one is to the radiation source or the greater the amount of radiation being emitted or both, and the greater the care that must be taken.

Instruments with pancake-type detection probes work well for measuring surface contamination. The response of a given instrument to surface contamination depends on the distance the detector is held from the surface and the speed at which the detector is passed over the surface. In assessing the potential hazard arising from localized spots, measurements are generally averaged over 100 cm^2. The distance from the surface should be kept constant during monitoring. A surface-to-probe distance of 0.5 cm or 0.5 in. is most common. Alpha detector probes are always placed directly on the surface of the item being checked, because alpha particles can travel only a few centimeters at most. (This restriction is considerably different than GM or ionization instruments, which may measure gamma or X-ray radiation at distances.) When moving a probe over rough surfaces such as splintered wood or soil, it is important not to allow any objects to touch the thin-window type probes. If there is a possibility of contaminating a probe, use a thin disposable glove or plastic wrap around the probe for protection against contamination.

Radiological surveys should be recorded and include the following common elements: date, time, and purpose of the survey: general and specific location of the survey; name and signature of the surveyor and analyst; pertinent information needed to interpret the survey results; reference to a specific radiological work permit if the survey is performed to support the permit; the instrument model and serial number; and results of the measurements of area dose rates. Contamination surveys should also include contamination levels (using appropriate units) and supporting parameters including counting efficiency, counting time, correction factors, type of radiation, and whether the contamination was fixed or removable. The location of areas found to contain hot particles or high concentrations of localized contamination should be noted. Follow-up survey results for decontamination processes should be cross-referenced to the original survey.

Sealed Sources

A sealed source is any radioactive substance intended to produce a radiation field. It is sealed in an inactive container or capsule or bound wholly within an inactive material so as to prevent dispersion of the radioactive substance during routine use (Fig. 9-3). In some cases, protection against heat and corrosion is also required. This type of design is commonly used in nuclear gauges that have a variety of applications including moisture detection, density measurement, and monitoring levels in tanks or bins. Gauges can be either permanently installed or used as portable instruments. A common use is soil density testing where the source is placed in a tube and inserted beneath the soil surface through a punched access hole. Radiation is then transmitted from the source to a detector on the base of the gauge. The density of the soil is determined by the radiation level at the detector.

Although sealed sources are physically quite small, they are often extremely powerful and highly radioactive and, as a result, are often required to be leak tested every 6 months. A common criterion for these leak tests is that they detect the presence of 0.005 μCi or removable contamination on a sealed source. An acceptable leak test for sealed sources for radiography licensees would be to test the nearest accessible point to the sealed source storage position, or other appropriate measuring point. Records of leak test results are to be kept in units of microcuries and maintained for six months or more after the next required leak test is performed or until the sealed source is transferred and disposed of. Other regulations require that records be kept for three years.

The state of Indiana considers any test that reveals the presence of 0.005 μCi or more of removable radiation to be considered evidence that the sealed source is leaking. The licensee must immediately withdraw the equipment involved from use to be decontaminated and repaired or disposed of. Leaks usually must be reported to the state health boards as well.

Certain sources are typically exempt from leak testing, including those containing either krypton or tritium. Tritium sources of more than 100 μCi of beta and/or gamma activity or 10 μCi of alpha must be tested. Some sources must be removed from their holders and the well inside wiped, as well as the top and sides of the source.

The usual method for locating a leaking source is to wipe the source with a cotton Q-tip or filter paper and check this for activity with an appropriate detector.

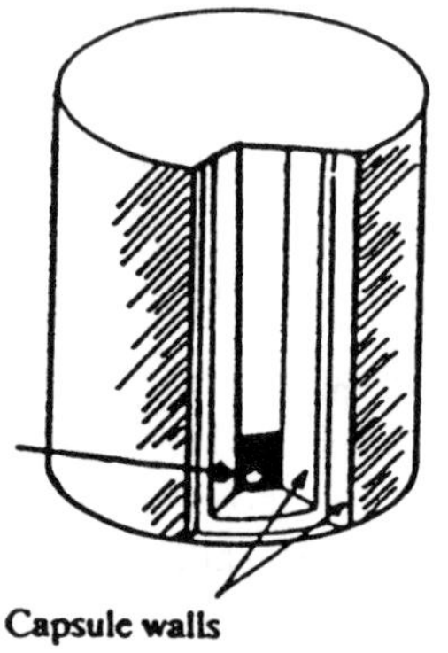

Figure 9-3. Sample configuration of a sealed source. A radioactive source in a special double capsule (as small as a pencil's eraser or as large as the tube inside a roll of paper towels) is inserted into a housing that shields the radiation emitted from the source.
Source: From NRC. n.d. *Working Safely with Nuclear Gauges*. NUREG/BR-0133. Washington, DC: U.S. Nuclear Regulatory Commission.

Procedure

1. Don gloves.
2. Dissolve the contents of the detergent package in approximately an ounce of water.
3. Wet tip of cotton swab on wooden stick with solution and wipe around all weldments of the source holder, source shutter, position handle, and all other corners and edges of the device.
4. Separate the identification tag from the swab and replace the swab in its packaging envelope.
5. Date and tie the tag to the source head being tested.
6. Put down the following information: person performing the test, date of wipe, source head manufacturer, source head model

number, source head serial number, type of isotype, quantity of radiation.

7. Remove gloves and put them into another plastic bag. Put both the swab and the gloves into the mailing envelope with the information and seal.
8. Survey the mailing package. Postal regulations require that the dose rate from any leak kits be less than 0.5 mR/hr at the surface when mailed.

Detecting Removable Contamination

In order to detect removable surface contamination, only methods that involve active contact with the surface are useful. The same variables that apply to wiping or swabbing surfaces for chemical contamination apply to radiation including the type of surface.

Smears

Smear (wipe) samples are taken in situations where direct instrument monitoring is impractical, or to show that as much loose contamination as possible has been removed during cleaning. Smears can be made with a dry or moist filter. In the case of moist wipes, the filter paper should have high wet strength and absorption capacity. They should be moistened with a solution that will not attack the material of which the container or source holder is made, and which under the conditions of this test has been demonstrated to be effective in removing the radioisotope involved. The entire exposed external surface of the object is wiped thoroughly. The paper is allowed to dry and then the radioactivity on the paper is measured. The results can vary depending on whether a dry or moist wipe is done (see, e.g., Table 9-4).

A filter paper disc with a 2.4 cm diameter is passed over a representative (usually 100 cm^2) portion of the surface in question by the tip of a thumb. Because the pressure-bearing portion of the filter paper disc is approximately 2 cm wide, the smear is about 50 cm long. The smear is applied in a "Z" or "S" pattern, and care is taken to avoid excess surface dirt. Duplicate smears are taken at one out of five locations. According to the NRC a 17 in. swipe in the shape of an "S" covers 100 cm^2.

For identifying removable material the NRC recommends that an area of 100 cm^2 be wiped with a dry filter or soft absorbent paper, applying moderate pressure, and measuring the amount of radioactive material on the wiping with an appropriate instrument of known efficiency. When removable contamination on objects of a surface area less than 100 cm^2 is determined, the activity per unit area should be based on the actual area and the entire surface should be wiped. It is not necessary to use wiping techniques to measure removable contamination levels if direct scan surveys indicate that the total residual surface contamination levels are within the limits for removable contamination; however, guidelines for

TABLE 9-4. Comparison of Removable Radiation Surface Contamination from Dry and Wet Wipes

		Percent of Deposited Contamination	
Surface	*Contaminant*	*Dry Swipe*	*Wet Swipe*
Shellstone	Na-acetate-H^3	5–10	7–19
	Paraffin-H^3	18–23	12–17
Fiberglass	Na-acetate-H^3	20–30	26–32
	Paraffin-H^3	15–30	5–6

Source: Data from Prince, J. R., and C. C. Wang. 1965. A method for evaluating surface contamination of soft beta emitters. In G. W. Royster and B. R. Fish (eds.), *Surface Contamination*. New York: Pergamon Press, pp. 179–183.

TABLE 9-5. Guidelines for Selecting Protective Clothing

	Removable Contamination Levels		
Work Activity	*Low (1–10 × Table 9-8 values)*	*Moderate (10–100 × Table 9-8 values)*	*High (> 100 times Table 9-8 values)*
Routine	Full set of PCs	Full set of PCs	Full set of PCs, double gloves, double shoe covers
Heavy work	Full set of PCs, work gloves	Double set of PCs, work gloves	Double set of PCs, work gloves
Work with pressurized or large volume liquids, closed system breach	Full set of non-permeable PCs	Double set of PCs (outer set non-permeable), rubber boots	Double set of PCs, non-permeable outer clothing, rubber boots

Source: Data from DOE. June 1992. *Radiological Control Manual.* DOE/EH-0256T. Washington, DC: U.S. Dept. of Energy, Assistant Secretary for Environment, Safety and Health.

selecting protective clothing for working in radiation contaminated areas are based on removable contamination levels (Table 9-5).

Tritium smears can be taken with a cotton tip swab and placed in contact with a liquid scintillation counting solution. A scintillation counter is used to analyze the sample in the laboratory.

Wipes are best when objects have awkward shapes. The area that is sampled may be 100 cm^2, 300 cm^2, or 1,000 cm^2. The largest area often provides the most consistent sampling results, but due to time and physical constraints the actual area sampled is usually 300 cm^2 or less. The amount of loose material removed by a single smear in a surface can range from 10% to 50%. Therefore, repeat wipes for radioactivity can prove useful. A 4 in. by 4 in. square of paper toweling was used for testing uranium alpha activity (Schultz and Becher, 1963). Measurements on wipe samples must always be made in an area away from any known radiation fields or in an area where background readings are considered normal.

Wipe surveys for removable contamination are reported in units of dpm/100 cm^2. For wipe surveys of small items covering less than 100 cm^2, the results are reported in units of dpm per area wiped. Large area wipes are encouraged and are used to supplement standard wipe techniques in areas generally assumed not to be contaminated, such as entrances to radiological buffer areas. If an evaluation indicates that a wiped area is contaminated, a thorough contamination wipe survey must be performed. Tape and large area wipes are used to collect highly radioactive particles.

Limitations of smear samples include variations of efficiency with different types of surfaces, variations in between surfaces of different shapes, pressure differences, and inability to identify fixed contamination.

Procedure Number 1

A 2.4-cm-diameter filter paper disc is required for this test (EPA, 1985). A 5 cm Whatman No. 1 filter has also been used.

1. Wipe the filter disc in a "Z" or "S" pattern over a representative portion of the surface to be sampled using firm, steady pressure with a finger or the tip of the thumb. The length of the wipe should be 50 cm. Since the pressure-bearing portion of the filter paper disc will be about 2 cm wide, the area of the surface sampled will be approximately 100 cm^2.
2. Avoid contacting excess dirt when wiping an area.

3. Test the sample with appropriate instruments for determining radiological contamination.

Procedure Number 2

Another method involves placing a Whatman No. 50 filter on the bottom of a No. 5 rubber stopper and rubbing over a 5–8-in.-diameter circular area in a rotary motion (Royster and Fish, 1965).

Adhesive Tape Sampling

This test is applicable to a device containing a sealed source in a source holder with an opening through which the radiation emerges. This opening is kept covered for a minimum of seven days with a piece of thin adhesive cellulose tape. The tape is removed carefully and the radioactivity that may have been deposited on its adhesive side is measured. Tape has been recommended for sampling radioactive particulates.

Air Impingement/Smair Sampling

The smair sampler is a conventional air sampler until the open end is placed against a surface. When the sampling head is pressed against a surface, the air intake is restricted to a series of small holes at angles so as to direct jets of air onto the surface to be sampled. Contamination, dispersed by air impingement, is collected on a filter paper like any other air sample.

Test Surface Method

The test surface method (Fig. 9-4) involves using a stationary detector and a fixed distance to the contaminated test material. This usually means attaching a piece of woven fabric to adhesive tape and gluing it down to the surface of interest (Anzai and Kikuchi, 1978). After a specific period of time the fabric is removed and any radioactivity deposited on it is counted with an appropriate instrument. This method measures the total amount of radioactivity deposited during that time (fixed plus removable). The fabric has also been used on the soles of workers' shoes and can be placed on surfaces of varying geometry. Fabric strips can be replaced on a regular basis to allow for regular monitoring. Fabric pieces have also been attached to complicated surfaces such as door handles, drawer knobs, and elevator buttons.

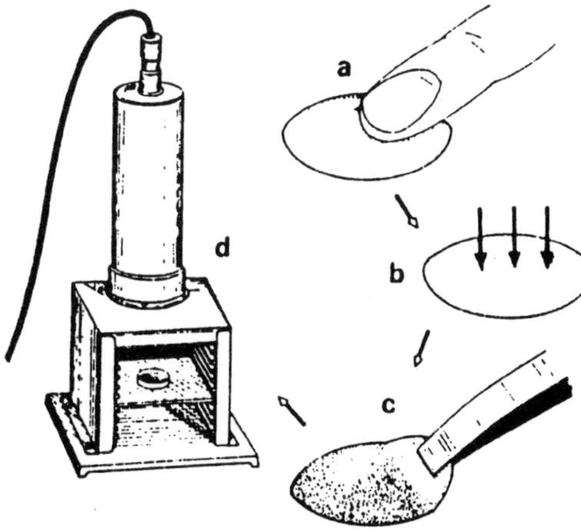

Figure 9-4. Procedure of the test surface method for monitoring surface contamination.
Source: From I. Anzai and T. Kikuchi. 1978. A new monitoring technique of surface contamination—the test surface method. *Health Physics* **34:**786. Reproduced with permission from the Health Physics Society.

Scrub Method

The object to be tested is immersed in a solution that will not attack the material of which the container or source holder is made, and that has been demonstrated to be effective in removing the radioisotope involved when the object is scrubbed with a brush under the surface of the liquid. All surfaces of the object are brushed thoroughly under these conditions. The total radioactivity is measured in the residue obtained by evaporation of the solution.

Immersion Test

The object to be tested is immersed in a solution that will not attack the material of which the container or source holder is made, and that, under the conditions of this test, has been demonstrated to be effective in removing the radioisotope involved. The solution is heated to 50°C ± 5°C and held at this temperature for 8 hours. The total radioactivity is measured in the residue obtained by evaporation of the solution.

Jar Method

This method works well for alpha emitters such as radon (Morris, Menker, and Dauer, 1968). The source to be tested is placed in a small glass jar and sealed for 24 hours. If the source is leaking, the radon gas will diffuse throughout the container and deposit its daughters uniformly on the inner surface of the jar and lid. At the end of 24 hours the lid is removed (inside a laboratory hood) and a check for alpha activity is made. It is essential that the lid seal tightly for this test to work. Alternatively an alpha detector such as a carbon canister can be left inside the jar for a longer period of time such as three to five days.

Skin Sampling

Some situations require regular monitoring of the skin and clothing of workers such as coveralls, lab coats, shoes, and shoe covers. Workers doing glove box work with radioactive sources should have arms and hands checked frequently as well as the glove ports as these often show early signs of contamination. The hands are the most commonly monitored area of the body and the highest single exposure to a portion of the hand, rather than an average exposure to the total area of the hand, sets the exposure limit. Faces are often monitored since they are usually uncovered. For the skin the average area of 100 cm^2, except for the hands where the entire area of one hand (300 cm^2) can be used. Radioactive contamination of the hands is most commonly monitored with an installed alpha proportional counter or beta proportional counter or a double scintillator. For other parts of the body an alpha scintillation probe on an installed monitor or a beta Geiger probe on an installed monitor is used.

Personnel should have a whole body frisk immediately upon exiting contamination areas, high contamination areas, and airborne radioactivity areas. In addition, personnel exiting a radiological buffer area containing contamination, high contamination, or airborne radioactivity should at a minimum perform a hand and foot frisk. This frisk is optional if the radiological buffer area exit is immediately adjacent to the location where the exiting worker has already performed a whole body frisk. Personnel frisking should be performed after removal of protective clothing and prior to washing or showering. Personal items, such as notebooks, papers, and flashlights, should be frisked as well.

Instructions for personnel frisking should be posted adjacent to personnel frisking instruments or monitors. Some radionuclides such as tritium cannot be detected by currently available handheld or automated frisking instrumentation; therefore, frisking is not useful and biological monitoring should be performed instead. People usually frisk themselves. Although the source-to-detector distance can be made very small, the user is unable to maintain this constant distance for the whole body survey. The frisking procedure with handheld survey instruments is as follows (DOE, 1992):

Procedure

1. Verify that the instrument is in service, set to the proper scale, and the audio output can be heard during frisking.
2. Frisk the hands before picking up the probe.
3. Hold probe less than 0.5 in. from surface being surveyed for beta and gamma contamination, and at approximately 0.25 in. for alpha contamination.
4. Move probe slowly over surface, approximately 2 in. per second.
5. Perform the frisk in the following order: head (pausing at the mouth and nose for ap-

proximately 5 seconds); neck and shoulders; arms (pause at each elbow); chest and abdomen; back, hips, and seat of pants; legs (pause at each knee); shoe tops; shoe bottoms (pause at sole and heel); personnel and supplemental dosimeters.

6. If the count rate increases during frisking, pause for 5–10 sec over the area to provide adequate time for instrument response.
7. If the count rate increases to a value greater than a preestablished contamination limit or the instrument alarms, remain in the area and notify radiological control personnel.
8. Return the probe to its holder and leave the area. The probe should be placed on the side or face-up to allow the next person to monitor his or her hands before handling the probe.
9. The whole body frisk should take at least 2–3 min.

For external exposure to the skin, especially when the distance to the source is short, or when the exposed area is very small, the dose should be averaged over 1 cm^2 in the region receiving the highest dose (ICRP, 1965). The dose averaged over 1 cm^2 of skin from the most active particle found in this study can therefore be compared with the maximum permissible dose for occupational exposure.

Survey techniques should be established to determine the extent of skin contamination before initiating decontamination procedures. Skin abrasion should be avoided during the decontamination process. Levels of skin contamination that trigger the need for dose assessments should be established for site-specific radionuclides. These trigger levels should not exceed 100 mrem (millirem). Personnel with skin contamination that triggers the need for dose assessment should be informed of the initial dose estimate to their skin as soon as practicable, preferably prior to the end of their workday. Table 9-6 provides limits for nonuniform exposure to the skin.

Clothing Monitoring

Cleaned personal protective equipment (PPE), such as face shields and respirators, that come into contact with the wearer's face and company issued nonpersonal protective clothing should be surveyed prior to use. Gloves are commonly monitored. It is not uncommon for dose rates on a single glove to vary by a factor of 100 from the highest reading to the lowest. Similarly laundered protective clothing should be surveyed using statistically representative sampling and should meet the following criteria prior to reuse:

TABLE 9-6. Nonuniform Exposure of the Skin

Area of Skin Irradiated	*Method of Averaging, Adding to Other Doses Received, and Recording Nonuniform Skin Dose*
≥ 100 cm^2	Averaged over the 100 cm^2 of skin receiving the maximum dose. Added to any uniform dose equivalent also received by the skin. Recorded as the annual extremity or skin (shallow) dose equivalent (H).
< 100 cm^2	Averaged over the 1 cm^2 of skin receiving the maximum dose (D), reduced by the fraction (f), which is the irradiated area in cm^2 divided by 100 cm^2 (i.e., $H = fD$). Added to any uniform dose equivalent also received by the skin. Recorded as the annual extremity or skin (shallow) dose equivalent.
< 10 cm^2	Averaged over the 1 cm^2 of skin receiving the maximum dose. Not added to any other dose equivalent, extremity or shallow dose equivalent (skin) recorded for the annual dose equivalent. Recorded in a person's radiation dose record as a special entry

Source: Data from DOE. June 1992. *Radiological Control Manual*. DOE/EH-0256T. Washington, DC: U.S. Dept. of Energy, Assistant Secretary for Environment, Safety and Health.

beta-gamma radioactivity less than 10,000 dpm/100 cm^2 and alpha radioactivity less than 1,000 dpm/100 cm^2. For measurements on clothing, an alpha scintillation probe or a beta Geiger probe on an installed or portable monitor is used.

Dosimetry

Whole dosimetry is primarily used to assess exposures to airborne radioactivity exposures, but it has also been used to measure skin dose. Personal dosimetry should be performed for personnel who are expected to receive an annual external whole body dose greater than 100 mrem or an annual dose to the extremities, lens of the eye or skin greater than 10% of the corresponding limits specified in Table 9-7. Neutron dosimetry must be provided when a person is likely to exceed 100 mrem annually from neutrons. The areas in which these doses are most likely to occur are radiation areas, high radiation areas, and radiological buffer areas. When dosimetry measurements are used to classify radiation areas, they are a distance of 30 cm from any surface through which radiation is penetrating.

Dosimeters should only be issued to personnel who have been formally instructed in their use and they should be worn on the chest area, or on or between the waist and neck. Film and thermoluminescent badges are most commonly worn this way. Wrist dosimeter badges are used to estimate the radiation exposure to the forearms and hands. Multiple dosimeters should be issued to personnel to assess whole body exposure in nonuniform radiation fields or as required on radiological work permits. Nonuniform radiation fields exist when the dose to a portion of the whole body will exceed the dose to the primary dosimeter by more than 50% and the anticipated whole body dose is greater than 100 mrem. Dosimeters should remain at the site and not be exposed to security X-ray devices, excessive heat, or medical sources of radiation.

INTERPRETATION OF RESULTS

Background radiation comes from naturally occurring radioactive materials often used in buildings such as granite; cosmic and natural terrestrial radiation; global fallout; and consumer products containing nominal amounts of radioactive material such as smoke detectors and static eliminators. Differences between radiation measurements outside and inside buildings are not uncommon and can be attributed to the natural radioactivity contained in building materials.

Typical levels of background radiation are below 0.05 mrem/hr. If levels such as these are measured the result would indicate that radiation is at

TABLE 9-7. Criteria for Posting Radiation Areas

Area	*Dose Rate Criteria*	*Posting*
Radiation area	> 0.005 rem/hr and ≤ 0.1 rem/hr	"CAUTION, RADIATION AREA" "TLD and RWP Required for Entry"
High radiation area	> 0.1 rem/hr and ≤ 500 rad/hr	"DANGER, HIGH RADIATION AREA" "TLD, Supplemental Dosimeter and RWP Required for Entry"
Very high radiation area	> 500 rad/hr	"GRAVE DANGER, VERY HIGH RADIATION AREA" "SPECIAL CONTROLS REQUIRED FOR ENTRY"
Hot spot	5 times general area dose rate and > 0.1 rem/hr	"CAUTION, HOT SPOT"

Source: Data from DOE. June 1992. *Radiological Control Manual.* DOE/EH-0256T. Washington, DC: U.S. Dept. of Energy, Assistant Secretary for Environment, Safety and Health.

normal background levels of less than 0.05 mrem because most survey instruments are not capable of making precise results below this level.

Resuspension factors are frequently calculated and applied to radioactivity measurements. The reader is referred to the discussion on these factors in Chapter 6.

Surface contamination can be related to increases in air activity. Areas having the greatest uranium alpha activity on the work surfaces have been found to have high alpha air activity in some studies (Becher, 1958). Other studies in uranium processing facilities have found a statistically significant, positive correlation between the average uranium alpha activity on work surfaces and the average urinary excretion rate of the employees (Schultz and Becher, 1963). The data also suggest that for continuous uranium release to the environment at the maximum permissible concentration for soluble natural uranium, the corresponding transferable surface contamination level would be about 40,000 dpm (disintegrations per minute) per 100 cm^2, or 9.2×10^{-5} $\mu c/cm^2$, and the corresponding urinary excretion rate for chronic exposure to this environment would be about 240 $\mu g/L$.

For skin the DOE standard for occupational workers is an annual dose equivalent (ADE) of 50 rem (0.5 sievert). Nonuniform exposures of the skin from X-rays, beta and or radioactive materials are based on an area of 100 cm^2. The dose is averaged over the 100 cm^2 of the skin that receives the maximum dose. Nonuniform exposures to the skin are to be added to uniform exposures with the sum being the skin (shallow) dose equivalent. For irradiated skin areas of less than 100 cm^2 but at least 10 cm^2, the formula $H = fD$ is used, where H is the dose equivalent averaged over the 1 cm^2 of the skin receiving the maximum dose, D is the maximum dose, and f is the irradiated area (in cm^2) divided by 100 cm^2 (f is at least 0.1). Also if the area of irradiated skin is less than 10 cm^2, the nonuniform dose equivalent is averaged over the 1 cm^2 of skin receiving the maximum dose.

The shallow-dose equivalent that applies to the external exposure of the skin or an extremity is taken as the dose equivalent at a tissue depth of 0.007 cm (7mg/cm^2) averaged over an area of 1 cm^2, which can also be stated as 50 rems to the skin or to any extremity. This measure should be applied to the part of the body receiving the highest exposure.

The allowable leak rate is usually specified in the specific license governing a particular operation. A common figure is 0.005 μCi. Certain medical sources have their own limits, for example, a teletherapy source is 0.05 μCi and a brachytherapy source is 0.001 μCi/24 hr.

When surface contamination is discovered, controls capable of precluding the inadvertent transfer of removable radioactivity to locations outside of the contaminated areas under normal operating conditions should be maintained and verified. When removable contamination found on indoor workplace surfaces located inside of radiological areas exceeds the levels specified in the radiation protection program for these surfaces, despite having these controls, the following actions should be taken:

1. Ad hoc controls should be established for the contaminated areas that are adequate to prevent further dispersal of the contamination and to ensure that personnel are not unknowingly exposed.
2. If the contamination levels exceed those specified in Table 9-8, the ad hoc controls should remain in effect until the levels no longer exceed these values.
3. The objective of the decontamination effort should be to restore the affected areas to preexisting conditions. The levels of fixed surface contamination specified in the table may be exceeded in areas within buildings, but outside of radiological areas only protective measures approved by the head of the DOE Field Organization are provided.
4. The area should be posted as a surface contamination area (values listed in Table 9-8) or a high surface contamination area (levels are ≥ 100 times the values in Table 9-8).
5. Exposures should be controlled in a manner commensurate with the physical and chemical characteristics of the contaminant, the radionuclides present, and the fixed and removable contamination levels.

6. Immediately before and after exit from a radiological area established to control surface and/or airborne radioactive contamination, personnel and personal property shall be monitored.
7. Protective clothing should be required for entry into areas in which removable surface contamination exists at levels exceeding those in Table 9-8. At the exits of such areas, control techniques should be provided to preclude the inadvertent transfer of contamination on protective clothing to other areas.

TABLE 9-8. Surface Radioactivity Values Recommended by OSHA and DOE

Nuclide	*Removable*[a, b] *(dpm/100cm^2)*	*Fixed + Removable*[a, c] *(dpm/100cm^2)*
U (nat'l), U^{235}, U^{238}, and associated decay products	1,000 alpha	5,000 alpha
Transuranics, Ra^{226}, Ra^{228}, Th^{230}, Th^{228}, Pa^{231}, Ac^{227}, I^{125}, I^{129}	20	300
Th (nat'l), Th^{232}, Sr^{90}, Ra^{223}, Ra^{224}, U^{232}, I^{126}, I^{131}, I^{133}	200	1,000
Beta-gamma emitters (nuclides with decay modes other than alpha emission or spontaneous fission) except Sr^{90} and others noted above[d]	1,000 beta, gamma	5,000 beta, gamma
Tritium organic compounds; surfaces contaminated by HT and metal tritide aerosols	10,000	10,000

Note: These values apply to radioactive contamination deposited on, but not incorporated into, the interior of the contaminated item. Where surface contamination by both alpha- and beta-gamma-emitting nuclides exists, the limits established for alpha- and beta-gamma-emitting apply independently.

[a]As used in this table, disintegrations per minute (dpm) means the rate of emission by radioactive material as determined by correcting the counts per minutes observed by, and appropriate detector for, background, efficiency, and geometric factors associated with the instrumentation.

[b]The amount of removable radioactive material per 100 cm^2 of surface area should be determined by wiping that area with a dry filter or soft absorbent paper, while applying moderate pressure, and then assessing the amount of radioactive material on the wipe with an appropriate instrument of known efficiency. (*Note:* The use of dry material may not be appropriate for tritium.) When removable contamination on objects of surface area less than 100 cm^2 is determined, the activity per unit area should be based on the actual area and the entire surface should be wiped. Except for transuranics and Ra^{228}, Ac^{227}, Th^{228}, Th^{230}, and Pa^{231}, and alpha emitters, it is not necessary to use wiping techniques to measure removable contamination levels if direct scan surveys indicate that the total residual surface contamination levels are within the limits for removable contamination.

[c]The levels may be averaged over 1 M^2 provided the maximum surface activity in any area of 100 cm^2 is less than three times the value specified. For purposes of averaging, any square meter of surface shall be considered to be above the activity value G if: from measurements of a representative number n of sections it is determined that $1/n\ Sn\ Si \geq G$, where Si is the dis/min 100 cm^2 determined from measurement of section i; or it is determined that the sum of the activity of all isolated spots or particles in any 100 cm^2 area exceeds 3G.

[d]This category of radionuclides includes mixed fission products, including the Sr^{90}, which is present in them. It does not apply to Sr^{90}, which has been separated from the other fission products or mixtures where the Sr^{90} has been enriched.

SURFACE RADIATION STUDIES

Contaminant	*Activity*	*Surface Methods*	*Other Sampling*	*Reference*
Uranium Radium	Closure of Frankford military arsenal	Filter paper wipes 2.4 cm in diameter of building and vent surfaces Initial and repeat sampling to verify decontamination	Area air samples for alpha radiation Sump samples of sludge and water	EPA, 1985
General radiation	Office building where three employees working on the 7th floor had developed cancer	Surface sampling of walls, desktops, chairs, floors, lamps, and other objects within offices, and other rooms for alpha and beta/gamma with direct reading instruments		NIOSH, August 1984 (HETA 84-270-1494)
General radiation	University concerned about a suspected cancer cluster among faculty and students in the Dept. of History	Wipe samples of building surfaces Beta/gamma measurements around the floor-wall interface of rooms, over all exposed piping in the rooms, and on selected sections of floor tiles with direct reading instruments		NIOSH, June 1992 (HETA 91-360-2226)
Uranium	Facility manufacturing uranium catalyst where employees had developed coughs, skin rashes, and nasal sores	Alpha and beta/gamma measurements on spray dryer surfaces including inaccessible areas where cleaning was difficult with direct reading instruments	General area survey measurements for alpha, beta, gamma in area near spray dryer	NIOSH, February 1985 (HETA 82-358-1558)
Uranium	Gaseous diffusion uranium enrichment plant	Measurements on workers' hands as they left the facility	Area air sampling Urine	Yu and Sherwood, 1991

Contaminant	*Activity*	*Surface Methods*	*Other Sampling*	*Reference*
Uranium Plutonium	DOE facility converting depleted or slightly enriched uranium into uranium metal	Measurements for alpha taken 0.5 in. from the surface in break rooms and in work areas with direct reading instrument	Skin contamination measurements with wrist badges	NIOSH, December 1985 (HETA 83-144-2001)
General radiation	Newspaper typographical facility	Measurements of the surfaces of VDTs for low energy X-ray beams taken as close to the surface as possible with direct reading instruments	RF and UV measurements	NIOSH, February 1982 (HETA 80-146-1044)
Radium 226 Tritium	Abandoned facility that manufactured (painted) watches and clock dials suspected of residual contamination	Wet smear surface tests for removable tritium Dry smearable surface tests for alpha Surface testing for gamma and alpha radiation with direct reading instruments Surfaces tested: floors, walls, ceilings, doors, windows, sinks, toilets, light fixtures, heating ducts, roof structures, and foundations	Area air samples for radium daughter products	EPA, 1985

REFERENCES

Anzai, I., and T. Kikuchi. 1978. A new monitoring technique of surface contamination—the test surface method. *Health Physics* **34:**271–273.

Becher, A. F. 1958. The development of surface alpha contamination limits. *Symposium in Occupational Health Experience and Practices in the Uranium Industry*. HASL-58. Washington, DC: U.S. Department of Energy.

DOE. 1992. *Radiological Control Manual*. DOE/EH-0256T. Washington, DC: U.S. Department of Energy, Assistant Secretary for Environment, Safety, and Health.

EPA. 1985. *Guide for Decontaminating Building, Structures and Equipment at Superfund Sites*. EPA 600/2-85-028. Washington, DC: EPA.

ICRP. 1965. *Recommendations of the International Commission on Radiological Protection*. ICRP Publication 9. Oxford, England: Pergamon Press.

Morris, J. O., D. F. Menker, and M. Dauer. 1968. A comparison of leak test procedures for sealed radium sources. *AIHA J*. **5/6:**279–284.

NIOSH, Health Hazard Evaluation Report. February 1982. *New York Post, NY*. HETA 80-146-1044. Cincinnati, OH: NIOSH.

NIOSH, Health Hazard Evaluation Report. August 1984. *Federal Energy Regulatory Commission, Washington, DC*. HETA 84-270-1494. Cincinnati, OH: NIOSH.

NIOSH, Health Hazard Evaluation Report. February 1985. *United Catalysts, Inc., South Plant, Louisville, KY*. HETA 82-358-1558. Cincinnati, OH: NIOSH.

NIOSH, Health Hazard Evaluation Report. December 1985. *Feed Materials Production Center, Westinghouse Materials Co. of Ohio, Fernald, OH*. HETA 83-144-2001. Cincinnati, OH: NIOSH.

NIOSH, Health Hazard Evaluation Report. June 1992. *University of Georgia, Athens, GA*. HETA 91-360-2226. Cincinnati, OH: NIOSH.

Royster, G. W., and B. R. Fish. 1967. Techniques for assessing "removable" surface contamination. In G. W. Royster and B. R. Fish (eds.), *Surface Contamination*. New York: Pergamon Press, pp. 201–207.

Schultz, N. B., and A. F. Becher. 1963. Correlation of uranium alpha surface contamination, air-borne concentrations, and urinary excretion rates. *Health Physics* **9:**901–909.

Spangler, G. W., and C. A. Willis. 1967. Permissible contamination limits. In G. W. Royster and B. R. Fish (eds.), *Surface Contamination*. New York: Pergamon Press, pp. 151–158.

Yu, R. C., and R. J. Sherwood. 1991. *A study of Human Exposure and Elimination of Uranium—A Reassessment of Past Field Data*. Salt Lake City, UT: American Industrial Hygiene Conference, Abstract.

CHAPTER 10

Decontamination

A good way to minimize contamination of surfaces is to have a program of routine wipe testing of equipment and building surfaces in work areas during the period of regular use. Potential sources of contamination could then be identified and remediated quickly, and additional contamination could be prevented. Closure operations could be simplified when time to sell or demolish a building. Contaminated equipment should be kept in the work area or other designated area until it can be decontaminated. Spills should be cleaned up and decontaminated promptly rather than allowing contaminants to build up over time. Similarly, leaking equipment should be identified through regular inspections and repaired.

Decontamination is best done in a segregated area to minimize the migration of contamination. A decontamination area is defined by the Occupational Safety and Health Administration (OSHA) as an area outside of, but as near as practical to, the regulated area, consisting of an equipment storage area, wash area, and clean change area used for the decontamination of workers, materials, and equipment. There can be several levels of decontamination depending on the type of usage planned for the affected chemical protective clothing (CPC) or building, and there are usually four phases to a decontamination project:

1. Determination of the nature and extent of contamination
2. Development and implementation of a site-specific decontamination plan
3. Decontamination
4. Evaluation of the effectiveness of the decontamination

DETERMINATION OF THE NATURE AND EXTENT OF CONTAMINATION

Development of an overall decontamination strategy revolves around the proper identification and evaluation of the contaminants present. Remedial site investigations of buildings and structures should include a records search, interviews with former employees, a visual inspection, and a sampling survey to determine the nature and level of contaminants present.

The visual inspection can identify areas of gross chemical contamination as well as the condition or soundness of a building or structure. This information is useful in determining whether a building or structure has any potential for future use or should be dismantled and disposed of. During the inspection, rafters, ventilation ducts, sumps, crawl spaces, window wells, and tanks are inspected for evidence of deterioration as well as suspected chemical residues or contaminated dust/particulate matter such as asbestos. Personnel involved in initial inspections and sampling should be thoroughly trained in appropriate safety precautions and hazard awareness. Equipment used to remove waste or collect samples should be routinely decontaminated before leaving the site to minimize the spread of contamination.

In some cases it is desirable to determine the extent of contamination due to a chemical release. Wipes are collected in the immediate vicinity of the release and at sites representing an incremental increase in distance from the site. Depending on the origin and size of the site contaminated by the release, samples could be collected in concentric circles as well.

A building that contained beryllium was cleaned with detergent and water to reduce the loose surface contamination, followed with wipe sampling; however, a large amount of beryllium remained embedded in the wood floor (Cohen and Kusian, 1967). It was determined that with the floor covered with linoleum tile, the building could be used as a laboratory without hazard to the lab employees; however, the building could not be sold or demolished without removal of the floor. In practice, because many decontamination projects involve industrial property transfer or long-term liability issues, leaving contaminants in place even under a protective surface coating is not always acceptable.

When testing buildings for contamination, it is good to sample different types of surfaces as the contaminant will interact with them differently. For example, in one facility there could be sheet metal walls, concrete foundations, and a wood framework. The type of surface may also dictate what method is to be used as noted in the previous recommendation to use adhesive tape for rough surfaces. The type of surface sampled should be documented on the sampling data sheet. In some cases, surfaces can be categorized as high skin contact—that is, prolonged direct dermal contact—such as desks, tables, counters, and file cabinets. Chemical permeation into porous surfaces makes decontamination very difficult and increases the likelihood that employees may be exposed. A good control is to paint concrete and wood surfaces in chemical work areas with a nonpermeable paint such as polyurethane or epoxy (Weeks and Dean, 1978).

DEVELOPMENT AND IMPLEMENTATION OF A SITE-SPECIFIC DECONTAMINATION PLAN

A detailed, site-specific decontamination plan should be developed and implemented before any cleanup personnel or equipment is allowed to enter areas where the potential for exposure to hazardous substances exists. The hazard evaluation is a decision-making process in which the benefits and risks associated with not treating the contaminated buildings, structures, or equipment are weighed against the potential benefits and risks of decontamination. Two types of hazards need to be evaluated: those associated with the contaminants themselves and those associated with the cleanup process.

This hazard evaluation consists of gathering information on the physical and chemical properties of the contaminants, the fire and explosion hazards, the toxicity and health hazards, and chemical reactivity. All existing exposure limits for particular contaminants must be included in the hazard evaluation. Health and safety aspects associated with the use of various cleanup techniques or processes must also be considered as part of the overall hazard evaluation. If two methods are considered equally effective in removing or treating a particular situation, the method that presents lower risks to the workers is preferable.

In most cases the decontamination strategy must be geared to meet the intended or potential future use of the site including buildings, structures, and equipment. There are three categories of use: unrestricted/public, restricted/industrial, and no future use. Buildings and structures that have no potential for future use will either be dismantled or demolished, or left standing, fenced, and guarded. Then decontamination target levels for all contaminants present should be established.

SURFACE DECONTAMINATION METHODS

Determining the most appropriate cleanup method or combination/sequence of methods to be used on buildings, structures, and equipment is central to the development of a decontamination plan. The first step in a decontamination program is to establish procedures that minimize contact with chemicals and thus the potential for contamination. These include work practices that minimize contact with hazardous substances such as remote sampling and handling techniques, and using disposable coverings for monitoring and other equipment not intended for direct contact with chemicals, contaminated soil, or water. Equipment that is difficult to decontaminate, such as air and water hoses and small tools, can be sealed in 6 mL plastic bags for removal from the site. These bags would not be reopened until they were placed into another containment work area (hot zone) at the next job site (Beaulieu, 1991). Another effective technique is the use of a dedicated decontamination chamber or pad (in the case of heavy equipment) at a central location for cleaning, reconditioning, and repainting of large equipment items. Table 10-1 describes the most common decontamination methods, while Table 10-2 provides a comparison of some of these techniques.

In general, gross decontamination is done using detergents in water combined with a physical scrubbing action. This process will remove most forms of surface contamination including dusts, many inorganic chemicals, and some organic chemicals. Soapy water scrubbing of protective suits may not be effective in removing oily or tacky organic substances. Furthermore, this form of decontamination is unlikely to remove any contamination that has permeated or penetrated the suit materials.

For certain surfaces decontamination is too difficult. An example is a wooden surface with 4,4'-methylene bis(2-chloroaniline) (MOCA) impregnated into it. In this case it would be better to seal the MOCA with urethane or isocyanate solutions. To minimize the need to decontaminate it is best for all concrete and wooden surfaces in chemical work areas to be painted with a nonpermeable paint, preferably oil base or epoxy. This action, along with regular cleaning and decontaminating, will minimize occupational health problems for workers in these areas.

Buildings that have become contaminated with polychlorinated biphenyls (PCBs) and tetrachlorodibenzodioxins (TCDDs) have been successfully decontaminated by scrubbing with brushes using a detergent solution and rinsing with high pressure water or steam cleaning (Perdek et al., 1991). This was preceded by scraping when necessary. The decontamination process was repeated until sampling and analysis showed that residual contamination was below the action levels. Contaminated wood may have to be incinerated.

EVALUATION OF THE EFFECTIVENESS OF DECONTAMINATION

Rationale

The extent of residual contamination following decontamination must be determined so the effectiveness of the cleanup methods can be assessed. A visual inspection and detailed sampling survey should be conducted in the same manner as described previously. The results of this survey should then be compared with the decontamination target levels. If the target levels have not been reached, the decontamination procedure or sequence must be repeated or amended as necessary. Once target levels have been achieved, the need for long-term monitoring to provide assurances that the target levels will be

(Text continues on page 257.)

TABLE 10-1. Summary of the Types, Advantages, and Disadvantages of Various Decontamination Methods

Method	*Description*	*Advantages*	*Disadvantages*
Asbestos containing material (ACM) abatement			
(a) Removal	Building materials are removed using physical, usually manual, labor with wet methods.	Permanently eliminates the source of asbestos fibers.	Costly and time-consuming if complex surfaces are involved; may require sealing of porous surfaces after removal.
(b) Encapsulation	A chemical penetrant or bridging type sealant is sprayed on ACM to bind together asbestos fibers and other material components for reduction of asbestos fiber release.	Initially, may be lower in cost than removal; does not require replacement of ACM.	More costly than removal over the long term because periodic reinspections are required to check for damage and deterioration. Subsequent repair of the encapsulated surface may be necessary; can decrease the fireproofing properties of the ACM. May make eventual removal more difficult.
(c) Enclosure	A permanent barrier is erected between the ACM and all portions of the occupied building. Release of asbestos fibers is contained behind the barrier.	Initially, may be lower in cost than removal.	More costly than removal over the long term due to periodic reinspections needed to check for damage and if subsequent repairs are needed. Require controlled access for maintenance or renovation activities as well as eventual removal of ACM.
Adsorption	Absorbent materials are used to pick up liquid contaminants. This method is most applicable immediately following liquid contaminant spills. Spills rapidly penetrate most surfaces, and absorbents act to contain contaminants and prevent such penetration. Depending on the surface and time elapsed since the spill, further decontamination procedures may have to be used.	Quickly contains gross contamination.	Normally requires secondary decontamination to clean up surface residues and subsurface contamination.

TABLE 10-1. *(continued)*

Method	*Description*	*Advantages*	*Disadvantages*
Demolition	The total destruction of a building, structure, or piece of equipment. Specific demolition techniques include complete burndown, controlled blasting, wrecking with balls or backhoe mounted rams, rock splinting, sawing, drilling, and crushing.	Decontamination is total since all contaminated building materials are removed, including structures and equipment.	Completely destroys the building, structure, or equipment; generates large quantities of contaminated debris for disposal; may expose workers or nearby residents to airborne contamination.
Dismantling	The physical removal of selected structures (such as contaminated piping, tanks, and other process equipment) from buildings or other areas. Dismantling can be the sole activity of decontamination efforts or it can be used in the initial stage of a more complex operation.	Less costly than complete demolition as only those structures that are contaminated are removed.	Generates large quantities of contaminated debris for disposal.
Dusting/vacuuming/ wiping	The physical removal of hazardous dust and particles from building and equipment surfaces by common cleaning techniques.	Generates small volumes of waste/wastewater, which are contained and easily disposed of in vacuum cleaner bags or on wipe cloths.	May spread contamination by creating fugitive dusts; may have to be repeated until the source of contamination is controlled.
Encapsulation/enclosure	Contaminants or contaminated structures are physically separated from building occupants and the ambient environment by a barrier. An encapsulating or enclosing physical barrier may take different forms; among them are plaster, epoxy resins, and concrete casts and walls. Acting as an impenetrable shield, a barrier keeps contaminants inside and away from clean areas.	Does not create large volumes of contaminated debris.	May render structures inaccessible or inoperable.
Grit blasting	A surface removal technique in which an abrasive material is used for uniform removal of contaminated surface layers from a building or structure.	Can simultaneously and readily remove paint and contaminants near the surface.	Generates large amounts of dust and debris; is slow and is effective only as a surface treatment; has the potential for detonating pockets of combustible contaminants.

TABLE 10-1. *(continued)*

Method	*Description*	*Advantages*	*Disadvantages*
Hydroblasting/water-washing	A high pressure (3,500 to 350,000 kPa) water jet is used to remove contaminated debris from surfaces. The debris and water are then collected and thermally, physically, or chemically decontaminated.	Relatively inexpensive, nonhazardous surface technique that uses off-the-shelf equipment; can easily incorporate variations such as hot or cold water, abrasives, solvents, surfactants, and varied pressures.	May not effectively remove contaminants that have penetrated the surface layer; requires collection and treatment of large amounts of contaminated liquids.
Painting/coating			
(a) Lead-based paint removal	Paint containing lead in excess of 0.5% is removed from building areas by commercially available paint removers and/or physical means (scraping, scrubbing, waterwashing).	Does not require large investments in equipment	Involves labor intensive operations that cannot be automated
(b) Fixative/stabilizer coatings	Various agents used as coatings on contaminated residues to fix or stabilize the contaminant in place and decrease or eliminate exposure hazards. The stabilized contaminants can be left in place or removed later by a secondary treatment.	Reduces the level of contamination to which building occupants are exposed; does not create hazardous wastes	Does not remove toxic contaminants; requires lifetime monitoring of the effectiveness of the barrier coating.
(c) Strippable coatings	Compounds that bind with contaminants and mixed with a polymer, applied to a contaminated surface and subsequently removed to achieve decontamination.	Physically holds or traps the contaminant for easier handling and disposal	May bind to the surface of the wall or item on which it is applied, resulting in large volumes of wastes or damage to the surface.
Scarification	A tool with pneumatically operated piston heads that strike the surface, causing concrete to chip off. The piston heads consist of multipoint tungsten carbide bits and are capable of removing up to 2.5 cm of surface layer from concrete or similar materials.	Can achieve a deeper penetration (removal) than most other surface removal techniques; is suitable for application to both large open areas and small areas.	Requires resurfacing of the treated surface; generates contaminant laden dust and substantial amounts of contaminated debris (water and concrete) that require further processing; presents a potential explosion hazard if pockets of combustible wastes are encountered; is restricted to use of concrete or concrete-like materials; can only be used in obstruction-free areas.

TABLE 10-1. *(continued)*

Method	*Description*	*Advantages*	*Disadvantages*
RadKleen	An example of a commercial process that uses fluorocarbon extraction of contaminants from building materials involving the pressure spraying of a fluorocarbon solvent onto the contaminated surface followed by collection and purification of the solvent.	Uses Freon 113 (a noncombustible chlorinated solvent), which permits rapid wetting of surfaces and easy particulate separation; allows for solvent recovery if used in a closed system.	Requires secondary treatment of used freon.
Solvent washing	An organic solvent is circulated across the surface of a building to solubilize contaminants. Spent solvent is either thermally or chemically treated to remove contaminants and recycled if no degradation of the solvent occurs during treatment.	Can remove contaminant as long as the proper solvent is selected.	Not suitable for intricate structures; may tend to carry contaminants farther into the wall before outward movement occurs; may require removal and/or decomposition of residual solvent in building materials.
Steam cleaning	A method of physically extracting contaminants from building materials and equipment surfaces in which steam is applied by handheld wands or automated systems, and the condensate is collected for treatment.	Relatively inexpensive and simple; depending on contaminant, may cause thermal decomposition and/or hydrolysis.	Known to be effective only for surface decontamination; is labor-intensive and costly if automated; generates large volumes of contaminated water.
Vapor-phase solvent extraction	An organic solvent with a relatively low boiling point (such as acetone) is heated to vaporization and allowed to circulate in a building. The vapors permeate into porous building materials, where they condense, solubilize contaminants, and diffuse outward.	Enhances solvent permeability and diffusibility; well suited to all areas of a building, including intricate structures; can remove contaminated paint if the proper solvent is selected.	May require long treatment times for outward diffusion of contaminant laden solvent.

TABLE 10-1. *(continued)*

Method	*Description*	*Advantages*	*Disadvantages*
Acid etching	Acid is applied to a contaminated surface to promote corrosion and removal of the surface layer. The resulting debris is then neutralized and disposed of. Thermal or chemical treatment of the removed material may be required to destroy the contaminant before disposal.	Certain contaminants are decomposed as they are removed from the surface.	Requires a large volume of acid and special application equipment; is applicable only to metals that will readily corrode.
Bleaching	Bleach formulations are applied to a contaminated surface, allowed to react with contaminants, and removed. Application usually occurs in conjunction with other decontamination efforts, such as the use of sorbents and/or water-washing.	Effective when used against metal surfaces.	Depending on the concentration and composition of the bleach slurry, may cause corrosion of application equipment and/or the surfaces being treated; may also cause periodic clogging of application equipment.
Flaming	Controlled high temperature flames are applied to noncombustible surfaces to thermally degrade all contaminants.	Provides complete and rapid destruction of all residues contacted.	Primarily a surface decontamination technique; would probably result in extensive damage to the material if used for subsurface decontamination; may detonate combustible residues; can involve high fuel costs.
Drilling and spalling	A technique that consists of drilling holes (2.5–4 cm diam) approximately 7.5 cm deep. The spalling tool bit is inserted into the hole and hydraulically spreads to spall off the contaminated concrete.	Can achieve deeper penetration (removal) of surfaces than other surface removal techniques; is good for large-scale application.	Requires resurfacing of the treated surface; may expose rebars; generates substantial amounts of contaminated debris.
K-20 sealant	The application of a material that penetrates a porous surface and immobilizes contaminants in place. K-20 is an example of a product being marketed for this purpose.	Immobilizes contaminants in situ; does not generate hazardous wastes.	In the developmental stages.

TABLE 10-1. *(continued)*

Method	*Description*	*Advantages*	*Disadvantages*
Microbial degradation	Contaminants are biologically decomposed by microbes capable of utilizing contaminants such as petroleum hydrocarbons as a nutrient source. Microbes are applied to the contaminated area in an aqueous medium and allowed to digest the contaminant over time. The microbes are then destroyed chemically or thermally and washed away.	Specific to targeted contaminants.	Requires a large development effort to achieve a workable system; would probably require supplementary treatment; may give rise to biological degradation products containing carcinogenic compounds.
Photochemical degradation	Intense UV light is applied to a contaminated surface for some period of time, the result being photodegradation of the contaminant. It has been shown to be useful for chlorinated dioxins. In order for it to work the contaminant must have the ability to absorb light energy, light of the proper wavelengths, and intensity must be available and a hydrogen donor must be present.	Can be relatively simple or scaled up (accompanied by increased technical efforts); is inexpensive when sunlight is used as the UV light source.	Will not work on contaminants embedded in dense particulate matter (such as thick carpet or deep soil) because UV light cannot penetrate through these surfaces; may result in exposure hazards from the use of intense UV radiation sources other than the sun (mercury and xenon-arc lamps) and from the use of flammable solvents as hydrogen donors.

TABLE 10-2. Gross and Final Decontamination Techniques and Their Effectiveness

Contaminated Surface	*Decontamination Techniques*	*Removal Effectiveness (%)*
Concrete floor	Scrubbing with detergent	50–95
	Acid etching	80–98
	Sandblasting/shotblasting	25–95
Unpainted cinderblock wall	High pressure water spraying	60–90
	Steam cleaning	90–99+
Galvanized painted ceiling and walls	High pressure water spraying	80–99+
Painted steel walls, ceiling, floor, and cabinets	High pressure water spraying	70–95
	Various methods	10–50

Source: From Woodyard, J. P., and Z. M. Zoratto. 1986. State-of-the-art technology for PCB decontamination of concrete. In J. Crine, (ed.), *Hazards, Decontamination, and Replacement of PCB: A Comprehensive Guide*. New York: Plenum Press.

maintained should be considered. This is especially important in situations where contaminants have been left in place behind protective coatings or barriers.

Also the conditions in the building or process must have remained essentially the same since contamination occurred unless the purpose of sampling is to determine if all contamination has been removed. For example, if extensive renovation in a building has resulted in the replacement or covering of most building surfaces, sampling would not be practicable. If the concern is surfaces that are most likely to contact the skin, and a large amount of the furniture and office equipment present in a building has been replaced since the contamination occurred, air sampling may be more useful than surface sampling.

Equipment reuse depends on demonstrating that adequate decontamination has taken place. Equipment used on jobs where carcinogens are present must be tested carefully to determine if decontamination was effective prior to removal from a site.

Assessing Residual Contamination

Decontamination methods vary in their effectiveness and unfortunately most methods for nondestructively evaluating contamination levels of CPC or equipment leave something to be desired as to their effectiveness. This shortcoming is especially true if only small areas are sampled and used to make assumptions as to the cleanliness of the whole item. However, such sampling is an improvement over the current reliance on visual inspections, and there are a number of methods that may assist in a determination of this type.

Wipe Sampling

Sampling methods for determining the nature and extent of contamination on building and equipment surfaces include dry and wet wipes. In some instances, it may be necessary to determine the depth of penetration of contaminants into porous materials such as wood, wallboard, or concrete. In these cases, small corings of the contaminated structural matter should be collected for analysis and handled as a solid waste. Representative samples should be collected and analyzed in accordance with EPA and NIOSH (National Institute of Occupational Safety and Health) methods. Several locations at the site should be sampled in order to identify all contaminated areas. The survey results should identify all contaminated substrates and report contaminant levels by sampling location. Wipe sampling of external and internal surfaces will provide information if the contaminants are suitable for collection using this procedure. Most tools, instruments, and other articles are too large to sample the entire surface, so wipe samples must be collected in places where penetration is most likely to occur.

It is particularly important to properly decontaminate rental equipment. Wipe sampling should be done on any frequently used equipment, especially equipment connected with the operation. One method to sample equipment is to make a grid using equidistant measurements. When repeating sampling of a surface after decontamination, position the sample grid 6 in. to the right of the initial sampling points, or if movement to the right is restricted, position 6 in. downward. The following is an EPA-recommended wipe sampling procedure (EPA, 1985).

Procedure

1. Use 27 mm glass fiber filters moistened with distilled water. Clean disposable surgical gloves (individual packaged powderless type) must be worn whenever the filters are handled. Care should be taken not to contaminate the exterior of the gloves when they are donned.
2. The wipe samples are to be shipped back to the lab in glass vials. Prior to the site visit, the vials are cleaned with Alconox and rinsed twice with deionized water. Several labels are made for each sample. Each set of labels must have a unique number. The sample vials are labeled using adhesive labels and placed inside plastic bags. Another

adhesive label is placed outside of the plastic bag.

3. At the sampling site, remove the filter from the packaging while wearing clean disposable gloves. Moisten the filter with distilled water. Gently wipe approximately 100 cm^2 of the surface to be sampled. Use a measured 100 cm^2 template as a guide to judge the size of the area to be wiped.
4. Without allowing the filter to contact any other surfaces, fold the filter with the exposed side in, then fold it again. Return the filter to the labeled glass vial and seal with a Teflon-lined cap.
5. Put a label for each sample on a sampling data sheet and record pertinent information concerning the site location and a complete description of the equipment that was wiped.
6. Seal the vials in their plastic bags and store them in a chest containing ice or blue ice packs for transport to the laboratory. Do not use dry ice. Ship the samples to the laboratory at the end of each sampling day using a next-day delivery service.

Tape Sampling

Tape sampling is a useful method for assessing surface contamination by fibrous dusts such as asbestos. As described in Chapter 7, a piece of cellophane tape is pressed on the surface to be sampled several times and then placed on a clean laboratory slide.

Typical equipment to be inspected on an abatement project would include respirators, hoses, vacuums, compressors, shower units, ladders and scaffolding, shovels, scrapers, and vehicles. One sampling strategy for a project utilizing this method is as follows: Sampling should be done prior to the start of the job after equipment has arrived to determine if contamination is present from work on other sites, periodically throughout the job, and at the end of the job in conjunction with final air clearance sampling. During each of these three sampling periods, a minimum of nine samples should be collected to ensure that representative sampling is performed on all equipment without incurring unreasonable cost. It is recommended that three samples be collected on equipment within the clean room area, focusing on personal respiratory protective equipment and room surfaces (Beaulieu, 1991). Three samples should be collected on support equipment outside the clean room, including ladders, negative air machines, and even air sampling equipment. Finally, the load-out chamber, the vehicles used for transporting asbestos waste to a landfill, should be evaluated with an additional three samples.

Rinseate Collection and Analysis

Rinseates can be collected as they drip off of the surface of the equipment being cleaned and are often easier to analyze than wipes and other media. However, the evaluation of used cleaning solutions cannot quantify the effectiveness of cleaning if the original contamination levels are unknown. This method can show if the cleaning solution is capable of removing a contaminant. Care must be taken to assure that cleaning agents do not pose an analytical interference with the contaminant.

Although methods are available to provide measurements of surface contamination visual inspection remains the most common method for verifying that decontamination is complete. While visual methods may be suitable for determining the removal of gross contamination they are unsuitable for many situations. Visual inspections are generally done under natural lighting if the materials are out-of-doors or in well lit areas if performed indoors. A limitation is that not all contamination results in visible stains. In the case of darkly colored objects, stains may be camouflaged. Rough surfaces and those with grooves or other indentations can be difficult to inspect. In the case of highly toxic contaminants, allowing even low levels to remain may produce significant exposures.

DECONTAMINATION OF CHEMICAL PROTECTIVE CLOTHING

It is not uncommon for CPC, such as gloves, to be reused for days or weeks without decontamination. What is often overlooked in such cases is that contaminants will continue to penetrate these items even during periods of storage and nonuse and, unless the contaminant has some sort of warning properties such as irritation or discoloration, it will not be detected when the worker is using the item. In a study on glove reuse issues, it was concluded that decreasing chemical contact time does not generally change the breakthrough time from that which would be measured for continuous exposure. Also, permeation continued for as long as 70 hr after ending a 4 hr chemical exposure test (Goydan and Schwope, 1992). Even liquid penetration is unlikely to be sensed because the use of gloves often causes the hands to perspire. Also, CPC generally does not show any identifiable change in appearance when breakthrough has occurred because degeneration occurs only after longer exposures.

Reuse of CPC should only be allowable under the condition that the effectiveness of decontamination or risk of exposure without decontamination in between uses has been fully evaluated under field usage conditions. In addition, an ongoing sampling program needs to be in place to verify that these methods continue to be effective. Any chemical and physical resistance tests should be repeated after the CPC has undergone a number of chemical exposures and decontamination cycles.

Often, the decision to decontaminate rather than dispose of CPC depends on the ability of the material to maintain its integrity not only against contaminant permeation but also on the decontamination methods. The primary concerns that must be evaluated for decontamination are whether the selected method is effective, does not adversely affect CPC, or does not produce exposures to decontamination personnel. Ease of decontamination or garment cleaning is also a factor for consideration in clothing selection. Materials that resist chemical permeation or penetration not only provide better protection but also generally require less decontamination of the garment (Smith and Burke, 1989). When CPC is contaminated by volatile chemicals, they will quickly evaporate from the surface but may remain detectable in the matrix for days (Perkins, 1991). Diffusion of the chemicals toward both surfaces will drive the molecules out, but the process is concentration dependent; therefore, as inner concentrations decrease or concentrations at the surface increase, outward diffusion shows. Alternatively, viscous, low volatility chemicals often will permeate the matrix quite slowly but will remain on the surface for long periods. Matrix contamination can change the character of a polymer, usually decreasing the time to steady-state permeation upon the next exposure. The best way to measure any effect is to subject the CPC to a number of exposure–decontamination cycles and to retest it using appropriate field tests.

There are two types of decontamination: (1) gross decontamination, to allow the end user to safely exit or doff their CPC, and (2) decontamination for reuse of CPC. Decontamination methods for CPC either physically remove contaminants, inactivate contaminants by chemical detoxification, disinfection/sterilization, or remove contaminants by a combination of both physical and chemical means. The RADKLEEN Model 1550 Clothing Decontamination System uses Freon 113 to extract contaminants. The used solvent is regenerated and purified by a built-in distillation process. Contaminants are removed from the system as still bottoms and materials trapped on replaceable filter-adsorbent cartridges. In some cases, decontamination procedures are specific for the type of chemical. For example, when working with color photographic developer solutions, gloves should be washed with an acid-type hand cleaner such as pHisoderm and then rinsed with water prior to removal.

The use of organic solvents such as hexane often provides for easier removal of heavy organic contamination, but may result in other problems. These problems include permeation into the clothing components pulling contaminant with it similar to problems that result when exposures to mixtures occur; spreading localized contaminant into other areas of the clothing; and generating large volumes of contaminated solvents that require disposal.

Due to the problems in using organic solvents for decontamination of CPC, other decontamination methods may prove more effective, such as washing with detergent or thermal desorption (Vahdat and Delaney, 1989). When the effectiveness of manually washing neoprene at 25°C was compared with washing in a dishwasher at 45°C, it was found that the 25°C was not effective in removing n-butyl acetate from this material (Berardanelli and Hall, 1988). Breakthrough times were significantly decreased (20–0 min). Thermal desorption must be applied with care as it has been shown that some CPC materials do not completely recover to their initial quality. Heating previously exposed Nytek gloves at 70°C or 100°C overnight led to only partial recovery of breakthrough values (75% of that expected) and still higher steady state permeation rates (increased permeation). Repeated thermal conditioning cannot be done for some materials. Forced circulation of heated air over clothing items for extended periods of time may prove a better method for removal in these cases. This method allows many organic chemicals to migrate out of the materials and evaporate into the heated air, and it does require that the contaminants be volatile. Additionally, low level heat may accelerate the removal of plasticizer from garment materials and affect the adhesives involved in garment seams.

The following points should be kept in mind when making decisions about decontaminating CPC:

1. Freon should not be used to decontaminate CPC as its effectiveness is <100%.
2. Air drying at 50°C was 100% effective for the volatile solvents tested.
3. When small amounts of solvents that have substantially different solubility properties are spilled on CPC, the chances of residual solvent remaining in the CPC are small and special decontamination should not be necessary (room temperature air drying is sufficient).
4. Priority should be given to decontamination when solvents having similar properties to polymer components have been spilled on the CPC.
5. Remove surface contamination from CPC whenever possible. Use hot water (50°C to 60°C) and detergents. Use a prewash on soiled spots or a solvent with similar polarity to the contaminant(s).
6. For matrix contamination, use heated (50°C to 60°C) air. Remember that at room temperature it will take much longer for a contaminant to "back out" of a garment than to move into the garment since the concentration gradients are usually much different.
7. For low toxicity contaminants, machine washing (40°C to 50°C) with a detergent, prewash additive, and/or bleach may suffice.
8. For higher toxicity contaminants, perform laboratory testing of the decontamination process.
9. If a number of garments have been contaminated, it may be advisable to sacrifice one garment for destructive testing by a qualified laboratory with analysis of contamination levels on and inside the garment.

All equipment used for decontamination of CPC—buckets, brushes, clothing, tools, and any other equipment intended for reuse the next day—must also be decontaminated and/or disposed of properly or CPC may be recontaminated. Also, all spent solutions and wash water should be collected and disposed of properly. CPC that is not completely decontaminated should be placed in plastic bags, pending further decontamination and/or disposal.

REFERENCES

Anonymous. 1983. Act II—How clean is clean? *Hazardous Waste Report* **5**(9):13.

Beaulieu, H. J. 1991. Asbestos contamination of abatement equipment surfaces. *Appl. Occup. Env. Hyg.* **6**(7):583–587.

Berardanelli, S. P., and R. Hall. 1988. Decontamination of chemical protective clothing exhibiting matrix release. In S. Z. Mansdorf, R. Sager, and A. P. Nielsen (eds.), *Performance of Protective Clothing*. Second Symposium. ASTM STP 989. Philadelphia, pp. 359–367.

Cohen, J. J., and R. N. Kusian. 1967. The significance of beryllium surface contamination to health. In B. R. Fish (ed.), *Surface Contamination*. London: Pergamon Press, pp. 345–348.

EPA. 1985. *Guide for Decontaminating Buildings, Structures and Equipment at Superfund Sites*. EPA 600/2-85-028. Washington, DC: EPA.

Goydan, R., and A. D. Schwope. 1992. Should protective gloves be used? An analysis of the potential for residual permeation during repeated use. *AIHA Conference Abstracts*. Boston.

Lunn, G., and E. B. Sansone. 1989. Decontamination of ethidium bromide spills. *Appl. Ind. Hyg.* **4**(9):234–237.

OSHA. 1991. *OSHA Technical Manual*, 2d ed. Washington, DC: OSHA.

Perdek, J. M., F. J. Freestone, D. Sandifer, and A. Sherman. 1991. Closure of a dioxin incineration facility. *Chemosphere* **23**(8/10):1295–1305.

Perkins, J. L. 1991. Decontamination of protective clothing. *Appl. Occup. Env. Hyg.* **6**(1):29–35.

Smith, I. D., and K. E. Burke. 1989. Decontamination of protective suit materials. In J. L. Perkins, and J. O. Stull (eds.), *Chemical Protective Clothing*. Philadelphia: ASTM, pp. 191–205.

Vahdat, N., and R. Delaney. 1989. Decontamination of chemical protective clothing. *AIHA J.* **50**(3):152–156.

Weeks, R. W., and B. J. Dean. 1978. Decontamination of aromatic amine cancer-suspect agents on concrete, metal, or painted surfaces. *AIHA J.* **39:**758–762.

PART IV

Dermal Sampling Techniques

CHAPTER 11

Introduction to Dermal Monitoring

Most dermal monitoring is done for chemicals; however, skin contamination from microbials that can enter through cuts or from radiation is also a concern. The direct evaluation of dermal exposure usually is far more complicated than that of airborne exposures due to variability in deposition rates onto the body, the effect of clothing, the duration of actual skin contact with the chemical, and the importance of time in the retention and permeation of the chemical through the skin. The first indication that a dermal problem has developed will frequently be in the form of reports from employees that a skin condition has developed. However, a skin condition may or may not be due to chemical irritation. Mechanical irritation and excessive washing of hands must be ruled out before initiating sampling for a chemical problem.

There are two types of methods for sampling dermal exposures: those that assess exposure indirectly by monitoring for surface contamination and those that assess the degree of contamination on the individual's skin (Table 11-1). Indirect methods (discussed in previous chapters) involve the use of filters, gauze pads, or swabs to wipe surfaces; instruments to "sniff" surfaces for volatile compounds; and adhesive tape to lift dust from surfaces. Direct methods are often experimental and have used cellulose, gauze, or charcoal pads; clothing for dosimetry; skin washes; and monitoring the skin for contaminants that fluoresce. Tracer methods may allow measurements to estimate dermal exposure to toxic contaminants without actually exposing the workers. Processes and tasks could be tested ahead of time to estimate exposure locations and the degree of overall body exposure. Controls would be implemented to minimize exposures prior to the toxicant actually being used. While the types of situations may be limited to those compatible with tracer chemicals, tracer methods represent a preventative approach.

CHEMICAL SELECTION

The most common groups of chemicals for which dermal monitoring has been performed are amines (3,3'-dichlorobenzidine, MOCA), metals (arsenic, lead, and mercury), polychlorinated biphenyls (PCBs), and pesticides. In many instances they were selected for monitoring for the same reasons described in Chapter 6 in situations where surface monitoring techniques are used as an indirect method of approximating dermal exposures.

TABLE 11-1. Dermal Methods

Method	*Description*	*Advantages*	*Limitations*	*Reference*
Pad	Layers of gauze or other material with backing attached to or under clothing	Specific site sampling of the body parts	Small sampling area Unlike skin Limited area of coverage	EPA, 1986
Skin wipes	Wetted filters, wipes or sponges used to wipe skin	Measures material in direct dermal contact	Does not measure absorbed material May not completely desorb material	Lees, Corn, and Breysse, 1987
Hand and body rinses	Solution of alcohol, surfactant or water in polyethylene bag	Collects material under nails and in skin crevices	Does not measure absorbed material May not completely desorb material	Sell and Maitlen, 1983
Cotton gloves/clothing/whole body dosimetry	Cotton clothing used to collect contaminant	Extension of sampling area over entire body part Provides good representation for dermal exposure	Clothing does not emulate skin absorption	WHO, 1986
Fluorescence measurements including fluorescent tracers and video imaging	Some compounds fluoresce naturally under UV light or fluorescent tracers are added to formulations where compounds do not fluoresce. Exposure patterns recorded by video imaging under longwave UV light	Low detection limits Qualitation and quantitative determinations of exposure are possible	UV light is carcinogenic and may be dangerous to both user and subject Tracer may not accurately represent target pollutant Tracer can be only added to specific sources	Fenske, 1988

Pesticide manufacture, formulation, and field application was one of the first situations where dermal monitoring was performed, and the use of dermal monitoring has been expanded to virtually all areas involving pesticides including field reentry, harvesting, greenhouse work, office buildings, and residences. As a result, the methodologies that have been standardized for the use of dosimetry pads and whole body dosimetry arose from pesticide monitoring. The only pesticides that cannot be sampled using these methods are gases and liquids with high vapor pressures because current techniques are inadequate to sample these. Field workers dislodge pesticide-laden particulate matter from foliage, fruit, and soils surfaces. These pesticide-containing particles settle on the worker's skin and clothing. Harvesters have been sampled extensively using dermal methods because most of their exposure is through contact with the foliage. Weeding is another activity that has been monitored. It has been found that weeding stirs up contaminated soil, creating an aerosol that will settle on all parts of the body (EPA, 1988). Both the Environmental Protection Agency (EPA) and the World Health Organization (WHO) have developed standardized protocols for the use of dermal monitoring for agriculture studies.

Acrylamide, polycyclic aromatic hydrocarbon (PAH) containing compounds, dinitrotoluene, pentachlorophenol, and certain hormones are examples of other compounds that have been successfully monitored, which indicates that dermal techniques can be expanded successfully to monitor for exposures to a wider variety of compounds in the future. However, whenever attempting to sample for any new compounds, validation of sample collection methods needs to be done.

DERMAL SAMPLING METHODS

Sampling professionals intending to monitor a worker's skin are cautioned that incorrect application or use of direct techniques may result in injury to the subject. Since dermal exposures are not currently assessed sufficiently, these methods are provided in the hope of finding improvements or alternatives to these methods.

Since the body is a much larger area to sample than the breathing zone, there are many challenges. For example, consider the face. The face is one of the most difficult areas to sample, yet, because it is always exposed, one of the most important. People are less likely to be receptive to having it touched or wiped or having some sort of sampler taped to it for many reasons including cosmetic concerns. Facial exposure has been estimated by placing two pads on the shoulders; however, because the orientation of the pads is different (horizontal rather than vertical), the measured exposure may be greater than the actual face exposure, especially for aerosols.

It has been proposed that sampling methods be selected based on the exposure pathway. Jobs requiring the skin to be immersed in chemicals would be sampled using washing or swabbing techniques. Where the exposure results from aerosol deposition or direct contact with the contaminated surfaces, swabbing, washing, dosimetry, and tracer techniques can be used depending on the body surface to be sampled (Brouwer and van Hemmen, 1992). Sampling must be done so that all skin surfaces with a potential for exposure are identified and monitored. The sampling duration will depend on the concentration of the contaminant as well as the collection characteristics of the monitoring method.

Skin Sampling

Skin sampling can be done using methods that require laboratory analysis or using methods that produce either color changes upon exposure or fluorescence under ultraviolet light (see Chapter 13). Chromate sensitivity in workers engaged in making color television screens was identified when an examination with a fluorescent lamp showed persistence of the fluorescent compounds on the hands and nail folds even after repeated washing of the hands (Stevenson and Morgan, 1983). Even though they wore nylon suits and hats and rubber overshoes, workers had eczema of the wrists and feet, most likely due to fluorescent wristwatches and protective rubber overshoes. The process used ammonium bichromate to produce cross-linking of light-sensitized polyvinyl alcohol (PVA), which in turn enabled fluorescent compounds (red, green, and blue) incorporated in the PVA to adhere to the screen.

Hands are the most common application for skin sampling methods when they are the primary source of exposure. Skin wipes would be useful if hands become blackened as a result of handling lead shielded copper grounding wire. Either the metal could be wiped or the hands or both. A similar situation may occur if workers handle soldering wire or lead-contaminated radiators. CPC may or may not be useful in these instances. For example, touching the exterior of cotton gloves during removal would contaminate the fingers and contact with moisture would allow the lead to permeate the material. Contamination of personal clothing can also lead to skin contamination. Tasks such as abrasive blasting of lead paint on a steel bridge will create a fine airborne dust, which then settles on the workers' clothing and surfaces in the workplace. In these situations a combination of both surface and skin sampling is useful.

Contaminated smoking materials may allow toxic materials, or their combustion products, to enter the body via the lungs (lead and mercury). Wiping of the skin that contacts cigarettes, such as hands and fingers, may be useful in evaluating this possible route of exposure. Another method is to wipe the inside surfaces or protective gear that may contact skin (OSHA, 1991).

Skin sampling is also useful to determine if cleaning methods are effectively removing skin contamination. For example, polyethelene glycol has been shown to be more effective at removing aromatic amine contamination than soap and water. In field testing with color change media, wipes found significant levels of aromatic amine (>20 μg/hand) on workers' skin after normal cleanup with soap and water (Klingner, 1992). Skin sampling, including wipes, is not recommended for compounds that absorb rapidly through the skin because it will most likely underestimate the exposure. Biological monitoring for these substances or their metabolites is one means of assessing absorption.

Sampling under gloves and other CPC can identify previously unsuspected exposures as well as estimate the degree of protection achieved during actual field use. Protection between different groups of workers can also be compared. Hand rinses were used in one study of Dicofol pesticide applicators and mixer-loaders who wore protective gloves (Edmont Solvex) (Nigg, Stamper, and Queen, 1986). It was determined that the applicators' hand exposure was reduced by wearing gloves (83 ± 8%, 86 ± 5%) while the mixer-loaders' exposures were actually increased (11 ± 19%, 58 ± 47%). The observed increase most likely resulted from work habit differences between applicators and mixer-loaders. Applicators seldom remove their gloves during the work period, whereas mixer-loaders often do so when loading. As a result, the hands of the mixer-loaders were in direct contact with contaminated machinery, and so forth; when the gloves were placed back onto the hand, the inside of the gloves were contaminated.

Pad Dosimetry

Of the techniques that have been developed to monitor for dermal exposure, pad or patch dosimeters have been used the most. Pad sampling techniques have been available since the late 1950s when they were first used for pesticides. With pad monitors, contaminants are entrapped or absorbed by the cloth mesh of the multilayered materials of which the pads are composed. A common method involves placing absorbent pads at various points on a worker's clothing or skin and exposing them for a carefully measured interval while the worker performs routine job functions (see Fig. 11-1). The pads are removed and transported to a laboratory, where the contaminant is extracted and analyzed. The amount of contaminant that comes into contact with the skin is calculated using an anatomical model that allows for extrapolation of the small area represented by the pad to one or more body parts.

Pads can measure the effectiveness of personal clothing for protection against chemicals, estimate skin exposure, and determine which parts of the body receive the highest exposures.

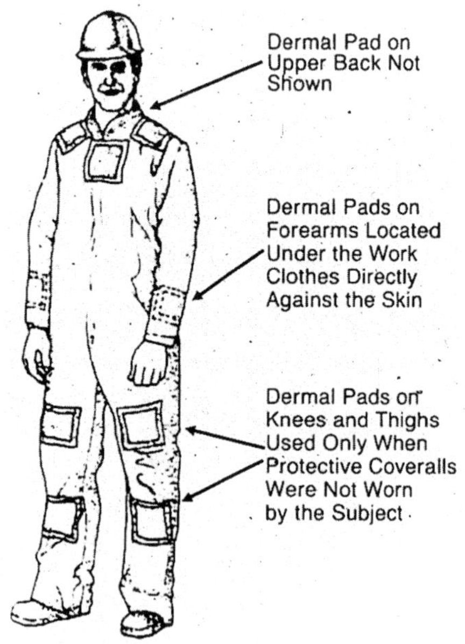

Figure 11-1. Badges attached to worker using EPA configuration.
Source: From EPA. 1987. *Acrylamide Grouting Study*. EPA 560/5-87-009. Washington, DC: EPA.

They fall into several categories. The most common have been developed to collect a contaminant in a specific physical form: spray or dust. Multiuse pads designed to collect either dusts or sprays have also been developed. More recently, chemical dopants and other materials such as polyurethane have been used to collect specific chemicals or chemical families. Alpha-cellulose is commonly used for measuring sprays and surgical gauze is used for measuring dusts. This type of cellulose is more adsorbent than conventional cellulose filter papers. In spray monitoring situations pads can easily saturate if they are not sufficiently adsorbent.

Pads have several advantages including their small size, portability, low cost, and passive sampling, which eliminates the need for pumps that require calibration and maintenance. They tend to absorb and retain materials like spray mists or particulates that have low vapor pressures.

There are differences in opinion as to the best way to measure dermal dose, whether pads should be worn outside or under the clothing or be taped to exposed skin. Considering whether normal work clothing can protect against skin exposure, another question is whether chemical protective clothing (CPC) should be worn during sampling to protect the worker if an excessive skin exposure is suspected.

The primary limitation of using absorbent pads is the assumption that exposures are uniform over various body parts. Since the pad technique collects a spot sample of the exposure to each body region, a potential source of error in using pads for sample collection is in the extrapolation from concentrations measured on a relatively small surface area compared to the entire body surface area (Fenske, 1990). Typically pads are only 26 cm^2 and therefore represent only a small fraction of the corresponding body regions: 0.73% of the chest/stomach or back, 1.4% of the thighs, 4.3% of the forearms (EPA, 1987). Since pads generally cover 6% or less of the body, exposures could be grossly over- or underestimated if droplets hit or miss the pad when spray applications are being monitored. Also, it is very difficult to monitor exposure to the scrotum, face, neck, or hands using pads. Another problem encountered when using external pads to monitor dermal exposure is the need to estimate how much of the material collected on the pads would have eventually penetrated clothing.

The biggest concern is how much the collection characteristics of the pads resemble the skin. In the case of wettable powder, which impinges on the skin and later drys and falls off, the resemblance may not be the same. Other factors depend on how moist the skin is with sweat. Because they do not physically resemble the skin, adsorption and retention of volatile or even nonvolatile materials by the cotton gauze may not be similar to the skin (Popendorf and Leffingwell, 1984). There are a wide range of skin variations both between and within individuals due to such factors as hairiness, ease of sweating, wrinkling, callouses, and smoothness.

Clothing for Dosimetry

A variation of the absorbent pad method involves knit cotton or other garments that cover the anatomical areas expected to have an exposure. These garments are then extracted in a laboratory for contaminants and the extract is analyzed. The most common method uses cotton gloves for collection and some studies have used long underwear. This type of monitoring is often used in conjunction with pads, but there are many variations and considerations involved that separate these methods from pad sampling. Table 11-2 contains data from a spray operation where both pads and whole body sampling were used.

Clothing samples fall into two categories: items deliberately prepared and selected to be used as monitoring media and items of normal work clothing that are identified during surveys as highly likely to contain contaminants, which are then collected and either sacrificed for sampling or a nondestructive method such as wiping, sniffing, or vacuuming is used as a qualitative determination of the presence of contaminants.

In some instances where dermatitis or other symptoms of disease are present, clothing contamination may be considered as the cause (Fig. 11-2). For example, although inhalation exposure as a result of improper drying of dry cleaned clothing has been a concern, especially to the customers and their residences, there have been

TABLE 11-2. Comparison of Potential Dermal Exposure to Paraquat of Spray Operators Using WHO Exposure Pad and Whole Body Sampling Methods

	Electrodyn Sprayer		*Micron Ulva Sprayer*		*Knapsack Sprayer*	
	Exposure Pads	*Whole Body*	*Exposure Pads*	*Whole Body*	*Exposure Pads*	*Whole Body*
	0.3	13.8	81.3	102.0	359.3	508.5
	0.3	26.6	51.2	262.9	238.4	52.4
	0.2	12.4	31.2	377.6	196.4	38.2
	0.1	11.3	824.8	402.5	275.5	58.5
	2.7	106.9	22.1	358.7	117.6	67.8
	0.1	17.5	120.8	595.5		
	0.1	5.6				
Mean	0.5	27.7	188.6	349.9	237.4	145.1
SD	1.0	35.5	313.8	163.1	89.9	203.4

Source: From Chester, G., and R. J. Ward. 1984. Occupational exposure and drift hazard during aerial application of Paraquat to cotton. *Arch. Env. Contamin. Toxicol.* **13**:551–563.
Notes: Potential dermal exposure (mg active ingredient/hr) of spray operators. SD = standard deviation.

instances where contact with this clothing has produced dermatitis including ulcers. An evaluation of genital ulcers suffered by several men in the same printing plant found that their coveralls, which were dry cleaned with stoddard solvent, were still damp, especially in the heavy seams of the crotch area. It was also determined that the drying process involved heat and was expensive; therefore, there was a tendency on the part of shops to decrease the time of this cycle as much as possible (Nethercrott et al., 1980). Similar findings have occurred with the use of perchloroethylene (PCE) for dry cleaning, although in the case of PCE ulceration has not been identified and significant percutaneous absorption is only known to occur in instances of occlusion (Kawauchi and Nishiyama, 1989). Therefore, taking a sample of actual clothing worn by workers can be useful in situations where an adverse effect or symptom is present.

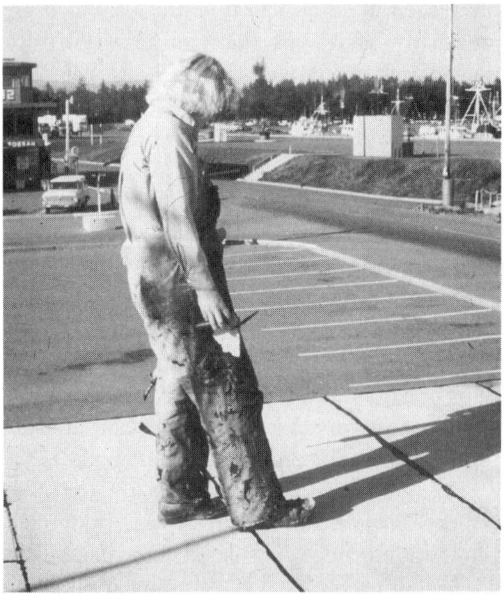

Figure 11-2. Roofer wearing contaminated clothing. Coal-tar based roofing compounds contain PAHs.

Sometimes the purpose of sampling is to determine the presence of a contaminant, rather than the degree of contamination, because the actual period of exposure cannot be determined. This was the case when electrical linemen's leather gloves were found to be contaminated with PCBs. Since these gloves are very specialized, there is a tendency to use them for a longer period of time and therefore small amounts of contaminant build up (Lees, Corn, and Breysse, 1987). Clothing items are sampled when it is suspected that they are creating a significant amount of contamination that is being spread from the workplace to the interiors of personal autos and workers' homes.

The whole body dosimetry method is best used for preventive sampling, that is, to determine if there is significant skin exposure and to what areas of the body it is occurring. It involves the use of clothing to cover the whole body and trap contaminants. There are two methods: (1) using undergarments of cotton, long underwear tops and bottoms, and socks to assess the amount of material penetrating outer clothing; and (2) using disposable overgarments such as Tyvek suits, which estimate exposure as if the skin were bare.

An alternative is to use portions of clothing to cut down on the bulk of material requiring analysis. This usually involves cutting away the most likely areas to show contamination either before monitoring or afterward. Cotton sleeves (covering the arm from the top of the arm to the wrists) and cotton leggings (covering the leg from the top part of the thigh to the ankle) washed before use have been used for sampling workers who were picking strawberries (Ritcey et al., 1987). In between these extremes lies the use of specific items of clothing, including gloves, T-shirts, and coveralls. If workers wear leather shoes it is possible for contamination to build up in them. In this case, foot exposure should also be assessed, which has been done by analyzing cotton socks.

A major obstacle is the lack of standard garments for sampling. In studies to date, garments have been selected for convenience rather than according to scientific criteria, and garment characteristics (fiber content, construction, finish, weight, thickness), of course, vary (Fenske, 1993).

INTERPRETATION OF RESULTS

With few exceptions, there are no standards related to dermal exposures; each situation must be handled on a case-by-case basis. The type of health effects caused, the contribution of skin absorption or ingestion to the total dose, and air sampling results (where appropriate) must be considered when evaluating sample results. The methods for calculating dermal exposure are fairly simplistic and frequently do not account for the use of protective clothing and its effectiveness. However, when measurements of dermal exposure are used to estimate absorbed dose, the amount of the contaminant penetrating clothing as well as estimates of dermal absorption data obtained in animal experiments should be incorporated into the result.

When interpreting results of dermal samples, it is generally assumed that 100% absorption unless the experimenter has enough information to adjust penetration using experimentally derived factors such as $K_{o/w}$. (For a discussion of these factors, see Chapter 2.) Another adjustment that must be considered is the permeability of the skin for a given area as there are wide variations in absorption. Due to the lack of standards for dermal exposure, risk assessments have been applied to determine acceptable levels. While much time can be spent attempting to extrapolate the results of dermal sampling for dose and body burden, usually simply showing significant dermal deposition is sufficient to indicate the need for controls.

The use of dermal absorption rates will enable more accurate estimates of exposure and improve the interpretation of dermal sampling results that are often criticized for oversampling. Dermal absorption rates are based on experimental data that may be derived from in vivo or in vitro experiments. For example, 10% is typically used as the dermal absorption rate for chlordane and heptachlor (Kamble et al., 1992; Feldman and Maibach, 1974). The use of dermal absorption rates to modify dermal testing must be done cautiously because there are many factors that can change them.

However, direct dermal absorption from contact with a treated surface or dermally deposited soil, dust, or liquids containing contaminants is difficult to assess. The rate of dermal absorption can differ dramatically between animals (even acceptable surrogate species) and humans. There can be dramatic differences in rates of absorption for contaminants on different areas of the body that need to be accounted for. It may also be difficult to extrapolate absorption rates measured directly in adult humans to a rate for children (Fenske et al., 1990).

Most early pesticide studies related dermal contact to the time the contaminant was applied; however, more recently the trend is to relate dermal contact to the amount sprayed due to varying concentrations used in formulations and differences in spraying speeds (Davis, 1980). This method assumes the back of the body receives a zero exposure and the exposure rate of the arms is similar to that of the chest. Using this method, one study determined that the differences in exposure results were due to differences in height of tea plants (Wan, 1990). One approach used to compare doses of different individuals is to divide each worker's dose by his or her weight and compare the results as µg/hr/kg. It is often assumed that workers all wear the same level (and types) of clothing for these calculations; for example, a shirt with short sleeves and open collar, long trousers, no hat or protective gloves. The assumption is also often made that personal work clothing provides complete protection to the area covered. In performing the calculations, the same assumptions would be applied to all workers in a study regardless of what was actually worn (Durham and Wolfe, 1962). Table 11-3 lists clothing assumptions used in selected studies. A review of this information illustrates the variability that can exist when comparing studies.

There are judgments the sampling professional must make regarding the pad sampling data. The amounts found on the pads may not be representative of the amount actually absorbed by the body. In one study of parathion exposure utilizing cellulose pads, it was found

TABLE 11-3. Differences in Clothing Assumptions in Selected Studies

Study Author	*Number of Replicates*	*Mean Exposure (mg/hr)*	*Clothing Assumptions*
Abbot et al., 1987	18	40.0	Long-sleeved shirt, long pants, 50% protection
Dubelman et al., 1982	12	0.93	Long-sleeved shirt, 50% protection Long pants, 100% protection
Maitlen et al., 1982	21	0.70	Short-sleeved shirt, long pants, 100% protection
Staiff et al., 1975	20	0.40	Short-sleeved shirt, long pants, 100% protection
Wojeck et al., 1983	23	72.0	Long-sleeved shirt, long pants, 100% protection
Wolfe, Durham, and Armstrong, 1967	7	9.4	Short-sleeved shirt, long pants, 100% protection
Lauer and Arras, 1981	2	0.15	Potential dermal exposure reduced by 80%

Source: From Lunchick, C., G. Burin, J. C. Reinert, and K. E. Warkentien. 1989. The Environmental Protection Agency's use of biological monitoring data for the special review of Alachlor. In *Biological Monitoring for Pesticide Exposure*. Washington, DC: American Chemical Society.
Note: All exposure estimates are based on an application rate of 1.0 lb active ingredient per acre.

Abbot, I. M., J. L. Bonsall, G. Chester, T. B. Hard, and G. J. Turnbull. 1987. Worker exposure to a herbicide applied with groundsprayers in the United Kingdom. *AIHA J.* **48**(2):167–175.
Dubelman, S., R. Lauer, D. D. Arras, and S. A. Adams. 1982. Operator exposure measurements during application of the herbicide Diallate. *J. Agric. Food Chem.* **30**:528–532.
Lauer, R., and D. D. Arras. 1981. Aerial and ground applicator exposure studies with Lasso herbicide under actual field conditions. Report no. MSL-1889, Monsanto Chemical Co.
Maitlen, J. C., C. R. Sell, and L. M. McDonough. 1982. Workers in the agricultural environment: Dermal exposure to carbaryl. In Plimmer, J. R. (ed.), *Pesticide Residues and Exposure*. Washington, DC: American Chemical Society, pp. 83–103.
Staiff, D. C., S. W. Comer, J. R. Armstrong, and H. R. Wolfe. 1975. Exposure to the herbicide, paraquat. *Bull. Env. Contam. Toxicol.* **14**(3):334–340.
Wojeck, G. A., J. F. Price, H. N. Nigg, and J. H. Stamper. 1983. Worker exposure to paraquat and diquat. *Arch. Env. Contam. Toxicol.* **12**:65–70.
Wolfe, H. R., W. F. Durham, and J. F. Armstrong. 1967. Exposure of workers to pesticides. *Arch. Env. Health* **14**:622–633.

that the amounts absorbed via the skin were two orders of magnitude lower than those found on the dosimeters (Durham, 1963). Thus, biological monitoring along with dosimetry is useful for interpretations. When comparing studies there are many factors that can account for variations, including formulation, rate of application (if the material is sprayed), location of dermal pads (and whether they are over or under clothing and/or CPC), composition of the pads used, environmental conditions (temperature, humidity, windspeed, and direction), use of controls such as closed cabs during spray applications, personal hygiene, personal work habits, and whether fresh work clothing was donned that day.

A large amount of material on a pad usually indicates the main part of the body exposed; however, if hands were habitually rubbed on a particular area to clean or dry them off, then this assumption could be misleading. Good observations throughout a survey are important. If concentrations on the lower legs are higher than expected, it is possible that moisture (dew) during the early morning hours caused the lower pant legs to become water soaked and contaminated with material. There are two ways that moisture contamination can affect pads and clothing. One is depletion of the material adsorbed yielding results that are lower than actual concentrations. High moisture levels such as rain, which will soak the media, can cause lower concentration numbers. The other is that high humidity may have a positive effect on contaminant transfer (such as pesticides from foliage) or adherence to gauze monitors.

Facial exposure is most often monitored using pads attached to outside of the clothing on the shoulders, chest, and back. In one case (apple thinning) the forearms were monitored with pads and the results were extrapolated to the face and neck (Davis et al., 1982). In this instance it was assumed that each worker's exposure was 14% of his forearm exposure. In a study of citrus harvesting, the exposure to forearms was extrapolated to represent the total body exposure (Popendorf and Leffingwell, 1982). In another instance of citrus harvesting, total body exposure was calculated from pads placed inside normal work clothing for the upper body, and outside pads for the lower body (Nigg and Stamper, 1984). Figure 11-3 provides an example of how skin exposure is extrapolated from monitoring sites.

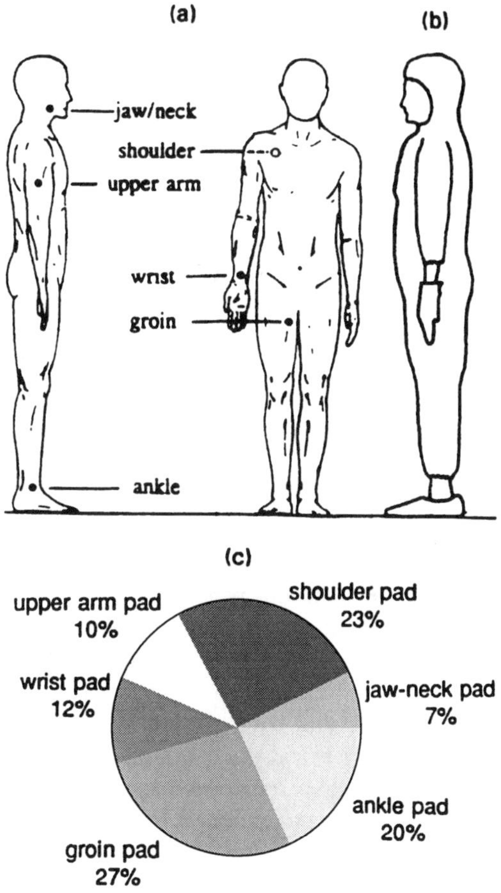

Figure 11-3. Skin sites where exposure pads were pasted for monitoring dermal polycyclic aromatic hydrocarbon contamination (*a*); the coveralls as worn to reduce skin contamination (*b*); and the percentage of the total body area that each pad was assumed to represent (*c*).
Source: From J. G. M. Van Rooij, E. M. A. Van Lieshout, M. M. Bodelier-Bade, and F. J. Jongeneelen. 1993. Effect of the reduction of skin contamination on the internal dose of creosote workers exposed to polycyclic hydrocarbons. *Scand. J. Work Env. Health* 19(3):202.

The results from glove monitoring are often used for hand exposure estimates and added into the dose. It is difficult to compare the residues observed in glove samples with pad results, since the analytical results of the two media are expressed in different units. One way of getting around this is to adjust glove results to units of square centimeters using an estimate of the surface area of the hands. A value of 820 cm^2 has been used (Davis, 1980). The results (usually in micrograms) for the gloves are divided by this value to get $\mu g/cm^2$. The importance of monitoring hands was demonstrated in one study of urban applicators. A significant correlation existed between the length of the application period and the amount of carbaryl recovered on the external pads and in the air sampling results, but not with the internal pads or hand washes. It was concluded that hand exposure occurring during the mixing and diluting of the formulated material overshadowed the exposure resulting from the actual application of carbaryl. Therefore, it is best to monitor different tasks separately even if performed by the same individual.

Pads have been used to evaluate the penetration of pesticides through fabric by placing them underneath workers' clothing. This approach assumes that there is a uniform distribution of exposure over each body region in order to directly compare inner and outer pads. Some of these studies using personal pad monitors placed beneath clothing of pesticide workers have shown that a significant proportion of the (calculated) dermal exposure may occur at anatomical sites that are covered by clothing. However, another source of exposure is deposition through openings such as the neck and cuffs (Fenske, 1988). In situations where individuals do not wear hoods or tape seams and breaks, such as those between gloves and coveralls, it is possible for deposition to be a significant contribution to exposure. In these cases, other methods such as skin washes and fluorescence may provide a better assessment of exposures at these points.

The interpretation of pads placed inside (or under) clothing is more complicated than when pads are on the outside because the types of fabric of disposable garments used to cover the subject can vary. Also, when placed under rubber aprons or rubber boots (on the shins), there is a vast difference between the permeability of materials designed to be protective and that of other materials. In the field, inside pads can become contaminated by other routes than directly through protective clothing or work garments (Table 11-4). In one study it was observed that when an applicator extended his arm, the sleeve of the coverall had a tendency to ride up, exposing the pad placed underneath the sleeve on the forearm (Stamper et al., 1989). Studies in which pads are worn both outside of and under workers' clothing can be even more difficult to interpret. In most cases, the percent of contaminant transmitted through a particular type (and weight) of fabric is unknown. Other factors such as perspiration and underclothing also have an impact.

The amount of contaminant on dosimeter clothing can be divided by the body surface area that the piece of clothing represents to arrive at the residue level (expressed as $\mu g/cm^2$) for each body part (EPA, 1986). Exposure results from clothing samples are often represented as a rate such as mg/hr; however, in some instances it is also good to present data in terms of production. In one study of measurements made when spraying liquid pesticides from hand-held lances or spray guns, and when applying dustable powders with a dust blower, the dermal exposure per hour for dustable powders was significantly higher than that for spraying even though the application rates for dustable powders were lower because spraying takes more time (Brouwer et al., 1992). However, when dermal exposure was expressed as the amount applied to a specific area during crop spraying (mg/1000 M^2), the exposure for dusting was seven times lower than for spraying.

In a study where cotton gloves were used to monitor the exposure of residents to pesticides applied to carpets in their homes, the following assumptions were used to compute dermal and daily air exposure doses for the applied compounds: 20 M^3 of air daily respired by a 70 kg adult; dermal absorption factors of 0.01 for granular and dust applications and 0.1 for liquid and spray applications.

When surface and dermal samplings are conducted simultaneously, dermal transfer coefficients can be calculated for a specific work activity. While principally applied to pesticides, this concept may prove useful for other compounds. The dermal transfer coefficient is a means of estimating the rate of surface contact frequency. It is calculated by dividing the dermal

TABLE 11-4. Mean Transmittance to Inside Pads

Location	*Fluvalinate*	*Chlorpyrifos*[a]	*Ethazol*	*Dicofol*
Chest, covered by:				
Tyvek® coverall only	0.005 ± 0.005 (7)	0.116 ± 0.084 (2)		0.012 ± 0.012 (9)
Tyvek® coverall plus butyl rubber apron	<0.001 ± 0 (20)	0.055 ± 0.026 (22)	0.451 ± 0.124 (19)	
Forearms, covered by:				
Tyvek® coverall only	0.016 ± 0.010 (26)	0.121 ± 0.057 (24)	0.344 ± 0.109 (18)	0.119 ± 0.054 (9)
Thighs, covered by:				
Tyvek® coverall only	0.021 ± 0.012 (7)	0.005 ± 0.003 (2)		0.003 ± 0.001 (9)
Tyvek® coverall plus butyl rubber apron	<0.001 ± 0 (20)	0.011 ± 0.008 (22)	0.126 ± 0.026 (19)	
Shins, covered by:				
Tyvek® coverall plus butyl rubber boots	0.038 ± 0.025 (27)	0.037 ± 0.028 (24)	0.015 ± 0.004 (18)	<0.001 ± 0 (9)

Source: From Stamper, J. H., H. N. Nigg, W. D. Mahon, A. P. Nielsen, and M. D. Royer. 1989. Pesticide exposure to greenhouse handgunners. *Arch. Env. Contam. Toxicol.* **18:**515–529.
Note: ± standard error, with number of replications in parentheses.
[a]Includes data for a subject who was acting as an assistant.

exposure by the transferable residue (Fenske, 1993):

$$\text{Dermal transfer coefficient (cm}^2\text{/hr)} = \frac{\text{Dermal exposure } (\mu\text{g/hr})}{\text{Transferable residue } (\mu\text{g/cm}^2)}$$

For residential studies the transferable or dislodgeable residue is usually measured using weighted rollers and cotton clothing. For agricultural workers contacting residue-bearing foliage (double sided leaf) 10,000 cm^2/hr has been determined to be a reasonable coefficient, based on a number of studies (Knaak, Iwata, and Maddy, 1989). Sampling methods for dislodgeable residues are described in Chapter 7.

Some studies have adopted the practice of providing the weight of the glove over a specified area, usually in mg/cm^2 (Fenske et al., 1989). This practice should be adopted by all as it provides a basis for comparing studies done with the same glove material. Substantially heavier gloves are likely to absorb higher levels of residues. When long-sleeved cotton gloves are used, the results are assumed to represent both the hands and the forearms (Brouwer et al., 1992).

When clothing has been used in residential studies to determine exposure to contaminants on rugs, a transfer coefficient is sometimes calculated (Ross et al., 1990). This coefficient is the percentage of contaminant on the floor that is physically transferred to the dosimeter clothing. It can be calculated by dividing the contaminant concentration (in μg/cm^2) on clothing by the concentration on the floor with which the person was in contact. Direct contact with surfaces is likely to result in higher exposures than contact from an aerosol.

An extrapolation using the threshold limit value (TLV), an airborne limit, has also been used to create a standard for glove permeation (Perkins and Knight, 1989). The calculation is as follows:

$$\text{(TLV) (20 L/min) (480 min)} = \text{Dose delivered to the lungs in mg}$$

This value is then compared to the results of the gloves expressed in total milligrams. Since the worst case is 100% absorption using this approach, it most likely will overestimate the danger level.

Dermal contact to the hands from a skin wash is the amount of contaminant found in all the hand rinses, divided by the exposure time. Handwash methods can vary. One solvent, such as 95% ethanol, may remove different pesticides with varying efficiency, and results from studies in which different solvents have been used may not be comparable. The use of gloves reduces the amount of contaminant found in handwash samples (taken under the gloves) by about 85% (Nigg and Stamper, 1985). For pesticide spray operations, handwash samples have been normalized for the spray rate (Table 11-5), the result being a measure of the applicators' mean exposure in mg deposited per kg sprayed (Stamper et al., 1989).

It is also true that not all hand monitoring methods will detect the same contamination. For example, extrapolating hand exposure from wrist patches will not identify high finger contamination. Skin wiping and washing techniques give information about individual exposures. However, skin absorption and binding cannot be accounted for and there is a time dependence wherein the most recent exposure will provide the highest contribution because there has not been enough time for normal weathering processes to deplete the residue. In situations where the individual spends time at more than one site over the monitoring period or handles materials which may be contaminated from exposure at other sites interpretation becomes even more difficult.

It can be difficult to get good correlation between air levels and dermal monitoring results, although they have been determined in some studies. As an example, the amount (ηg) of PAH (either as total or individual compounds) found in skin wipes collected post–work shift significantly correlated with that in air samples (μg/M^3) (see Table 11-6.)

SETTING VALUES FOR COMPOUNDS USING TOXICITY TESTING DATA

The first values used in dermal exposure assessments were LD_{50}s. Respiratory and dermal exposures given in mg/hr were expressed as percentage of toxic dose using these LD_{50} values often for male white rats (Durham and Wolfe, 1962). In a study comparing exposures while ap-

TABLE 11-5. Handwash Data Normalized for Spray Rate

Compound	*Subj. No.*	*Spray Rate (kg a.i./hr)*	*Handwash (Left Hand)*	*Handwash (Right Hand)*	*Normalized Total Handwash*
Fluvalinate	1	0.016 ± 0.001 (3)	10 ± 6 (3)	13 ± 6 (3)	1.92 ± 0.38
	2	0.040 ± 0.005 (10)	26 ± 8 (10)	71 ± 31 (10)	
	3	0.037 ± 0.007 (9)	28 ± 9 (9)	32 ± 10 (9)	
	4	0.055 ± 0.003 (5)	38 ± 8 (5)	43 ± 7 (5)	
Chlorpyrifos	1	0.076 ± 0.007 (7)	55 ± 53 (7)	280 ± 278 (7)	1.60 ± 1.30
	2	0.118 ± 0.008 (7)	11 ± 3 (7)	14 ± 5 (7)	
	3	0.083 ± 0.011 (9)	25 ± 7 (9)	14 ± 4 (9)	
Ethazol	1	0.020 ± 0.003 (2)	0 ± 0 (2)	0 ± 0 (2)	0.10 ± 0.03
	2	0.039 ± 0.003 (7)	1 ± 1 (7)	4 ± 2 (7)	
	3	0.029 ± 0.002 (10)	1 ± 0 (10)	1 ± 1 (10)	
Dicofol	4	0.044 ± 0.002 (9)	20 ± 10 (9)	19 ± 9 (9)	0.86 ± 0.39

Source: Adapted from Stamper, J. H., H. N. Nigg, W. D. Mahon, A. P. Nielsen, and M. D. Royer. 1989. Pesticide exposure to greenhouse handgunners. *Arch. Env. Contam. Toxicol.* **18:**515–529.
Note: ± standard error, with number of replications in parentheses.

TABLE 11-6. PCBs and PAHs in Skin Wipes and Air Samples from Workplaces

Air Levels ($\mu g/M^3$)	*Skin Wipes ($\mu g/cm^2$)*	*Air Dose*[a] *($\mu g/day$)*	*Skin Dose*[b] *($\mu g/day$)*	*Skin:Air*	*Chemical/Wipe*
80–275 (178)	2–22 (12)	1,424	2,400	1.7:1	PCB, hands
0–264 (132)	0.1–7 (3.5)	1,056	700	0.7:1	PCB, face
0.4–9 (4.7)	0.05–5 (2.5)	38	500	13:1	PCB, face
0.5–6.1 (3.3)	0.008–1.08 (0.54)	4–48.8 (26)	1.2–215 (108)	4:1	PCB, hands (approx.)
<100 (50)	0.002–0.019 (0.011)	400	2.2	0.006:1	PCB, forehead preshift
2–34 (18)	0.004–0.13 (0.067)	141	13.4	0.09:1	PAH, forehead preshift
10.2	0.008	82	1.6	0.02:1	PAH, forehead preshift
10.2	0.097	82	19.4	0.24:1	Forehead, postshift

Source: Adapted from Wolff, M. S., R. Herbert, M. Marcus, M. Rivera, P. J. Landrigan, and L. R. Andrews. 1989. Polycyclic aromatic hydrocarbon (PAH) residues on skin in relation to air levels among roofers. *Arch. Env. Health* **44**(3):157–163.
Note: Numbers in parentheses are midpoints.
[a]Air dose = $\mu g/M^3 \times 8\ M^3/day$.
[b]Skin dose = $\mu g/cm^2 \times 200\ cm^2$.

plying carbaryl with a telescoping pole and a high-pressure hydraulic sprayer, the total mg of exposure from each worker's pads was calculated (Haverty et al., 1983). All trials were summed and an average was determined for each type of application. It was assumed that the average worker weighs 65 kg and that an acute dermal LD_{50} for carbaryl was 2,000 mg/kg. The average mg of exposure was divided by 65 kg, giving a value in mg/kg. This value was then divided by the dermal LD_{50} to come up with percentages. In this instance, it was calculated that a worker would receive 0.05% of an acute dermal LD_{50} while applying carbaryl with the telescoping pole and 0.001% of the dose with the high-pressure hydraulic sprayer.

Risk assessments have been used to determine acceptable limits for dermal exposure studies. Where the no-observed-effect level (NOEL) or lowest-observed-effect level (LOEL) for a compound by any route of entry (usually oral) is known, it can be compared to the results. For the worst case the exposure intake is 100% (LaGoy, Bohrer, and Halvorsen, 1992). One technique uses the margin of safety (MOS), which can be determined as follows (Severn, 1984):

MOS =
NOEL/(dermal exposure)(absorption rate) + (respiratory exposure)(1.00*)

where

NOEL = No observed effect level in mg/kg/day
Dermal exposure is in mg/kg/day
Dermal absorption rate is selected from the literature for that compound
Respiratory exposure is in mg/kg/day
*Respiratory absorption rate is usually set at 100%

The rat ED_{10} has also been used to set a dermal exposure limit (Knaak, Jacobs, and Wang, 1986). The dose inhibiting 10% of the red cell cholinesterase activity in rats following skin application was determined. This was considered the no effect level. In order to extrapolate this value to humans, the exposure in both rats and humans was expressed in the form of total body surface area. This was done by dividing the total amount of the contaminant, fenamiphos, collected on the hands and body over an 8 hr workday by the total body surface area. The ED_{10} value was found to be 4.33 μg/cm² of body surface area for the rat. The exposure levels for the worker ranged from 0.037 μg/cm² to 0.267 μg/cm² of body surface. Thus, exposures as compared to the extrapolated ED_{10} were considered to be safe by a margin of at least 20.

COMPARISON OF DERMAL MONITORS WITH BIOLOGICAL MONITORING DATA

The simultaneous application of pad dosimetry, skin washing, and biological monitoring has been incorporated into exposure studies by several groups. Attempts have been made to establish a correlation of exposure measurements by both methods. Pad dosimetry has been combined with urinary metabolite determinations to compare worker exposure as a function of pesticide application method (Wojeck et al., 1983; Carmen et al., 1982), formulation plant worker exposure (Comer et al., 1975), and homeowner exposure (Staiff et al., 1975). Numerous other studies have similarly attempted to correlate exposure estimates obtained by the use of patches with urine levels of pesticide and/or its metabolite(s). In most of these studies, no clear-cut correlation was found between exposure estimated by both methods. One reason may be that by definition the dermal dosimeters trap materials and do not make allowances for the amount of contaminant that would pass into the skin through absorption, while biological monitoring measures only what has passed into the body.

A set of studies on 2,4,5-trichlorophenoxyacetic acid (2,4,5-T) exposure found that urinary excretion provided a more reliable measure of dose than the pads worn by the workers (Leng et al., 1982). A comparison of external 2,4,5-T exposure as measured on pads with that measured in urine indicated that exposure predictions from pads were much higher than those measured in the urine (Table 11-7).

In some older studies where good correlations were identified for biological and pad samples there was no statistical analysis; there-

TABLE 11-7. Apparent External Exposure Compared to Actual Dose of 2,4,5-T Absorbed by Forest Workers

		mg 2,4,5-T per kg body weight	
Job Description	*Number of Exposures*	*Gauze Patches*[a]	*Excreted in Urine*[b]
Mixers	7	0.04–1.62	0.011–0.127
Backpack sprayers	11	0.20–2.54	0.017–0.093
Mistblower crew (excludes mixer)	5	0.20–1.58	0.029–0.042
Helicopter crews (excludes mixers and pilots)	12	ND–0.02	<0.001–0.004
Pilots	4	ND–0.11	<0.001–0.039

Source: From Leng, M. L., J. C. Ramsey, and W. H. Braun. 1982. Review of studies with 2,4,5-trichlorophenoxyacetic acid in humans including applicators under field conditions. In *Pesticide Residues and Exposure*. Washington, DC: American Chemical Society.

Note: Leng, Ramsey, and Braun cite the following sources of data for their table: T. L. Lavy, J. S. Shepard, and J. D. Mattice, 1980, Exposure measurements of applicators spraying 2,4,5-trichlorophenoxyacetic acid in the forest, *J. Agric. Food Chem.* **28:**626–630, and T. L. Lavy, J. S. Shepard, and D. C. Bouchard, 1980, Field worker exposure and helicopter spray pattern for 2,4,5-T, *Bull. Env. Contam. Toxicol.* **24:**90–96.

[a]Based on average 2,4,5-T found on six patches per subject for each exposure, and estimated total skin area exposed on each subject as calculated by the method of Wolfe, H. R., J. F. Armstrong, D. C. Staiff, S. W. Comer, and W. F. Durham. 1975. Exposure of apple thinners to parathion residues. *Arch. Env. Contam. Toxicol.* **3:**257–267.

[b]Excluding amount found in urine on day 0 before spraying, possibly due to wearing contaminated clothing.

fore, the results may or may not have been significant (Fenske et al., 1989). Another problem when comparing studies where biological monitoring was performed with studies of pad samples is whether interfering exposures are controlled. For example, if a respirator is not worn, inhalation will contribute to the exposure and the resulting biological samples will reflect both inhalation and dermal exposure. A similar argument can be made for the placement of pads on top of clothing. On the other hand, if pads are placed under clothing the variation due to different fabric penetrabilities makes it impossible to compare studies.

In one study on lead exposure to children from house dust, an attempt was made to determine whether or not hand and blood lead were related (Que Hee et al., 1985). It was determined that this outcome depended on (1) the efficiency and representativeness of the washing or handwiping method, (2) whether the hands are deliberately washed by the child and the care taken prior to sampling (which is often beyond the investigators' control), (3) which parts of the hand are placed most often in the mouth, (4) whether the lead is evenly distributed over the surface of the hand, and (5) if wiping varied from investigator to investigator.

Concerns have been expressed that performing certain types of dermal monitoring and biological monitoring at the same time will invalidate the biological sampling data (Nigg and Stamper, 1989). As an example, suppose workers who normally work ungloved and do not customarily wash their hands participate in an exposure study. Requiring that they wear gloves in order to monitor hand exposure might reduce their total dermal exposure, and, hence their urinary metabolite level, by 21%. This is assuming that hand exposure originally constituted 50% of the total dermal exposure and that the gloves, worn for 1.2 hr of the workday, gave 85% protection. Requiring handwashes might lead to a similar reduction. However, for workers who normally wear gloves or who regularly wash their hands, hand rinses or cotton glove monitors may not affect the experimental outcome.

DERMAL MONITORING COMPOUNDS AND MEDIA*

Compound	*Media*	*Source*
Acetone	Solvent Permatec Pad Pt. No. 3050 (skin, CPC)	CLI Labs
Acid ions		NIOSH, August 1983*b* (HETA 83-417-1357)
Acrylamide	α-Cellulose pad dosimeters	EPA, 1990
Acrylamide	37 mm glass fiber filter moistened with deionized or distilled water (skin, CPC)	Cummins et al., 1992
Acrylamide	Skin wash with 50 mL of deionized water	Cummins et al., 1992
Aluminum trihydrate	Cotton gloves	NIOSH, June 1977 (HHE 77-39-400)
Aluminum trihydrate	37 mm 0.8 μm MCE filter, dry (skin)	NIOSH, June 1977 (HHE 77-39-400)
Aniline	Permatec Breakthrough Indicator Pt. No. 3001 (skin, CPC)	CLI Labs
Arsenic	Whatman 40 filters, dry	NIOSH, February 1976 (HHE 75-8-263)
Arsenic	Skin wash of 500 mL 0.1 N nitric acid	Roels et al., 1980
Arsenic	Skin wash of 500 mL of 0.1 HCI	Polissar et al., 1990
Arsenic acid	100% cotton overalls as dosimeters	Miller, Hoover, and Culver, 1980
Asbestos	Vacuum sampling with personal sampling pump and 25-mm 0.8-μm MCE filter (clothing)	NIOSH, March 1990 (HETA 87-126-2019)
Beclomethasone		Phillips, 1982
Benzene solubles	Filter moistened with acetone or isopropanol (skin)	Cheng, 1981
Benzene solubles	Skin wash with cyclohexane using aerosol spray apparatus with collection cup	Cheng, 1981
Benzene solubles	Gauze pad (5 cm) wetted with 70% isopropanol (skin)	DOE, 1979
Benzo-α-pyrene	Spill Spotter (UV) instrument (skin)	Hill, 1984
Benzo-α-pyrene	Black light (UV) lamp (skin)	Hill, 1984
3,4,-Benzpyrene	UV lamp with 253.7 ηm light (skin)	Ketcham and Norton, 1960
Bismuth	Whatman 40 filters, dry (skin)	NIOSH, February 1976 (HHE 75-8-263)
Cadmium	Skin wash of 500 mL 0.1 N nitric acid	Roels et al., 1980
Carbon graphite fibers	37-mm 0.8-μm MCE filter, dry (skin)	NIOSH, August 1985 (HETA 82-289-1496)
Chlordane	Cotton puff, soaked with 0.5 mL of 70% ethanol, 0.25 cm^2 area (skin)	Hirai and Tomokuni, 1993
Chloroform	Solvent Permatec Pad Pt. No. 3050 (skin, CPC)	CLI Labs
Chromic acid. *See* Cr VI		
Chromium VI	Spot test using (skin)	NIOSH, September 1975 (HHE 74-87-221)

*For pesticides, see Appendix D.

Compound	*Media*	*Source*
Chromium VI	Whatman smear tab, wetted with distilled water used to wipe followed up with drops of 0.5 normal sulfuric acid and 1% alcoholic diphenylcarbazide solution for visualization (skin, CPC, clothing)	NIOSH, June 1981 (HETA 81-85-889)
Coal tar. *See* PAHs		
Copper fungicide	Carefree sanitary pad dosimeters	Machado Neto, Matuo, and Matuo, 1992
Copper oxide dust	Double-sided adhesive tape (clothing)	
Crude oil	Luminoscope (UV) instrument (skin)	NIOSH, 1992 (HETA 89-200-2111)
Cyanide	Silver membrane filters (CPC)	NIOSH, March 1987 (HETA 86-30-1785)
DEF	Flannel cloth (4×4) pad dosimeters	Kilgore et al., 1984
Dibutyl phthalate	Cotton gloves	NIOSH, May 1982 (HETA 81-275-1122)
Dichlorobenzidine	Gauze pad dosimeter (25 cm^2) with and without aluminum foil backing	NIOSH, November 1985 (HETA 80-35-1635)
Dichlorobenzidine	Whatman smear tab moistened with cyclohexane (skin)	NIOSH, November 1985 (HETA 80-35-1635)
Diethyl amine	Solvent Permatec Pad Pt. No. 3050 (skin, CPC)	CLI Labs
Diethyl phthalate	Cotton gloves	NIOSH, May 1982 (HETA 81-275-1122)
Diglycidyl ether of bisphenol A	Cotton gloves	NIOSH, September 1984 (HETA 83-132-1508)
Dimethylpolysiloxane	Whatman smear tabs, dry (skin)	NOISH, May 1982*b* (HETA 81-396-1118)
Dinitrotoluene	Cotton gauze moistened with isopropanol for wipes (skin)	Levine et al., 1985
Dioctyl adipate	Cotton gloves	NIOSH, May 1982*a* (HETA 81-275-1122)
Dipropylene glycol monomethyl ether	Whatman filters, dry (skin)	NIOSH, August 1983*a* (HETA 81-304-1361)
Elements (Al, As, Ba, Be, Ca, Cd, Co, Cr, Cu, Fe, Li, Mg, Mn, No, Ni, Pb, Pd, K, Pt, Se, Ag, Na, Sn, Te, Th, Ti, W, Va, Yt, Zn, Zr)	Whatman smear tabs moistened with distilled water (CPC)	NIOSH, February 1992 (HETA 91-51-2177)
Ethylene thiourea (ETU)	Whatman smear tabs, dry (skin, clothing, CPC)	NIOSH, 1978 (HHE 77-67-499)
2-Ethylhexanoic acid	Dosimeter pads (10×10 cm) of filter papers	Korger et al., 1990
Fiberglass	Transparent tape (skin)	NIOSH, April 1984*b* (HETA 83-409-1450)

Compound	*Media*	*Source*
HDI	Permatec Breakthrough Indicator Pt. No. 3003 (CPC, skin)	CLI Labs
HMDI	Permatec Breakthrough Indicator Pt. No. 3003 (CPC, skin)	CLI Labs
Hydrazine	Permatec Breakthrough Indicator Pt. No. 3004 (CPC, skin)	CLI Labs
Hydrogen peroxide	Litmus paper (skin, hair)	NIOSH, May 1980 (HHE 79-105-687)
Isodecanes	Cotton gauze pad saturated with alcohol (skin)	NIOSH, January 1980 (HHE 78-77-659)
Lead	Whatman 40 filters, dry (skin, CPC)	NIOSH, February 1976 (HHE 75-8-263)
Lead	Skinwash of 500 mL 0.1 N nitric acid	Roels et al., 1980
Lead	37-mm 0.8-μm MCE filter moistened with isopropanol (skin, clothing, CPC)	NIOSH, 1991 (HETA 91-290-2131)
Lead	Premoistened baby wipes (skin, clothing, CPC)	NIOSH, 1991 (HETA 91-290-2131)
Lead	Whatman filter moistened with acetic acid to wipe followed by drops of sodium sulfide for visualization (skin)	Askin and Alvarez, 1993
Lead	Whatman filter, dry (CPC)	NIOSH, February 1979 (TA 78-59)
Lead	Sections of trouser bottoms analyzed	Winegar et al., 1977
Lead	Water bath with 0.0042% sodium sulfide, turns lead on skin brownish to black (skin)	Lerner and Hogan, 1985
Lead	Whatman smear tab, dry (skin)	NIOSH, January 1988 (HETA 87-339-1863)
Lead	Commercial premoistened paper towelettes (skin)	Sayre et al., 1982
Lead arsenate	Gauze pad 16-ply dosimeters (10.2 in. by 10.2 in.) backed with filter paper	Wojeck et al., 1983
Manganese	Skinwash of 500 mL 0.1 N nitric acid	Roels et al., 1980
Mercury	Whatman 40 filters, dry (skin)	NIOSH, February 1976 (HHE 75-8-263)
Mercury	Jerome Model 411 Gold Film Mercury analyzer (skin, clothing, CPC)	NIOSH, 1977 (HETA 76-77-52)
4,4'-Methylene bis(2-chloroaniline)	Gauze pad dosimeters (1 in. by 1 in.)	Clapp, 1991
4,4'-Methylene bis(2-chloroaniline)	Gauze pad dosimeters moistened with glycerine	NIOSH, September 1985 (HETA 84-508-1626)
Methylene chloride	Permatec Solvent Pad Part No. 3050 (skin, CPC)	CLI Labs
Methylene dianiline (MDA)	Cotton gloves	NIOSH, September 1984 (HETA 83-132-1508)
MDA	Permatec Breakthrough Indicator Pt. No. 3001 (skin, CPC)	CLI Labs

Compound	*Media*	*Source*
Methylene diisocyanate (MDI)	Permatec Breakthrough Indicator Pt. No. 3002 (skin, CPC)	CLI Labs
Methyl ethyl ketone	Solvent Permatec Pad Pt. No. 3050 (skin, CPC)	CLI Labs
Methyl Isobutyl ketone	Solvent Permatec Pad Pt. No. 3050 (skin, CPC)	CLI Labs
Nitrobenzene		NIOSH, February 1983 (HETA 82-338-1266)
Organic vapors	Whatman smear tabs moistened with distilled water (CPC)	NIOSH, April 1984*c* (HETA 82-284-1456)
PAHs. *See also* Benzene solubles, Benz-α-pyrene, 3,4,-Benzpyrene		
PAHs	Spill Spotter (UV) instrument (skin)	Hill, 1984
PAHs	Polypropylene pad dosimeters (1.77 cm^2) (skin)	Jongeneelen et al., 1988
PAHs	Black light (UV) lamp (skin)	Hill, 1984
PAHs	Filter moistened with acetone or isopropanol	Cheng, 1981
PAHs	Skin wash with cyclohexane using aerosol spray apparatus with collection cup	Cheng, 1981
PAHs (cyclohexane solubles)		NIOSH, October 1985 (HETA 82-309-1630)
PCBs	Cotton puffs moistened with petroleum ether: acetone (4:1)	Maroni et al., 1981
PCBs	Whatman smear tabs No. 50 (skin)	Smith et al., 1982
PCBs	Whatman smear tabs moistened with (skin, CPC)	NIOSH, April 1984*a* (HETA 83-281-1457)
PCBs	37-mm 0.8-μm MCE filter or backup pad, dry (skin)	NIOSH, May 1978 (HHE 77-7A-7B-486)
PCBs	Whatman smear tabs moistened with distilled water, 75–100 cm^2 area (skin, CPC)	NIOSH, June 1984 (HETA 80-212-1474)
PCBs	Whatman No. 40 filters dry and moistened with xylene (skin, CPC)	NIOSH, October 1984 (HETA 80-7-1520)
Pentachlorophenol	Whatman smear tabs moistened with distilled water (skin)	NIOSH, April 1986 (HETA 84-53/425-1680)
Pentachlorophenol	Whatman smear tabs, dry (skin)	NIOSH, 1985 (HETA 83-90-1326)
Pentachlorophenol, sodium salt	Fluorescent tracer (disodium fluorescein) added to spray mix and visualization under UV lamp (skin, clothing)	Bentley, Horstman, and Morgan, 1989
m-Phenylene diamine	Cotton gloves	Gunderson et al., 1989
Pyridene		NIOSH, February 1983 (HETA 82-338-1266)
Stainless steel fibers	37-mm 0.8-μm MCE filter, dry (skin)	NIOSH, August 1985 (HETA 82-289-1496)
2,4,5-T	Gauze pad dosimeter (10 cm^2 by 10 cm^2) 9-ply, backed with two layers of Whatman No. 1 filter paper	Lavy, Shepard, and Bouchard, 1980

Compound	*Media*	*Source*
2,3,4,6-Tetrachlorophenol	Fluorescent tracer (disodium fluorescein) added to spray mix and visualization under UV lamp (skin, clothing)	Bentley, Horstman, and Morgan, 1989
Tetrachlorophenol	Fluorescent tracer (4-methyl-7-diethylamino-coumarin) added to treating formulation and visualization under UV light using video imaging system (skin)	Fenske, Horstmann, and Bentley, 1987
Tetrachlorophenol	Cotton gloves	Fenske, Horstmann, and Bentley, 1987
Thiophene		NIOSH, February 1983 (HETA 82-338-1266)
Toluene	Solvent Permatec Pad Pt. No. 3050 (skin, CPC)	CLI Labs
Toluene diisocyanate (TDI)	Permatec Breakthrough Indicator Pt. No. 3002 (skin, CPC)	CLI Labs
o-Toluidine	Permatec Breakthrough Indicator Pt. No. 3001 (skin, CPC)	CLI Labs
Tris 2,3-dibromopropyl phosphate	Cotton gloves	NIOSH, June 1977 (HHE 77-39-400)
Tris 2,3-dibromopropyl phosphate	37-mm 0.8-µm MCE filter, dry (skin)	NIOSH, June 1977 (HHE 77-39-400)
Xylene	Solvent Permatec Pad Pt. No. 3050 (skin, CPC)	CLI Labs
Zeranol	Cotton gauze pad dosimeters (25 cm^2) with aluminum foil backings	Aw et al., 1989

REFERENCES

Aw, T. C., A. B. Smith, R. L. Stephenson, and C. J. Glueck. 1989. Occupational exposure to zeranol, an animal growth promoter. *Brit. J. Ind. Med.* **46:**341–346.

Bentley, R. K., S. W. Horstman, and M. Morgan. 1989. Reduction of sawmill worker exposure to chlorophenols. *Appl. Ind. Hyg.* **4**(3):69–74.

Brouwer, D. H., and J. H. van Hammen. 1992. Elements of a sampling strategy for dermal exposure assessment [abs.]. International Occupational Hygiene Association First International Scientific Conference. Brussels, Belgium, December 7–10.

Brouwer, D. H., R. Brouwer, G. DeMik, C. L. Maas, and J. J. van Hemmen. 1992. Pesticides in the cultivation of carnations in greenhouses: Part I—Exposure and concomitant health risk. *AIHA J.* **53**(9):575–581.

Carmen, G. E., Y. Iwata, J. L. Pappas, J. R. O'Neal, and F. A. Gunther. 1982. Pesticide applicator exposure to insecticides during treatment of citrus trees with oscillating boom and airblast units. *Arch. Env. Contam. Toxicol.* **11:**651–659.

Cheng, R. 1981. *The Industrial Hygiene Occupational Medicine Program for the SRC-II Project.* Proceedings of a workshop on industrial hygiene and occupational medicine in coal conversion projects. DOE/CONF-801143, pp. 65–68.

Clapp, D. E., G. M. Piacitelli, D. D. Zaebst, and E. Ward. 1991. Assessing exposure to 4,4'-methylene bis(2-chloroaniline) (MBOCA) in the workplace. *Appl. Occup. Environ. Hyg.* **6**(2):125–130.

Comer, S. W., D. C. Staiff, J. F. Armstrong, and H. R. Wolfe. 1975. Exposure of workers to carbaryl. *Bull. Env. Contam. Toxicol.* **13**(4):385–391.

Cummins, K., D. Morton, D. Lee, E. Cook, and R. Curtis. 1992. Exposure to acrylamide in chemical sewer grouting operations. *Appl. Occup. Env. Hyg.* **7**(6):385–391.

Davis, J. E. 1980. Minimizing occupational exposure to pesticides: Personal monitoring. *Res. Rev.* **75:**34–49.

Davis, J. E., V. H. Freed, H. F. Enos, R. C. Duncan, A. Barquet, C. Morgade, L. J. Peters, and J. X. Danauskos. 1982. Reduction of pesticide exposure with protective clothing for applicators and mixers. *JOM* **24:**464–468.

DOE. 1979. Solvent-refined coal (SRC) process—Health programs, Research and Development Report No. 53, Interim Report No. 28, Vol. III. Pilot plant development work, Pt. 4. *Industrial Hygiene, Clinical and Toxicological Programs for the Period July 1, 1977 through June 30, 1978,* Publ. No. FE/496-T19. U.S. Dept. of Energy, Division of Coal Conversion and Utilization.

Dubelman, S., R. Lauer, D. D. Arras, and S. A. Adams. 1982. Operator exposure measurements during application of the herbicide Diallate. *J. Agric. Food Chem.* **30:**526–532.

Durham, W. F. 1963. An additional note regarding measurement of the exposure of workers to pesticides. *Bull. World Health Organ.* **29:**279–281.

Durham, W. F., and H. R. Wolfe. 1962. Measurement of the exposure of workers to pesticides. *Bull. World Health Organ.* **26:**75–91.

EPA. 1986. *Pesticide Assessment Guidelines Subdivision U, Applicator Exposure Monitoring.* EPA 540/9-87-127. Washington, DC: Office of Pesticide Programs.

EPA. September 24, 1986. Guidelines for exposure assessment. *Fed. Reg.* **51:**34042.

EPA. 1988. *Pesticide Hazard Assessment Project: Harvester Exposure Monitoring Studies (1980–1986),* vols 1 and 2. Washington, DC: EPA.

EPA. 1990. *Acrylamide Grouting Exposure Study.* EPA 560/5-87-009. Washington, DC: EPA.

Feldmann, R. J., and H. I. Maibach. 1974. Percutaneous penetration of some pesticides and herbicides in man. *Toxicol. Appl. Pharm.* **128:**126–132.

Fenske, R. A. 1988. Comparative assessment of protective clothing performance by measurement of dermal exposure during pesticide applications. *Appl. Ind. Hyg.* **3**(7):207–213.

Fenske, R. A. 1988. Correlation of fluorescent tracer measurements of dermal exposure and urinary metabolite excretion during occupational exposure to malathion. *AIHA J.* **49:**438–448.

Fenske, R. A. 1990. Nonuniform dermal deposition patterns during occupational exposure to pesticides. *Arch. Env. Contam. Toxicol.* **19:**332–337.

Fenske, R. A. 1993. Dermal exposure assessment techniques. *Ann. Occup. Hyg.* **37**(6):687–706.

Fenske, R. A., S. J. Hamburger, and C. L. Guyton. 1987. Occupational exposure to Fosetyl-Al fungicide during spraying of ornamentals in greenhouses. *Arch. Environ. Contam. Toxicol.* **16:**615–621.

Fenske, R. A., S. W. Horstmann, and R. K. Bentley. 1987. Assessment of dermal exposure to chlorophenols in timber mills. *Appl. Ind. Hyg.* **2:**143–147.

Fenske, R. A., S. G. Birnbaum, M. M. Methner, and R. Solo. 1989. Methods for assessing fieldworker hand exposure to pesticides during peach harvesting. *Bull. Env. Contam. Toxicol.* **43:**805–813.

Fenske, R. A., K. G. Black, K. P. Elkner, C. Lee, M. M. Methner, and R. Soto. 1990. Potential exposure and health risks of infants following indoor residential pesticide applications. *Am. J. Publ. Health* **80:**689–693.

Fletcher, T. E., J. M. Press, and D. S. Wilson. 1959. Exposure of spray-men to dieldrin in residual spraying. *Bull. WHO* **20:**15–25.

Franklin, C. A., R. A. Fenske, R. Greenhalgh, L. Mathieu, H. V. Denley, J. T. Leffingwell, and R. C. Spear. 1981. Correlation of urinary pesticide metabolite excretion with estimated dermal contact in the course of occupational exposure to Guthion. *J. Tox. Env. Health* **7:**715–731.

Gunderson, E. C., B. A. Kingsley, C. L. Witham, and D. C. Bomberger. 1989. A practical study in laboratory and workplace permeation testing. *Appl. Ind. Hyg.* **4**(12):324–329.

Haverty, M. I., M. Page, P. J. Shea, J. B. Hou, and R. W. Hall. 1983. Drift and worker exposure resulting from two methods of applying insecticides to pine bark. *Bull. Env. Contam. Toxicol.* **30:**223–228.

Hill, R. H. 1984. Ultraviolet detection of synthetic oil contamination of skin. *AIHA J.* **45**(7):474–484.

Hirai, Y., and K. Tomokuni. 1993. Levels of chlordane, oxychlordane, and nonachlor on human skin and in human blood. *Bull. Env. Contam. Toxicol.* **50:**316–324.

Jongeneelen, F. J., P. T. J. Scheepers, A. Groenendijk, L. A. G. J. M. Van Aerts, R. B. M. Anzion, R. P. Bos, and S. J. Veenstra. 1988. Airborne concentrations, skin contamination, and urinary metabolite excretion of polycyclic aromatic hydrocarbons among paving workers exposed to coal tar derived road tars. *AIHA J.* **49**(12):600–607.

Kamble, S. T., C. L. Ogg, R. E. Gold, and A. D. Vance. 1992. Exposure of applicators and residents to Chlordane and Heptachlor when used for subterranean termite control. *Arch. Env. Contam. Toxicol.* **22:**253–259.

Kawauchi, T., and K. Nishiyama. 1989. Residual tetrachloroethylene in dry-cleaned clothes. *Env. Res.* **38:**296–301.

Ketcham, N. H., and R. W. Norton. 1960. The hazards to health in the hydrogenation of coal. *Arch. Env. Health* **1:**28/194–41/207.

Kilgore, W., C. Fischer, J. Rivers, N. Akesson, J. Wicks, W. Winters, and W. Winterlin. 1984. Human exposure to DEF/merphos. *Res. Rev.* **91:**71–101.

Klingner, T. 1992. *New Developments in Surface Contamination Monitoring for Aromatic Amines.* Proceedings of the conference on advanced composites. Cincinnati, OH: ACGIH, pp. 43–46.

Knaak, J. B., K. C. Jacobs, and G. M. Wang. 1986. Estimating the hazard to humans applying nemacur-3EC with rat dermal-dose ChE response data. *Bull. Env. Contam. Toxicol.* **37:**159–163.

Knaak, J. B., Y. Iwata, and K. T. Maddy. 1989. The worker hazard posed by reentry into pesticide-treated foliage: Development of safe reentry times, with emphasis on chlorthiophos and carbosulfan. In D. J. Paustenbach (ed.), *The Risk Assessment of Environmental and Human Health Hazards: A Textbook of Case Studies.* New York: Wiley.

Kroger, S., J. Liesivuori, and A. Manninen. 1990. Evaluation of workers' exposure to 2-ethylhexanoic acid (2-EHA) in Finnish sawmills. *Int. Arch. Occup. Env. Health* **62:**213–216.

LaGoy, P. K., R. L. Bohrer, and F. H. Halvorsen. 1992. The development of cleanup criteria for an acutely toxic pesticide at a contaminated industrial facility. *AIHA J.* **53**(5):298–302.

Lavy, T. L., and J. D. Mattice. 1986. Progress in pesticide exposure studies and further concerns. *Toxicol. Letters* **33:**61–71.

Lavy, T. L., J. S. Shepard, and D. C. Bouchard. 1980. Field worker exposure and helicopter spray pattern of 2,4,5-T. *Bull. Env. Contam. Toxicol.* **24:**90–96.

Lees, P. S. J., M. Corn, and P. N. Breysse. 1987. Evidence for dermal absorption as the major route of body entry during exposure of transformer maintenance and repairmen to PCBs. *AIHA J.* **48**(3):257–264.

Leng, M. L., J. C. Ramsey, W. H. Braun, and T. L. Lavy. 1982. Review of studies with 2,4,5-trichlorophenoxyacetic acid in humans including applicators under field conditions. In *Pesticide Residues and Exposure.* Washington, DC: American Chemical Society, pp. 133–156.

Lerner, S. I., and D. J. Hogan. 1985. Detection of inorganic lead contamination with sodium sulfide. *JOM* **27:**293–294.

Levine, R. J., M. J. Turner, Y. S. Crume, M. E. Dale, T. B. Starr, and D. E. Rickert. 1985. Assessing exposure to dinitrotoluene using a biological monitor. *JOM* **27**(9):627–638.

Machado Neto, J. G., T. Matuo, and Y. K. Matuo. 1992. Dermal exposure of pesticide applicators in staked tomato (*Lycopersicon esculentum miii*) crops: Efficiency of a safety measure in the application equipment. *Bull. Env. Contam. Toxicol.* **48:**529–534.

Maroni, M., A. Colombi, S. Cantoni, E. Ferioli, and V. Foa. 1981. Occupational exposure to polychlorinated biphenyls in electrical workers. I. Environmental and blood polychlorinated biphenyls concentrations. *Brit. J. Ind. Med.* **38:**49–54.

Miller, C. S., W. L. Hoover, and W. H. Culver. 1980. Exposure of pesticide applicators to arsenic acid. *Arch. Env. Contam. Toxicol.* **9:**281–288.

Nethercott, J. R., J. M. Pierce, G. Likwornick, and A. A. Murray. 1980. Genital ulceration due to stoddard solvent. *JOM* **22:**549–552.

Nigg, H. N., and J. H. Stamper. 1984. Exposure of spray applicators and mixer loaders to chlorobenzilate miticide in Florida citrus groves. *Arch. Env. Contam. Toxicol.* **12:**477–482.

Nigg, H. N., and J. H. Stamper. 1989. Biological monitoring for pesticide dose determination. In *Biological Monitoring for Pesticide Exposure.* Washington, DC: American Chemical Society.

Nigg, H. N., J. H. Stamper, and R. M. Queen. 1986. Dicofol exposure to Florida citrus applicators: Effects of protective clothing. *Arch. Env. Contam. Toxicol.* **15:**121–134.

NIOSH, Health Hazard Evaluation Report. September 1975. *Industrial Platers, Inc., Columbus, OH.* HHE 74-87-221. Cincinnati, OH: NIOSH.

NIOSH, Health Hazard Evaluation Report. February 1976. *Hestrom Union Co., Bedford, PA*. HHE 75-8-263. Cincinnati, OH: NIOSH.

NIOSH, Health Hazard Evaluation Report. 1977. *St. Claire Rubber Co., Marysville, MI*. HETA 76-77-52. Cincinnati, OH: NIOSH.

NIOSH, Health Hazard Evaluation Report. June 1977. *Fisher Body No. 2 Plant, Grand Rapids, MI*. HHE 77-39-400. Cincinnati, OH: NIOSH.

NIOSH, Health Hazard Evaluation Report. 1978. *St. Clair Rubber Co., Marysville, MI*. HHE 77-67-499. Cincinnati, OH: NIOSH.

NIOSH, Health Hazard Evaluation Report. May 1978. *Union Electric Co., St. Louis, MO*. HHE 77-7A-7B-486. Cincinnati, OH: NIOSH.

NIOSH, Technical Assistance Report. February 1979. *Minerals Reclamation Corporation, Adell and Milwaukee, WI*. TA 78-59. Cincinnati, OH: NIOSH.

NIOSH, Health Hazard Evaluation Report. January 1980. *R. L. Pok Co., Cincinnati, OH*. HHE 78-77-659. Cincinnati, OH: NIOSH.

NIOSH, Health Hazard Evaluation Report. May 1980. *RCA Corp., Marion, IN*. HHE 79-105-687. Cincinnati, OH: NIOSH.

NIOSH, Health Hazard Evaluation Report. July 1980. *Commonwealth of Massachusetts, Dept. of Labor and Industries, Div. Occupational Hygiene, Boyleston, MA*. TA 90-19. Cincinnati, OH: NIOSH.

NIOSH, Health Hazard Evaluation Report. June 1981. *Valley Chrome Platers, Bay City, MI*. HETA 81-85-889. Cincinnati, OH: NIOSH.

NIOSH, Health Hazard Evaluation Report. May 1982*a*. *General Telephone Company, York, PA*. HETA 81-275-1122. Cincinnati, OH: NIOSH.

NIOSH, Health Hazard Evaluation Report. May 1982*b*. *Keebler Co., Cincinnati, OH*. HETA 81-396-1118. Cincinnati, OH: NIOSH.

NIOSH, Health Hazard Evaluation Report. February 1983. *Center for Molecular Nutrition and Sensory Disorders, Washington, DC*. HETA 82-338-1266. Cincinnati, OH: NIOSH.

NIOSH, Health Hazard Evaluation Report. March 1983. *Swissvale Auto Surplus Parts, Inc., Pittsburgh, PA*. HETA 82-246-1275. Cincinnati, OH: NIOSH.

NIOSH, Health Hazard Evaluation Report. August 1983*a*. *Robertson Paper Box Company, Monteville, CT*. HETA 81-304-1361. Cincinnati, OH: NIOSH.

NIOSH, Health Hazard Evaluation Report. August 1983*b*. *U.S. Environmental Protection Agency, Triangle Chemical Site, Bridge City, TX*. HETA 83-417-1357. Cincinnati, OH: NIOSH.

NIOSH, Health Hazard Evaluation Report. April 1984*a*. *Holley Electric Corporation, Jesup, GA*. HETA 83-281-1457. Cincinnati, OH: NIOSH.

NIOSH, Health Hazard Evaluation Report. April 1984*b*. *King Kwit Minit Market, Inc., Cincinnati, OH*. HETA 83-409-1450. Cincinnati, OH: NIOSH.

NIOSH, Health Hazard Evaluation Report. April 1984*c*. *Port Authority of NY and NJ, Elizabeth Industrial Park Site, Elizabeth, NJ*. HETA 82-284-1456. Cincinnati, OH: NIOSH.

NIOSH, Health Hazard Evaluation Report. June 1984. *Pacific Gas and Electric Company, San Francisco, CA*. HETA 80-212-1474. Cincinnati, OH: NIOSH.

NIOSH, Health Hazard Evaluation Report. September 1984. *Grand Gulf Nuclear Power Plant, Port Gibson, MS*. HETA 83-132-1508. Cincinnati, OH: NIOSH.

NIOSH, Health Hazard Evaluation Report. October 1984. *GSA Switchgear Shop, Washington, DC*. HETA 80-7-1520. Cincinnati, OH: NIOSH.

NIOSH, Health Hazard Evaluation Report. November 1985. *Bofors-Nobel/Lakeway Corporation, Muskegon, MI*. HETA 80-35-1635. Cincinnati, OH: NIOSH.

NIOSH, Health Hazard Evaluation Report. 1985. *Fort Stanwix National Monument, Rome, NY*. HETA 83-90-1326. Cincinnati, OH: NIOSH.

NIOSH, Health Hazard Evaluation Report. August 1985. *Schlegel Corp., Rochester, NY*. HETA 82-289-1496. Cincinnati, OH: NIOSH.

NIOSH, Health Hazard Evaluation Report. September 1985. *Steinmetz & Sons, Moscow, PA*. HETA 84-508-1626. Cincinnati, OH: NIOSH.

NIOSH, Health Hazard Evaluation Report. October 1985. *Inland Steel, East Chicago, IN*. HETA 82-309-1630. Cincinnati, OH: NIOSH.

NIOSH, Health Hazard Evaluation Report. April 1986. *Montana Log Home Residents, Kalispell, MT*. HETA 84-53/425-1680. Cincinnati, OH: NIOSH.

NIOSH, Health Hazard Evaluation Report. March 1987. *Vimar Corp., Boulder, CO*. HETA 86-30-1785. Cincinnati, OH: NIOSH.

NIOSH, Health Hazard Evaluation Report. January 1988. *St. Francis–St. George Hospital, Cincinnati, OH*. HETA 87-339-1863. Cincinnati, OH: NIOSH.

NIOSH, Health Hazard Evaluation Report. March 1990. *Chrysler Chemical Division, Trenton, MI*. HETA 87-126-2019. Cincinnati, OH: NIOSH.

NIOSH, Health Hazard Evaluation and Technical Assistance Report. 1991. *New England Burning Co. (NELCO), Eaton Metals, Salt Lake City, UT*. 1991. HETA 91-290-2131. Cincinnati, OH: NIOSH.

NIOSH, Health Hazard Evaluation Report. 1992. *Exxon Valdez Alaska Oil Spill*. HETA 89-200-2111. Cincinnati, OH: NIOSH.

NIOSH, Health Hazard Evaluation Report. February 1992. *AVX Corp., Myrtle Beach, SC*. HETA 91-51-2177. Cincinnati, OH: NIOSH.

Perkins, J. L., and V. B. Knight. 1989. Risk assessment of dermal exposure to polychlorinated biphenyls permeating a polyvinyl chloride glove. *AIHA J.* **50:**A-171–A-172.

Phillips, B. L. D. 1982. Effects of beclomethasone exposure in industry. *J. Soc. Occup. Med.* **32:**196–200.

Polissar, L., K. Lowry-Coble, D. A. Kalman, J. P. Hughes, G. van Belle, D. S. Covert, T. M. Burbacher, D. Bolgiano, and N. K. Mottet. 1990. Pathways of human exposure to arsenic in a community surrounding a copper smelter. *Env. Res.* **53:**29–47.

Popendorf, W. J., and J. T. Leffingwell. 1982. Regulating OP pesticide residues for farmworker protection. *Res. Rev.* **82:**125.

Que Hee, S. S., B. Peace, C. S. Cleark, J. R. Boyle, R. L. Bornschein, and R. B. Hammond. 1985. Evolution of efficient methods to sample lead sources such as house dust and hand dust in the homes of children. *Env. Res.* **38:**77–95.

Ritcey, G., R. Frank, F. L. McEwen, and H. E. Braun. 1987. Captan residues on strawberries and estimates of exposure to pickers. *Bull. Env. Contam. Toxicol.* **38:**840–846.

Roels, H. A., J. Buchet, R. R. Lauwerys, P. Bruaux, F. Claeys-Thoreau, A. Lafontaine, and G. Verduyn. 1980. Exposure to lead by the oral and the pulmonary routes of children living in the vicinity of a primary lead smelter. *Env. Res.* **22:**81–94.

Ross, J., T. Thonsinthusak, H. R. Fong, S. Margetich, and R. Kriger. 1990. Measuring potential dermal transfer of surface pesticide residue generated from indoor fogger use: An interim report. *Chemosphere* **20**(3/4):349–360.

Sayre, J. W., E. Charney, J. Vostal, and I. B. Pless. 1974. House and hand dust as a potential source of childhood lead exposure. *Am. J. Dis. Child* **127:**167–170.

Sell, C. R., and J. C. Maitlen. 1983. Procedure for the determination of residues of (2,4-dichlorophenoxy)acetic acid in dermal exposure pads, hand rinses, urine and perspiration from agricultural workers exposed to the herbicide. *J. Agric. Food Chem.* **31:**572–575.

Severn, D. J. 1984. Use of exposure data for risk assessment. In S. Siewierski (ed.), *Determination and Assessment of Pesticide Exposure*. Studies in Environmental Science 24. New York Elsevier, p. 13–19.

Smith, A. B., J. Schloemer, L. K. Lowry, A. W. Smallwood, R. N. Ligo, R. Stanaka, W. Stringer, M. Jones, R. Hervin, and J. Glueck. 1982. Metabolic and health consequences of occupational exposure to polychlorinated biphenyls. *Brit. J. Ind. Med.* **39:**361–369.

Staiff, D. C., S. W. Comer, J. R. Armstrong, and H. R. Wolfe. 1975. Exposure to the herbicide, paraquat. *Bull. Env. Contam. Toxicol.* **14**(3):334–340.

Stamper, J. H., H. N. Nigg, and K. M. Queen. 1986. Prediction of pesticide dermal exposure and urinary metabolite level of tree crop harvesters from field residues. *Bull. Env. Contam. Toxicol.* **36:**693–700.

Stamper, J. H., H. N. Nigg, W. D. Mahon, A. P. Nielsen, and M. D. Royer. 1989. Pesticide exposure to greenhouse handgunners. *Arch. Env. Contam. Toxicol.* **18:**515–529.

Stevenson, C. J., and P. R. Morgan. 1983. Investigation and prevention of chromate dermatitis in color television manufacture. *J. Soc. Occup. Med.* **33:**19–20.

Wan, H. 1990. Pesticide exposure of applicators working in tea plantations. *Bull. Env. Contam. Toxicol.* **45:**459–462.

WHO. 1986. Field surveys of exposure to pesticides: Standard Protocol. Pesticide Development and Safe Use Unit, Division of Vector Biology and Control. *Toxicol. Letters* **33:**223–235.

Winegar, D. A., B. S. Levy, J. S. Andrews, P. J. Landrigan, W. H. Scruton and M. J. Krause. 1977. Chronic occupational exposure to lead: An evaluation of the health of smelter workers. *JOM* **19**(9):603–606.

Wojeck, G. A., J. F. Price, H. N. Nigg, and H. J. Stamper. 1983. Worker exposure to paraquat and diquat. *Arch. Env. Contam. Toxicol.* **12:**65–70.

CHAPTER 12

Skin Sampling Methods, Part I: Wiping, Swabbing, and Washing

SKIN PREPARATION

When planning to sample the skin, it is extremely important that the skin is clean before the day's exposure begins, and following exposure, skin cleaning is even more important. Since there is a binding capacity for certain chemicals in layers of the skin, including the stratum corneum, which in some cases has preferential binding, skin contamination may not be effectively removed by washing with soap and water (Thomas, 1986). Some compounds are poorly soluble in water. A splash of a resinous material on the skin such as styrene or methylene dianiline (MDA) may not come off with just water and a solvent may be necessary. The solvent should be selected carefully so as not to increase the absorption of the contaminant(s). Certain surfactants in water have been used to rinse or clean hands prior to sampling. Polyethylene glycol (PEG) has been suggested as a good skin cleanser for many contaminants and has been incorporated into D-TAM skin cleanser from CLI Laboratories.

Skin sampling has been used to determine the effectiveness of various skin cleansers. One study suggested PEG was preferable to soap and water for MDA because MDA is highly soluble in PEG and PEG in turn is soluble in water. The addition of a surfactant to the PEG assisted with removal of extraneous dirt (Groth, Housel, and Klingner, 1992).

In the workplace if proper cleaning techniques are not used workers can have increased exposures. Many soaps and waterless hand cleaners contain lanolin because of its skin softening effects. Lanolin, however, is absorbed through the skin and contaminants entrained in the lanolin may have increased absorption. Abrasive cleansers do abrade the skin and remove protective oils from it, making the skin more vulnerable to contaminants.

Some hand cleansers designed for health care personnel contain antiseptics. These cleansers are primarily used when it is not feasible to wash with soap and water; however, the additives may interfere with analysis for contaminants. Other workers who might use these preparations are housekeepers in health care facilities, employees assigned to provide emergency first aid, clinic employees, home health care workers, laundry workers, medical lab personnel, firefighters, paramedics, medical equipment repair personnel, and sanitary waste handlers.

Pre- and postshift skin sampling will assist in determining if there are additional sources of contamination in a work vehicle or residence provided the employee washes daily. Note that many outdoor sites where construction, hazardous waste remediation, and investigation and agricultural work are performed have limited water available for cleaning.

Prior to surveys where wiping, swabbing, or washing will be used to sample the skin, subjects should be requested not to apply lotions or creams that day as they may interfere with the analysis or interact with the contaminant being sampled. Many lotions, similar to soaps, contain lanolin and other skin softeners that may enhance the ability of contaminants to penetrate the skin. Workers should also be requested not to use barrier creams on the sampling day. If there is access to a cleansing facility, note what type of cleanser is used. If portable water stations are used, determine if bactericides are added to the water.

SAMPLING STRATEGIES

Sampling strategies most commonly attempt to identify whether a particular region of the body is being contaminated. Occasionally more than one area is sampled at a time such as the forehead and hands. Most often skin samples are collected before lunch and at the end of a work shift, or in the case of community monitoring, on a onetime basis. However, another strategy that can be used in the workplace is to collect samples that reflect the exposure presented by specific tasks. This strategy can be useful in developing specific recommendations for controls. Table 12-1 provides an example of how this strategy was used in a dinitrotoluene (DNT) manufacturing plant. Several sequential samples can be collected on a single worker or several workers performing the same task for comparison.

Dermal exposure studies of pesticide workers have demonstrated the important contribution of hand exposure to overall dermal contact, so it is not surprising that hands are the most frequently sampled area of the body (see Table 12-2). In one study of pesticide spraying by plane where pilots' hands were monitored, it was found that pilots received 73% of dermal exposure to the hands, which was attributed to the adjustment of spray nozzles on the aircraft without wearing gloves (Wojeck et al., 1982). Depending on their specific tasks, specialized studies have shown pesticide workers to experience 12% to 43% of their total exposure through their hands, approximately 20% to 23% through their heads and necks, and 36% to 64% through their torsos and arms, despite the use of protective gloves and clothing.

The neck is generally exposed and is not washed during the course of the day; thus, it is a

TABLE 12-1. Skin Wipe Samples in a DNT Manufacturing Plant

Sample No.	*Personnel*	*Task*	*2,4-D Result (μg)*
1	Operator	Both hands after performing DNT analysis	ND
2	Operator	Hands and forehead after collecting a sample	44.9
3	Operator	Hands and forehead after analyzing a sample	50.1
4	Operator	Hands and face after collecting and analyzing a sample	179.5
5	Loader	Hands and forehead after returning from the tank farm	122.3
6	Laboratory analyst	Hands and forehead following analysis in the central plant lab	46.0

Source: From Levine, R. J., et al. 1985. Assessing exposure to dinitrotoluene using a biological monitor. *JOM* 27(9):627–638.
Note: ND = no data.

TABLE 12-2. Comparison of Hand Exposure to Total Dermal Exposure

Activity	*Hand Exposure as % of Total Dermal*	*Reference*
Drivers of tractors equipped with canopies during air blast spraying of citrus	41	Wojeck et al., 1982
Bulk spray suppliers for above application	52	Wojeck et al., 1982
Drivers of ordinary tractors during boom spraying of tomatoes	25	Wojeck et al., 1983
Applicators using hand guns to spray aquatic weeds from airboats	47	Wojeck et al., 1983
Drivers for airboats for above application	89	Wojeck et al., 1983
Aerial applicators	55	Maddy, Wang, and Winter, 1983
Flaggers for above application	39	Maddy, Wang, and Winter, 1983
Applicators spraying lawns, trees, and gardens with power sprayers	37	Leavitt et al., 1982
Applicators spraying lawns with hose-end sprayers	98	Davis et al., 1983

Davis, J. E., E. R. Stevens, D. C. Staiff, and L. C. Butler. 1983. Potential exposure to diazinon during yard applications. *Env. Monit. Assess.* **3**(1):23–28.

Leavitt, J. R. C., R. E. Gold, T. Holcslaw, and D. Tupy. 1982. Exposure of professional pesticide applicators to carbaryl. *Arch. Env. Contam. Toxicol.* **11**(1):57–62.

Maddy, K. T., R. G. Wang, and C. K. Winter. 1983. *Dermal Exposure Monitoring of Mixers, Loaders, and Applicators of Pesticides in California.* Worker Health and Safety Unit Report HS-1069. Sacramento, CA: California Department of Food and Agriculture, 7p.

Maddy, K. T., R. I. Drieger, L. O'Connell, M. Bisbiglia, and S. Margetich. 1989. Use of biological monitoring data from pesticide users in making pesticide regulatory decisions in California. In *Biological Monitoring for Pesticide Exposure.* Washington, DC: American Chemical Society, pp. 338–353.

Wojeck, G. A., H. N. Nigg, R. S. Braman, J. H. Stamper, and R. L. Rouseff. 1982. Worker exposure to arsenic in Florida grapefruit spray operations. *Arch. Env. Contam. Toxicol.* **11**:661–667.

Wojeck, G. A., J. F. Price, H. N. Nigg, and J. H. Stamper. 1983. Worker exposure to paraquat and diquat. *Arch. Env. Contam. Toxicol.* **12**:65–70.

good sampling area. The forehead may have a higher exposure potential because chemical absorption may be increased due to the reduced skin thickness of this area. The forehead has been reported to have a skin permeability that is four times greater than the forearm for parathion and certain other chemicals (Webster and Maibach, 1989).

The Occupational Safety and Health Administration (OSHA) recommends that its compliance officers wipe only hands and fingers if doing skin wipes (OSHA, 1991). Before any skin wipe is taken, the compliance officer must explain why the sample is necessary and ask the employee about any possible skin allergies to the chemicals in the sampling filter or media. A strategy for hand rinses is to rinse only the hand of preference (Cummins et al., 1992; Boleij et al., 1991). Either only a portion such as the fingers or palm or the entire hand can be wiped.

SAMPLING METHODS

A problem with any skin sampling procedure is finding a solvent that will provide adequate removal of residues without causing injury to the skin or increased absorption of a contaminant. Most often the solvent used to sample direct skin is water. Solvents should be selected that are not irritating, do not cause drying or cracking of the skin, and are not readily absorbed by the skin. In addition, they should not facilitate skin penetration of the material being sampled. There have been several instances of problems with degradation of pesticide residues and interference with analyses due to the solvent used for washing (EPA, 1986). If detergent solutions are used, it is usually necessary for the laboratory to extract the contaminant from this solution into a suitable solvent for analysis.

Commonly used solvents to rinse contaminated workers' hands are 95% ethanol, 10% isopropanol, acetone, distilled water, or water containing detergent, or some combination of these three materials such as 50:50 ethanol:water (Maddy, Wang, and Winter, 1983). A sodium bicarbonate solution has been used to remove 2,4-D from hands (Grover et al., 1986). Vegetable oils have been used to remove coal tars for analysis. Dilute nitric acid has been used to rinse hands to measure lead levels on the skin of children, however compounds such as nitric acid must be used on human skin with great care (Roels et al., 1980). Ten percent isopropyl alcohol in distilled water has been used for skin wipes (Fenske, Hamburger, and Guyton, 1987). OSHA directs its compliance officers not to use any solvents on the skin other than water (OSHA, 1991). Surfactants, because of their low toxicity and corrosiveness, may prove a better choice. Two percent Igepal and 1% Surten, another surfactant, have been used for hand wipes and washing. Dioctyl sulfosuccinate, an anionic surfactant, at a concentration of 0.008% has been used to simulate the emulsifiers in human saliva that would be expected on children's hands. Hexane has been used as a hand wash solvent for parathion; however, due to the toxicity of this solvent it is not recommended (Richter et al., 1980). Most often skin sampling is done at breaks, lunch, and postwork.

Wipe Methods

Wiping methods for skin use the same types of media as are used for surfaces, such as filters, gauze, and commercial premoistened wipes. Given the concerns regarding solvent selection in the previous section, the simplest option is to wipe the skin with a dry filter. In some instances the skin will be moist with perspiration and the use of a solvent will only dilute the sample. Depending on the compounds for which analysis will be performed, perspiration can present problems. For a discussion of perspiration and sampling factors, see Chapter 2.

Similar to surface wipes, skin wipes should be done on equal-size areas so that comparisons can be made not only of different areas on the same individual, but also of different individuals. However, estimating area size can be difficult. Another approach used to qualitatively identify areas with the highest exposure is to wipe the fingers separately from the palms, allowing specific identification of the portion(s) of the hand receiving the greatest exposure. The neck is useful because it is rarely washed during the day.

One way to determine if the source of a contaminant on skin is related to the immediate environment is to wipe controls (who are in a known lead-free environment) and compare skin samples. In one study of battery plant workers, exposures were 40 to 50 times greater than the controls (hand leads). Facial wipes tended to correlate with higher airborne levels, while hand wipes correlated with both higher surface levels and airborne levels. Table 12-3 lists lead levels in environmental and biological samples.

There may be a limitation to the number of times a hand can be wiped or washed per day because skin moisture and oils can be depleted, thus changing the sampling characteristics of the skin.

A disadvantage of wipe methods to detect semivolatile mixtures such as polycyclic aromatic hydrocarbons (PAHs) is their inability to collect the most volatile fraction. In the PAH study on roofers (Wolff et al., 1989), anthracene was detected on the sorbent tube to back up the filter used for air sampling, but was not detected in the filter or the skin wipe.

Whatman Smear Tabs

Skin wipes were collected for polychlorinated biphenyl (PCB) exposure to workers involved in capacitor processing and transformer mainte-

TABLE 12-3. Lead Levels in Environmental and Biological Samples

Measurement	*Group/Location*	*Results*	*SD*
Airborne lead (mg/M³)	Control	1.6–2.1 (1.8)	0.2
	Assembly Dept.	16.1–164.8 (71.2)	46.1
	Pasting Dept.	90.6–114.2 (99.9)	8.9
Hand lead (mg)	Control	38.2–155.6 (72.0)	36.9
	Assembly Dept.	1,523–14,023 (5,227)	4,190
	Pasting Dept.	1,956–8,381 (5,510)	2,598
Facial lead (mg)	Control	—	—
	Assembly Dept.	25.1–187.0 (81.0)	48.7
	Pasting Dept.	106–603 (298)	183
Work surface (mg/100 cm²)	Control	2.2–11.9 (7.1)	4.3
	Assembly Dept.	353–2,809 (1230)	837
	Pasting Dept.	218–7,465 (3,885)	2,818
Blood lead (mg/100 mg)	Control	<10–17.0 (12.2)	3.3
	Assembly Dept.	25–51 (34.4)	7.2
	Pasting Dept.	38–49 (41.0)	4.6
Blood ZPP (mg/100 mg)	Control	11–35 (19.2)	11
	Assembly Dept.	39–382 (122.4)	7.2
	Pasting Dept.	38–49 (41.0)	4.6
Hemoglobin (%)	Control	13.1–16.1 (14.6)	1.2
	Assembly Dept.	12.7–15.2 (13.7)	0.7
	Pasting Dept.	14.1–15.2 (14.7)	0.4

Source: From Chavalitnitikul, C., L. Levin, and L. Chen. 1984. Study and models of total lead exposures of battery workers. *AIHA J.* **45**(12):802–808.
Note: Mean is in parentheses.

nance using Whatman Smear Tabs (No. 50). (Smith et al., 1982). In this study, forehead, nose, cheeks, and hands of selected workers were wiped. The wipe samples were analyzed using the same procedure as that used on the filter wipes for surface contamination.

Smear tabs were also used in a study on PAH exposure from roofing materials during removal of an old coal tar pitch roof and installation of a new asphalt roof (Table 12-4; Wolff et al., 1989). A 3 cm by 3 cm area of the forehead (defined by a stencil) was wiped both preshift and postshift on the same workers. The wearing of hats or bandanas was recorded. A sample was also collected on a nonexposed person for technique evaluation and for blank reference. Air samples were also collected for PAHs using filters and backup sorbent tubes. Skin wipes were analyzed by the same extraction/filtration technique described in the NIOSH air sampling method. It is most likely that both surface contamination and skin oils would be sampled with this method.

Area air samples are sometimes also included in these studies in order to identify as many compounds in the air as possible. These samples are usually collected in a position that is most likely to have maximum contaminant levels. In an evaluation of synthetic oils, the relative concentration of individual PAHs in all personal and area air samples was the same: fluoranthene > pyrene > benzanthracene > benzo(a)pyrene > benzo(b)fluoranthene > benzo(ghi)perylene > benzo(k)fluoranthene (Hill, 1984). A similar pattern was observed in the matching skin wipe samples. All postshift PAH skin residues were higher than those collected preshift. Monday morning preshift wipes had approximately one-

TABLE 12-4. PAH Levels in Personal Air Samples and Skin Wipes from Roofers

	Skin Wipes (ηg)		*Personal Air (μg/M³)*	
PAH	*Preshift (N = 10)*	*Postshift (N = 10)*	*Day 1 (N = 9)*	*Day 2 (N = 9)*
Anthracene			1.5 (0.6)	0.5 (0.2)
Fluoranthene	20 (18)	282 (298)	7.0 (2.2)	3.1 (1.2)
Pyrene	17 (16)	171 (197)	5.4 (1.7)	2.6 (1.0)
Benzo(α)anthracene[a]	13 (11)	124 (127)	2.5 (0.7)	1.3 (0.5)
Benzo(bf)fluoranthene	7 (6)	93 (85)	1.2 (0.3)	0.8 (0.3)
Benzo(k)fluoranthene	4 (4)	55 (50)	0.7 (0.2)	0.4 (0.2)
Benzo(α)pyrene	9 (9)	83 (88)	1.5 (0.4)	0.9 (0.4)
Benzo(ghi)perylene[b]	8 (6)	68 (62)	0.9 (0.3)	0.6 (0.3)
Total	75 (69)	876 (901)	21 (5.1)	10.2 (3.9)

Source: Adapted from Wolff, M. S., R. Herbert, M. Marcus, M. Rivera, P. J. Landrigan, and L. R. Andrews. 1989. Polycyclic aromatic hydrocarbon (PAH) residues on skin in relation to air levels among roofers. *Arch. Env. Health* **44**(3):157–163.
Note: Numbers in parentheses are the standard deviation.
[a]For preshift skin wipes, *N* = 9.
[b]For preshift skin wipes, *N* = 8.

tenth of the PAHs of Monday postshift wipes, which indicates significant dermal retention of PAHs from work the previous week. However, unless the exact amount of materials (coal tar pitch versus asphalt) to which workers were exposed can be measured, the significance of this indication cannot be determined.

Prepackaged Wipes

A variety of premoistened commercial materials have been used to perform skin wipes. Several different types of prepackaged hand wipes were evaluated in one study for their ability to sample for lead contamination of the hands (Que Hee et al., 1985). These included Wash 'n' Dri Soft Cloths, Moist Towelettes No. 634910, Abco Nice Clean Towelettes, Washkin's Hospital Packettes, Walgreen's Brand Wet Wipes, Lehn and Fink's Wet Ones, and Baby Size Wet Ones. Wash 'n' Dri Soft Cloths, Moist Towelettes, and Walgreen's Brand Wet Wipes were the most effective in removing and retaining lead contamination from the hands. Three to five wipes (repeated over the same hand using the same wipe) were required for precision in results and to supply enough material to satisfy detection level requirements of analytical methods for lead. Therefore, the effectiveness of hand wipes depended not only on the type of wipe but on the number of repetitive wipes. Walgreen's Brand Wet Wipe, at 322 cm², is typical of most of these wipes in size and composition, containing water, SD alcohol 40, propylene glycol, sorbic acid, sodium nonoxynol-9-phosphate, Oleth 20, PEG/75, lanolin, disodium phosphate, citric acid, and fragrance.

Hand and face wipes for lead exposure have been performed with a commercially available paper towel (14 cm by 20 cm) premoistened with benzalkonium (1:750) and alcohol (20%) using the following methodology (Chavalitnitikul, Levin, and Chen, 1984). Each battery plant worker was requested to open the paper towel packages, unfold the moistened towel, and wipe his or her hands thoroughly including the palms, the back of the hand, and each finger. Sampling was conducted each afternoon and the hand wipes were placed in sealed plastic bags. The facial wipe began at the right corner of the participant's forehead and was moved to the left, down to the left cheek, the chin, and then up to the right cheek, down the nose, and finally around the mouth.

The method that is frequently being used to perform hand wipes uses premoistened commercial baby wipes and is as follows (NIOSH,

1992): The first wipe in the package is discarded. The subject is asked to pull the second wipe from the package. The subject is then instructed to thoroughly wipe both hands for one minute, after which time the used baby wipe is placed into a clean labeled Zip-Loc™ bag. It is not necessary to wear gloves during this procedure because the sample wipe only comes in contact with the subject.

Swabbing or Wiping with Solvents

As an alternative to premoistened wipes, cloth towels or cotton puffs moistened with solvent have also been used, as has surgical gauze. Any part of the body can be wiped or swabbed, and a study by Ware and Morgan (1976) describes swabbing the torso using ethanol saturated gauze pads 2 in. by 2 in.

Swabbing or wiping the hands with solvent is not as effective as rinsing methods because of difficulties in adequately removing residues from between the fingers and around the fingernails (EPA, 1990). One swab may be insufficient, and up to four swabs may be needed to remove 90% of a contaminant such as parathion from an area of skin the size of the back of a man's hand (Durham and Wolfe, 1962). The procedure can be tedious and time-consuming and will not remove residues that are absorbed into the skin during the exposure period. Therefore, for substances that can rapidly penetrate the skin, wipes or swabs are not recommended; instead, biological monitoring is the prescribed method.

Procedure Using Gauze

1. Prior to exposure, the area of the skin to be monitored must be cleansed.
2. Swabs must consist of two 8-ply 10 cm by 10 cm surgical gauze squares that have been extracted with the same solvent to be used for analyses. The squares are folded twice to form 5 cm by 5 cm squares and then stapled near the folded edge.
3. Place the swabs in a glass jar saturated with 95% ethanol (do not use 99.95 ethanol as it may contain benzene). The lid of the jar should be lined with Teflon to prevent contamination of the gauze with residue on the lid. The jar should be kept shut until ready to use.
4. In the field, open the jar and grasp a swab at the stapled edge using ring forceps or another similar device. Allow the excess ethanol to be squeezed off by rubbing the pad against the interior of the jar.
5. Continuing to hold the pad using forceps, the skin area selected is rubbed back and forth over the surface with light pressure. Each area selected should be swabbed up to four times.
6. Alternatively, the gauze can be handed to the subject and wetted with 10 mL of solvent. The square is opened and the subject then performs his or her own hand wipe with the gauze and deposits it inside a jar to minimize outside contamination of the sample.
7. Pads for the same area can be combined into a clean, labeled jar as a single sample. The Teflon lid should be replaced promptly.

Skin Washing Methods

The Environmental Protection Agency (EPA, 1986) recommends skin washing for hand exposure estimations. Skin washing is considered most appropriate for chemicals that have low rates of dermal absorption. Therefore, it is inappropriate for use with organophosphate pesticides, unless used in conjunction with other sampling methods such as dermal dosimetry and biological samples (Popendorf and Leffingwell, 1982).

Skin washing has been used for the hand, wrist, arm, foot, and ankle, but most commonly the hands are washed. Some studies have rinsed the entire arm (wrist bone to shoulder), the torso, and portions of the legs, but swabs are usually used for larger parts of the body. Sometimes the skin is also brushed. In general, washing techniques can be used when it is necessary to sample a larger body surface area.

Rinsing techniques may be more representative of actual exposure than surface (pad, cotton glove) methods because the skin is subjected to more variables such as sweating and changes in body temperature. However, the effectiveness of this method is severely limited by the rapid rate at which the skin absorbs and retains certain compounds, such as organophosphates. Therefore, skin rinsing may underestimate the potential dose, because only the unabsorbed or slowly absorbed fractions of a contaminant may be collected (Webster and Maibach, 1983). Also, hand rinsing requires that workers stop their labors for several minutes after each exposure period; thus, further monitoring may become objectionable to the workers or their supervisor.

The physical form or formulation of a chemical mixture may influence the effectiveness of a hand rinse. Oil in liquids may enhance binding to the skin, which would reduce the recovery amount. Powders or colored compounds may be easily identifiable and therefore more likely to be washed from the skin. Correction factors should be generated to adjust data for incomplete removal of residues using hand rinses. Factors that can influence recoveries include time, type of rinsing solution, and formulation.

If hand rinses are to be carried out using one particular solvent with subsequent partition into a second solvent for analysis, then a determination of the efficiency of the second solvent to extract the contaminant should be done. If EPA protocols are followed, this process would involve performing seven determinations (EPA, 1986). The mean ± the standard deviation for recovery should be determined. If the lower limit of the 95% confidence interval is less than 70%, the extraction procedure is considered unsatisfactory. If hand rinses are to be stored, a study of stability should be conducted for each hand. The period of exposure that the rinses represent must be recorded. After returning to the laboratory, both right hand rinses are combined into one sample; the same is done for the left hand.

Bag Method

The bag rinse procedure is the most common rinsing method and involves the use of polyethylene bags containing a suitable solvent, such as distilled water, for washing the contaminant from the hands (Durham and Wolfe, 1962). The most common intervals to select for rinse samples are morning break, lunch, afternoon break, and after work. Sometimes a sample is collected before the start of work to determine if there is residual contamination.

Bags are selected that are sturdy enough to hold 200 mL of solvent. One type of bag found to be satisfactory is the ½ gallon frozen food plastic Zip-Loc™ bag. Bags less than 1 mL thick will puncture too easily to be useful. A thickness of at least 0.001 in. (0.025 mm) has been recommended (Davis, 1980). It is best to use the heaviest available material that is still pliable enough to be wrapped in a tight seal around the wrist. Prior to field use for a new solvent, plastic bags must be shaken with that solvent to determine whether it degrades the bag material. After shaking, an analysis of this material must be done to identify any potential interferents.

The bag rinse is faster than the swabbing technique; however, it will not remove residues that are absorbed into the skin during the exposure period, and it cannot be used to sample large body surface areas. It is a relatively slow process and therefore cannot be done at short intervals, such as hourly, without impacting the productivity of the workers. Bag sampling is not satisfactory if the toxicant is insoluble or if it is degraded by solvents that will not harm the hands (Davis, 1980). Also, skin washes require more liquid to carry into the field. If the weather is cold, the subject can be uncomfortable during collection as well as changing sampling efficiency. For this reason skin wipes are often more acceptable for sampling subjects.

The bag rinse can be more effective than the swab method for removing hand contamination. In one study it was found that approximately twice as much residue could be removed from a worker's hands using the bag rinse method rather than the swab method (Durham and Wolfe, 1962). The percentage of extractable parathion pesticide using the hand rinse method ranged from 77% to 94% for the first rinse and 89% to 98% for the second rinse in one study (or an average of 96% for the two bag rinses). The amount of parathion recovered in the third rinse was usually less than 5% of the total recovered (Durham and Wolfe, 1962). Therefore, three rinses have been shown to be optimum to assure that most of the contaminant has been removed from each hand.

For analysis, rinses of the same hand are usually composited. If total hand exposure is needed, all rinses can be combined as one sample.

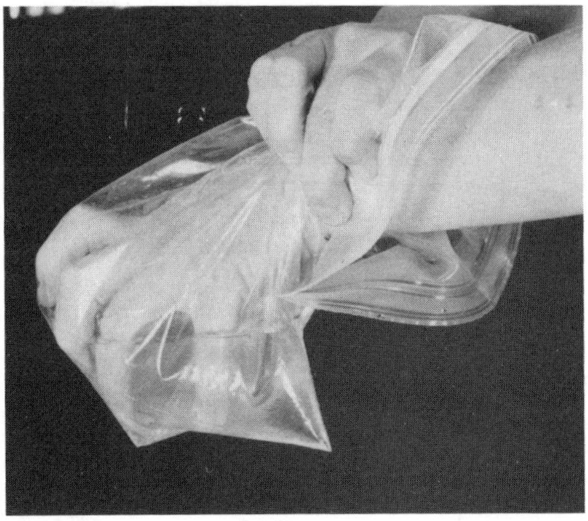

Figure 12-1. Bag rinse.
Source: Photo by Ed Wesly.

Procedure

This procedure should be performed prior to and immediately following the task or operation where the exposure is expected to occur and after the workers remove their protective clothing at break periods and at the end of the day.

1. Prior to sampling, rinse a 5 ½ in. by 15 in. polyethylene bag with 100 mL of distilled water. Discard this water. Also prepare several number 402 mason jars by washing with Alconox followed by two rinses with deionized water. Seal the jars with a Teflon lined lid.
2. Fill a labeled polyethylene bag with 50 mL of distilled water. An alternative is to use 200 mL of 95% ethanol.
3. Separate samples are collected on each hand using different bags and rinse solutions.
4. Insert one of the worker's hands and hold the bag around the worker's wrist tightly (Fig. 12-1). The person should cup the hand slightly and hold the fingers a short distance apart during most of the shaking operation to allow for thorough rinsing around the fingers. Occasionally, the thumb and fingers should be rubbed against one another and against the palm to help loosen adhering material and thus increase efficiency of the washing process.
5. Have the worker vigorously shake his or her hand about 50 times.
6. Allow the hand to drain above the solvent for 10 sec before removal from the bag.
7. Transfer the rinse to a 4 oz sterile widemouth jar. The bag is then rinsed with a second 25 mL of solvent, which is added to the previous amount in the jar.
8. Wipe the worker's hand with a paper towel unless additional rinses (to determine recovery efficiency) are planned.
9. Repeat a second time for each hand using fresh ethanol and put this into a new labeled jar. After the sample is collected, the area between the lid and the jar should be taped for protection.
10. Seal each jar in a plastic bag and place them in a chest containing ice or blue ice packs for transport to a laboratory. Do not use dry ice. Ship the samples to the laboratory at the end of each sampling day using a next-day delivery service.

Cup Method

The cup method (Fig. 12-2) utilizes a modified aerosol spray delivery system (tin-coated steel can) with nonreactive materials (Viton stem gasket, stainless steel spring, Teflon dip tube) (Keenan and Cole, 1982). The propellant used was carbon dioxide. The actuator button was fitted with a spray extension tube to permit introduction of the solvent into the sampling cap. A spacer made from rubber tubing was used to maintain a fixed distance between the end of the extension tube and the surface of the skin. The cup has a small bottle as a side extension to collect the sample. The bottles are replaceable.

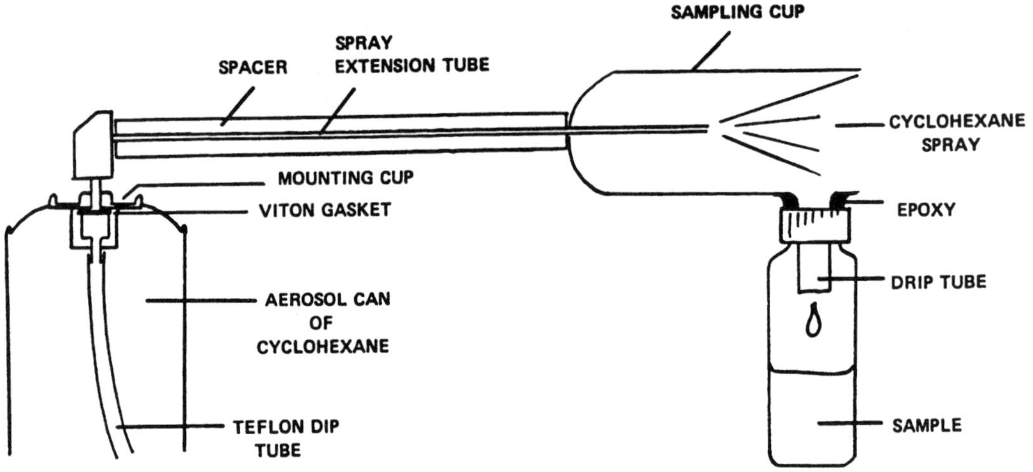

Figure 12-2. Skin wash sampling cup.
Source: From R. R. Keenan and S. B. Cole. 1982. A sampling and analytical procedure for skin contaminant evaluation. *AIHA J.* 43:474.

The system samples a 5.0 cm^2 area of skin. If samples with this system are to be compared with hand washes or those taken from other body surfaces, then a more accurate result would be obtained by taking several samples and averaging them. If a comparison is to be made with a palm wipe, then only the palm area would be sampled.

Procedure

1. A prelabeled 12 mL vial is affixed to a sampling cup and the cup is held against the surface of the skin.
2. Cyclohexane is sprayed through the cup onto the skin from an aerosol can. The cup will drain the skin washings into the sample bottle.
3. Sampling is terminated when the level of cyclohexane in the 12 mL vial reaches the sampling cup drip tube. This process happens very fast, in approximately 10 sec.
4. The vial is then removed and sealed with a Teflon-lined screw cap and labeled. The cup is cleaned between samples by rinsing with a small amount of solvent from the can, and the rinse is discarded into a waste container.
5. A blank is also created by spraying 10 mL of solvent directly into a vial.

Pouring Method

Hand washes can be performed as simply as releasing 250 mL of distilled water or other solvent from a separatory funnel or other container held over the hands, and collecting it in a stainless steel bowl (Knaak, Jacobs, and Wang, 1986). The wash water is transferred to glass jars that were covered and sealed. Washing the hands in a stream of solvent or in a basin containing solvent is faster than shaking the hands in plastic bags containing solvent, but is not as standardized or as convenient as the bag rinse.

A variation is to have the subject place one hand at a time into a 1000 mL beaker and pour 90 mL of a suitable solvent such as ethanol over the hand. The subject is asked to wash each hand for 1 min. The sample is transferred to a glass vial with a Teflon-lined screw cap. The beaker is washed twice with 5 mL of solvent, which is also transferred to the vial (Kangas et al., 1993).

Another variation of this technique involved pouring 500 mL of 0.1 N nitric acid slowly over the palm of the dominant hand while the fingers were slightly spread to collect lead and other metallic contamination (Roels et al., 1980). The diluted nitric acid was collected in a metal-free polyethylene bottle (500 mL) by means of a metal-free polyethylene funnel. After each rinse the funnel was rinsed with 500 mL 0.1 N nitric acid and analysis was done using atomic absorption. While the use of nitric acid in any concentration to wash the skin is debatable, the technique is applicable to other solvents, including distilled water. The nitric acid rinse can be more effective than a soap solution. Similar to wipes and swabs, three to five rinses are necessary to approach a high efficiency.

Yet another variation of this method involves using a polyethylene squeeze bottle (Fig. 12-3) to direct a stream of solvent over the hands (about 200 mL), which is then collected through a funnel into a 450 mL glass bottle, which is then stoppered with a polyseal cap and labeled (Atallah, Cahill, and Whitacre, 1982). In some tests 250 mL of solution have been used in this manner.

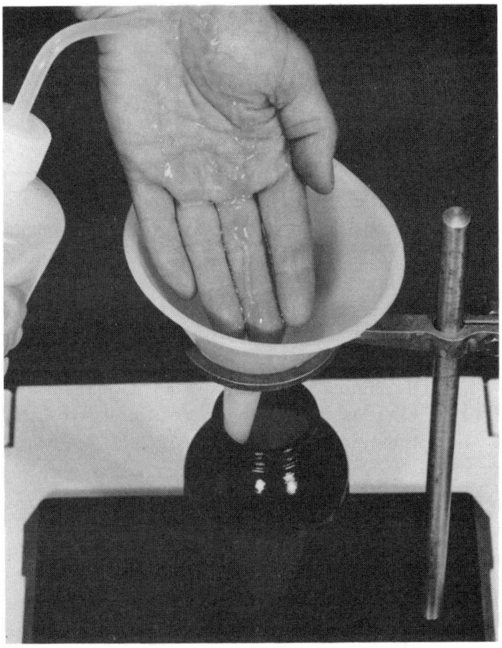

Figure 12-3. A variation of the pouring method of skin washing using a polyethelene squeeze bottle to direct a stream of solvent over the hands, which is collected through a funnel into a glass bottle. *Source:* Photo by Ed Wesly.

Washing with Oil

Sunflower oil has also been used to wash hands for PAH exposure. This may also be suitable to other oil-soluble, sticky materials which will not rinse off easily with a solvent.

Procedure

1. Pipet 5 mL of refined sunflower oil onto the worker's hands and ask worker to rub for 1 min.
2. Wearing disposable nitrile gloves, wipe the hands with a paper tissue(s).
3. Place tissue in a labeled, glass vial.
4. Pipet a second 5 mL aliquot onto the worker's hands and repeat the procedure.
5. Place second tissue(s) into same glass vial. Change gloves in between each worker's samples.
6. After collecting samples, take a clean tissue with a clean pair of disposable gloves and pipet 5 mL of sunflower oil on it. Place into a clean, labeled vial and send along with samples as a field blank.
7. Store in a chest at 4°C prior to analysis.

Adhesive Methods

Preweighed self-adhesive labels (Avery #5615, 1⁄16 in. by 3.5 in. [21.5 cm^2] have been used to sample a standard area on the palms of children for lead exposure from contaminated soil (Lepow et al., 1975). Information was kept concerning the subject who was sampled. The preweighed labels were pressed once on a single area, although it was often necessary to press several times over the palm to obtain an adequate sample. The sample was placed in a wax bag and stored away from the sun to prevent dehydration, and was delivered to the lab within two to three days. This method may not be adequate for hands since only a small fraction of the dirt actually present on the hands was captured. Much of the dirt may be trapped in skin folds and creases; moreover, the distribution of contamination may be patchy rather than evenly spread out.

Tape has been used to collect fibers directly from skin when employees in a data processing computer room were complaining of itching and localized rashes (NIOSH, 1984). Transparent tape was applied either to skin lesions or to the normal exposed skin of workers. If no skin lesions were present, the tape was applied to the volar (inside) surface of the elbow or wrist of one arm.

ANALYSIS OF SKIN WASHES AND SWABS

Hand rinse solutions can be quantitatively transferred to volumetrics and diluted to a 100 mL volume for analysis. Another method of preparation for hand wash samples is to transfer the rinse solution (in this case, 95% ethanol) to a separatory funnel with deionized water; hexane is added and the funnel is shaken (Stamper et al., 1989). The ethanol will partition into the water and most pesticides will go into the hexane. The hexane fraction is then evaporated to dryness on a rotary evaporator and is reconstituted with more hexane, which is then analyzed.

In some cases, an aliquot of the rinse solution is analyzed rather than extracting the entire amount (Fenske, Hamburger, and Guyton, 1987). Hand wash samples (95% ethanol) have been extracted in separatory funnels into a different solvent (e.g., hexane; Stamper et al., 1989).

Glove and hand wash samples have been analyzed for metabolites as well as the contaminant in order to determine if either excretion of the metabolite in sweat or conversion to a metabolite on the skin was occurring (Nigg and Stamper, 1983).

REFERENCES

Atallah, Y. H., W. P. Cahill, and D. M. Whitacre. 1982. Exposure of pesticide applicators and support personnel to 0-ethyl O-(4-nitrophenyl) phenyl phosphonothioate (EPN). *Arch. Env. Contam. Toxicol.* **11:**219–225.

Boleij, J. S. M., H. Kromhout, M. Fleuren, W. Teileman, and G. Verstappen. 1991. Reentry after Methomyl application in greenhouses. *Appl. Occup. Env. Hyg.* **6**(8):672–676.

Chavalitnitikul, C., L. Levin, and L. Chen. 1984. Study and models of total lead exposures of battery workers. *AIHA J.* **45**(12):802–808.

Cummins, K., D. Morton, D. Lee, E. Cook, and R. Curtis. 1992. Exposure to acrylamide in chemical sewer grouting operations. *Appl. Occup. Env. Hyg.* **7**(6):385–391.

Davis, J. E. 1980. Minimizing occupational exposure to pesticides: Personal monitoring. *Res. Rev.* **75:**43–49.

Durham, W. F., and H. R. Wolfe, 1962. Measurement of exposure of workers to pesticides. *Bull. WHO* **26:**75.

EPA. 1986. *Pesticide Assessment Guidelines Subdivision U, Applicator Exposure Monitoring*. EPA 540/9-87-127. Washington, DC: Office of Pesticide Programs.

EPA. 1990. *Acrylamide Grouting Study*. EPA 560/5-87-009. Washington, DC: EPA.

Fenske, R. A., S. J. Hamburger, and C. L. Guyton. 1987. Occupational exposure to Fosetyl-Al fungicide during spraying of ornamentals in greenhouses. *Arch. Env. Contam. Toxicol.* **16:**615–621.

Groth, K., T. Housel, and T. Klingner. 1992. *Strategy for the Development and Testing of an Effective Dermal Decontamination Procedure for Aromatic Amines*. Boston, MA: American Industrial Hygiene Conference, Abstract.

Grover, R., C. A. Franklin, N. I. Muir, A. J. Cessna, and D. Riedel. 1986. Dermal exposure and urinary metabolite excretion in farmers repeatedly exposed to 2,4-D amine. *Toxicol. Letters* **33:**73–83.

Hill, R. H. 1984. Ultraviolet detection of synthetic oil contamination of the skin. *AIHA J.* **45**(7):474–484.

Kangas, J., S. Laitinen, A. Jauhiainen, and K. Savolainen. 1993. Exposure of sprayers and plant handlers to mevinphos in Finnish greenhouses. *AIHA J.* **54**(4):150–157.

Keenan, R. R., and S. B. Cole. 1982. A sampling and analytical procedure for skin contaminant evaluation. *AIHA J.* **43:**473–476.

Knaak, J. B., K. C. Jacobs, and G. M. Wang. 1986. Estimating the hazard to humans applying Nemacur 3EC with rat dermal dose ChE response data. *Bull. Env. Contam. Toxicol.* **37:**159–163.

Lepow, M. L., L. Bruckman, M. Gillette, et al. 1975.

Investigations into sources of lead in the environment of urban children. *Env. Res.* **10:**415–426.

Maddy, K. T., R. G. Wang, and C. K. Winter. 1983. *Dermal Exposure Monitoring of Mixers, Loaders, and Applicators of Pesticides in California.* HS-1069, Worker Health and Safety Unit, State of California, pp. 1–7.

Nigg, H. N., and J. H. Stamper. 1983. Exposure of spray applicators and mixer-loaders to chlorobenzilate miticide in Florida citrus groves. *Arch. Env. Contam. Toxicol.* **12:**477–482.

NIOSH, Health Hazard Determination Report. 1977. *Ottenheimer and Sons, Inc., Dawson Springs, KY.* HHE 77-74-720. Cincinnati, OH: NIOSH.

NIOSH, Health Hazard Evaluation Report. April 1984. *King Kwit Minit Market, Inc., Cincinnati, OH.* HETA 83-409-1450. Cincinnati, OH: NIOSH.

NIOSH, Health Hazard Evaluation Report. August 1992. *Independence Police Department, Indoor Range, Independence,* MO. HETA 90-168-2248. Cincinnati, OH: NIOSH.

Popendorf, W. J., and J. T. Leffingwell. 1982. Regulating OP pesticide residues for farmworker protection. *Res. Rev.* **82:**125.

Que Hee, S. S., B. Peace, C. S. Clark, J. R. Boyle, R. L. Bornschein, and P. B. Hammond. 1985. Evolution of efficient methods to sample lead sources, such as house dust and hand dust, in the homes of children. *Env. Res.* **38:**77–95.

Richter, E. D., B. Cohen, M. Curia, J. Schoenberg, E. Weisenberg, and M. Gordon. 1980. Exposures of aerial spray workers to parathion. *Israel J. Med. Sci.* **16:**96–100.

Roels, H. A., J. P. Buchet, R. R. Lauwenys, P. Branx, F. Claeys-Thoreau, A. Lafontaine, and G. Verduyn. 1980. Exposure to lead by oral and pulmonary routes of children living in the vicinity of a primary lead smelter. *Env. Res.* **22:**81–94.

Smith, A. B., J. Schloemer, L. K. Lowry, A. W. Smallwood, R. N. Ligo, S. Tanaka, W. Stringer, M. Jones, R. Hervin, and C. J. Glueck. 1982. Metabolic and health consequences of occupational exposure to polychlorinated biphenyls. *Brit. J. Ind. Med.* **39:**361–369.

Stamper, J. H., H. N. Nigg, W. D. Mahon, A. P. Neilsen, and M. D. Royer. 1989. Pesticide exposure to greenhouse handgunners. *Arch. Env. Contam. Toxicol.* **18:**515–529.

Thomas, A. 1986. Skin absorption: A potential contributing factor to the BEI. *Appl. Ind. Hyg.* **1**(2):87–90.

Ware, G. W., and D. P. Morgan. 1976. Worker reentry safety. IX. Techniques of determining safe reentry intervals for organophosphate-treated cotton fields. *Res. Rev.* **76:**191–226.

Ware, G. W., D. P. Morgan, B. J. Estesen, and W. P. Cahill. 1975. Establishment of reentry intervals for organophosphate-treated cotton fields based on human data: III. 12 to 72 hours post-treatment exposure to monocrotophos, ethyl- and methyl parathion. *Arch. Env. Contam. Toxicol.* **3:**289–306.

Webster, R. C., and H. I. Maibach. 1983. Cutaneous pharmacokinetics: Ten steps to percutaneous absorption. *Drug. Metab. Rev.* **14:**169–205.

Webster, R. C., and H. I. Maibach. 1989. Regional variation in percutaneous absorption. In R. L. Bronaugh, and H. I. Maibach (eds.), *Percutaneous Absorption*, 2nd ed. New York: Marcel Dekker.

Wojeck, G. A., H. N. Nigg, R. S. Braman, J. H. Stamper, and R. L. Rouseff. 1982. Worker exposure to arsenic in Florida grapefruit spray operations. *Arch. Env. Contam. Toxicol.* **11:**661–667.

Wolff, M. S., R. Herbert, M. Marcus, M. Rivera, P. J. Landrigan, and L. R. Andrews. 1989. Polycylic aromatic hydrocarbon (PAH) residues on skin in relation to air levels among roofers. *Arch. Env. Health* **44**(3):157–163.

Wolff, M. S., R. McConnell, L. Cedillo, and M. Rivera. 1992. Dermal levels of methyl parathion, organochlorine pesticides, and acetylcholinesterase among formulators. *Bull. Env. Contam. Toxicol.* **48:**671–678.

CHAPTER 13

Skin Sampling Methods, Part II: Direct Reading

Direct reading methods are available for skin monitoring for polycyclic aromatic hydrocarbons (PAHs), amines, and metals. At the simplest, monitoring can be examination of a worker's skin for obvious discoloration since certain compounds such as methylene dianiline (MDA) may be the cause. Another option is to put a testing device on the skin, which will become discolored if it comes into contact with the chemical to be tested. The most well known direct reading method is fluorescence, which has been used to identify dermal contamination in two situations: when compounds such as PAHs possess a natural fluorescence and when fluorescent compounds have been deliberately added to contaminants so that their contamination can be visibly traced. An ultraviolet (UV) light is used to visualize the contamination in both cases. Eye damage from excessive exposure to UV radiation both to the sampling professional and to the worker is a concern when using this technique and therefore protective glasses must be worn. Interferences include deodorants, coal-tar shampoos, and other cosmetic preparations that can also fluoresce.

Video imaging has been integrated with fluorescent tracers, and although it is not yet widely used, it may be a primary method in the future since air sampling studies have also incorporated this technique. An obstacle to widespread use is the current unavailability of nontoxic fluorescent tracers, which would be compatible with a wide range of agricultural formulations (Dubelman and Cowell, 1989). The technique quantifies dermal deposition, which is often the major component of an exposure, but does not account for the portion of the dose resulting from inhalation or ingestion. Estimates of dermal penetration are still necessary for calculation of body doses.

An important advantage of the technique is its ability to provide a visual qualitative assessment of the affected body areas. Tracers are particularly useful in detecting spills, splashes, and other exposures that are not homogeneously distributed over the body surface (Franklin et al., 1981).

Scanning a surface with a UV light for fluorescence has been done for detecting PAH exposure derived from raw synthetic crude oils and their distillate fractions and coal tars at active coal gasification facilities and their cleanup sites. The use of UV light as a screening procedure for skin contamination by synthetic oils has been subject to academic debate due to the potential for biological activity enhancement of irradiated PAHs by UV. Therefore, this technique is likely to be replaced with fluorescent tracers due to the potential problems related to the deliberate exposure of humans to carcinogenic UV light, as well as.the synergistic effects of UV and PAHs.

However, UV screening was used extensively at a Union Carbide Corp. coal hydrogenation pilot plant in Institute, West Virginia, that operated in the 1950s to monitor skin contamination, and to devise and evaluate worker clothing and showering programs (Hill, 1984). The technique was also used to evaluate skin contamination and to educate workers at the solvent refined coal pilot plant. No apparent health effects due to UV usage have been documented at these two facilities.

FLUORESCENCE

Qualitative Methods

Black lights have been used to screen workers' skin for fluorescence from both naturally fluorescing compounds such as PAHs and mixtures in which fluorescing compounds have been added. The technique consists of scanning the body of a worker with a handheld UV lamp and examining the fluorescence in a dark room. The contaminated areas generally exhibit a fluorescence signal brighter than that of the skin. The Wood's lamp, a UV type of lamp, has also been used by dermatologists to detect depigmentation.

In one plant, a booth to detect skin contamination was constructed for employee use (JRB Associates, 1979). The booth operated at 320–400 ηm with an approximate exposure time of 15–30 sec. A person standing inside the booth under UV light could observe fluorescent material on the body by looking into mirrors on all four walls, enabling the worker to detect contamination that might otherwise go unnoticed. Contamination may occur from sitting or leaning on contaminated surfaces or from not washing hands before using sanitary facilities. When the booth was used, eye protection was required and employees were instructed to keep exposure time to a minimum. The medical personnel at this facility used contour marking charts to rate fluorescent intensity of the skin on a numeric scale. Because of the possible risk associated with excessive use of a UV booth, UV examination for skin contamination should only be conducted under medical supervision.

Although UV light has been used in several plants to detect skin contamination, there is concern about the risk of skin sensitization and carcinogenic effects. Skin sensitization may be wavelength dependent. In one study, UV radiation at 330–440 ηm but not at 280–320 ηm in combination with exposure to coal tar pitch was found to induce a photosensitive reaction (NIOSH, 1977).

Quantitative Methods

Two developmental instruments, called the Spill Spotter and the Lightpipe Luminoscope, utilize the UV excitation principle for quantitating surface and/or skin fluorescence (Schuresko, 1980; Vo-Dinh and Gammage, 1981). Both of these instruments produce a beam of low intensity, long wave UV light to cause emissions in the visible range from excited PAHs. The emissions are then detected by the instruments, which quantitate the fluorescence as a voltage response. It is not necessary to provide a darkened environment in order to use these instruments for measurements.

The Luminoscope

The Luminoscope, which uses a 125 watt mercury lamp as an excitation source, has a background-nulling feature that allows it to compensate for normal skin variations, providing a direct reading of the net fluorescence signal has been used in some studies. Interchangeable filters can be placed in the instrument. A fiber optics wave guide is used to channel the excitation light into the surface being scanned and to retransmit the luminescence of the contaminants back into the entrance slit of the detection system. Luminescence signals are detected by a photomultiplier that operates in the digital single-photon counting mode (Vo-Dinh, 1987). The records developed for each individual can be used for calibration prior to measurement. The best use of this instrument is in qualitative detection of contamination or to verify that decontamination procedures are adequate (Fig. 13-1).

An evaluation of the response of this instrument to coal distillate contamination on filter paper and mouse skin was conducted (Vo-Dinh, 1987). The excitation wavelength was selected by an optical filter at 313 ηm. The emission wavelength was set by the monochromator at 350 ηm. The intensity levels given in photon counts per second represent the net fluorescence (background subtracted) integrated over 1 sec periods. For surface contaminant concentrations between 0.2 ηm/cm^2 and 25 ηg/cm^2, the fluorescence intensity varied linearly with the amount of surface materials. For the concentration range between 25 ηg/cm^2 and 600 ηg/cm^2, a quantification was not possible. At >600 ηg/cm^2, the fluorescence intensity started to decrease, possibly due to quenching effects, filter effects, and energy transfer processes.

In practice, the decrease of fluorescence intensity at high surface concentrations is not a problem because heavy surface contamination is detected readily by visual examination and subsequently can be removed by washing. The differences in fluorescence analytical curves for coal liquid on filter paper and on mouse skin indicated the need to use calibration data for the type of surfaces to be monitored in order to calculate quantitative estimates of surface contaminants. Because of gradual absorption of the coal distillate into the mouse skin, less and less material was left on the skin surface. As a result, the quenching process decreased, causing an increase in the fluorescence signal of the 50% coal distillate spot after 1.5 hours.

Figure 13-1A. *Below:* Use of Luminoscope in the field. *Right:* Close up of Luminoscope in the laboratory.
Source: From T. Vo-Dinh. 1987. Evaluation of an improved fiberoptics luminescence skin monitor with background correction. *AIHA J.* **48**:595.

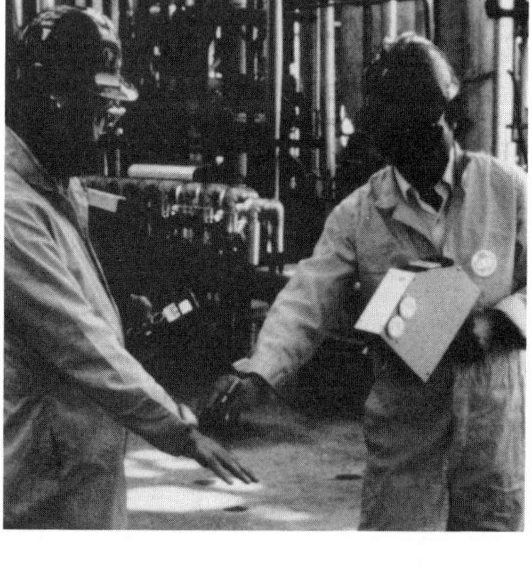

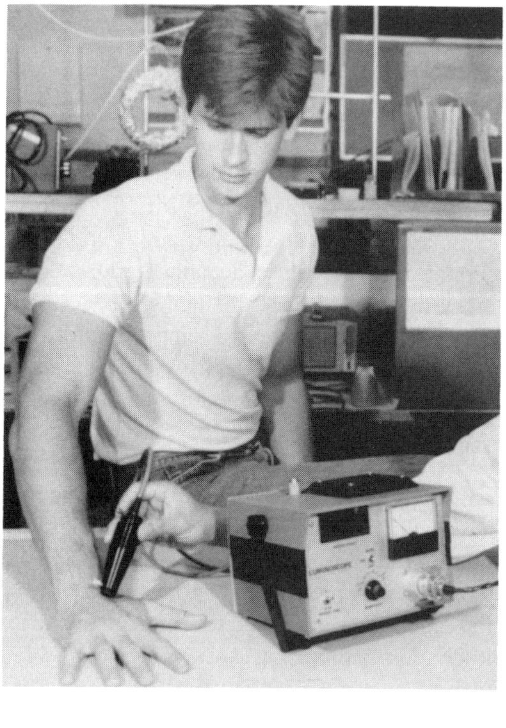

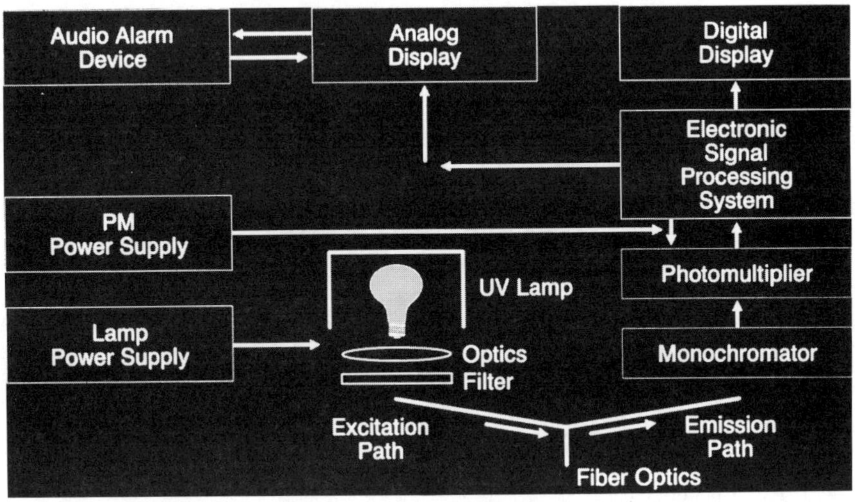

Figure 13-1B. Block diagram of the electronic design of the Fiberoptics Luminoscope II.
Source: From NIOSH, Health Hazard Evaluation Report. 1991. *Exxon Valdez Alaska Oil Spill*. HETA 89-200/273-211. Cincinnati, OH: NIOSH.

Most recently the Luminoscope was used during the Exxon/Valdez oil spill cleanup by NIOSH for the detection of contamination on the hands and forearms of workers (NIOSH, 1991). Results were not interpretable because of the inability to properly monitor important issues such as the types of soaps and shampoos used. Ten workers, all from the same beach work crew, were examined with the Luminoscope preshift before they donned their chemical protective clothing (CPC) in the morning, postshift but before cleanup (showering) upon return to the berthing vessel, and postshift after cleanup. However, the use of the method was terminated due to problems with interpretation of initial field data because more experience needs to be gained when using these types of instruments for this application. The data obtained from the workers, considered typical, are presented in Figure 13-2.

Figure 13-2 data from employee #1 show that the highest reading was the preshift measurement for all four body locations (palm of right hand, back of right hand, right forearm, and right side of neck). The reading on the palm decreased significantly upon return from the beach but increased almost to the original reading after cleanup. Figure 13-2 data from employee #7 show that the postshift after cleanup was significantly higher than the preshift or the postshift before cleanup values. Figure 13-2 data from employee #9 show that the preshift reading was the highest; however, it was expected that the preshift reading and the postshift after cleanup readings would be the lower values, and that the postshift before cleanup would either be about the same (if the CPC was effective) or higher (if the CPC was not effective or not worn).

A possible explanation for the low readings (relative to the preshift readings) from skin that was visibly contaminated with "weathered crude oil" may be that there was a "quenching" effect. That is, the UV energy may have been absorbed by the oil. Although there were problems with interpretation of the Luminoscope data, NIOSH determined that the technique deserved more evaluation. It was suggested that a more successful situation would occur if workers were monitored for several days in a row, with closer monitoring of frequency of washing and types of soaps used.

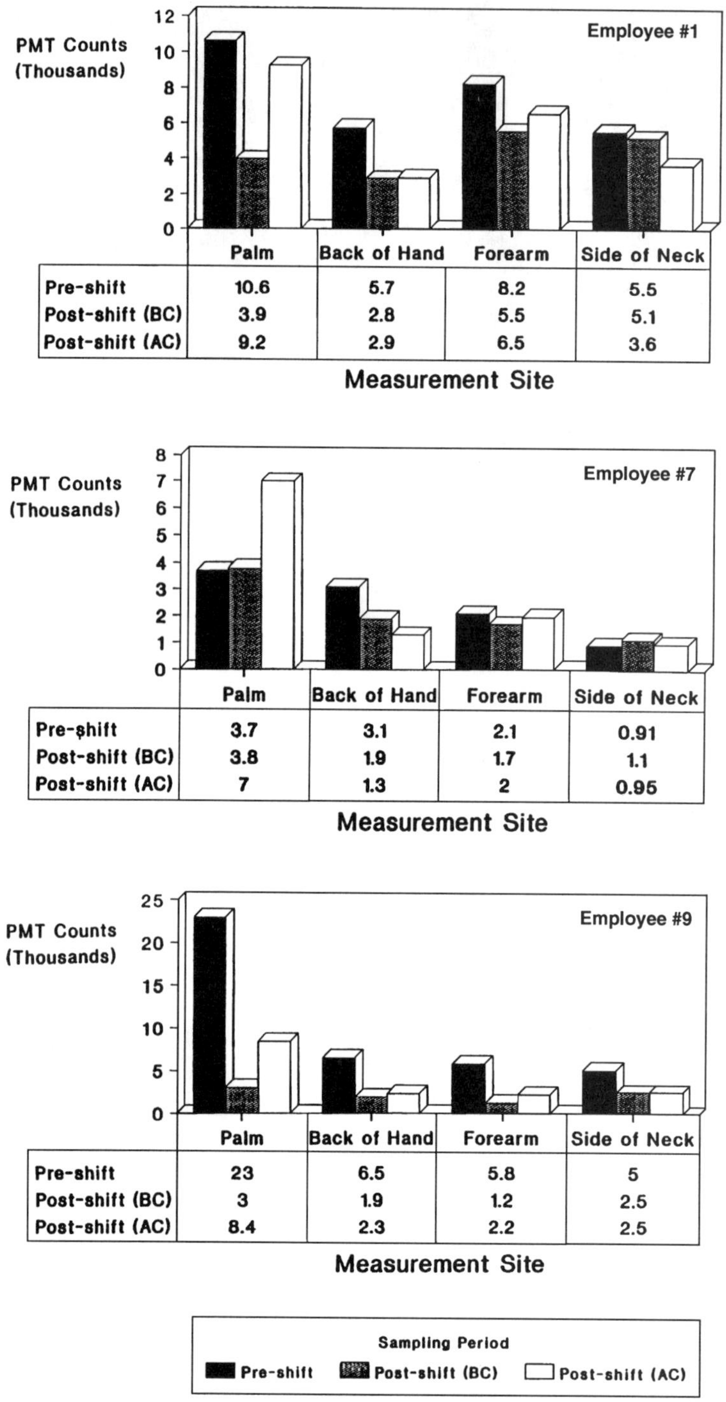

Employee #1

	Palm	Back of Hand	Forearm	Side of Neck
Pre-shift	10.6	5.7	8.2	5.5
Post-shift (BC)	3.9	2.8	5.5	5.1
Post-shift (AC)	9.2	2.9	6.5	3.6

Employee #7

	Palm	Back of Hand	Forearm	Side of Neck
Pre-shift	3.7	3.1	2.1	0.91
Post-shift (BC)	3.8	1.9	1.7	1.1
Post-shift (AC)	7	1.3	2	0.95

Employee #9

	Palm	Back of Hand	Forearm	Side of Neck
Pre-shift	23	6.5	5.8	5
Post-shift (BC)	3	1.9	1.2	2.5
Post-shift (AC)	8.4	2.3	2.2	2.5

(BC)=Before Cleanup/(AC)=After Cleanup

Figure 13-2. Exxon/Valdez oil spill luminescence measurements for three employees.
Source: From NIOSH, Health Hazard Evaluation Report. 1991. *Exxon Valdez Alaska Oil Spill.* HETA 89-200/273-211. Cincinnati, OH: NIOSH.

The Spill Spotter

The Spill Spotter (Fig. 13-3) was used by Ashland Synthetic Fuels, Inc., personnel at the H-Coal Pilot Plant in Catlettsburg, Kentucky, for quantitatively evaluating skin contamination among process workers (Hill, 1984). For comparison, a handheld black light was also used to validate the presence, location, and degree of synfuels material contamination on a qualitative basis for a number of the process workers monitored with the Spill Spotter. The

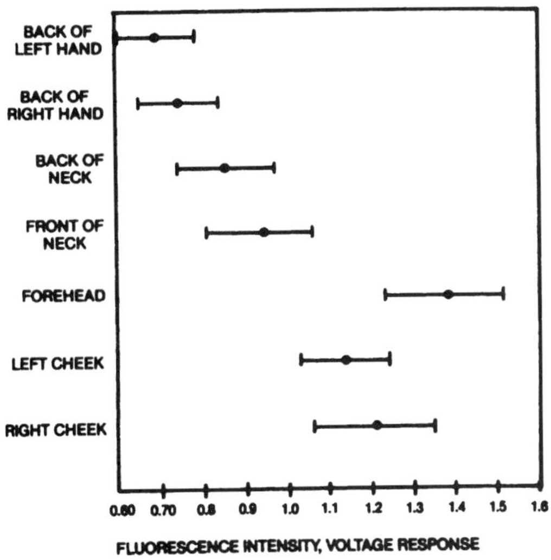

Figure 13-3. The Spill Spotter (*below*) and the means and 95% confidence intervals for white male control group skin fluorescence measured by the Spill Spotter (*left*).
Source: From R. D. Hill. 1984. Ultraviolet detection of synthetic oil contamination of skin. *AIHA J.* **45**(7):475, 477.

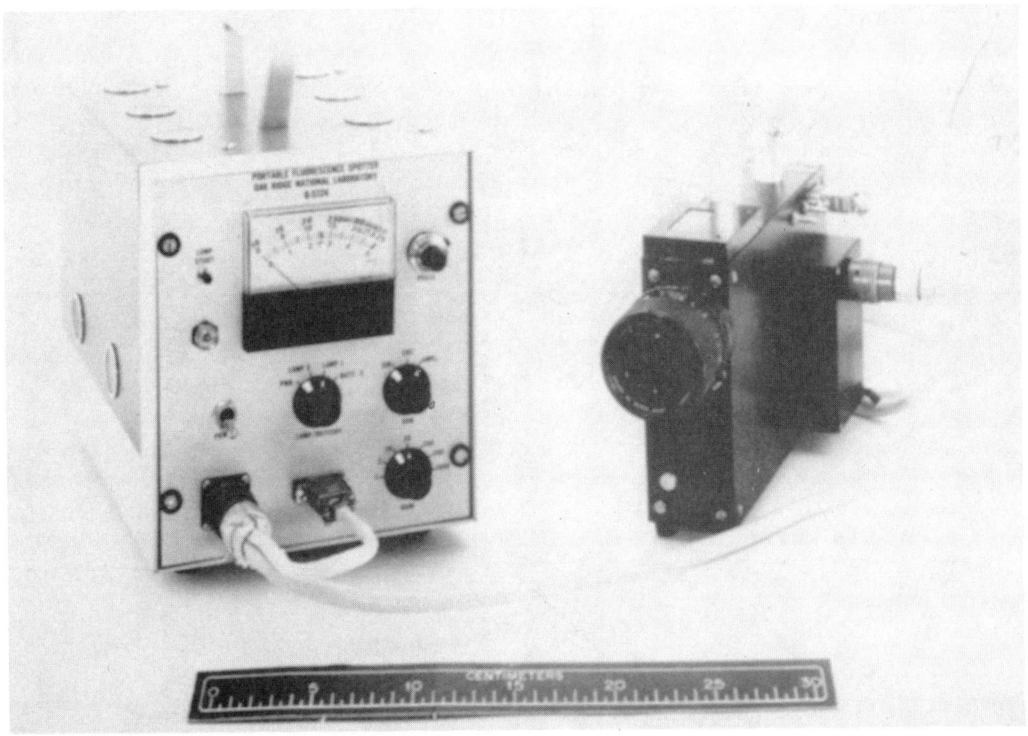

instrument was calibrated with a 1 ppm concentration of benzo(a)pyrene (BaP) in an optical epoxy disk to produce a 1 volt response. All measurements were taken at 10 cm from the Spill Spotter lens, with distance being held constant by using a 10 cm cone attached to the lens. At this distance the UV beam was 1.5 cm in diameter, covering an area of 1.8 cm^2. The BaP standard's response was 1 volt ± 10% at a distance of 10 cm. A gain of 20 was typically used, and data at other gain settings were standardized to 20 gain for reporting the results. For all measurements, the Spill Spotter lens (a commercially available 50 mm lens from a single lens reflex camera) was set at an aperture of 2.8 and focused to infinity.

Background luminescence of human skin has to be accounted for. Natural background skin fluorescence can vary from 10% to 15% among individuals. Calluses, dried skin, and fingertips usually exhibit a fluorescence intensity greater than other parts of the hands (Fig. 13-4). Also,

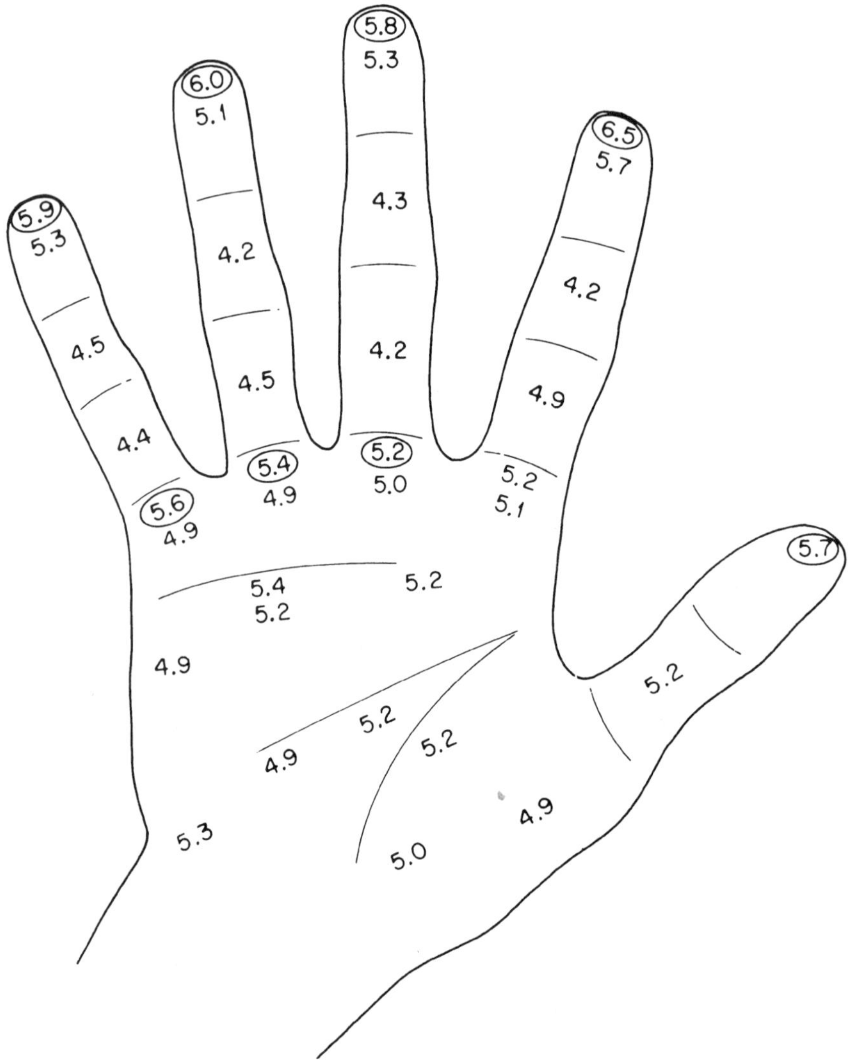

Figure 13-4. Fluorescence intensity levels from various locations on a person's hand. *Source:* From T. Vo-Dinh and R. B. Gammage. 1981. The lightpipe luminoscope for monitoring occupational skin contamination. *AIHA J.* **42**(2):117.

body location, sex, and pigmentation will cause fluorescence variability (Hill, 1984). Black males tend to have the lowest skin fluorescence readings. Since females generally have fairer complexions and smoother skin than males, a higher fluorescence reading would be expected, as seen by readings on the neck area and hands in one study. However, facial makeup worn by females caused quenching of the fluorescence signal to the detector. Deposits of coal dust and coal tars can decrease luminescence of the skin. These deposits and other dark, grimy deposits on the skin that are easily visible to the naked eye will absorb UV and quench the response of these instruments. The result is an indication of less fluorescence than is actually there. If this type of monitoring is done, a data file should be developed for each individual based on a background fluorescence scan (Vo-Dinh and Gammage, 1981).

During the study at the H-Coal Pilot Plant, workers selected from four different job categories were monitored. The job categories (Table 13-1), including hydrogenation operators, solids/liquids separation workers, sample technicians, and boilermakers, were chosen to include both operations and maintenance personnel performing substantially different job functions at the plant. The workers selected were those with relatively high potential for skin contact with process material based on field observation of job duties by industrial hygiene personnel, and on industrial hygiene air monitoring data to identify workers having the relatively highest exposure to airborne aerosols.

TABLE 13-1. Description of Work Activity for Selected Job Categories

Job Category	*Work Activity*
Hydrogenation operators	Operate process equipment in the coal hydrogenation and liquid and gas recovery units. Due to the high operating pressures (up to 3,000 psi), equipment is tightly constructed and well maintained.
Solids/liquids separation workers	Operate process equipment that recovers a high solids content vacuum bottoms oil by solidification on a water-cooled conveyor belt. Activities also include materials handling for storage of solidified oil.
Sample technicians	Collect gaseous, liquid, and solid samples from process equipment.
Boilermakers	Perform maintenance and repair on exterior and interior of process vessels.

Source: From Hill, R. H. 1984. Ultraviolet detection of synthetic oil contamination of skin. *AIHA J.* **45**(7): 474–484.

Workers were monitored before starting work in process areas, after completing the work shift, and after showering. Areas of the body that were monitored included the forehead, neck, cheeks, and back of hand. Selected workers were also monitored using a handheld, low intensity (850 $\mu w/cm^2$), long wave (365 nm) black light. The facial area of these workers was monitored after working in process areas, and also after showering, or after washing the facial area, to determine the extent of removal of fluorescent material. The time of UV exposure during monitoring was only a few seconds and was conducted in a darkened office. Workers were instructed to keep their eyes closed during this observation period. Fluorescence ratings, based on intensity and area of facial fluorescence as subjectively determined by the monitoring technician, ranged from none detected to marked fluorescence (0–5).

It was noted that two of the groups of workers had higher fluorescence ratings in the preshift measurements than when measurements were taken on the prior day after their showers. This complication was attributed to the fact that workers with heavy deposits on their skin may shower more thoroughly—that is, with longer and harder rubbing—than other groups to remove obviously visible grime. This aggressive washing could cause the skin to become more flushed and reddened, lowering its fluorescence. By the next morning, the skin fluorescence would be increased since the skin would be less irritated and less gorged with blood.

It was concluded that it would be advantageous to use a process material to calibrate the Spill Spotter rather than the 1 ppm benzo(a)pyrene. A comparison of a distillate to benzo(a)pyrene indicated the distillate was much more fluorescent than the benzo(a)pyrene standard (5.2:1).

Skin Wash

A method for rinsing fluorescent compounds such as PAHs off of the skin with a solvent and then using UV to analyze the solvent has also been proposed (Keenan and Cole, 1982). This method has the advantage of not exposing the skin to UV and the disadvantage of diluting the contaminant in the solvent as well as the need to verify that the solvent selected will successfully remove the contaminant. It also allows for specific analysis for the contaminants of interest. This specific method, which uses an aerosol spray and cup to deliver and collect the solvent, is described in detail in Chapter 12.

Tracer Methods

The addition of fluorescent compounds to mixtures has been used during pesticide application to "trace" leaf coverage, equipment efficiency, droplet size, and "drift" of spray clouds. The Environmental Protection Agency (EPA) has used fluorescent compounds to investigate visual warning methods for farmworker exposure to pesticide residues (Johnson, Adams, and Millar, 1975).

Methods have also been developed for the measurement of fluorescent tracers as quantitative indicators of pesticide exposure to workers during mixing and application, as well as to determine the effectiveness of CPC. One approach uses gauze pads, which are discussed in Chapter 14, to collect the material, and then the pads are monitored with UV light rather than the worker. Another uses a rinse and a third method is direct examination of the workers' clothing and skin. Tracers have also been proposed as a method for evaluating the effectiveness of CPC (Vo-Dinh and White, 1987; Fenske, 1988*b*). A concern is that a tracer may not permeate the CPC in the same manner as the solvent, so prior evaluation of its appropriateness is essential (Perkins, 1987).

The use of fluorescent compounds can be coupled with photography or video imaging measurements to estimate exposures to the entire body. This approach requires pre- and post-exposure images of skin surfaces under longwave UV illumination, development of a standard curve relating dermal fluorescence to skin-deposited tracer, and chemical residue sampling to quantify the relationship between the tracer and the chemical substances of interest as they are deposited on the skin (Fenske, 1993).

The basis for using fluorescence tracers assumes quantitatively similar behavior of the two compounds from mixing to deposition on the skin surface. A concern is compatibility of the tracer and the formulation being applied due to solubility and mixing characteristics. Compatibility will determine the likelihood of partitioning of the tracer from the rest of the formulation during the application process. Problems will most likely be the result of solubility differences and incomplete mixing by the spray apparatus. This procedure has the potential to quantify worker exposure as well as to evaluate the effectiveness of protective clothing under actual field conditions. Quantitative studies are best for applications involving controlled spraying or routine surface contact rather than spills and splashes (Fenske, 1993). They provide a measure of the effect of personal hygiene and work practices upon exposure. Qualitative use of tracers can be helpful for worker training in order to enhance awareness of the ramifications of not using the correct handling procedures (Fenske et al., 1986).

These techniques were used in a study of exposure beneath CPC and ordinary clothing. Fluorescent Whiting Agent (4-methyl-7-diethylaminocoumarin) was added to a spray mixture of azinphos-methyl. After removing their clothing each applicator was examined with UV light. Unclothed areas such as the face and neck were not monitored with pads, but the tracer revealed that these were significant areas of exposure. The tracer was also found beneath the protective and ordinary clothing, confirming the concept that there may have been penetration of the pesticide (Franklin et al., 1981).

Fluorescent tracers were also used to see if workers could be motivated to use good work practices that minimize the potential for skin contamination if they could actually see the contamination on their skin. Sawmill employees involved in treating lumber with chlorophenols or handling the treated wood were monitored (Bentley, Horstman, and Morgan, 1989). Disodium fluorescein was added daily to the mixing tanks supplying Permatox, a chlorophenol containing wood preservative. Participants were given protective glasses (UV products, Blakray No. UVC-303) before being placed in front of two sets of four long wavelength UV lamps (Sylvania Blacklight blue F 40/BLB) and given the opportunity to visualize areas of their body that were contaminated. Close inspection of areas with low fluorescence was done using a long wavelength UV spotlight (UV products 100 watts). All areas of skin and clothing contaminated with the Permatox fluoresced bright green when placed under the UV lighting. Exposure prevention practices were discussed. As a result, it was concluded that employees were motivated to practice better hygiene and work practices while on the job: their levels of exposure, as measured during urine monitoring, decreased over the period of the study.

Photographic Analysis

Photographic analysis is often referred to as qualitative analysis. The photographic method was used in one study as follows: Subjects were examined in a darkened room under long wave UV light (320–400 ηm) prior to work and immediately following the exposure period (Fenske, 1990). Photographs of the greenhouse workers' exposed body regions were collected with a tripod-mounted single lens reflex camera equipped with a 2E Wratten filter (Kodak) mounted on a 50 mm lens (Fig. 13-5). Camera-to-subject distance was 90 cm. Optimal photographic parameters were ASA 400 film, 1/15 sec shutter speed, and f/2.0 aperture. It is best if workers wear only black shorts during the examination.

Video Imaging Analysis

Video imaging analysis is often considered a quantitative method. A study of airblast spray pesticide applicators involved using video imaging (Fenske, 1990). The imaging system divides the skin surface into discrete units known as picture elements (pixels). Each pixel represents a portion of the surface area of the skin: for example, one pixel represents 0.113 cm^2 with a camera-to-subject distance of 85 cm. Each pixel is assigned a gray level value based on the amount of fluorescence emitted from the portion of skin represented by the pixel. Pixels in the postexposure image with gray level values that exceed corresponding values in the preexposure image are designated "exposed," producing a measure of total area exposed and total tracer exposure for each body region. It is best if subjects wear only black shorts during the examination.

Four video images were normally recorded for each body region (Table 13-2). The forearm was sampled by segmenting the surface into four wrist-to-elbow images, with each image recorded as the worker held his arm in a vertical position and rotated 90 degrees. Before and after image segments were superimposed to reduce background effects, exposure was quantified based on a standard curve. The standard curve was developed by spotting small areas of skin with a range of tracer concentrations and recording the fluorescence on the skin with the imaging system.

The lighting system for the video camera consisted of black light bulbs with filters. The intensity of the UVA light to which subjects were exposed was evaluated prior to examination with a UVX Radiometer. With a light-to-subject distance of 90 cm, the maximum long wave UV illumination was 210 μwatts/cm^2. Both pre- and postexposure images were taken of all body regions above the waist for each subject, resulting in a total of 30 pairs of video images per subject. The camera-to-subject distance varied between 70 cm and 80 cm and at times the camera was moved up or down to accommodate the location of the body part. A fixed aperture of f/1.4 was used throughout the study (Fenske, Leffingwell, and

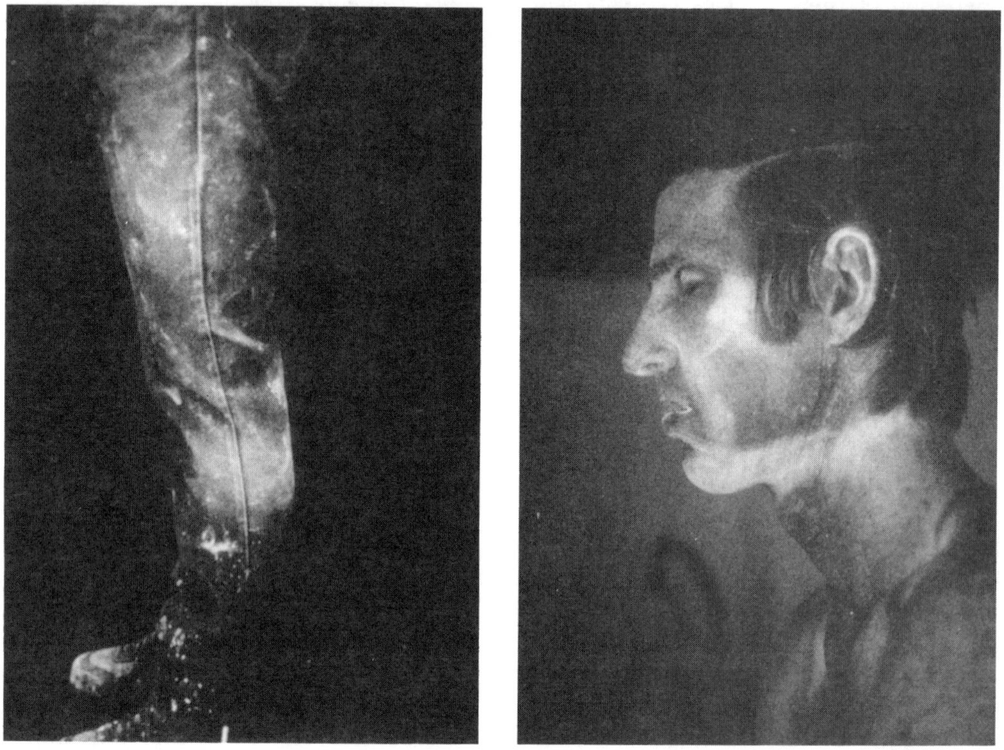

Figure 13-5. *Left:* Exposure to side of greenhouse applicator pants due to contact with hand-held spray canister. *Right:* Facial exposure to greenhouse applicators: spraying at bench height results in high deposition on neck but little exposure to forehead.
Source: From: R. A. Fenske. 1990. Nonuniform dermal deposition patterns during occupational exposure to pesticides. *Arch. Env. Contam. Toxicol.* **19:**334, 335.

Spear, 1985). A variable background reflectance from the skin is commonly observed with this system. Images of the various body parts must be recorded prior to the worker's exposure to provide baseline data. Thus, the area of interest for quantification on the after image (postexposure) is outlined and superimposed onto the before image, and background variability is eliminated. Images are then corrected for lens distortions and changes in distance and also adjusted for the nonplanar characteristics of the various body parts. Ratios of pesticide tracer based on environmental samples allow calculation of pesticide exposure (Table 13-3). The gauze pads provide a means of calculating the ratio of contaminant and tracer as they reach the worker. Laboratory studies have demonstrated that pesticides and tracer compounds penetrate cotton coverall fabric at different rates (Fenske, 1984).

The video imaging analysis of deposition patterns beneath protective clothing indicated that exposed surface areas were a relatively small fraction of the total surface areas. A higher proportion of the forearm was exposed (22%) than either the upper arm (12%) or torso (4%). Furthermore, the percent of each body region exposed was highly variable, ranging from 3% to 50% for the forearms, 1% to 35% for the upper arms, and <1% to 24% for the torso. The conclusion was that exposure is not distributed uniformly over the individual body regions during orchard/air blast mixing and application. The need for ancillary studies involving chemical extraction and analysis to make sure the tracer and contaminant are transferred uniformly to some extent undermines the primary advantage of video imaging, which is the rapid collection and analysis of samples (Fenske, 1993).

TABLE 13-2. Body Parts for Video Imaging Analysis

Body Part	*No. Images Recorded*	*Anatomical Boundaries*
Hands (1)	4	Up to the wrists
Forearm (2)	8	Wrists to the elbow
Upper arm (2)	6	Elbow to the shoulder (excludes insides of arms)
Head (1)	4	Includes neck, face, sides and back of head
Upper torso (1)	4	Neck to breast (includes front of neck)
Lower torso (1)	4	Breast to waist

Source: From Fenske, R. A., J. T. Leffingwell, and R. C. Spear. 1985. Evaluation of fluorescent tracer methodology for dermal exposure assessment. In *Dermal Exposure Related to Pesticide Use*. Washington, DC: American Chemical Society.

Case Studies

In a pesticide mixing and application study it was noted that the mean deposition ratios for applicators and mixers calculated from pads were 14.12 and 6.12, respectively. The mixer ratio was similar to the 5.7 initial tank ratio, but the applicator ratio was much higher. The deposition ratio for applicators increased because of a lower water solubility of the tracer relative to the wettable powder formulation (Fenske, 1988*a*).

Another study involved the use of the tracer 4-methyl-7-diethylaminocoumarin added to bags of diazinon 50% wettable powder. The tracer concentration on exposure pads and on the subjects was evaluated through a scanning television apparatus. There was a discrepancy in the amount of tracer actually found on the face and the amount that had been estimated. The pad technique estimated much more exposure to the head than the tracer indicated (Fenske, Leffingwell, and Spear, 1984).

Tracer Problems

Fluorescent tracers are not yet widely used. One problem is a lack of nontoxic fluorescent tracer compounds that would be compatible with a wide variety of contaminants. The major disadvantage of this technique when compared to the patch method is its high cost. The stability of the UV illumination and the instrument's performance must be monitored (Fenske, 1989). The ratio of contaminant and tracer deposition on the skin's

TABLE 13-3. Tracer Deposition Ratio

	Mean ($\mu g/cm^2$)	*Range*	*C.V.*[a] *(%)*	*Corr.*[b] *Coeff.*
Applicators (N = 14)				0.957[c]
Malathion[d]	59.94	4.3–178	87	
Tracer[d]	5.32	0.64–19.1	104	
Ratio[e]	14.12	7.9–29.9	39	
Mixers (N = 7)				0.168
Malathion	3.93	1.46–7.3	56	
Tracer	1.07	0.30–2.1	58	
Ratio	6.12	2.0–11.4	51	

Source: From Fenske, R. A. 1988. Correlation of fluorescent tracer measurements of dermal exposure and urinary metabolite excretion during occupational exposure to malathion. *AIHA J.* **49**(9):438–444.
[a]C.V. = coefficient of variation (std. dev./mean × 100%).
[b]Pearson correlation coefficient of malathion and tracer.
[c]F-test; $p < 0.001$.
[d]Mean = average levels of malathion or tracer deposited on eight gauze pads.
[e]Ratio = mean of malathion/tracer ratio for each worker.

surface must be determined through field sampling in each survey. Also, the behavior and stability of the tracer once it reaches the skin must be validated. In some cases, clothing penetration may be different for the two compounds, requiring a correction factor.

Degradation can occur when the tracer deposited on the skin is exposed directly to sunlight, as portions of the head and neck were in one study (Fenske, 1988*b*). Previous studies with field targets determined that such degradation was no more than 20% over the study period (Fenske, 1990). When sunlight intensity is high, however, degradation will be highly variable among workers. This variability, as well as quenching, can underestimate exposure.

The problem of quenching is inherent to any method measuring dermal fluorescence. When excess fluorescent material is deposited on the skin, the fluorescence produced is no longer proportional to deposition. Therefore, areas of high concentration may be underestimated (Fenske, 1989).

Comparison of Fluorescence Monitoring with Other Techniques

A comparison of the fluorescence and pad methods was done in a study of head and neck exposure to malathion. Exposure of worker number 1 was 1,026 μg by the tracer method while the estimate of the exposure for the same areas derived from the pad technique was 10,069 μg, or ten times greater (Table 13-4). The pad estimate of 9,926 μg for worker number 2 was quite similar to that of worker number 1, while the tracer estimate of 163 μg was much lower (Fenske, 1989) (Table 13-5).

DIRECT EXAMINATION FOR DISCOLORATION

Some chemicals or formulations produce a visible discoloration of the skin under normal light (Table 13-6). Inspection can be done when a compound is deliberately dyed, such as tetraethyl lead, tetramethyl lead, or when discoloration is a unique property of the chemical such as silver or copper. In its proposed method for methylene dianiline (MDA), the Occupational Safety and Health Administration (OSHA) has included a recommendation for a visual skin examination because this material discolors the skin. Toluene diamine is also known to cause skin and surface discoloration. The discoloration associated with this material is considered to be due to oxidation products since aromatic amines are very easily oxidized by air.

Greenish hair and beard discoloration have been known to occur in bronze and copper workers since the 1700s. It has been reported in workers at copper smelters, burnishers, and fillers. It has also been produced from brass hair pins and on the fingers from rings. Such sporadic observations have been poorly documented but several reports have described deposits of bluish-green copper "crystals" apparently observed by light microscopy of hair strands. Water, which has been acidified by fluoridation processes, can leech excessive copper from household water pipes and has been reported to cause green hair when used for bathing. Similarly, chlorine in swimming pools has produced a greenish tint in swimmers' hair.

The pesticide DNOSBP also stains the skin. In one study where dermal exposure measurements were made using pads and hand rinses, it was noted that staining occurred in areas that were not being directly measured in some cases (Wolfe, Durham, and Batchelor, 1961). A flagman for airplanes (crop sprayers) had visible staining of the face, neck, and hands from spray drift. Stained pads had much higher concentrations than those that were not stained.

In the case of 1-fluoro-2,4-dinitrobenzene, a chemical used in biochemical research for the characterization of amines and other laboratory tests, the first and most obvious effect was the characteristic yellow staining of the fingertips and nails (Thompson and Edmonds, 1980). This effect was followed by tiny sago-grain type vesicular lesions on the inner aspects of the fingers, which often produced blisters.

The yellow-brown discoloration of metaphenylene diamine (MPDA) with exposure to air was the clue that indicated gloves were not providing adequate protection for workers in a process using epoxy resin and MPDA in the

TABLE 13-4. Comparison of Malathion Dermal Exposure Measured by Fluorescent Tracers and Urinary Excretion Levels

	Mean (mg)	*Range (mg)*	*C.V.*[a] *(%)*	*% Total Exposure*
Applicators (N = 13)				
Total exposure	7.62	0.81–26.4	95	100.0
Hands	0.95	0.07–3.12	99	12.4
Head/neck	1.81	0.45–3.97	56	23.8
Torso/arms	4.86	0.30–19.4	113	63.8
Urinary excretion	1.27	0.16–5.01	97	—
Mixers (N = 6)				
Total exposure	4.25	1.37–7.26	46	100.0
Hands	1.84	0.64–3.22	34	43.3
Head/neck	0.87	0.24–1.84	64	20.5
Torso/arms	1.54	0.50–2.64	50	36.2
Urinary excretion	0.98	0.26–1.78	63	—

Source: From Fenske, R. A. 1988. Correlation of fluorescent tracer measurements of dermal exposure and urinary metabolite excretion during occupational exposure to malathion. *AIHA J.* **49**(9):438–444.
Note: Dermal exposure = tracer measurements × tracer deposition ratio (14.12 for applicators; 5.7 for mixers).
[a]C.V. = coefficient of variation (std. dev./mean × 100%).

amine hardener. Workers using this material had persistently stained hands (Gunderson et al., 1989).

Ubiquitous discoloration throughout a work area and change areas in a process using this type of chemical would indicate widespread contamination with a significant potential for both dermal and inhalation exposures. In these areas mapping out the physical contamination and verifying that the material is present in the stains is sufficient to demonstrate a dermal hazard. For example, in a manufacturing facility producing 4,4'-diaminostilbene-2,2'-disulfonic acid (DAS), an intermediate in the manufacture of a wide variety of optical brightening agents, a fine yellowish film was observed on surfaces throughout the work area such as handrailings, equipment, and the floor where DAS was put into metal drums for transport (Quinn et al., 1990). This film was visible on the hands and forearms of some of the workers. Therefore, even though the airborne exposures were relatively low, there was evidence

TABLE 13-5. Dermal Exposure Estimation by Patch and Tracer Techniques

Worker No.	*Body Part*	*Surface Area (cm²)*	*Patch Exposure (µg/cm²)*	*Calculated Exposure (µg/part)*	*Tracer Exposure (µg/part)*
1	Face	650	12.45	8,092	996[a]
	Back of neck	110	0.99	109	
	Front of neck	150	12.45	1,868	30
			Total	10,069	1,026
2	Face	650	11.94	7,761	146
	Back of neck	110	3.40	374	
	Front of neck	150	11.94	1,791	17
			Total	9,926	163

Source: From Fenske, R. A., J. T. Leffingwell, and R. C. Spear. 1985. Evaluation of fluorescent tracer methodology for dermal exposure assessment. In *Dermal Exposure Related to Pesticide Use*. Washington, DC: American Chemical Society.
[a]Head region for tracer technique includes sides and back of neck.

TABLE 13-6. Changes of Skin Color as Markers of Occupational Exposure

Color	*Compound*	*Groups Affected*	*Reference*
Orange	Tetryl (trinitrophenylmethylnitramine)	Explosives workers	
	Chlorine gas	Chemical workers Bleachers Laundry workers Swimming pool maintenance	
	Phenothiazine	Insecticide workers Dye and pharmaceutical workers Nurses	
Yellow	Picric acid and picrates	Explosives and dye workers	Schwartz, 1944
	Dinobuton 2-(1-methyl-2-propyl)-4,6-dinitrophenyl isopropylcarbonate	Acaricide and fungicide exposures to agricultural workers	Wahlberg, 1974
	Acrex	Acaricide and fungicide exposures to agricultural workers	Wahlberg, 1974
	Dessin	Acaricide and fungicide exposures to agricultural workers	Wahlberg, 1974
	Dinofen	Acaricide and fungicide exposures to agricultural workers	Wahlberg, 1974
	4,4'-Methylenedianiline	Plastics (epoxy and urethane resins) workers	Cohen (pers. comm., 1981)
	Dichromate	Electroplaters Leather tanners Lithographers	
	Fluorescein dye	Machinists Metal flaw detection	
	Glutaraldehyde	Nurses Dental personnel Hemodialysis technicians	
	Sodium nitrite	Machinists performing etching	Fregert, Poulsen, and Trulsson, 1980
	Nitric acid		
Green	Copper dust	Electrical workers Machinists Copper smelters	
Blue	Silver nitrate	Photographers	Buckley, Oster, and Fassett, 1965
	Sulfadiazine silver (Silvadene)	Pharmaceutical workers Nurses in burn units	Pariser, 1978
	Oxalic acid	Automobile radiator cleaners Dye makers and dryers Metal cleaners	
Blue-gray	Bismuth		
	Gold		
	Lead salts		
Brown	Chrysarobin	Pharmacists Nurses	

TABLE 13-6. *(continued)*

Color	*Compound*	*Groups Affected*	*Reference*
	Anthralin	Pharmacists Nurses	
	p-Phenylenediamine	Dye manufacturers Color photography developers	
	Permanganates	Bleach makers Dye makers Water purifiers Paper pulp bleachers	
	Phenothiazines	Agricultural workers Veterinarians Nurses	
Bronze	Arsenic (pigmentation on the trunk)		
Black	Osmium trioxide Toxicodendron radicans resin	Histology technicians Incandescent lamp makers Organic chemical synthesis Platinum hardeners	Guin, 1980 Mallory, Miller, and Tyler, 1982
Slate gray	Mercury (most pronounced in skin folds)	Cosmetologists Veterinarians	

Buckley, W. R., C. F. Oster, and D. W. Fassett. 1965. Localized argyria. II. Chemical nature of the silver-containing particles. *Arch. Dermatol.* **92:**697–705.
Fregert, S., J. Poulsen, and L. Trulsson. 1980. Yellow stained skin from sodium nitrite in an etching agent. *Cont. Derm.* **6:**296.
Guin, J. D. 1980. The black spot test for recognizing poison ivy and related species. *J. Am. Acad. Dermatol.* **2:**332–333.
Mallory, S. B., D. F. Miller, and W. B. Tyler. 1982. Toxicodendron radiacans dermatitis with black lacquer deposit on the skin. *J. Am. Acad. Dermatol.* **6:**363–368.
Pariser, R. J. 1978. Generalized argyria. *Arch. Dermatol.* **114:**373–377.
Schwartz, L. 1944. Dermatitis from explosives. *JAMA* **125:**186–190.
Wahlberg, J. E. 1974. Yellow staining of hair and nails and contact sensitivity to dinobuton. *Cont. Derm. Newsletter* **16:**481.
Source: From Adams, R. M. 1983. *Occupational Skin Disease*. New York: Grune & Stratton.

for potential dermal exposure to the fine DAS powder.

Sometimes the discoloration is unexpected. Five employees developed methemoglobinemia while working at a rubber manufacturing company (NIOSH, 1987). Their job included manually placing adhesive coated metal parts into rubber molds without using gloves. They experienced yellow hands, cyanosis of the lips and nailbeds, headache, dizziness, nausea, chest pain, confusion, and difficulty in concentration. Chemical analysis of the most recent shipment of the adhesive being used identified dinitrobenzene at 1% by weight. This adhesive had been used at the company for several years without incident but had recently been reformulated. After the company switched to a different adhesive that did not contain dinitrobenzene the symptoms ceased.

In another example, men working with cores and molds noted that their hands were being stained a very dark color and that this pigment was extremely difficult to remove (Arndt, Perone, and Tubich, 1968). Neither soap nor solvents would remove the discoloration; apparently the soil came off only as the skin was sloughed off. A new process had been introduced into foundries to improve the production of castings: an oil-base no-bake binding system that eliminated the need for baking sand cores and molds prior to filling them with molten metal. Three components were involved: an air curing oil such as modified linseed oil; a metal drier catalyst such as cobalt naphthenate; and an aromatic polyisocyanate, methylene diphenyl diisocyanate (MDI). The usual procedure was to premix the oil and drier and then mix this with the sand. The introduction of the MDI causes the curing reaction to begin cross-linking the oil and the process continues as the piece "air cures." The investigation determined that the adhesive properties of the binding system were causing carbon black in the soil to bond to the skin of the workers' hands.

Photographic Examination

Color photographs of the skin of workers will demonstrate that their skin is contaminated. It will also assist in comparing skin contamination from one visit to the next. In a study of the effects of silver exposure in silver reclamation workers (photographic film, paper, and liquid wastes), facial photographs were used to determine whether the silver workers had more facial discoloration than a group of matched controls, and if so, whether it was judged to be cosmetically objectionable (Pifer et al., 1989). In order to prevent color reflection from clothing and to avoid identification of an employee's job based on the work clothes, a neutral colored cloth was draped over the neck and shoulder area. As an additional constraint during the photographic review, each portrait was covered with a paper mask allowing only the subject's face to be visualized.

Panels of laypeople and physicians evaluated color photographs of the faces of each matched pair of study subjects for the presence of skin discoloration. After the judges read a brief instructional statement, they were given a card describing the categories to be used for ranking the individuals according to the extent of their cosmetic impairment. Each pair of portraits was then examined in sequence. The reviewers were first asked to select the person with facial discoloration and then to score that individual on a scale of one to five; the second photograph was scored as zero. The study subjects were reviewed in pairs rather than individually because of the strong association between age and the presence of acne, nevi, and other facial blemishes.

A more simplistic method was used on painters (Sparer et al., 1988). Each worker was rated at the end of the workday as to whether he looked "clean" or and "little," "moderate," or "lots" of paint on him.

Color Change Tests on Skin

Spot tests that have been used most often on surfaces to detect contamination have also been used on workers' skin, usually the hands or fingers. The best known test detects chromium VI, a carcinogen, although recently an application for lead has been used. The skin is either wiped with a filter and the test is performed on the filter (the preferable method) or the reagents are swabbed directly on the skin. The reaction of the reagents with the contaminant causes a distinct color to form. The latter method may cause irritation depending on the reagents involved and must be done very cautiously. If a chemical reaction will not harm the skin this condition, too, can be used to detect exposures. As an example, dilute sodium sulfide baths have been used to assist lead workers in identifying skin contamination so they can make sure they are clean before leaving work.

Color Change Patches

Perma-tec pads are small Band-Aids that contain color change media that will stick on the skin without harming it. The sensor is on the back of the pad. If a worker encounters one of the detectable chemicals, a color change will take place. The main application is for detecting contamination under CPC; however, the pads can be worn over the day to determine if any unsuspected contamination of the worker's skin is occurring. They can also be placed directly under work clothing. See Chapters 3 and 6 for more detail. A number of different pads are available for specific chemical families.

Color Change Paper

Impact sensitive chart recorder paper has been attached to the chest and back of an operator to estimate skin exposure during spraying pyrethroid on cotton (Prinsen and Van Sittert, 1980). The impact of the spray droplets created a color change on the paper. For compounds with a high or low pH, litmus paper can be used. This technique was used to identify hydrogen peroxide deposition on factory workers manufacturing picture tubes for televisions who had problems with their hair turning green (NIOSH, 1980). Monitoring has also been done using 25 mm wide, water-sensitive, paper strips that stain blue when exposed to moisture (Lengerich and Burroughs, 1989). The paper is sensitive to droplets as small as 50 μm (CIBA-GEIGY, Ltd., 1985). Prior to the use of this paper in the study it was determined that 98% of the droplets generated from the spray nozzles of herbicide sprayers were larger than 100 μm.

The strips show a symmetrical dot if a droplet is collected and smears if wiped against something such as wet (from herbicide spray) vegetation. This allows for a qualitative evaluation of the relative contributions from air and surface exposures to various parts of the body.

The strips can be clipped to elastic bands to put around ankles, forearms, thighs, and calves. They can also be directly attached to clothing such as a waistband or pocket. In this study the strips were cut to specific lengths for each body region, accommodating not only the various sizes of the body parts but also making each strip readily identifiable by its length. After each spraying trial, the exposed strips were placed into a plastic bag along with the corresponding data sheet. Bags were then stored in a covered box in an air conditioned room until analysis. Because of their extreme sensitivity to moisture, the strips should be handled at all times with latex gloves.

Analysis of strips is done through a combination of objective and subjective methods. Controls containing various droplet densities were analyzed by an Artek colony counter designed for use as a petri dish colony counter. Comparison of the field strips to these strips by technicians allowed a quantitative estimation of their concentration.

REFERENCES

Arndt, K., V. Perone, and G. E. Tubich. 1968. Stained hands in the foundry: An undesirable effect of oil-base no-bake binders. *Arch. Env. Health* **16:**256–257.

Bentley, R. K., S. W. Horstman, and M. S. Morgan. 1989. Reduction of sawmill worker exposure to chlorophenols. *Appl. Ind. Hyg.* **4**(3):69–74.

CIBA-GEIGY, Ltd. 1985. *Product Manual for Water Sensitive Paper for Monitoring Spray Distribution.* Basel, Switzerland: CIBA-GEIGY, Ltd.

Dubelman, S., and J. E. Cowell. 1989. Biological monitoring technology for measurement of applicator exposure. In *Biological Monitoring for Pesticide Exposure.* Washington, DC: American Chemical Society, pp. 240–250.

Fenske, R. A. 1984. *A Fluorescent Tracer Technique for Assessing Dermal Exposure to Pesticides.* Northern California Occupational Health Center Report No. NCOHC 84-B-1, Berkeley, CA, 270 p.

Fenske, R. A. 1988*a*. Comparative assessment of protective clothing performance by measurement of dermal exposure during pesticide applications. *Appl. Ind. Hyg.* **3**(7):207–213.

Fenske, R. A. 1988*b*. Correlation of fluorescent tracer measurements of dermal exposure and urinary metabolite excretion during occupational exposure to malathion. *AIHA J.* **49**(9):438–444.

Fenske, R. A. 1989. Validation of environmental monitoring by biological monitoring. In *Biological Monitoring for Pesticide Exposure.* Washington, DC: American Chemical Society.

Fenske, R. A. 1990. Nonuniform dermal deposition pattern during occupational exposure to pesticides. *Arch. Env. Contam. Toxicol.* **19:**332–337.

Fenske, R. A. 1993. Dermal exposure assessment techniques. *Ann. Occup. Hyg.* **37**(6):687–706.

Fenske, R. A., J. T. Leffingwell, and R. C. Spear. 1985. Evaluation of fluorescent tracer methodology for dermal assessment. In R. C. Honeycutt, G. Zweig, and N. Ragsdale (eds.), *Dermal Exposure Related to Pesticide Use.* ACS Symposium Series 273, pp. 377–393.

Fenske, R. A., et al. 1986. A video imaging technique for assessing dermal exposure. II. Fluorescent tracer testing. *AIHA J.* **47**(12):771–775.

Franklin, C. A., R. A. Fenske, R. Greenhalgh, L. Mathieu, H. V. Denley, J. T. Leffingwell, and R. C.

Spear. 1981. Correlation of urinary pesticide metabolite excretion with estimated dermal contact in the course of occupational exposure to guthion. *J. Toxicol. Env. Health* **7**(5):715–731.

Gunderson, E. C., B. A. Kingsley, C. C. Witham, and D. C. Bomberger. 1989. A practical study in laboratory and workplace permeation testing. *Appl. Ind. Hyg.* **4**(12):324–329.

Hill, R. H. 1984. Ultraviolet detection of synthetic oil contamination of skin. *AIHA J.* **45**(7):474–484.

JBR Associates. 1979 (June). *Summary Plant Observation Report and Evaluation.* McLean, VA. Under NIOSH Contract No. 210-78-0017.

Johnson, D. E., L. M. Adams, and J. D. Millar. 1975. *Sensory Chemical Pesticide Warning System, Pt. I. Experimental, Summary and Recommendations.* San Antonio, TX: Southwest Research Institute, EPA 540/9-75-029.

Keenan, R. R., and S. B. Cole. 1982. A sampling and analytical procedure for skin-contamination evaluation. *AIHA J.* **43**(7):473–476.

Lengerich, S. K., and F. G. Burroughs. 1989. Near real-time monitoring of potential dermal exposure during backpack herbicide spraying. *AIHA J.* **50**(10):516–519.

NIOSH. 1977. *Exposure Tests for Organic Compounds in Industrial Toxicology.* NIOSH Pub. No. 77-144. Cincinnati, OH: NIOSH.

NIOSH. 1978. *Criteria for a Recommended Standard—Occupational Exposure to Coal Tar Products.* Cincinnati, OH: NIOSH.

NIOSH, Health Hazard Evaluation Report. May 1980. *RCA Corp., Marion, IN.* HHE 79-105-687. Cincinnati, OH: NIOSH.

NIOSH, Health Hazard Evaluation Report. July 1987. *Barr Rubber Corp., Sandusky, OH.* HETA 86-350-1815. Cincinnati, OH: NIOSH.

NIOSH, Health Hazard Evaluation Report. 1991. *Exxon Valdez Cleanup.* HHE 89-200/273-2111. Cincinnati, OH: NIOSH.

Perkins, J. L. 1987. Chemical protective clothing. Vol. I. Selection and use. *Appl. Ind. Hyg.* **2**(6):222–230.

Pifer, J. W., B. R. Friedlander, R. T. Kintz, and D. K. Stockdale. 1989. Absence of toxic effects in silver reclamation workers. *Scand. J. Work Env. Health* **15**:210–221.

Prinsen, G. H., and N. J. Van Sittert. 1980. Exposure and medical monitoring study of a new synthetic pyrethroid after one season of spraying on cotton in Ivory Coast. In W. F. Tordoir and E. A. H. van Heemstra (eds.), *Field Worker Exposure During Pesticide Application.* Amsterdam: Elsevier, pp. 105–120.

Quinn, M. M., D. H. Wegman, I. A. Greaves, S. K. Hammond, M. J. Ellenbecker, R. F. Spark, and E. R. Smith. 1990. Investigation of reports of sexual dysfunction among male chemical workers manufacturing stilbene derivatives. *Am. J. Ind. Med.* **18**:55–68.

Schuresko, D. D. 1980. Portable fluoromatic monitor for detection of surface contamination by polynuclear aromatic compounds. *Anal. Chem.* **52**:371–373.

Sparer, J., L. S. Welch, K. McManus, and M. R. Cullen. 1988. Effects of exposure to ethylene glycol ethers on shipyard painters: I. Evaluation of exposure. *Am. J. Ind. Med.* **14**:497–507.

Thompson, J. S., and O. P. Edmonds. 1980. Safety aspects of handling the potent allergen FDNB. *Ann. Occup. Hyg.* **23**:27–33.

Vo-Dinh, T. 1987. Evaluation of an improved fiberoptics luminescence skin monitor with background correction. *AIHA J.* **48**(6):594–598.

Vo-Dinh, T., and R. B. Gammage. 1981. The Lightpipe Luminoscope for monitoring occupational skin contamination. *AIHA J.* **42**:112–119.

Vo-Dinh, T., and D. A. White. 1987. Development of luminescence procedures to evaluate permeation of multi-ring polyaromatic compounds through protective materials. *AIHA J.* **48**(4):400–405.

Wolfe, H. R., W. F. Durham, and G. S. Batchelor. 1961. Health hazards of some dinitro compounds: Effects associated with agricultural usage in Washington state. *Arch. Env. Health* **3**:468–475.

CHAPTER 14

Pad Dosimetry Methods

Dermal sampling using small pads or patches attached to various areas of the skin or clothing is one of the most standardized methods for collecting chemicals. Pad samplers of cellulose materials such as filter paper and multilayered gauze are appropriate for sampling contaminants with low vapor pressures, when exposure is the result of airborne mists or dusts. For volatile materials, pads containing charcoal have been developed, and for certain semivolatile materials, polypropylene pads have been used. Although they are not as well tested as the cellulose pads, their use is promising because it may provide for greater collection efficiency and a broader number of compounds for sampling. Other variations include the use of multiple materials and adding chemical dopants to enhance collection. This variety is needed because it is unlikely that any one material or combination of materials will collect all contaminants. Similarly a wide variety of media and variations have been developed to collect compounds using integrated air sampling techniques.

Pads must be absorbent enough to retain all the liquid that contacts them, or, if used for collecting dusts or dried residues, must be porous enough to collect these materials. The pads must be strong enough to hold up under the abuse they will receive in the field. They must not contain additives such as sizing that will interfere with the chemical analysis of the extracted chemicals. Additives can usually be removed by preextraction of the pads; however, some interfering compounds cannot be adequately removed to allow analysis of low levels of contaminants. The following are variables in pad use:

- Size
- Type of media
- Combinations of media
- Backing(s)
- Number of layers
- Preextracted versus not extracted
- Holder
- Means of attachment
- Number of pads used for monitoring
- Sampling locations: top of and under CPC, top of and under work clothing, top of underclothing, on top of skin
- Overlapping versus adjacent pads
- Sampling period
- Combined or analyzed separately

This chapter was coauthored by William Popendorf, Ph. D. (Institute of Agricultural Medicine, Iowa City, Iowa), and Shirley A. Ness.

In most of the initial studies on dermal exposure, the assumptions behind the use of pads were the same: that the contaminant (pesticide) would adhere to the pad in the same manner as it would to the skin, that the distribution of the contaminant would be uniform over the body surface area represented by the pad, and that dermal contact would occur only on exposed skin surfaces and not on skin covered by clothing. However, recognition that there can be penetration of clothing as well as concerns as to how well skin collection is mimicked by these pads has produced some changes in these assumptions. Existing data indicate extreme variability in permeation and/or penetration of clothing and the skin by chemicals (Table 14-1).

To accommodate clothing issues, a different pad system was devised. Pads are placed on the outside of work clothing, with a second set inside. The amount of contaminant collected by the interior pads is then used to adjust the exposure estimate of the outside pad deposits (Nigg et al., 1991). In the Nigg study, although there were fewer interior pads than exterior pads, the amounts extracted from these pads suggested that about 5% of the outside deposit penetrated the clothing. The outside exposure values were adjusted by this amount. It has been found that the ratios of inside to outside pads are higher for dry than for wet deposits (Popendorf, 1989).

TABLE 14-1. Degree of Protection Provided by Ordinary Work Clothes and Coveralls to Three Body Regions

Body Region	*Dermal Exposure* ($\mu g/kg$)[a]	*Amount on Coveralls* ($\mu g/kg$)[a]	*Percent Protection*
Chest	19.0	58.1	67
Back	14.2	30.7	53.7
Forearm (right)	4.9	12.1	59.5

Source: From Hussain, M., K. Yoshida, M. Atiemo, and D. Johnston. 1990. Occupational exposure of grain farmers to Carbofuran. *Arch. Env. Contam. Toxicol.* **19:**197–204.

Note: Percentage protection was calculated according to the following:

$$\text{Percent protection} = \frac{(\text{Amount on coveralls} - \text{Dermal exposure})}{\text{Amount on coveralls}} \times 100$$

[a]Microgram of active ingredient per kilogram of carbofuran used.

Another way to express exposures is to call those based on outer pads "potential" exposures, since they estimate the amount of contaminant deposited on the clothing, and exposures based on inner pads may be called "actual" exposures since the contaminant penetrates the clothing. Outside pad estimates are useful for comparison of exposure levels from study to study (Fenske et al., 1991). Inside pads cannot be compared between studies unless identical conditions existed including the type of overcovering; however, they will provide a better approximation of actual dermal exposure.

The primary advantages of pad sampling methods are that they are simple to perform; less expensive to analyze than dosimeter clothing; allow for differentiation of routes of exposure and identification of locations of high exposure; can provide an evaluation of the protection provided by clothing during field useage; and allow for specific tasks to be sampled. The limitations are the small area sampled relative to the surface area of the body to which it is extrapolated; lack of uniformity of deposition density; the requirement for some user intervention; and the requirement for a controlled dose database for proper interpretation.

TYPES OF PADS

α-Cellulose

The Environmental Protection Agency (EPA) recommends that pads be constructed from papermaking pulp or a similar material, approximately 1 mm thick, which is commonly called α-cellulose. It resembles blotter paper. A good grade of this material will absorb a considerable amount of spray without disintegrating and hopefully will not require preextraction to remove substances that interfere with contaminant analysis, which must be determined before exposure tests begin. This material usually must be purchased in bulk, which can be cut in sizes other than 2 in. by 2 in. or 3 in. by 3 in. pads, such as is sufficient to be wrapped around the ankles or used as a headband (Culver, Caplan, and Batchelor, 1956).

Papers

Many different types of cellulose based papers have been used in studies. These include blotter paper (102 mm by 102 mm by 0.5 mm), Whatman Grade 542 filter papers (80 cm^2), Postlip Filter Paper (grade: soft 160; 0.08 cm thick; 430 g/M^2), and preparative chromatography paper (17 Chr or Whatman Grade 3 MM). Benchkote®, which is Whatman 542 filter paper backed with polyethylene, has also been used. Multiple layers of filter paper (12.5 cm) are often used.

Sheets of chromatography paper are cut into 4 in. by 4 in. (10.2 cm by 10.2 cm) squares, which are then stapled to the center of a 5 in. square protective backing of glassine paper or aluminum foil.

Gauze

Gauze pads are recommended for dust collection. They can be assembled from individually cut layers of material or used as off-the-shelf medical supplies, such as surgical dressings or sponges. The dressings are available in sterile 2 in. by 2 in. (8 ply), 3 in. by 3 in. (12 ply), and 4 in. by 4 in. (12 ply) sizes while the sponges come as 4 in. square pads and either can be purchased in pharmacies as sterile or nonsterile. The sterile pads are individually packaged. Sterility is not necessary except to avoid interference.

The composition of a typical gauze pad for dermal sampling is layers (often 8, 9, 16, or 32) of surgical gauze with an impervious backing. Early backing material was a single sheet of 4 in. by 4 in. filter paper, to prevent loss of material, with masking tape overlapping the gauze on all four edges to hold the pad together. Once bound with tape, the sampling surface is about 2.5 in. on each side. Laboratory tests have shown that gauze pads retain approximately 90% of the dust applied to them, even if they are inverted and shaken (Durham and Wolfe, 1962). Aluminum foil or polyethylene are more impervious backings, and most recent tests use a glassine-coated aluminum paper envelope (see Fig. 14-3).

Other Cellulose Materials

Table cloth paper (27 cm by 23 cm) has been fixed to both arms and the breast of a worker operating a clearing saw that sprayed MCPA (Hattula, Wasenius, and Arstila, 1979). The sheets were wrapped in aluminum foil after removal and kept frozen until analysis. Women's Carefree™ sanitary pads from Johnson & Johnson have also been used for sampling (Neto et al., 1992). While these materials may be a somewhat unlikely choice for sampling media, they demonstrate the wide variety of media that has been used.

Glass Fiber Filters

Glass fiber (GF) filters (47 mm diameter) (AP40 microfiber glass discs, Millipore or 37 mm Whatman) have been mounted in a sandwich of coarse surgical gauze and backed by a piece of cardboard to protect them from mechanical damage and to reduce accidental loss (Grover et al., 1986). GF filters are used for sampling compounds that can be analyzed using high pressure liquid chromatography (HPLC).

Fabrics

Fabric by itself has also been used as a collection medium. One hundred percent white cotton cloth pieces (28 cm by 30 cm) have been used to monitor for exposure to paraquat. The large patches were wrapped around the arms and legs (Bandara et al., 1985). Muslin (4 in. by 4 in.) squares have also been attached to the clothing of spray applicators and fieldworkers (Winterlin et al., 1984). Flannel was used to collect DEF in a study on applicators, harvestors, and cotton gin workers (Kilgore et al., 1984). Cloth patches of cotton chambray, cotton knit jersey, or 1:1 Avril (rayon) polyester may be better since these materials are representative of shirt fabrics (Knaak et al., 1978). Pads (gauze or α-cellulose) have been covered with fabric similar to the work clothing typically worn by the worker to simulate the degree of protection provided by this material (Kurtz and Bode, 1985). An example is the use of denim to cover a pad placed on the lower leg. However, it is unlikely that such a physical arrangement accurately parallels penetration or permeation of real work clothing.

There are also problems associated with the use of commercial fabrics. Type of fabric, thickness, pretreatment, and special finishes can influence the collection, retention, and penetration of residues. Since laundering removes finishes over time, this fact must be considered when making assumptions about whether the results are representative of the protectiveness of work clothing. Because the fabric characteristics vary widely among studies, comparisons of exposures are difficult. In general, there is not standardized type of work clothing. Also, fabric pads only provide simulation of the penetration of residues through freshly laundered clothing during the first exposure period of the day. In a study to compare their collection efficiency during reentry into an orange grove sprayed with Phosalone, the data suggested that the fabric, the finish, or alteration of surface morphology, governed the amount of surface residue retained. Although not conclusive, it appeared that washing decreased the ability of a fabric to retain pesticide residues.

An advantage of fabric is that it can be cut to various sizes to accommodate the anatomical area being sampled. For estimation of exposure to the wrist area, a 2.5 cm by 15 cm strip of fabric can be stapled to each shirt cuff. For estimation of exposure to the bare skin of the head and neck, a 2.5 cm by 40 cm strip can be stapled to the collar of the shirt, and another strip similarly attached to the hat band, extending from the front and around both sides toward the back. Tubular support (elasticized knit) bandages (Tubigrips®) have been used to measure the dermal exposure of the legs beneath clothing (Chester and Woolen, 1981; Chester and Ward, 1984). The bandage was located adjacent to the skin from the top of the right thigh to the ankle.

Plastics

Soft polypropylene (Fig. 14-1) has been used as an adsorbing material for polycyclic aromatic hydrocarbons (PAHs) and may also be useful for sampling other semivolatile materials (Jongeneelen et al., 1988). A circular piece of material with a diameter of 25 mm is punched from the polypropylene and placed on top of a self-adhesive stretch bandage material cut in a 40 mm diameter circle. A second circular (40 mm diameter) piece of self-adhesive material with a circular interior opening (16 mm diameter) cut into the center is placed over the polypropylene. The effective monitoring surface is 1.77 cm^2. For analysis of PAHs, the self-adhesive is removed and the polyethylene was extracted ultrasonically

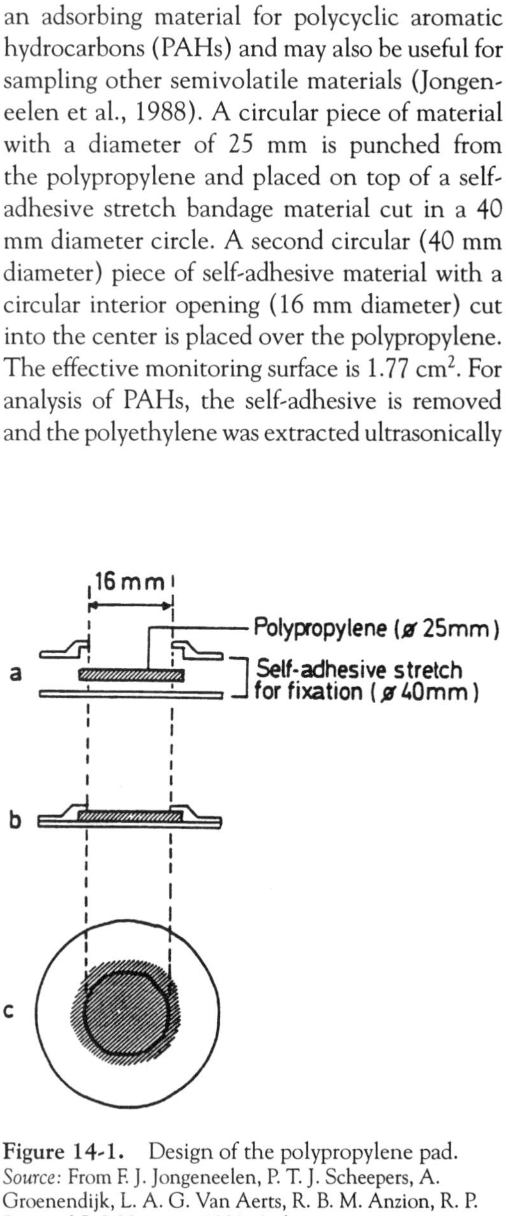

Figure 14-1. Design of the polypropylene pad. *Source:* From F. J. Jongeneelen, P. T. J. Scheepers, A. Groenendijk, L. A. G. Van Aerts, R. B. M. Anzion, R. P. Bos, and S. J. Veenstra. 1988. Airborne concentrations, skin contamination, and urinary metabolite excretion of polycyclic aromatic hydrocarbons among paving workers exposed to coal-tar derived road tars. *AIHA J.* **49**(12):601.

with 10 mL dichloromethane for 15 min and dried under a gentle flow of nitrogen at 40°C. The residue is dissolved in 2 mL methanol and centrifuged. The supernatant is analyzed using HPLC.

Pads made out of polyurethane foam have also been tried (Nigg and Stamper, 1985). Polyurethane foam (6 mm thick) with a surface area of 100 cm^2 was fastened to protective clothing with Velcro strips.

Tegaderm is a thin, transparent, synthetic plastic film (3M Co.) that was used to monitor carbofuran by attaching an 8 cm by 8 cm piece of film to the adhesive-backed side of a 12 cm by 8 cm brown dressing tape (Hussain et al., 1990). A 3.3 cm by 3.3 cm portion of the dressing tape was cut away in the center to expose a 10 cm^2 area of the Tegaderm for sampling. Laboratory studies conducted prior to the survey indicated that over a 5 hr period more than 98% of the carbofuran adhered to the plastic film. The pad was attached to the skin or coveralls with the adhesive side of the dressing tape.

Aluminum Foil

Aluminum foil by itself can be used for oily formulations (WHO, 1986). It has been used to sample for synthetic pyrethroid spray (Prinsen and Van Sittert, 1980). After sampling it is rinsed in the laboratory with an appropriate solvent to remove the contaminant. An advantage is that it does not require extensive extraction.

Charcoal Pads

Charcoal pads had been proposed for monitoring for dermal exposure to volatile compounds, such as organic solvents and fumigants (Cohen and Popendorf, 1989). The pads consist of a commercially available charcoal cloth cut into 8 cm by 5 cm squares. Four layers are then sewn together and a protective covering of a thin polyester fabric is applied; then a backing of a strong polyethylene coated belting material is attached. Collection techniques are similar to those used for gauze pads; however, sample handling following exposure is different. The units must be stored at –20°C or lower until analysis to minimize evaporation.

Materials with vapor pressures of 10 mm Hg and greater should be monitored only where ventilation effectively reduces vapor concentration, or vapor concentrations must be monitored separately and used to adjust dosimeter measurements for passive vapor absorption (Cohen and Popendorf, 1989). Chemical volatility also affects the usefulness of these dosimeters in that a liquid deposit on the skin is subject to air evaporation as well as absorption by the skin. The more volatile a compound, the shorter the contact period on the skin. Charcoal impregnated cloth has also been used to measure hand exposure to 1,3-dichloropropane (Popendorf, Leffingwell, and Cohen, 1983). A smaller charcoal strip designed to be used under gloves to detect permeation has also been developed. It is described in more detail in Chapter 15.

Impregnated Pads

A variation on selecting the media most likely to adsorb a contaminant is doping a material with a chemical that will stabilize or otherwise enhance collection of the contaminant on the media. Gauze pads have been doped with glycerin to enhance collection of 4,4'-methylene bis(2-chloroaniline) (MOCA) (NIOSH, 1985). The use of lanolin in α-cellulose pads was explored on the theory that it may simulate the slightly greasy surface of the skin (Fletcher, Press, and Wilson, 1959). Filter paper pads were impregnated with an emulsion made from 20 g lanolin in 100 mL isohexane at the rate of 1.8 g lanolin per 100 cm^2 and had a slightly greasy texture. When used to monitor sprayers for dieldrin, the results indicated much greater variation than when plain filter pads were used. It was found that lanolin can interfere with the analysis depending on the method (in this case colorimetric). Also, since lanolin is absorbed by the skin, the blank value varied from one part of the body to another depending on the amount of sweating that had occurred.

Collection of parathion and dimethoate on

gauze has been improved by immersing pads in a solution of 10% ethylene glycol (in acetone) for 10 minutes and then allowing them to air-dry in a laboratory hood (Carman et al., 1982). The collection of parathion can be improved by as much as a factor of three (30% to 90%) using this approach (Serat, Van Loon, and Serat, 1982). Similarly to improve collection of 2,4-D amine salt, GF filters were impregnated with ethylene glycol (Grover et al., 1986). This approach shows promise for improving specificity of pad sampling media.

PREPARATION AND CONSTRUCTION OF PADS

It is a matter of discussion as to whether or not pads must be extracted beforehand, usually in a Soxhlet apparatus (Fig. 14-2), with the same solvent that is later used to analyze them. Another extraction method is to place the materials into a wide mouthed plastic bottle fitted with a screw cap and to add solvent. The bottle is then shaken on a reciprocal shaker for 2 hr or more. The solvents chosen will depend on the contaminant being sampled.

The other option is to use the materials as purchased. The choice must be made prior to use by analysis of samples of the media for interferents with the compound(s) to be studied. Pads and gauze should be free of ink, oils, and other potentially interfering markings prior to use.

If extraction is selected, it is best to preextract with the same solvent to be used during analysis. Both prepared pads and gauze bundles have been extracted.

The size of pads can vary, although commonly used sizes are 3 in. by 3 in., 4 in. by 4 in., and 2 in. by 2 in. Different size pads may be used for monitoring different size body parts. In one study, 10.2 cm by 10.2 cm pads were attached to the chest, lower leg, and forearm, and 5.1 cm by 5.1 cm pads were attached to the hands (Putnam et al., 1983). Since the amount of contaminant on a pad is multiplied by a specific body area, this procedure may lead to considerable error if pads are too small. Thus, it is desirable to maximize the size of the pads (Honeycutt, 1986).

The purpose of backings is to prohibit contamination of pads by skin oils and perspiration from beneath the dosimeter. Glassine (weighing) paper, polyethylene plastic (4–10 mL), filter paper, brown wrapping paper, and aluminum foil are commonly used as backings. Glassine backings are common in EPA studies. In some cases, two different backings are used such as glassine paper with chromatographic paper or filter paper on top of it if heavy soaking is a concern (Kamble et al.,

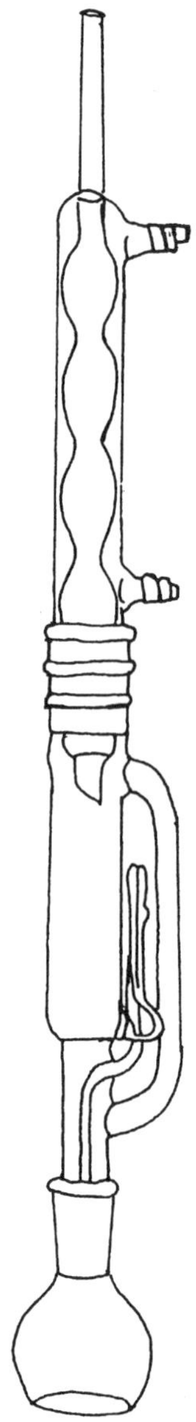

Figure 14-2. Soxhlet extraction apparatus.
Source: Drawing by Renea Joslin.

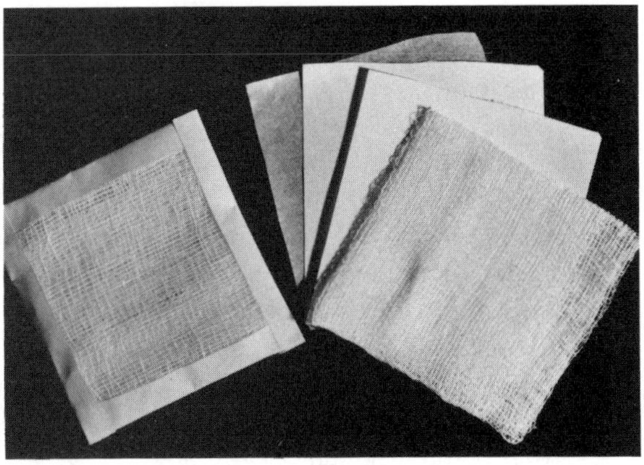
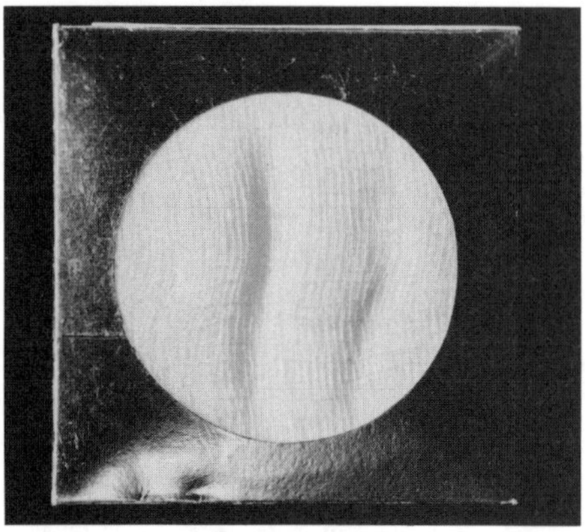

Figure 14-3. Examples of different types of pad constructions (*left*) and a pad holder (*right*).
Source: Pad holder courtesy of Western Paperbox Co., Hayward, CA. Photos by Ed Wesly.

1992). Aluminum foil provides the best protection when a subject's clothing is very wet. Another advantage of backings is that they provide stiffness to a pad. After sampling, the backings are usually discarded.

A multiuse pad for situations where both dusts and sprays are being generated either at the same time or sequentially, such as when pesticides are mixed and then applied by the same person, consists of one or more layers of filter paper covered with multiple layers of gauze, for example, 8-ply surgical gauze (4 in.^{2} by 4 in.^{2}) stapled to a double layer of filter paper (4 in.^{2} by 4 in.^{2}) with a backing of manila poster paper (4 in.^{2} by 5 in.^{2}) (Maitlen, Sell, and McDonough, 1982). The filter paper readily absorbs liquids while the gauze collects impinging dry residues and poster paper provides extra mechanical strength. When gauze is used outside α-cellulose, it helps maintain the shape of the pads and minimizes separation within the filter if the pads get wet.

To hold the pad together during sampling there are a number of options ranging from a simple staple in the center to surrounding it with tape or placing the pad inside of a specially made holder (Fig. 14-3). The most common style offers a smooth silver exterior with a circular 5.5 cm diameter hole facing the outside (away from the skin). Holders have been made by cutting a hole (60 mm diameter) in one side of a glassine paper envelope. The finished pad should be bound so that a maximal sampling area is exposed.

Cardboard lantern slide mounts (40.32 cm^2 exposed area) have been used to hold gauze pads with plastic backings. The advantage was that when used under clothing it kept the gauze slightly recessed, allowing contact with the backing only when the clothing pressed against the skin (Franklin et al., 1981). Filters can be placed in round holders specially sized to hold them.

In some instances the configuration of a pad can be customized to fit better over the body part being sampled, which is especially important for difficult areas such as the head, hands, and feet. Headbands have been used for the forehead: either the band itself is constructed of material that can be desorbed or the band is used to hold a pad. Gauze pads have been stapled to both ends of an elastic strap loop, which is then slipped over the hand so that one pad is on the dorsal portion of the hand and the other is on the palm (Fig. 14-4). In this instance, the pads were only 1 in. squares. For analysis they could be extracted together or separately, depending on what information is of interest (Clapp et al., 1991). Another option for hands is to tape or staple a gauze pad to the backs and palms of cotton gloves. The pad is removed from the glove after sampling. This configuration may be more comfortable to the worker than others such as taping the pads directly to the skin. The feet are the most difficult to sample. One option is to

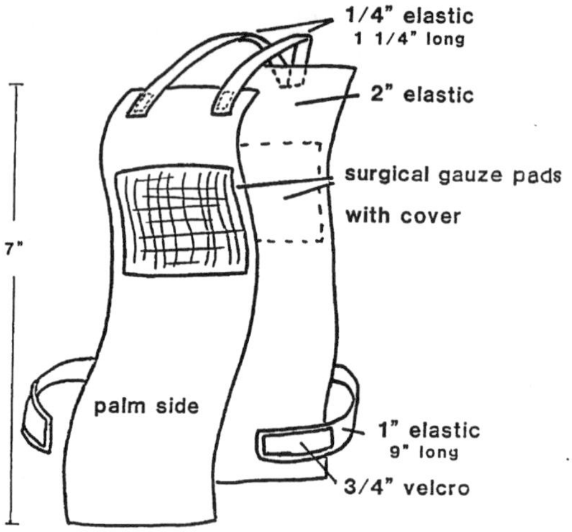

Figure 14-4. NIOSH design for a gauze hand monitoring pad.
Source: NIOSH, Health Hazard Evaluation. September 1985. *Steinmetz and Sons, Moscow, PA*. HETA 84-508-1626. Cincinnati, OH: NIOSH.

place a pad on the tongue of a work boot. Socks can also be used as samplers. They are described in Chapter 15.

Where only a portion of a pad is to be analyzed, one technique is to mark this area prior to sampling. At the end of sampling, the pads are removed and the marked square is cut out of the center of the pad.

Contaminant Recovery Determination

Once the construction of the pads is chosen, prior to performing the sampling study a determination of recovery of the contaminant should be carried out in the lab (EPA, 1986). To 5 cm by 5 cm squares cut from exposure pads, add carefully measured 0.05 mL and 0.1 mL aliquots of the concentrated contaminant as well as the formulation in which it is used in the operation. The pads are then extracted and recovery is determined.

Since different compounds are going to be absorbed and retained on pads in different efficiencies, an evaluation of loss of material from the pads should be done whenever monitoring for a new compound in order to determine the optimum exposure (sampling) period. One method is to fortify the pads with the same mixture being sampled and to process them in the same manner as the pads being used for collection (Davis, 1980). The other is to do preliminary sampling with unfortified pads during the operation to be sampled (Nigg and Stamper, 1985). Pads are left on the worker for different periods of time (1 hr or longer). The shortcoming of this method is that it assumes that the exposure concentration to the pads is equal for all exposure periods and ignores temperature and humidity effects. Another approach is to place fortified pads in an outdoor holding device and remove and analyze these pads at intervals to determine the degree of loss of material from the pads.

Prelabeling and Storing Dosimeters

For storage prior to use, paper envelopes, glass or plastic jars, or freezer bags may be used. Check containers for any material that will interfere with analysis, since any portion of the containers that will be in contact with stored exposure pads can contaminate the pads. Pads can also be placed between folds of Whatman filter paper. These filter paper envelopes are contained in individual Zip-Loc bags, which also protect against contamination.

The pads should be labeled prior to the site visit. One method is to use bar code labels that identify the samples and track them through the sampling and analytical procedures. Sample numbers are then logged with a laptop computer and light pen using bar code software. Labels can be placed on the pad backing as well as on the sample container.

SAMPLING STRATEGIES

A protocol should be developed prior to the start of the study that sets the criteria for collecting samples taking into account the goals of the survey. In order to eliminate the contribution of previous contamination from workers' clothing to a new sampling day, a standardized set of laundered clothing can be issued to all subjects at the start of each day's operation (Grover et al., 1986). A typical set consists of cotton work pants, a short-sleeved cotton T-shirt, and a long-sleeved cotton coverall of heavy material. In another study clothing consisted of cotton pants, a thin, short-sleeved cotton shirt, and a thick, long-sleeved coverall (Franklin et al., 1981). At the end of the exposure period the clothing is collected along with the pad samplers. When pads are used on top of disposable clothing, this clothing is also replaced between applications.

Other aspects can be standardized as well. While spraying ornamentals in greenhouses with Fosetyl-Al, the same backpack sprayer was used for all applications, each worker completed the same number of work cycles, and the amount of pesticide mixed or applied was the same for all workers (Fenske, Hamburger, and Guyton, 1987). The major uncontrolled variables were the actual use of protective clothing (e.g., removal of gloves), the performance of the spraying equipment, and the work practices of the individual subjects.

The number of workers selected to be sampled and, where multiple sites are involved, the number of sites selected to develop a representative sample must also be decided. The EPA recommends that for aircraft pilots a minimum of three individuals per site (or the same individual over three days) and three different sites performing the same operation be sampled. All other occupations involved should have five different individuals at a minimum of three sites monitored. However, in general it is best to monitor as many different individuals as practicable at any given time.

Sample Locations

There are four basic strategies for locating pad dosimeters: (1) measuring dermal exposure or deposition onto the body due to the environment only, in which case dosimeters are placed outside the work clothing only; (2) measuring dermal dose to skin, in which case dosimeters are placed on the skin under the clothing; (3) measuring both skin and work clothing exposure, which also allows one to measure the protection afforded certain clothing; and (4) measuring the degree of protection provided by chemical protective clothing (CPC), in which case sometimes three layers of pads are used.

As for standardized methods, the EPA has two different pad location scenarios: one for sampling workers not wearing impervious CPC and another for when CPC is worn. The World Health Organization (WHO) and National Agricultural Chemicals Association (NACA) have also developed protocols (Table 14-2).

TABLE 14-2. Comparison of EPA, NACA, and WHO Sampling Locations

Body Region Represented	*U.S. EPA (1987)*	*NACA (1986)*	*WHO[a] (1982)*
Head	Shoulder, back, and chest	Front and back	Head
Face	Chest	—	—
Back of neck	Back	—	—
Front of neck	Chest	—	—
Chest/stomach	Chest	Chest	Sternum
Back	Back	Back	Back
Upper arm	Shoulder and forearm/upper arm	Upper arm	—
Forearm	Forearm	Lower arm	Midway between elbow and wrist
Thigh	Thigh	Upper leg	Thigh
Lower leg	Shin	Lower leg	Lower leg
Feet	—	—	—

Source: From Curry, P., and S. Iyengar. 1992. Comparison of exposure assessment guidelines for pesticides. *Rev. Env. Contam. Toxicol.* **129:**79–93.

[a]In WHO guidelines, pads for lower leg, thigh, and lower arms are placed on only one side, depending on whether the subject is right- or left-handed.

Each one varies according to recommended pad locations and by the amount of surface area each pad is considered to monitor for (Table 14-3). When only work clothing and no impervious CPC is worn, the EPA recommends that at least 10 dermal pads be attached at the following locations: in front of the legs just below the knees, in front of the thighs, in back of the forearms, on top of the shoulders, in back of the neck at the edge of the collar, and on the upper chest near the jugular notch (Table 14-4) (EPA, 1986).

If only a CPC suit is being worn, 6 pads are attached. Figure 14-5 shows both pad attachment configurations. If the purpose of sampling is to estimate how much contaminant will penetrate the clothing, extra pads can be attached under the appropriate clothing (Fig. 14-6). The most common placement is to offset the interior pad so that it is right next to the pad on top of the clothing so that both pads sample similar exposures. These extra pads should be attached to areas of the body that are expected to receive the highest exposure.

TABLE 14-3. Comparison of Surface Areas (cm^2) by Body Surface Area

Body Region	*U.S. EPA (1987)*	*NACA[a] (1986)*	*WHO[b] (1982)*
Head	1,300	1,080	1,100
Neck	260	228	
Upper arm	2,910	1,840	
Forearms	1,210	1,270	1,200
Hands	820	1,310	800
Shoulders		1,290	
Chest	3,550	1,520	
Back	3,550	1,520	
Hips		1,730	
Thighs	3,820	3,420	3,500
Calves/lower leg	2,380	2,570	2,300
Feet	1,310	1,220	
Face	650		

Source: From Curry, P., and S. Iyengar. 1992. Comparison of exposure assessment guidelines for pesticides. *Rev. Env. Contam. Toxicol.* **129:**79–93.
Note: Canadian guidelines will recommend body surface areas similar to those of EPA.
[a]From Popendorf (1976).
[b]In WHO guidelines, the V of neck, top of shoulders near neck, and back just below neck total 650 cm^2.

TABLE 14-4. Locations of Dermal Exposure Pads That Represent Different Regions of the Adult Body for EPA Monitoring

Body Area of Concern	*Exposure Pads Representative of the Body Area*
Totally unprotected head[a]	Shoulder, chest, and back[b]
Face	Chest
Neck	Chest and back
Upper arms	Shoulder and forearm/upper arm
Forearms	Forearm
Hands	Total of residues in the hand rinses, or monitoring gloves is used without regard for surface area
Chest	Chest
Back	Back
Thighs	Thigh
Calves	Shins
Feet	If necessary, total of contaminant in socks can be used without regard for surface area

Source: From EPA. 1986. *Pesticide Assessment Guidelines, Subdivision U, Applicator Exposure Monitoring.* EPA 540/9/-87-127. Washington, DC: Office of Pesticides Programs.
[a]Includes face.
[b]Exposure to the head may be estimated by using the mean of the shoulder, back, and chest patches or by using a head patch.

If pads are placed both inside and outside of normal work clothing, the ability of the fabric to protect against the contaminant can be determined by comparing outer and inner monitor values. This technique has also been applied to different types of fabrics (Fenske, Hamburger, and Guyton, 1987; Popendorf, 1989; Popendorf et al., 1979; Spear et al., 1977).

It is important to note that the workers' shirts and trousers are often constructed of different materials, and therefore, comparisons of penetration between workers may be difficult. However, since the most likely routes of penetration are either permeation through the fabric or penetration around it through openings such as at the neck, cuffs, or in between button closures (which, especially for dry contaminants, are affected strongly by movement of the outer clothing with respect to the dosimeter), placing the

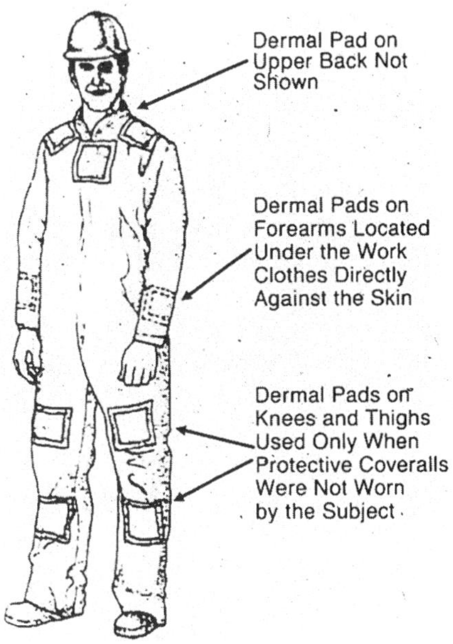

Figure 14-5. Badges attached to worker using the EPA configuration.
Source: EPA. 1987. *Acrylamide Grouting Exposure Assessment*. EPA 560/5-87-009. Washington, DC: EPA.

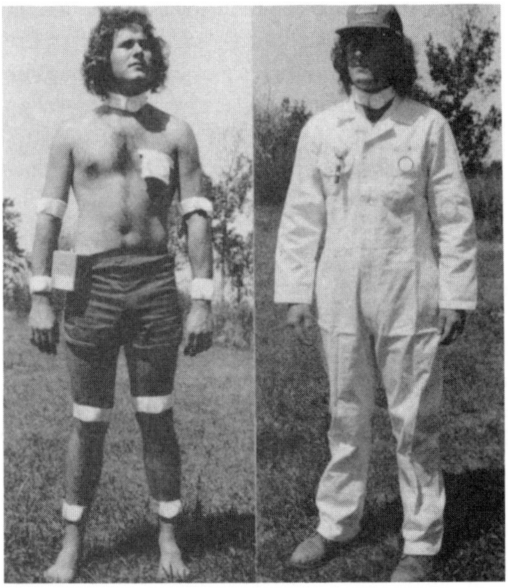

Figure 14-6. Worker being monitored with pads underneath clothing (*left*) and on top of clothing (*right*).
Source: R. Grover and A. J. Cessna et al. 1986. Factors affecting the exposure of ground-rig applicators to 2,4-D dimethylamine salt. *Arch. Env. Contam. Toxicol.* **15:**679.

inner dosimeter on the protective clothing is likely to underestimate penetration and thus overestimate the magnitude of protection provided by the clothing. Even when work clothing is shown to be adequate to protect skin from contaminant absorption, the clothing itself becomes a form of contamination and should not be reused until laundered. If significant contamination has occurred, the worker's clothing should not be laundered with family clothing.

Another variation of this technique involves using a protective suit, typically of Tyvek, over standardized work clothing and placing pads at three levels (Nigg, Stamper, and Queen, 1986). In this case, pads offset from one another so that they do not overlap, are placed on top of the Tyvek, on top of the work clothing under the Tyvek, and pinned under the work clothing.

While the standardized methods for pad placement are useful, the specific needs of the survey may require other variations. If the workers are engaged in some activity that is likely to result in extraordinary exposure to regions of the body that are not well represented by the usual pad locations, extra pads should be included to assess these additional exposure areas. The thigh can be a critical area to sample given the high permeability of the scrotum and high exposure levels in package handling or while seated on open tractors (Popendorf, 1989). In a study of diazinon application to turfgrass, the body pads with the greatest amount of exposure contamination were those on the wrist and on the inner thigh just below the scrotal area, because when applying the liquid spray the applicator would walk at a brisk pace and the handheld nozzle releasing the spray would swing from side to side in a rhythmical motion (Freeborg, Daniel, and Konopinski, 1985).

The final selection of sites will depend on the potential for exposure during a specific activity. If exposure is expected to be limited to the arms, and it has been demonstrated in prior studies of the same task, then there is no benefit to sampling the head, chest, back and so forth (Fig. 14-7). For example, during the picking of sweet corn, the forearms, thighs, head, and shoulders were monitored, whereas picking peas only required forearm and leg pads (EPA, 1988*a*). An-

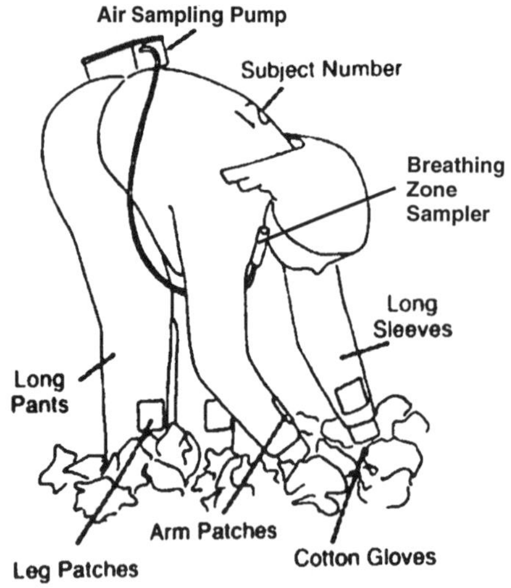

Figure 14-7. Sampling configuration for worker performing hand harvesting.
Source: EPA, Pesticides Hazard Assessment Project. 1988. *Harvestor Exposure Monitoring Studies (1980–1986)*, Vol. I, *Thirteen Studies*. EPA 540/09-88-036. Washington, DC: EPA.

other rationale where the number of dosimeters is reduced has been applied in situations where the pattern of exposures to one chemical is well identified and subsequent studies are conducted on different chemicals (Popendorf, 1980). In this instance the indicator pads are used to adjust for differences in concentrations over the entire body. This can be a cost savings. In some cases, pads have even been taped on the face or attached to the tongue of work shoes. The shoes are laced up so that only a portion of the pad is exposed.

When CPC such as aprons or boots are used, additional decisions must be made as to where to place pads. In one study where all pads were placed outside clothing, if an apron or boot covered any of the exposure sites, pads were placed on the outside of the apron or boot at the same level the pad would be located if the apron or boot were not there (Stamper et al., 1989). When hard hats are required, pads have been placed both under and outside of the hat (Gold and Holcslaw, 1985). Pads have also been taped to the top front of boots. If pants are normally worn over the boot, this position is not changed.

SAMPLING PROCEDURES

Pad Attachment

There are a variety of ways to attach pads to clothing. Some studies have utilized specially designed harnesses or lightweight vests fitted with open-front pockets to hold the shoulder, chest, and back pads in position. Chest pads have also been placed inside shirt pockets. Tabs made from Scotch filament tape can be improvised in the field so the tans can be used to pin pads to the clothing. For arms and legs, the pad can be attached to an elastic band and slid on. Strips of gabardine with Velcro at the ends have been pinned to pads and used for attachment to arms and legs. Velcro has also been attached to the pad backings. For the head, pads are usually pinned to each side or under the brim of a baseball cap, or stapled to a headband. Surgical tape, masking tape, zinc oxide, and safety pins have also been used for attachment.

When pads are placed under garments, various approaches are to tape the pad to the skin under the garment, pin the pad under the same clothing to which the outer pad is attached, or pin or tape the pad to a T-shirt underneath the clothing. Additional methods that can speed up pad replacement are described in a later section.

Pads are also attached directly to the skin. Extreme caution is needed when doing so because of the sensitivity of skin and potential discomfort if the wrong techniques are used. Surgical tape used to attach pads directly to skin is generally nonirritating to perspiring skin and tolerable by the wearer.

Procedure

1. Secure the pad or pad holder with surgical tape to the area where monitoring is to be done.
2. After use, each pad should be placed in an airtight, labeled glass container.
3. For analysis, the tape is cut away from the pad, leaving a 5 cm by 5 cm square. This 25 cm^2 piece is put through a Soxhlet extraction, and the extractant is analyzed. Results are reported in $\mu g/cm^2$.

Monitoring Duration

Monitoring media should be changed during some natural break in the worker's schedule. However, it is difficult to specify in advance the optimal exposure period to monitor for a given contaminant. This period will depend on the nature of the material being used and the activity being studied. The ideal period is long enough to collect sufficient contaminant for analysis but not so long that there is significant loss of material through evaporation, absorption, or chemical conversion. The range of periods used in monitoring studies ranges from 1 hr to 8 hr.

Significant losses of both parathion and Dicofol occurred in one study after fortified fabric patches, including cotton gauze, were exposed to ambient conditions for 4–6 hr (Serat, Van Loon, and Serat, 1982). Therefore, it appears that there is a finite time for collection, which must be determined ahead of time, and other variables such as humidity and workers' perspiration must be considered. Two hours has commonly been used to monitor harvesters, especially when gross contamination is a concern. Pads have also been left on for the entire workday (6–8 hr).

Although it might seem that the longer the monitoring period, the greater likelihood of assessing the true exposure, it has been found that a negative correlation is obtained between the relationship of hours worked and dermal exposure (mg/hr) (EPA, 1988*b*). This result may be due to the dosimeters becoming saturated. Therefore, it is best to change them at regular intervals. Pads are generally removed after no more than 4 hr. If the work requires more time, the pads must be replaced.

Pad Replacement

Removing and replacing pads can be time consuming and therefore must be done as efficiently as possible in order to minimize work interruptions. Pad replacement is done when different tasks are to be monitored, when heavy buildup is suspected, or when gathering information on morning versus afternoon exposures. Unless several people are available to assist in performing sampling, it is best to identify a pad replacement method to cut down on this time. Workers are often in a hurry to eat lunch or take their break and may balk at wearing an extra jacket with pads attached to it or waiting for 10 pads taped to their skin and/or clothing to be removed.

Attaching pads to disposable jackets, coveralls, and hats minimizes the time required for changeovers for resampling. Pads can be attached to coveralls that are donned over existing clothing and worn for the workday. Tape and staples work well for attaching dosimeters to these jackets. When using disposable clothing as a means to attach pads, it should not be assumed that this method will prevent contaminants from reaching the skin. In one study where pads were used on top of and underneath Tyvek coveralls, the Tyvek protected 99 ± 1% from fluvalinate, 89 ± 5% from chlorpyrifos, 96 ± 2% from dicofol, but only 66 ± 11% from ethazol (Stamper et al., 1989). Forearm pad changing can be expedited by the use of pads preattached to a day's supply of elastic wristbands designed for racquet sports (Davis, 1980).

Another way to speed up pad exchange is to staple pads to the outside of fresh white cotton T-shirts and put the shirts on the subjects over their work clothing at the beginning of the exposure period. Following sampling, remove the entire shirt, cutting it away from the body if necessary. T-shirts with pads can also be placed under normal work clothing to account for the ability of the work clothing to deflect and absorb the contaminant before it reaches the skin. If a T-shirt is worn next to the skin of the subject, the dosimeters are exposed to only that portion of the contaminant that would end up on the skin.

Exposure Conditions

Once pads are attached, workers should be instructed not to purposely touch them. One field member should be in charge of recording start and stop times and for calling off the operation if conditions change so as to interfere with getting good samples. For example, when sampling outdoors, heavy winds and extreme cold can significantly change exposures. When interruptions due to weather halt sampling, it is best to change media before workers restart. Mechanical breakdowns should be treated similarly. The circumstances and the time worn will determine if the pads in use prior to the interruption are analyzed.

A photo of each worker in sampling garb is useful for estimating the amount of skin exposed, type of work clothing worn, and CPC worn. Extensive notes (Fig. 14-8) should be taken during sampling including temperature; humidity; wind velocity and direction; duration of sampling; type, concentration, and amount of chemicals present; type of equipment used; and any other parameters relevant to the process. Typical observations often made of the individuals being sampled are physical characteristics (sex, age, weight, height, and body surface) as well as individual productivity. It has been suggested that age correlates positively with productivity, possibly because older workers are more experienced and motivated (EPA, 1988*b*).

Workers need to be observed during monitor-

Revision No.: 1
Date: April 3, 1986
Page 5 of 13

Company Name	Contract Number 68-12-3929	Date (Mo/Da/Yr)
Site ID	Work Assignment No 47	Substance Monitored ACRYLAMIDE

EMPLOYEE AND WORK AREA DATA	
Employee Name	Job Title/Work Duties:
PERSONAL PROTECTIVE EQUIPMENT	
Eye Protection	NOTE: Specify type, material, brand, etc.
Boots/Shoes	Head Protection
Respirator	Gloves
Protective Suit/Coveralls	

DERMAL SAMPLING DATA

Dermal Pad Media: WHATMAN CHROMATOGRAPHY PAPER No. 17 (4 X 4 inch Pads)	Lot No.

Body Region	Start Time	Stop Time	Duration	Sample Numbers	
Back					
Chest					
Forearms				Left	Right
Shoulders				Left	Right
Thighs				Left	Right
Shins				Left	Right
Hand Rinses Solvent:				Left	Right
DISTILLED WATER				Left	Right
				Left	Right

Signature	Date	Checked by:

Figure 7-2. Dermal assessment data sheet

Figure 14-8. Dermal assessment data sheet.
Source: EPA. 1986. *Pesticide Assessment Guidelines, Subdivision U, Applicator Exposure Monitoring*. EPA 540/9-87-127. Washington, DC: Office of Pesticide Programs.

ing since problems during pad sampling can occur. Pads and/or their holders (such as harnesses) can get snagged on branches or equipment. Extremely heavy loading of contaminant or moisture can disintegrate pads. High heat and humidity promote perspiration, which can saturate pads in a short period of time. If a subject's clothing is wet from perspiration, a second backing of aluminum foil should be added to the next set of pads. As with any sampling media, if saturation occurs there may be too much contaminant to do an analysis; therefore, whenever there are heavy deposits of contaminant and extraneous materials (soil, moisture), pads should be removed and replaced (Popendorf and Selin, 1994).

Blanks and Spikes

On the day of sampling, field blanks and spiked samples are prepared. Field blanks of the dermal pads should be handled in the same manner as the exposed pads except they are not attached to the worker. An absorbent pad is removed from the plastic bag container and immediately returned to the bag and resealed. One field blank may be prepared at the beginning of the sampling period and one at the end. Field blanks are stored and shipped with the exposed samples.

Pads are spiked with a known quantity of the material being sampled at the approximate concentration expected to occur. The pads should be spiked with the contaminant(s) to be monitored and extracted. The EPA requires that the mean ± the standard deviation for recovery be determined using seven determinations. If the lower limit of the 95% confidence interval is less than 70%, the extraction procedure is considered unsatisfactory. If extracts are to be stored, a study of stability should be conducted.

One spiked sample is prepared at the beginning of the sampling period and exposed to the same weather conditions as the exposed samples for the duration of the sampling period. The other spiked sample is prepared at the end of the sampling period. Both spiked samples are handled, stored, and shipped in the same manner as the exposed samples.

EPA PROCEDURE FOR SAMPLING WORKERS WITHOUT IMPERVIOUS CPC

The locations of the pads are shown in Figure 14-9 and described in detail as follows (EPA, 1986):

1. On the right and left forearms, midway between the wrist and elbow, on the side of the arm opposite the palm, a pad shall be positioned face-up with the glassine backing flush against the outside of the worker's street clothing using safety pins. If the worker is wearing a short sleeve shirt, attach the pad directly against the skin using surgical tape.
2. On the subject's upper back immediately below the collar, the pad shall be positioned face-up on the outside of the worker's street clothing using safety pins.
3. On the upper chest near the jugular notch, the pad shall be positioned face-up on the

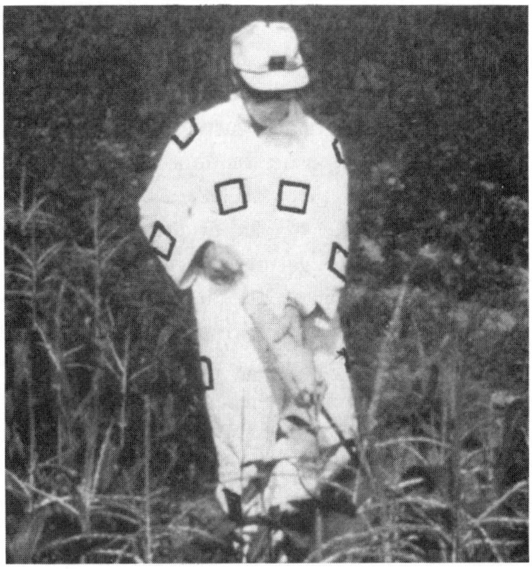

Figure 14-9. Worker wearing pads for EPA procedure for sampling workers without impervious protective clothing.
Source: From D. A. Kurtz and W. M. Bode. 1985. Application exposure to the home gardener. In R. C. Honeycutt, G. Zweig, and N. N. Ragsdale (eds.), *Dermal Exposure Related to Pesticide Use*. Washington, DC: American Chemical Society, p. 142. Reprinted with permission; copyright © 1985 by the American Chemical Society.

outside of the worker's street clothing using safety pins.

4. On the top of the right and left shoulders, a pad shall be positioned face-up with the glassine backing against the outside of the worker's street clothing using safety pins.
5. On the right and left front thighs, a pad shall be positioned face-up with the glassine backing against the outside of the worker's street clothing using safety pins.
6. On the right and left front shins just below the knee, the pad shall be positioned face up with the glassine backing against the outside of the worker's clothing using safety pins. If the worker is wearing shorts, the pad shall be attached directly against the skin using surgical tape.

EPA PROCEDURE FOR SAMPLING WORKERS WEARING IMPERVIOUS CPC

There are certain situations where workers are required to wear protective clothing. Extra pads are often needed in these situations to assess penetration. These pads should be located in regions that are expected to receive maximum exposure such as beneath garment seams. Since the maximum exposure or area of penetration cannot always be accurately anticipated, additional pads may be needed under unseamed areas of protective garments in all the same locations as specified for dermal exposure monitoring of workers not wearing protective clothing. Pads under protective garments should be near, but not covered by, any pads on the outside of the clothing. Even if the label specifies that protective gloves must be worn, hand exposure under the gloves must be assessed. The locations of the pads (EPA, 1986) are:

1. On the right and left forearms midway between the wrist and elbow, on the side of the arm opposite the palm, a pad shall be positioned face-up with the glassine backing taped flush against the skin. Attach the pad with surgical tape applied only to the glassine backing.
2. On the subject's upper back immediately below the collar, the pad shall be positioned face-up on the outside of the protective clothing using safety pins.
3. On the upper chest near the jugular notch, the pad shall be positioned face-up on the outside of the protective clothing using safety pins.
4. On the top of the right and left shoulders, a pad shall be positioned face-up with the glassine backing against the outside of the worker's protective clothing using safety pins.

WHO PROCEDURE USING PADS

The WHO procedure varies somewhat from the EPA's and is commonly used in European studies. Pads are prepared of α-cellulose, 10 cm by 10 cm, backed with glassine paper or aluminum foil (WHO, 1986). WHO stresses prior extraction of pad material so that there will be no interference with the analysis of residues of a particular contaminant.

Pads should be fixed with masking tape covering the edges of the pad only, and attached to clothing with safety pins through the edge of the pad. On each day of application, four workers from the group being surveyed should be chosen serially to wear exposure pads for at least 1 hr, except for the pad attached to the skin, which should be worn the entire day. The attachment of the pads should be checked frequently and corrected if necessary. Pads should be applied as explained below, on clothing (where worn) or on skin. The following applies to a right-handed person; if left-handed people are sampled, opposites apply:

1. Arm: upper surface of left forearm held with elbow bent at right angle across body, midway between elbow and wrist.
2. Leg: front of left leg, above ankle; front of left leg, mid-thigh.
3. Trunk: over sternum; on back between shoulder blades.
4. Head: if head not covered, forehead as high as possible to give good adhesion; if head covered, on hat as close as practicable to top of forehead.
5. In addition, one pad is applied to the skin under clothing to the upper abdomen at ap-

proximately the same height as the arm pad and below the sternal pad but not shielded by it.

Upon removal at the end of the day, a 5 cm by 5 cm square should be cut from the pad. Care should be taken that the scissors or other cutting instruments are not contaminated. Decontamination can be carried out by swabbing with cotton balls soaked in an appropriate solvent.

STORAGE AND HANDLING

At the end of the sampling period, the pads are carefully removed from the worker. Care should be taken not to touch the sampling portion of the absorbent pad. Samples can be handled by their outside perimeters, or clean latex gloves worn or forceps used to remove them. When feasible, fold the dosimeter onto itself before sliding the pad into its original prelabeled plastic bag, and seal or place two dosimeters into the bag face-to-face if they are to be analyzed as one sample. Place all the bags from a single test subject in a sealed container such as a wide-mouth jar or another plastic bag. Seal the jar inside another plastic bag and store the samples in an ice chest at 4°C. Test tubes with covers can also be used to contain pads for transport from the field to the lab and interim storage. Another technique is to use a box with individual compartments spaced close enough so that pads can stand on edge. The compartments should be labeled for the portions of the body to which the pads are attached. After pads have been collected and replaced, the exposed pads can be placed in bags and labeled.

The procedure for handling exposed pads will depend on the stability of the material being studied. There are two methods recommended by the EPA: one for stable contaminants and the other for unstable contaminants (EPA, 1986).

For stable contaminants, remove the tape used to attach the pad to the test subject and also remove the protective backing from the pad. Slide the prelabeled protective envelope just far enough out of the sandwich bag to insert the pad, then carefully put it back into the bag. Staple together all bags containing exposed pads from one exposure of a single test subject without puncturing the area of the bag containing the samples and store in a chest containing ice or an appropriate frozen plastic gel. Refrigerate the bags until they reach the laboratory.

For unstable contaminants, remove the tape used to attach the pad to the test subject. Place a template of a convenient size (25 cm^2 has been used) in the center of the pad and trim away the excess material around the template. Discard the protective backing and place the sample obtained from the center of the pad in a labeled wide mouth jar or other appropriate container filled with a convenient volume of a suitable solvent and close with a Teflon lined lid. Refrigerate these samples.

When glass jars containing up to 400 mL of the solvent that will be used for extraction are used, some precautions are required (Lavy et al., 1980*a*). If a bottle containing solvent is used, the cap of the bottle should have an aluminum or Teflon liner inserted, and the bottle should be closed and shaken gently to ensure that the whole pad is wetted with the solvent. The exterior of the bag or bottle should be labeled clearly with the date, worker's name, site of the pad, and whether it was attached to clothing or skin. A suggested labeling system uses D for date, C for clothing, and S for skin, so that a sample for person number 6 might be labeled D3 6 Thigh C.

Transport of pads in solvent has been successful in situations where losses occurred from dry pads. Dimethoate applied to cellulose decreased by 90% after three weeks' storage; when benzene was added to pads in bottles and used for transport and storage, 89% of the original amount was recovered (Copplestone et al., 1976). If pads are taped, the tape should be cut from the edges prior to immersion into any solvent for transport or analysis, since the glue from the tape may interfere with analyses. If light sensitivity is an issue, amber jars should be used. This technique may not be appropriate for samples shipped by air.

Storage times must be determined ahead of time if pads will not be analyzed within 48 hours. Dimethoate applied to cellulose diminished to approximately 10% after three weeks' storage. Ten mL benzene added to pads in bottles and used for transport and storage produced 89% recovery. If exposed pads are to be stored pending extraction, then a study must be done beforehand to determine the stability of the material on spiked exposure pads similar to those previously discussed. The pads and their protective bags are to be stored for a time period chosen so that the longest period corresponds to the greatest projected storage period for field samples. At the end of each time period, samples are extracted and analyzed by the methods that will be used for field studies. A decay curve can then be constructed that will allow extrapolation of contaminant levels found in field samples back to the time of collection. These results can also be used to determine the length of time acceptable for pad storage prior to analysis. This is particularly important where the stability of the contaminant to be collected is unknown or if the material is volatile or subject to degradation.

ANALYSIS

Cellulose and Gauze Pad Samples

The analytical procedure used for the dosimeters should be capable of quantitative detection of material on exposure pads at a level of 1 μg per cm^2 or less to meet EPA criteria (EPA, 1986). Results are reported as μg per cm^2 of patch area. The efficiency of the extraction method is also important.

There are two different ways of analyzing pads. One method is to combine pads from opposite sides of the body prior to extraction. For example, both forearms would be combined as well as both legs. However, if exposure values from particular pads are needed for calculations, these pads must be extracted individually. Examples of pads that should not be combined are those from the chest and back and exterior pads adjacent to pads under clothing that will be used to estimate penetration. Also, if there is a concern that a specific work practice or piece of equipment may impact exposure, then individual pad analysis may be desirable.

Pads can be extracted in the same jars in which they are shipped (if this is the case) so long as they are the proper size. Otherwise, in the laboratory each pad is removed from its container and the margins including tape of each pad are cut away with a paper trimmer, leaving a central area. Backings are removed. The portion of the pad is then extracted with a solvent and analyzed. Another method is to cut the edges off of the exposed pad using a cutting board, for example, a 4 in. by 4 in. pad would be cut into a 2.5 in. by 2.5 in. pad (Nigg, Stamper, and Mahon, 1990). The center portion is then quartered and extracted. Sometimes only a portion of a pad is extracted. One methodology recommends that a 2 in. by 2 in. section (5 cm by 5 cm) be cut from a 4 in. by 4 in. (10 cm by 10 cm) cellulose pad and this smaller section is extracted for analysis. If pads are cut prior to analysis, then the paper cutter, knife, or scissor should be decontaminated in between each pad with the same solvent to be used for extraction.

If the pad has been stored in a paper envelope inside a plastic bag or between filter papers, the envelope or filters can be treated as part of the sample and analyzed along with the pad (Herman, Hunt, and Sheets, 1985). If a gauze pad is attached to an α-cellulose layer, the two can be extracted together. Pads can be placed in a separatory funnel for extraction.

If pads are not preextracted, cleanup is sometimes required before the samples can be analyzed. This is done by taking the extracts and running them through a nondestructive procedure such as HPLC. If the compound of interest has a metallic constituent, such as lead arsenate, pads are often analyzed for just the metal, rather than the specific compound, because specific methods for metals are standardized and this type of analysis is widely available.

Charcoal Pads

Following collection, a correction must be made, because charcoal has a much higher adsorptive surface area than human skin, and the amount of vapors adsorbed onto the charcoal pad will be several times higher than the amount that could be adsorbed onto a similar area of human skin (Cohen and Popendorf, 1989). Also, the total amount of chemical collected on the dosimeter

TABLE 14-5. Estimated Retention Efficiencies for Charcoal Cloth Pads as a Function of Vapor Pressure, Retained Liquid, and Humidity

VP (mmHg):	0.3				1.0				4.0				10				15			
RL (μL):	10	25	60	100	10	25	60	100	10	25	60	100	10	25	60	100	10	25	60	100
RH(%)																				
30	94	93	92	92	92	90	89	88	87	85	83	82	83	81	77	75	81	78	75	72
50	91	90	89	88	88	86	84	83	81	78	75	73	75	71	66	63	72	67	61	58
70	89	87	85	84	84	82	79	77	75	72	67	64	67	62	55	51	62	56	49	43
90	87	84	82	81	81	78	74	72	70	75	60	56	60	52	44	38	53	45	34	26

Source: From Cohen, B. M., and W. Popendorf. 1989. A method for monitoring dermal exposure to volatile chemicals. *AIHA J.* **50**(4):216–223.

would include depositions from both the liquid phase and the vapor phase in the case of materials that are being sprayed. The following calculation can be used to determine the initial liquid deposit to the charcoal pad:

$$\text{Initial liquid deposit} = \frac{\text{Total amount} - \text{adsorbed vapors}}{\text{RE}/100}$$

where the total amount is obtained from the desorption and analysis of the cloth in the dosimeter, RE is the retention efficiency, and the amount of adsorbed vapors is unknown (Table 14-5).

If the deposition rate is less than the adsorption rate, the deposition rate will be the limiting factor. Under these conditions, it might be expected that the majority or a high fraction of the deposition would be adsorbed, depending on the adsorption rate coefficient. If the deposition rate is greater than the adsorption rate, the adsorption rate will be the limiting factor, for example, immersion of the skin into chemicals with low adsorption potential, or deposition of larger quantities of these chemicals by splashing (Cohen and Popendorf, 1989).

CALCULATION OF RESULTS

The resulting measured levels of contaminant can be used in several ways as presented in the example shown in Table 14-6. Most of the following calculations would apply equally well to pads placed either inside or outside of clothing. The example given in Table 14-6 is for dose inside the clothing, but the following discussion uses the more generic term *deposition*. The first step may be to calculate the dermal deposition density. To do this, the total micrograms of contaminant found during analysis (column B), which may or may not be adjusted for collection efficiency, is divided by the surface area of the pads (column C), usually expressed in cm^2.

$$\text{Dermal deposition density } (\mu g/cm^2) = \frac{\text{Chemical mass}}{\text{Dosimeter area}}$$

In the example selected, pairs of 28 cm^2 dosimeters were used, except for the chest and back (which had only one pad) and the hands, which used gloves. Glove dosimeters are treated like full-body dosimeters; the areas of the dosimeters correspond to the body areas covered as shown near the bottom of columns C and D. (See also Chapter 15 for a further discussion of whole body monitoring.) Note that the anatomic areas in Table 14-6 were those reported and do not correspond to those listed in Table 14-3. Dermal deposition density (column E) is useful without further modification to assess the risk of dermatitis. However, there is no rationale for adding these density values.

Several assumptions are used to estimate the worker's total dermal deposition (column F).

TABLE 14-6. Example of Dermal Dosimeter Result Calculations for a Pesticide Mixer-Loader

A	B	C	D	E	F	G	H
Dosimeter Location	*Chemical Mass (μg)*	*Dosimeter Area (cm^2)*	*Anatomic Area (cm^2)*	*Dose Density (μg/cm^2/h)*	*Total Dose (mg)*	*Dose Rate (mg/hr)*	*Equivalent Dose of Dust (mg)*
Head	22.2	56	1300	.099	.704	.176	.88
Chest	1.45	28	2190	.013	.112	.028	.14
Back	0.56	28	2190	.005	.044	.011	.055
Upper leg	57.6	56	3460	.257	5.024	1.256	6.28
Lower leg	5.15	56	2600	.023	.244	.061	.31
Upper arm	4.70	56	1860	.021	.176	.044	.22
Lower arm	17.2	56	1290	.077	.424	.106	.53
Hand	22.36	2150	2150	5.59	22.36	12.15	27.9
Totals					29.09	13.83	36.3

Source: Adapted from data reported by Popendorf (1988) for mixer-loader dermal doses to an 80% AI solid formulation (sprills) of captafol for 4 hours.

First, it is necessary to extrapolate the amount of material found on each unit area of pad to the amount that would have been deposited on the total body region represented by the pad:

$$\text{Dermal deposition (mg)} = \text{Chemical mass}\ \frac{\text{Anatomic area}}{\text{Dosimeter area}}$$

This calculation assumes that the dermal deposition of the chemical reaching each pad represents the mean of that reaching the corresponding region of the body. The validity of this assumption can be qualitatively judged based on observation of the setting. A set of standard body surface areas is typically used (see Table 14-3 for adults other than column D). If dosimeters were only placed outside the clothing, then an assumption would also need to be made as to how much of the residue found on a pad would have penetrated the worker's clothing. Some assumed values are listed in Table 11-3, although they are much higher than the 3–7% penetration measured in the cited example (the results of outside pads is not shown herein). The results of hypothetical changes in the work practices or use methods can be predicted by varying the assumptions as suggested below.

At this stage, the distribution of deposition by body location is usually readily apparent. As can be seen in Table 14-6, hands were the major site of deposition because no gloves were worn. The data also indicates that had protective gloves been worn (assume for the moment that hand doses were near zero), the upper legs would have been the next major site of skin deposition. This scenario suggests the next most important change in work methods or protective clothing beyond gloves.

It is also only at this stage and beyond that the set of dermal depositions at each location can be meaningfully added to yield a total. The total dose to the cited mixer-loader is 29 mg of the measured chemical. In practice, both the distribution and the measured total dermal depositions can vary quite widely among people or settings. Geometric deviations in low total doses of antimicrobial chemicals applied in industrial settings ranged from 4× to 9× (Popendorf, Selim, and Lewis, 1994). However, geometric deviations less than 2× have also been reported between repeated measures on the same person when the mechanism of exposure was more uniform (Popendorf, 1988). While variability can be useful to identify important interpersonal differences in work practices, it may require some replication in measurements to establish a reliable central tendency such as a mean or geometric mean or an estimate of clothing penetration.

One additional common step is to compare the dermal dose to the airborne dose. This comparison can include adjustment factors for both dermal adsorption (as discussed in Chapter 2 and other references cited therein) and/or for respiratory retention, which is usually also well less than 100% either for particles (where the site of deposition and retention varies by particle size) or for gases and vapors (where retention varies by chemical). As a first approximation, nominal doses or dose rates are often compared without adjustments. The nominal airborne dose can be calculated by multiplying airborne concentration (C, mg/m^3) times respiratory minute volume (RMV, Lpm, or the equivalent m^3/hr) times exposure duration. Typical respiratory minute volumes are 20.8 Lpm (corresponding to 10 m^3/8-hours for light work rates; see also Table 2-8) or 29 Lpm for moderate work as recommended by EPA (1987). Thus far, most reported comparisons have involved low volatility compounds and nominal dermal doses predominate by a ratio on the order of 100:1 over airborne doses (some exceptions are noted in Table 11-6).

The remaining steps are various options to adjust or normalize the data for some denominator common across multiple settings. One option is to divide by the amount of material applied or used during the assessment, for instance mg dose per kg or pound applied (Franklin et al., 1981). A more common practice, used particularly in the agricultural pesticide sector, is to divide by the duration of the assessment to calculate the dose rate (column G in Table 14-6):

$$\text{Dermal deposition rate (mg/hr)} = \frac{\text{Dermal deposition}}{\text{Task or exposure time}}$$

The final option, if the measured chemical is part of a mixture, is to adjust from the amount of measured chemical to the amount of the entire solution or solid matrix deposited:

$$\text{Equivalent dermal deposition (mg or g)} = \frac{\text{Dermal deposition}}{\text{Contaminant concentration}}$$

Equivalent dose is very useful to compare results if data is collected in settings in which the solution concentrations vary or to apply results from one mixture to another at a different concentration (Table 14-7). In the latter case, the equivalent dermal deposition would be multiplied times the new concentration to yield exposures or doses expected in the new setting (Popendorf, Selim, and Lewis, 1994). The equivalent dose of formulated product for mixer-loaders (labelled "dust" in column H) is not much different than the dose of active ingredient because in this case 80% of the compound being deposited was the measured chemical. However, the measured chemical comprised only 0.12% of the aqueous mixture to which the associated spray applicator was exposed (either as a mist or on contaminated surfaces), resulting in equivalent doses expressed most appropriately in grams.

TABLE 14-7. Example of Dermal Dosimeter Result Calculations for a Pesticide Applicator

A	B	C	D	E	F	G	H
Dosimeter Location	*Chemical Mass (µg)*	*Dosimeter Area (cm²)*	*Anatomic Area (cm²)*	*Dose Density (µg/cm²/h)*	*Total Dose (mg)*	*Dose Rate (mg/hr)*	*Equivalent Dose of Mist (g)*
Head	19.2	56	1300	.215	1.59	.319	1.32
Chest	2.38	28	2190	.017	.185	.037	.154
Back	1.40	28	2190	.010	.135	.027	.112
Upper leg	34.4	56	3460	.123	2.36	.473	1.97
Lower leg	4.20	56	2600	.015	.290	.058	.242
Upper arm	12.9	56	1860	.046	.495	.099	.412
Lower arm	44.5	56	1290	.159	1.55	.310	1.29
Hand	126	2150	2150	11.6	126	25.2	105
Totals					132.6	25.31	110.4

Source: Adapted from data reported by Popendorf (1988) for spray applicator dermal doses to a 0.12% AI aqueous mixture of captafol for 5 hours.

FUTURE APPLICATIONS

Since the trend is to apply pad sampling to techniques to industrial contaminants, validations will be necessary to determine the behavior of new chemicals when sampled with pads. The procedure used for new pesticides may be applicable in this instance. The EPA requires that each exposure situation for new pesticides be evaluated using at least 15 replicates. Each replicate is a measure of the exposure to one worker for one exposure period. To obtain a single "typical" exposure for the situation being studied, one must include individual values obtained under as many different conditions expected to significantly affect exposure as possible. Three variables expected to have the most significant effect on exposure are differences in application equipment, wind conditions during outdoor applications, and most importantly, different work practices and attitudes toward safety of the study subjects. The EPA also recommends that there be a minimum of five replicates from each of three different application sites. It is recommended that the replicates be obtained using as many different workers as possible.

Another method that may prove useful for estimating exposures to mineral and metallic dusts is the use of double-face adhesive tape. This method has been used to measure the deposition of particles onto various parts of clothing in a dust resuspension study with CuO (Fish et al., 1965). The average rate of transfer in terms of concentration of particles per cm^2 of tape compared with the particles per cm^2 of floor surfaces was determined after two people swept floors (Fig. 14-10).

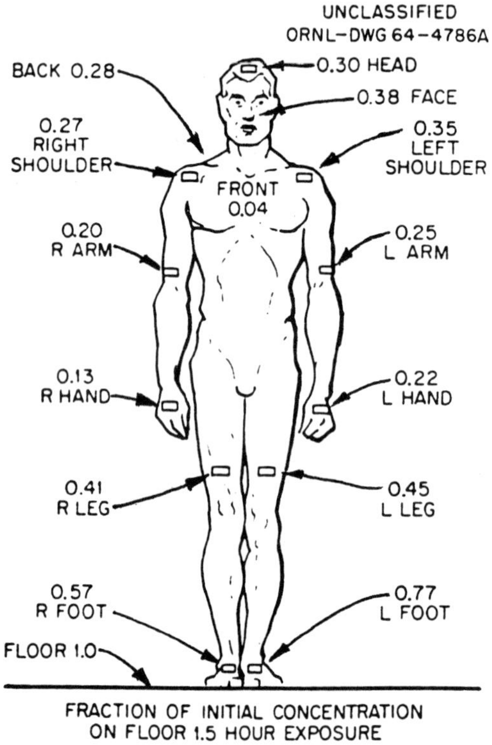

Figure 14-10. Deposition of redispersed CuO particles on clothing.
Source: From B. R. Fish, R. L. Walker, G. W. Royster, and J. L. Thompson. 1965. Redispersion of settled particulates. In G. W. Royster and B. R. Fish (eds.), *Surface Contamination*. London: Pergamon Press, p. 80.

REFERENCES

Al-Jaghbir, M. T., A. S. Salhab, and F. A. Hamarsheh. 1992. Dermal and inhalation exposure to methoate. *Arch. Env. Contam. Toxicol.* **22:**358–361.

Bandara, J. M. R. S., P. C. Kearney, P. G. Vincent, and W. A. Gentner. 1985. Paraquat: A model for measuring exposure. In R. C. Honeycutt, G. Zweig, and N. N. Ragsdale (eds.), *Dermal Exposure Related to Pesticide Use*. Washington, DC: American Chemical Society, p. 279–285.

Berkow, J. 1931. Surface area of the human anatomy. *Am. J. Surgery* **2:**315.

Carman, G. E., Y. Iwata, J. L. Pappas, J. R. O'Neal, and F. A. Gunther. 1982. Pesticide applicator exposure to insecticides during treatment of citrus trees with oscillating boom and air blast units. *Arch. Env. Contam. Toxicol.* **11:**651–659.

Chester, G., and R J. Ward. 1984. Occupational exposure and drift hazard during aerial application of paraquat to cotton. *Arch. Env. Contam. Toxicol.* **13:**551–563.

Chester, G., and B. H. Woolen. 1981. Studies of the occupational exposure of Malaysian plantation workers to paraquat. *Brit. J. Ind. Med.* **38:**23–33.

Clapp, D. E., G. M. Piacitelli, D. D. Zaebst, and E. Ward. 1991. Assessing exposure to 4,4'-methylene bis(2-chloroaniline) (MBOCA) in the workplace. *Appl. Occup. Env. Hyg.* **6**(2):125–130.

Cohen, B. M., and W. Popendorf. 1989. A method for monitoring dermal exposure to volatile chemicals. *AIHA J.* **50**(4):216–223.

Copplestone, J. F., Z. I. Fakhri, J. W. Miles, C. A. Mitchell, Y. Osman, and H. R. Wolfe. 1976. Exposure to pesticides in agriculture: A survey of spraymen using dimethoate in the Sudan. *Bull. WHO* **54:**217–223.

Culver, D., P. Caplan, and G. S. Batchelor. 1956. Studies of human exposure during aerosol application of malathion and chlorthion. *Arch. Ind. Health* **32:**37–50.

Davis, J. E. 1980. Minimizing occupational exposure to pesticides: Personal monitoring. *Res. Rev.* **75:**34–49.

Devine, J. M., G. B. Kinoshita, R. P. Peterson, and G. L. Picard. 1986. Farm worker exposure to Terbufos (phosphorodithioic acid, S-(tert-butylthio) methyl O,O-diethyl ester) during planting operations of corn. *Arch. Env. Contam. Toxicol.* **15:**113–119.

Dubelman, S., R. Lauer, D. D. Arras, and S. A. Adams. 1982. Operator exposure measurements during application of the herbicide Diallate. *J. Agric. Food Chem.* **30:**526–532.

Dubois, D., and E. F. Dubois. 1916. Clinical calorimetry. Tenth paper. A formula to estimate the approximate surface area if height and weight be known. *Arch. Int. Med.* **17:**863–871.

Durham, W. F., and H. R. Wolfe. 1962. Measurement of the exposure of workers to pesticides. *Bull. World Health Organ.* **26:**75–91.

EPA. 1986. *Pesticide Assessment Guidelines Subdivision U, Applicator Exposure Monitoring*. EPA 540/9-87-127. Washington, DC: Office of Pesticide Programs.

EPA. 1987. *Acrylamide Grouting Exposure Assessment*. EPA 560/5-87-009. Washington, DC.

EPA Pesticide Hazard Assessment Project. 1988*a*. *Harvester Exposure Monitoring Studies (1980–1986)*, vol. 1. EPA 540/09-88-036. Washington, DC: EPA.

EPA Pesticide Hazard Assessment Project. 1988*b*. *Harvester Exposure Monitoring Studies (1980–1986)*, vol. 2. EPA 540/09-88-037. Washington, DC: EPA.

Fenske, R. A. 1990. Nonuniform dermal deposition patterns during occupational exposure to pesticides. *Arch. Env. Contam. Toxicol.* **19:**332–337.

Fenske, R. A. 1993. Dermal exposure measurement techniques. *Ann. Occup. Hyg.* **37:**687–706.

Fenske, R. A., S. J. Hamburger, and C. L. Guyton. 1987. Occupational exposure to Fosetyl-Al fungicide during spraying of ornamentals in greenhouses. *Arch. Env. Contam. Toxicol.* **16:**615–621.

Fenske, R. A., P. B. Curry, F. Wandelmaier, and L. Ritter. 1991. Development of dermal and respiratory sampling procedures for human exposure to pesticides in indoor environments. *J. Exp. Anal. Env. Epidemol.* **1**(1):11–29.

Fish, B. R., R. L. Walker, G. W. Royster, and J. L. Thompson. 1965. Redispersion of settled particulates. In G. W. Royster and B. R. Fish (eds.), *Surface Contamination*. London: Pergamon Press.

Fletcher, T. E., J. M. Press, and D. B. Wilson. 1959. Exposure of spray-men to dieldrin in residual spraying. *Bull. Wld. Health Org.* **20:**15–25.

Franklin, C. A., R. A. Fenske, R. Greenhalgh, L. Mathieu, H. V. Denley, J. T. Leffingwell, and R. C. Spear. 1981. Correlation of urinary pesticide metabolite excretion with estimated dermal contact in the course of occupational exposure to guthion. *J. Toxicol. Env. Health* **7**(5):715–731.

Freeborg, R. P., W. H. Daniel, and V. J. Konopinski. 1985. Applicator exposure to pesticides applied to turfgrass. In R. C. Honeycutt, G. Zweig, and N. N. Ragsdale (eds.), *Dermal Exposure Related to Pesticide Use*. Washington, DC: American Chemical Society.

Gold, R. E., and T. Holcslaw. 1985. Dermal and respiratory exposure of applicators and residents to dichlorovos-treated residences. In R. C. Honeycutt, G. Zweig, and N. N. Ragsdale (eds.), *Dermal Exposure Related to Pesticide Use*. Washington, DC: American Chemical Society, pp. 253–264.

Grover, R., H. J. Cesona, N. I. Muir, D. Riedel, C. A. Franklin, and K. Yoshida. 1986. Factors affecting the exposure of ground rig applicators to 2,4-dimethylamine salt. *Arch. Env. Contam. Toxicol.* **15:**677–686.

Hattula, M. L., V. Wasenius, and A. U. Arstila. 1979. The exposure to MCPA in the use of clearing saw. *Chemosphere* **7:**473–476.

Hayes, W. J. 1975. *Toxicology of Pesticides*. Baltimore, MD: Williams & Wilkins Co.

Herman, N. D., T. W. Hunt, and T. J. Sheets. 1985. Hand harvester exposure to maleic hydrazide in flue-cured tobacco. *Bull. Env. Contam. Toxicol.* **34:**469–475.

Honeycutt, R. C. 1986. NACA overview on assessment of mixer-loader-applicator exposure to pesticides. *Toxicol. Letters* **33:**175–182.

Hunt, T. W., G. W. Wojeck, and T. J. Sheets. 1985. Applicator exposure to maleic hydrazide (MH) in flue-cured tobacco. *Bull. Env. Contam. Toxicol.* **34:**403–406.

Hussain, M., K. Yoshida, M. Atiemo, and D. Johnston. 1990. Occupational exposure of grain farmers to carbofuran. *Arch. Env. Contam. Toxicol.* **19:**197–204.

Jongeneelen, F. J., P. T. J. Scheepers, A. Groenendijk, L. A. G. J. M. Van Aerts, R. B. M. Anzion, R. P. Bos, and S. J. Veenstra. 1988. Airborne concentrations, skin contamination, and urinary metabolite excretion of polycyclic aromatic hydrocarbons among paving workers exposed to coal tar derived road tars. *AIHA J.* **49**(12):600–607.

Kamble, S. T., C. L. Ogg, R. E. Gold, and A. D. Vance. 1992. Exposure of applicators and residents to chlordane and heptachlor when used for subterranean termite control. *Arch. Env. Contam. Toxicol.* **22:**253–259.

Kilgore, W., C. Fischer, J. Rivers, N. Akesson, J. Wicks, W. Winters, and W. Winterlin. 1984. Human exposure to DEF/merphos. *Res. Rev.* **91:**S71–101.

Knaak, J. B., K. T. Maddy, M. A. Gallo, D. T. Lillie, E. M. Craine, and W. F. Serat. 1978. Worker reentry study involving phosalone application to citrus groves. *Tox. Appl. Pharm.* **46:**363–374.

Kurtz, D. A., and W. M. Bode. 1985. Application exposure to the home gardener. In R. C. Honeycutt, G. Zweig, and N. N. Ragsdale (eds.), *Dermal Exposure Related to Pesticide Use.* Washington, DC: American Chemical Society, pp. 139–161.

Lavy, T. L., J. S. Shepard, and D. C. Bouchard. 1980*b*. Field worker exposure and helicopter spray pattern of 2,4,5-T. *Bull. Env. Contam. Toxicol.* **24:**90–96.

Lavy, T. L., J. S. Shepard, and J. D. Mattice. 1980*a*. Exposure measurements of applicators spraying (2,4,5-trichlorophenoxy)acetic acid in the forest. *J. Agric. Food Chem.* **28**(3):626–630.

Maddy, K. T., R. G. Wang, and C. K. Winter. 1983. *Dermal Exposure Monitoring of Mixers, Loaders, and Applicators of Pesticides in California.* HS-1069, Worker Health and Safety Unit, State of California, pp. 1–7.

Maitlen, J. C., C. R. Sell, and L. M. McDonough. 1982. Workers in the agricultural environment: Dermal exposure to carbaryl. In *Pesticide Residues and Exposure.* Washington, DC: American Chemical Society, pp. 83–103.

Neto, J. G. Gachado, T. Matuo, and Y. K. Matuo. 1992. Dermal exposure of pesticide applicators in staked tomato (*Lycopersicon esculentum mii*) crops: Efficiency of a safety measure in the application equipment. *Bull. Env. Contam. Toxicol.* **48:**529–534.

Nigg, H. N., and J. H. Stamper. 1985. Field studies: Methods overview. In R. C. Honeycutt, G. Zweig, and N. N. Ragsdale (eds.), *Dermal Exposure Related to Pesticide Use.* Washington, DC: American Chemical Society.

Nigg, H. N., J. H. Stamper, and R. M. Queen. 1986. Dicofol exposure to Florida citrus applicators: Effects of protective clothing. *Arch. Env. Contam. Toxicol.* **15:**121–134.

Nigg, H. N., J. H. Stamper, and W. D. Mahon. 1990. Handgun applicator exposure to ethion in Florida citrus. *Arch. Env. Contam. Toxicol.* **45:**463–468.

Nigg, H. N., J. H. Stamper, S. N. Deshmukh, and R. M. Queen. 1991. 4,4'-Dichlorobenzilic acid urinary excretion by dicofol pesticide applicators. *Chemosphere* **22**(3/4):365–373.

NIOSH, Health Hazard Evaluation Report. September 1985. *Steinmetz and Sons, Moscow, PA.* HETA 84-508-1626. Cincinnati, OH: NIOSH.

Noel, M. E., G. Zweig, and W. J. Popendorf. 1983. Abstract Papers, 185th National Meeting. American Chemical Society. CHAS 27. Washington, DC.

Popendorf, W. J. 1976. An Industrial Hygiene Investigation into the Occupational Hazard of Parathion Residues to Citrus Harvesters. Ph.D. dissertation, University of California, Berkeley, CA.

Popendorf, W. J. 1980. Exploring citrus harvesters exposure to pesticide contaminated foliar dust. *AIHA J.* **41**(9):652–659.

Popendorf, W. J. 1989. Mechanisms of clothing exposure and dermal dosing during spray application. In *Second International Symposium on the Performance of Protective Clothing.* Philadelphia: ASTM Publications.

Popendorf, W. J., J. T. Leffingwell, and B. Cohen. 1983. *Nematocide Exposure Assessment Field Studies 1981–1982.* Pesticide Hazard Assessment Project, University of California and University of Iowa, Final Report.

Popendorf, W. J., M. Selim, and M. Q. Lewis. 1994. Exposure while applying antimicrobial pesticides. *AIHA J.* (in press).

Popendorf, W. J., R. C. Spear, J. T. Leffinwell, Y. Yager, and E. Kahn. 1979. Harvester exposures to Zolone® (Phosalone) residues in peach orchards. *JOM* **21**(3):189–194.

Prinsen, G. H., and N. J. Van Sittert. 1980. Exposure and medical monitoring study of a new synthetic pyrethroid after one season of spraying on cotton in Ivory Coast. In W. F. Tordoir, and E. A. H. van Heemstra (eds.), *Field Worker Exposure During Pesticide Application.* Amsterdam: Elsevier, pp. 105–120.

Putnam, A. R., M. D. Willis, L. K. Binning, and P. F. Boldt. 1983. Exposure of pesticide applicators to Nitrofen: Influence of formulation, handling systems, and protective garments. *J. Agric. Food Chem.* **31:**645–650.

Serat, W. F., A. J. Van Loon, and W. H. Serat. 1982. Loss of pesticides from patches used in the field as pesticide collectors. *Arch. Env. Contam. Toxicol.* **11:**227–234.

Spear, R. D., W. J. Popendorf, J. T. Leffingwell, T. H. Milby, J. E. Davies, and W. F. Spencer. 1977. Fieldworkers' response to weather residues of parathion. *JOM* **19:**406–410.

Spittler, T. D., and J. B. Bourke. 1985. Potential exposure in the application of pesticides to orchard and field crops. In R. C. Honeycutt, G. Zweig, and N. N. Ragsdale (eds.), *Dermal Exposure Related to Pesticide Use.* Washington, DC: American Chemical Society.

Stamper, J. H., H. N. Nigg, and R. M. Queen. 1986. Prediction of pesticide dermal exposure and urinary metabolite level of tree crop harvesters from field residues. *Bull. Env. Contam. Toxicol.* **36:**693–700.

Stamper, J. H., H. N. Nigg, W. D. Mahon, A. P. Neilsen, and M. D. Royer. 1989. Pesticide exposure to greenhouse handgunners. *Arch. Env. Contam. Toxicol.* **18:**515–529.

WHO. 1986. Field surveys of exposure to pesticides: Standard protocol. Pesticide Development and Safe Use Unit. Division of Vector Biology and Control, WHO Headquarters, Geneva. *Toxicol. Letters* **33:**223–235.

Winterlin, W. L., W. W. Kilgore, C. R. Mourer, and S. R. Schoen. 1984. Worker reentry studies for captan applied to strawberries in California. *J. Agric. Food Chem.* **32:**664–672.

CHAPTER 15

Clothing for Dosimetry and Protection

Whole items of clothing used as samplers eliminate the need to extrapolate an exposure from a smaller collecting device such as a pad over the body surface. Clothing items are usually prepared and placed on the subject for the specific purpose of sampling although workers' personal clothing has also been collected for analysis. A typical situation where this might be done is shown in Figure 15-1. The worker dumping bags of lead pigment could contaminate his personal vehicle and his residence by wearing this clothing home. Cotton clothing is often used for dosimetry because of its high absorbency and minimal penetration by sprays and dusts. Testing of chemical protective clothing (CPC) is often done before it is issued to workers after being selected for field suitability. Testing can also be useful in determining CPC service life, the cycle over which it can be reused, and the appropriateness and effectiveness of decontamination methods.

Gloves have been used for the hands, short sleeve undershirts for the upper part of the body, socks for the feet, and the tops of socks for both ankles and wrists. Work clothing has also been analyzed after laundering to determine the effectiveness of laundering. In the case of polycyclic aromatic hydrocarbons (PAHs) and pesticides, significant residuals have been identified after the use of common laundering techniques.

Whole items of clothing usually contain material that must be extracted prior to use and require large amounts of solvent for extraction of contaminants. Since they often contain interfering materials, these must also be preextracted prior to use, requiring additional solvents, although in some cases washing with detergent several times has been sufficient. The adequate preextraction of interfering additives can necessitate extensive extraction equipment and lengthy extraction periods. Most commercial labs are not set up to do this type of analysis; therefore, people performing studies either need access to their own laboratory and analytical personnel or special arrangements need to be made with an outside laboratory. The solvent to be used for extracting clothing should be tested for its effectiveness. One solvent may extract different compounds with varying efficiency, and results from studies in which different solvents have been used may not be comparable.

It is very difficult to change clothing or underclothing after each exposure period without interfering with the work pace. Also, it is nearly impossible to remove these garments without contaminating them with residues from other

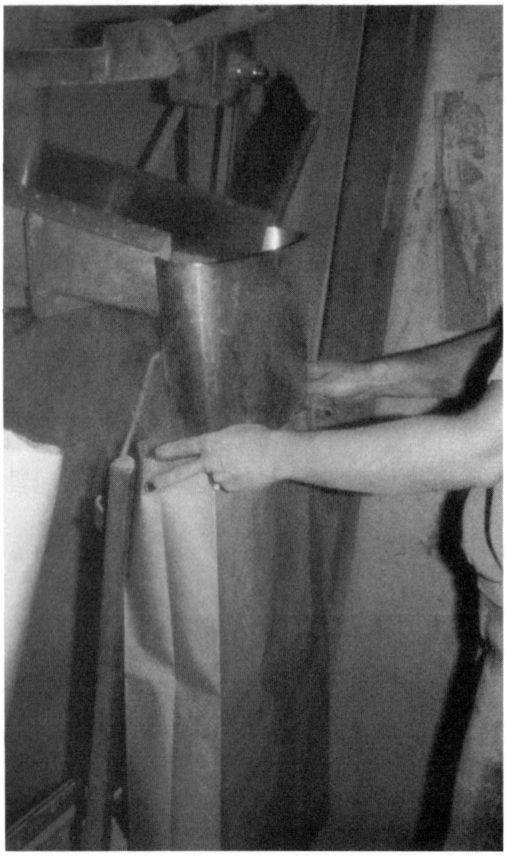

Figure 15-1. Worker filling bags with lead pigment. Note contamination on hands and clothing.

areas of the body, especially those on the workers' hands and hair unless special precautions are taken. Occasionally a garment may have to be cut off the subject in order to avoid its contamination by some part of the body. T-shirts fall into this category. However, the upper portion of a sock that has been used to measure exposure of the lower arm and wrist may be removed by slipping it over a plastic bag used to cover the hand. Clean disposable gloves should always be worn when removing and handling items of clothing used for sampling. Clothing used as samplers has the advantage of decreasing exposure to the skin; however, it can saturate and, once contaminated, become a source of continuing exposure. Lastly, covering contamination already present on the hands or body with dosimeter clothing may result in an increased exposure of the test subjects due to occlusion, so hygiene is important.

HANDS

Most studies agree that the hands generally experience the greatest exposure in many different operations. Absorbent gloves are a popular method for measuring contaminants contacting the hands. The Environmental Protection Agency (EPA) has recommended their use for pesticide reentry studies (EPA, 1986). Two types of lightweight absorbent gloves are used most frequently: white 100% cotton gloves (also known as "pallbearer's gloves," photographic-darkroom gloves, or electronics assembly gloves), which are white cotton twill work gloves with knit wristlets and seamless palms, and white nylon gloves similar to those used for fruit picking. Nylon gloves are lint-free and some studies have found them easier to extract than cotton gloves (EPA, 1988*a*). When both cotton and nylon gloves were used to monitor workers (at separate times) who were involved in thinning apples sprayed with Phosalone it was determined that there was no significant difference in the amount of Phosalone collected on either type of glove (Davis et al., 1982). Therefore, their collection characteristics were very similar for this application. Although short-sleeve gloves are the most commonly used, long-sleeve gloves have been used when both hand and forearm exposures were expected to be significant, for example, during crop harvesting. Glove samplers can be worn either in place of or underneath protective gloves, such as nitrile, to estimate permeability.

The amount of time that each subject wears the gloves should be recorded. A typical period of time for gloves to be worn is 1–2 hr. Often a second pair of gloves is put on in the afternoon for a similar time period. Gloves should be replaced whenever obvious staining or moisture has soaked into them. The best exposure period for gloves can be determined through pilot studies before actual monitoring is performed in order to improve field accuracy. One method is to expose gloves in the laboratory to varying concentrations of contaminant for specified periods of time and use washes of the subjects' hands to determine the degree of breakthrough (Brouwer et al., 1992). For chlorothalonil it was determined to be 5% after 1 hr, so during the actual monitoring the gloves were replaced hourly over the entire day. Breakthrough can also be determined in field studies; however, interpretation can be difficult and will require follow-up studies for better quantitation.

Studies have examined both the amount of material collected and retained by gloves as well as the likelihood of breakthrough during the monitoring period. Nylon gloves collected 90–95% of the organophosphate residue that workers contacted on citrus trees (Popendorf et al., 1979). It remained on the surface of the gloves and did not penetrate to their skin. Captan residues recovered from the hands beneath the gloves indicated that breakthrough occurred within the 0.5 hr sampling interval and increased with sampling time. Glove exposure was equal to bare hand (hand rinse) exposure for the 1 hr sampling interval and exceeded bare hand exposure for longer sampling times. The decrease in glove collection rates was due to buildup of residues on the hand beneath the glove. The study indicated that cotton gloves used as monitors produce significantly higher estimates of exposure than hand washing for short sampling periods only (<1.5 hr). When used for sampling, cotton gloves can be worn over uncontaminated latex surgical gloves if there is a concern regarding breakthrough (Fenske, Horstman, and Bentley, 1987).

One way of minimizing contamination when removing gloves is to peel gloves from the hands inside-out (Fig. 15-2). When removing fitted gloves, grasp the cuff of the glove and pull it inside-out. Avoid pulling on the fingers, as pulling can weaken the area of the glove. It is best to have a technician wearing latex gloves performing this procedure.

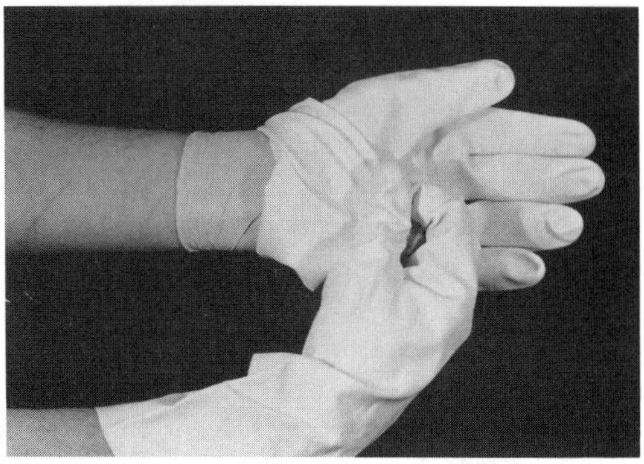

Figure 15-2. Proper way to remove gloves without spreading contamination.
Source: Photo by Ed Wesly.

Prior to use, gloves are usually prepared in a manner similar to dosimetry pads to remove interferents. They may be laundered one or more times with detergent, bleached, and then extracted with a solvent such as acetone or a solvent blend (hexane-acetone) one or more times depending on the level of analytical detection required. Sometimes following laundering they are rinsed in distilled water prior to extraction. Gloves should be handled using an instrument such as solvent rinsed forceps in between each extraction procedure and never by a laboratory technician's hands. The gloves are then loosely wrapped in solvent rinsed aluminum foil to air dry and stored until needed. Regardless of what preparatory procedure is chosen, blanks should be processed in exactly the same manner as the other gloves to be sent to the laboratory for analysis along with the samples. After sampling, exposed cotton or nylon gloves are processed in the same manner as exposed dermal pads. In the field, each pair of exposed gloves is either placed directly into a container of solvent or into a protective envelope inside a zip-lock bag. Another method is to wrap them in aluminum foil. Often the foil is rinsed beforehand with the solvent to be used for extraction. When long-sleeve gloves are used and the areas are to be analyzed separately, the gloves are separated at the wrist before storage.

Gloves should be stored in a refrigerated container (4°C) until analysis. At the laboratory, both gloves are thawed, then extracted by an appropriate method. As with dosimetry pads, the gloves can be composited or extracted individually. Sometimes only sections (1–2 cm^2) are cut from the back and palm of lightweight absorbent gloves for analysis (EPA, 1988*b*). Gloves can also be cut into pieces ranging in size from 1–2 cm^2 to 6.45 cm^2 prior to extraction. Then the volume of the sample extract is reduced and analysis proceeds. During analysis the gloves should be handled with forceps that are often rinsed with the extraction solvent first. Both clean and spiked gloves are analyzed along with the exposed ones as controls or blanks.

Leather horsehide gloves have been used for sampling, especially if they were typically used in the operation. The following examples show different approaches: one using the workers' own gloves and the other utilizing prepared gloves for sampling. The regular work gloves of electric utility linemen with an exposure to polychlorinated biphenyls (PCBs) were collected on a periodic basis. For analysis, three areas measuring 0.64 cm^2 were stamped out from the thumb, index finger, and palm of the right glove of each pair (Thind, Karmali, and House, 1991). The glove material was extracted in toluene for 10 min, diluted, and then analyzed. New leather gloves were used as samplers for paraquat by placing them over rubber gloves to protect the workers from exposure in the event of breakthrough (Bandara et al., 1985). The entire glove was cut into small pieces (3 cm by 3 cm) with a razor blade and then refluxed with 100 mL of sulfuric acid in a wide mouth 1,000 mL boiling flask fitted with a water cooled condenser for 3 hr. Separate razor blades were used for each glove to minimize contamination. Gloves from the right hand and left hand were analyzed separately to determine if the exposure on one hand was greater than the other.

Gloves are often used when hand rinses are not acceptable. Lightweight absorbent gloves also provide several advantages over rinsing or swabbing for the assessment of hand exposure. It is easy to exchange gloves in between monitoring periods. Absorbent gloves are the only method for monitoring the hands that will collect residues that would otherwise be absorbed into the skin during the exposure period, although if the exposure period is too long or concentrations are too great then breakthrough could occur (Fig. 15-3). In general, gloves accumulate a significant amount of a contaminant with only low concentrations reaching the hands underneath.

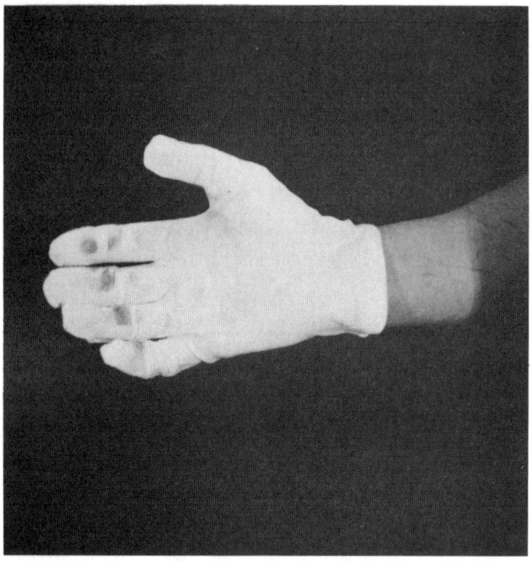

Figure 15-3. Cotton gloves on a worker's hands for sampling.
Source: Photo by Ed Wesly.

Hand rinses are sometimes done in conjunction with the use of absorbent gloves. At the end of the workday, after the final pair of gloves is removed, the hands are rinsed using the procedures described in Chapter 12. Towels can also be used to wash hands in conjunction with absorbent glove use, the purpose being to determine the amount of contaminant that permeates the gloves and reaches the skin.

The use of gloves may have certain disadvantages. Cotton and nylon gloves have absorption characteristics that differ from skin. They can get in the way and impede work where high dexterity is required. The wide variety of hand shapes found in the population (palm widths, finger lengths) makes it difficult to get a smooth fit in many instances because the sizes of gloves are limited. Gloves may absorb more material than would be retained by the skin, thus overestimating hand exposure (Davis, Stevens, and

Staiff, 1983). Even the smooth surfaced nylon gloves may retain several times more residue than would have adhered to flesh. Gloves also contain foreign materials such as sizing that may be difficult to remove by preextraction and may interfere with chemical analysis of low levels of contaminants. This problem can be reduced by preextraction of gloves with an appropriate solvent.

Gloves are more prone to moisture buildup than most monitoring devices since the hands are in contact with so many objects. If cotton gloves become wet, such as can happen when they are used to monitor harvesting of produce, they tend to saturate and are not reliable as collectors. Rain or moisture on surfaces during sampling may also result in loss of sample on gloves (EPA, 1988*b*). Gloves are also prone to buildup materials that might be sloughed off by skin, namely oils and dirt, which may reduce the amount of contaminant absorbed by the glove during the exposure period. For harvesters, fruit juice and organic buildup is a concern, especially the stickiness of the fruit juice as it attracts these other materials. A concern is that extraneous materials that build up may interfere with the extraction procedure or introduce interferents into the analysis. When this is a problem, hand rinses can be substituted for gloves.

The alternative to using gloves to monitor hand exposures is hand washes. When hand exposures using cotton and nylon gloves were compared with ethanol hand rinses over two days of monitoring, higher exposures occurred with the gloves (Davis, Stevens, and Staiff, 1983; Table 15-1). When compared at the 95% confidence level, hand exposures obtained by rinsing were significantly lower than those obtained by using either type of glove. However, there was no significant difference between exposures obtained by using the different types of gloves. When mean exposures were compared, those obtained by using cotton and nylon gloves were approximately five and four times larger, respectively, than those obtained by using the hand rinses.

In harvesting studies, hand washing and glove exposure measurements have correlated better with worker picking rates than with time worked (Table 15-2). Glove accuracy was dependent on sampling time, with the 0.5 hr result significantly higher than the 1.5 hr and 3 hr estimates. These results indicated that the absorptive capacity of the glove was greater at the outset of exposure and that the glove collection rates did not become constant until sampling was extended beyond 1.0 hr. Hand wash exposure rates were significantly lower than glove rates for the 0.5 hr and 1.0 hr sampling intervals, but were not significantly different for the 1.5 hr and 3 hr intervals. Loading of 30–50 mg modified the absorptive capacity of the glove. Bare hand exposure rates remained constant over time within each picking category, although average rates differed significantly among the picking categories (22.5 mg/hr, 16.4 mg/hr, 6.4 mg/hr) for high, medium, and low respectively.

TABLE 15-1. Comparison of Apple Thinners' Hand Exposures Monitored with Ethanol Rinses or Absorbent Gloves

	Rate of Exposure to Azinphos-methyl (μg/hr)[a]		
Days After Application	*Ethanol Rinses*	*Cotton Gloves*	*Nylon Gloves*
2	1,800 ± 300 (6)	8,500 ± 1,700 (5)	7,000 ± 2,000 (5)
9	960 ± 340 (6)	5,200 ± 2,200 (11)	3,900 ± 900 (11)

Source: From Davis, J. E., E. R. Stevens, and D. C. Staiff. 1983. Potential exposure of apple thinners to azinphosmethyl and comparison of two methods for assessment of hand exposure. *Bull. Env. Contam. Toxicol.* **31:**631–638.

[a]Mean ± standard deviation for the number of replicates indicated in parentheses.

TABLE 15-2. Glove and Hand Wash Exposure Rates by Sampling Time

	Glove Exposure Rate (mg/hr)			*Hand Exposure Rate (mg/hr)*			
Time (hr)	*Mean*	*Median*	*SD*	*Mean*	*Median*	*SD*	*G/H Ratio*
0.5	43.6[a]	43	28	18	17	9	2.4[b]
1.0	32.5	31	18	15.5	15	8	2.1[b]
1.5	23.2[a]	25	8	16.6	16	8	1.4
3.0	21.0[a]	19	9	14.7	13	9	1.4

Source: From Davis J. E., E. R. Stevens, and D. C. Staiff. 1983. Potential exposure of apple thinners to azinphosmethyl and comparison of two methods for assessment of hand exposure. *Bull. Env. Contam. Toxicol.* **31**:631–638.
[a]Glove rate at 0.5 hr significantly different than 1.5 hr and 3.0 hr rates.
[b]Glove rates significantly different than hand rates.

FEET

Cotton or nylon socks are used to measure the amount of contaminant that enters the shoes in a method similar to using gloves for measuring hand exposure. Socks can show contamination that is transported home. Socks with the feet cut off have been used for measuring exposure around the forearms, lower legs, and ankles. In one study where workers had their personal underwear and socks laundered at home, socks were analyzed for lead exposure (Bach et al., 1983). There was a correlation between increasing levels in the socks and airborne exposure. The number of days worn was less important than the individual's exposure. Perspiration may be a greater concern when using socks to sample than when using gloves because boots will trap perspiration. Therefore, if the boot material is suitable, rinses of the boot interiors may be more useful than monitoring socks.

White cotton socks were used to determine if the pesticide DNOSBP penetrated shoes (Wolfe, Durham, and Batchelor, 1961). The socks were worn during spraying operations for 2.5 hr to 10 hr. The highest value was for a sprayer who wore low-cut canvas shoes. The others who wore leather shoes had lower, although detectable, exposures.

Many parts of shoes have been wiped or "sniffed" with a direct reading instrument, depending on the contaminant. Soles are frequently tested to determine if there is carryover into other areas. Liquid proof poly-D disposable boots have been analyzed for exposure to paraquat during harvesting of treated plants (Bandara et al., 1985). The disposable plastic boots were refluxed in 50 mL of sulfuric acid and combusted in an oxidizer for analysis. To evaluate the potential for exposure to workers, wipes of work-shoe exteriors and interiors are often performed. The tongues and tips are frequently wiped. Leather shoes, similar to leather gloves, can be "punched" to collect a sample. However, this method is destructive and does not allow for reuse. Boots of rubber and other polymers can have their interiors rinsed.

FACE AND SCALP

Paper caps (0.44 ft^2 in area) have been used to measure head (scalp) exposure to 2,4-D from a hand sprayer held at hip level (Taskar et al., 1982). The results indicated that exposures were greater to the head than the chest or back (which were measured using gauze pads). This finding is of interest because the head is rarely monitored for exposure. Disposable paper respirators have been used to estimate facial exposures and will provide an estimate of contamination to the nose, chin, and cheeks. An advantage of this method is that the shape of these masks results in their only touching the face around the edges where the face seal is made. This eliminates the problem with sweating and picking up potentially eliminated contaminants that may have been stored in the skin, as well as that of getting the sampler damp. A disadvantage is the mask surface area is much larger than the portion of the face that is covered, so estimates of the actual surface area being sampled may be difficult. This measurement is different from when respirators are used to collect samples representing inhalation exposures.

LEGS

Legs are another part of the body rarely monitored even though some activities may produce significant exposures. Fabric tights (footless, white) made of 54% cotton, 36% polyester, and 10% spandex have been used for monitoring dermal exposure to carpet residue produced by indoor pesticide foggers when subjects performed exercises on carpets that had been exposed to the fogger (Ross et al., 1990). Subject also wore long-sleeve T-shirts of 100% cotton, thin 100% cotton gloves, and white athletic socks of 100% cotton. Prior to entering the room where the fogger was used, the subjects wore foot covers over their socks. At the end of the exercise class the subjects removed their cotton gloves, placed them in Zip-Loc bags, and covered their hands with polyvinyl chloride (PVC) gloves. They then removed their socks, recovering their feet with the foot coverings, placed the socks in plastic bags, and exited the room. The subjects returned to an untreated room where they removed the remaining dosimeter clothing. They then discarded their PVC gloves and dressed in fresh clothing for the next exposure period. It is likely that more studies of this type will be done in the future because of increasing concerns regarding exposures to community use of pesticides in homes. Similar to the studies required on workers to register pesticides, home applications will be reviewed as well if the material is to be sold to consumers.

Blue jeans have been analyzed for exposure to pesticides (ethyl and methyl parathion) during field reentry (Ware et al., 1974). Analysis was done by washing the jeans separately three times in hexane, soaking them for 10 minutes during each wash. The extracts were combined and concentrated or diluted, as required, for gas chromatography (GC) analysis. All jeans were purchased from the same manufacturer. Prior to use the jeans were laundered twice.

TORSO

Short sleeve T-shirts have been used to measure the amount of a contaminant that penetrates through outer work clothing, both ordinary work garb and CPC (Hayes, 1975; Chester and Ward, 1984). Underpants may be useful for studying exposures to compounds known to produce scrotal cancer such as PAHs.

In a study of 2,4-D exposure, workers wore T-shirts as undergarments and changed them every 24 hr (Sell and Maitlen, 1983). Before use, the shirts were laundered with soap and water, extracted with methanol in a Soxhlet for 18 hr, and then dried in a household clothes dryer. In another study using T-shirts for exposure to ethyl and methyl parathion, the shirts were extracted three times in a total of 2.5 liters of hexane for a period of 15 min and the extract analyzed (Ware et al., 1974). All T-shirts purchased were from the same manufacturer. Prior to use the T-shirts were laundered twice.

WHOLE BODY MONITORING

Overalls and coveralls can be used along with gloves to approximate the total body exposure. As with other clothing, there is the option to either analyze a worker's existing clothing or to purchase and prepare clothing to use specifically for sampling. One application in which it is best to use the worker's personal clothing is when there is a question as to whether contamination is remaining in the clothing. This technique was used to evaluate the clothing of a group of workers exposed to dioxin who washed their work overalls after use every day (Rappe et al., 1985). After being used for 14 days an overall was found to have 28 ηg of 2,3,7,8-tetrachlorodibenzofuran/M^2 and about 100 ηg/M² of all tetrachlorodibenzofurans. Another pair of overalls used and washed for one month followed by dry cleaning had almost the same levels. A set of underwear also used for one month had less than 5 ηg of 2,3,7,8-tetrachlorodibenzofuran/M². Therefore, in order to avoid dermal exposure when wearing one's own clothing for work around dioxins, double layers of protective clothing should be worn.

Using the alternative approach, 10 oz 100% cotton coveralls with long sleeves were purchased specifically for monitoring the exposure of pesticide applicators to arsenic acid (Miller, Hoover, and Culver, 1980). The individuals wore them during loading and spraying operations. The coveralls were collected and placed in sealed plastic bags for subsequent shipment to the laboratory. For analysis, a complete pair of dry coveralls was placed in a 7.6 L plastic tray that contained 2 L of 1.6 N nitric acid, which provides a good example of the quantities of solvent often required for extraction of large items of clothing. The coveralls were allowed to soak in the acid for 30 min and then they were squeezed and resoaked in the same acid three times for a total of 2 hr, so analytical preparation times are often increased as well. The solution was then squeezed from the coveralls into the soaking tray, a somewhat difficult task. The solution from the tray was analyzed by atomic absorption.

The current trend is to use long underwear, sometimes called a union suit, or disposable body suits such as Tyvek (Fig. 15-4). When worn under regular clothing, a body suit covers the entire trunk and the extremities; alternatively disposables can be worn over regular clothing. When used as underwear, the suits are often worn for 4 hr and then collected. Removal must be done carefully so as not to disturb collected material. After removal the underwear is often placed in Zip-Loc bags and stored on dry ice until processing. Clothing can be cut up in order to identify exposures to specific parts of the body. In some instances after an observation period a decision is made to analyze only portions of the long underwear such as arms and legs. A disadvantage of this method is the potential for heat stress to workers due to the additional layer of clothing.

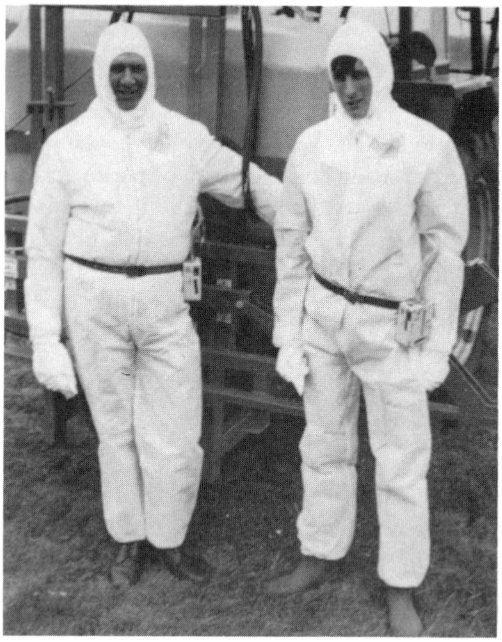

Figure 15-4. Spray operators wearing disposable body suits according to WHO protocol.
Source: From I. M. Abbott, J. L. Bonsall, G. Chester, T. B. Hard, and G. J. Turnbull. 1987. Worker exposure to a herbicide applied with groundsprayers in the United Kingdom. *AIHA J.* **48**(2):170.

When using disposable coveralls to perform whole body dosimetry the material should be checked first to determine its ability to collect the contaminant of interest. For example, some compounds such as Ethazol will readily penetrate Tyvek® (Stamper et al., 1989). Disposable Tyvek suits were used to estimate the exposure that might occur if a bystander were accidentally sprayed by a helicopter overhead using a boom sprayer to apply 2, 4-D (Frank, Campbell, and Sirons, 1985). After exposure the disposable suits were cut off the subjects and divided into four portions: hoods, arms, torso, and legs. Each portion was placed in a container of 500 mL methanol for transport to the laboratory.

Clothing dosimetry is currently the only technique that can be used to measure contamination to the total body surface without having to use extrapolation from a smaller sampling area. Monitoring times may be limited by the potential for heat stress in many environments as well as by perspiration buildup. However, concerns still exist as to how accurately the residues picked up by the disposable suits or long underwear reflect the ability of the skin to collect and retain contaminants. As shown by the arsenic acid study, the size of the sample matrix makes for a complicated and potentially expensive analysis. It is difficult to get good reproducibility because large numbers of samples are difficult and expensive to collect. Extraction techniques are not standardized and this can produce significant variability between laboratories as well.

WHO Method for Total Body Dosimetry Using Disposable Body Suits

Disposable body suits have been recommended as a collection medium for contaminants during spraying operations and a procedure has been developed by the World Health Organization (WHO, 1982). In theory all contaminant is collected that otherwise might contact the skin and clothing of the worker. This method differs from the pad method in that it does not require a surface area extrapolation since the majority of the body is covered and the surface area of the clothing can be considered the same as the skin.

Each worker is required to wear a new disposable overall and gauntlets for a minimum period of 1 hr or more during any one day of spraying (WHO, 1986). The tight fitting underwear (long sleeve top and bottoms) is worn under regular clothing. If significant head exposure is likely, then a head pad or a disposable hat should also be used. Care should be taken to ensure that the overall or gauntlets do not become saturated; should this occur, a fresh overall and gauntlets must be worn. The exact periods of time and amount of contaminant used during the period that each overall/gauntlet is worn must be recorded. The exposure time can vary.

Upon completion of each assessment period the overalls and gauntlets are carefully taken off by a technician to avoid cross-contamination. Prior to analysis each gauntlet should be placed in a separate plastic or polyethylene bag and stored in a place out of direct sunlight and as cool as is practicable. All bags should be labeled separately to include the following information: worker's number/name, date, location of survey.

The overalls are immediately sectioned into the following parts: legs—above and below the knees; arms—above and below the elbows; torso—front and back. Care should be taken to make sure that the instrument used for sectioning the overall is not contaminated. Decontamination can be performed by swabbing with cotton balls soaked in an appropriate solvent. Each body part sample is then stored separately under identical conditions as are the gauntlets.

In one study using this method, Strentex Corovin disposable coveralls, Strentex Tyvek gauntlets and hoods, and white nylon socks were selected as the dermal sampling media (Abbott et al., 1987). The trouser legs of the body suits were worn over (outside) the worker's boots or shoes. At the end of the sampling period, the gauntlets, socks, coverall, and hood were removed and turned inside-out. Each gauntlet, sock, or hood was wrapped in aluminum foil and placed in a separate polyethylene bag, labeled appropriately. The coveralls were sectioned into the following portions: arms, body front and back, and both legs above and below the knees. Each portion was treated in the same way as the gauntlets, socks, or hood. The scissors used for sectioning must be washed with an appropriate solvent in between each cut in order to minimize carryover. Each set of samples from each individual for each sampling period were placed in a single large polyethylene bag and stored in a cooler out of direct sunlight until sent to the laboratory for analysis.

Calculation of Exposure for Disposable Suits

The potential dermal exposure is found by adding the quantity of contaminant (in mg) found in all sections of the overall covering parts of the body not normally covered by working clothes, plus the quantity of contaminant in the head pad (if worn) relating the mg/cm^2 to a figure of 1,100 cm^2. If a head pad was not used, the total is body exposure plus 10%. The total exposure is then related to the time the suit was worn:

$$\frac{\text{Total quantity in mg} \times 60}{\text{Total time (in minutes)}} = \text{Total exposure (mg/hour)}$$

In cases where disposables fit tightly on the subject being monitored, the surface area of the disposable has been assumed to be equal to the body area (Frank, Campbell, and Sirons, 1985). When suits were very baggy some studies have recalculated body surface area by measuring the surface areas of various parts of clothing on life size front view photos. The surfaces of arms, legs, and torso are assumed to be cylindrical to simplify calculations so that three-dimensional surface areas can be calculated by multiplying the cross-sectional areas by pi (π). Impervious gear such as respirators and goggles (the area they cover) is generally deducted from the surface area assumed to be available for deposit, however, since this is often not true for actual practice, this may not be the best practice.

Pad Variation for Disposable Suits

A variation on this method involves using a coverall body suit, but only analyzing selected areas similar to what would be done with pads. The worker wears a Tyvek suit for a designated interval. It might be the entire shift or a specific activity. If several tasks are performed over a shift, such as mixing-loading, and pesticide applications using different techniques are performed, such as boom application and handgun spraying, a new suit should be donned for each. At the end of the monitoring period the suit is cut off each individual and stored in a plastic bag in a cooler. Square sections (112 cm^2) are cut from strategic areas in the suit following exposure (Reed, Hall, and Krueger, 1990). For analyses the sections are rinsed with a solvent such as ethanol and the rinseate is analyzed.

Vacuum Method for Dusts and Fumes on Clothing

When the concern is exposure of the worker's personal clothing to dusts, the vacuuming method can provide a good qualitative estimate. If the area sampled is measured, it may be possible to make some quantitative exposure assumptions. The vacuuming method works well for any inorganic dusts, such as metals or fibers, and has been used for some organic dusts as well, such as pesticides. Inert dusts have been sampled off clothing using a vacuuming technique similar to that used to collect samples off of carpets and as settled dust. If the interest is in collecting metals or fibers in a plastic cassette, a filter such as a mixed cellulose ester is attached via a short piece of tubing to a personal air sampling pump. A second piece of tubing is attached to the inlet of the cassette. This is used to vacuum dust off of the clothing. Shirts and pants have been sampled for asbestos fibers using this method (NIOSH, March 1990). The cassette was 25 mm with a 0.8 μm MCE filter, the same as is used for asbestos air sampling. In another instance the dust from cuffs of work pants worn home by a worker in a lead smelter was vacuumed to determine if there was carryover to the home and family. In this instance the cuffs would be most likely to retain the highest concentration of dust (Winegar et al., 1977).

Sniffing Methods for Volatile Chemicals

In situations where the source of contamination is volatile enough to be measured with a direct reading instrument, such as stoddard solvent, formaldehyde, perchloroethylene, or mercury, the sniffing method can be used. Special attention should be paid to heavily seamed areas where material may be prone to buildup. Garments can also be placed inside a container, allowing gases and vapors to build up to higher concentrations and be detected through a hole made in the container. This method may be especially useful for difficult to sample items such as leather work boots. For more information on direct reading instruments and sampling volatiles inside containers, see Chapter 7.

Field Sampling Methods for Chemical Protective Clothing

Since there are still many chemicals for which testing information is not available, it is useful to run a field visual and tactile degradation test on CPC prior to use to screen unsuitable products cheaply. During use gloves can be wiped, rinsed, or tested using commercial pads that change color. Care should be used in selecting field methods because certain plasticizers and additives can be removed by surface sampling methods or migrate out of the materials over time.

Finger Cot Test

The finger cot test can be used in the field to supplement laboratory testing of CPC for evaluating breakthrough times when exposed to a constant liquid hazard. All measurements are in millimeters. The samples are weighed, soaked overnight, patted dry, immediately reweighed, visually inspected, and compared with an unexposed sample for properties such as stretchability. Three individuals should perform actual tasks similar to those in their regular jobs using the gloves. Each individual compares the cut resistance of the gloves by making slices in the material with a razor blade and subjectively rating each sample material. Products with fewer visual, weight, and other physical property changes generally provide longer protection against chemical permeation.

In addition to the equipment in Figure 15-5, the following was used to construct this cell: standard taper outer joint (Pyrex, No. 24/40, length 150 mm [Corning 6580]); standard taper inner joint No. 24/40; PID detector; ring stand and two clamps; chart recorder (optional); timer; 50 mL beaker and micrometer.

Procedure

1. Review the PID manual to ensure that it will respond to the chemical being tested.
2. Place 1 mL of the liquid in question into a 50 mL beaker. Using the PID, sample the vapor near the top of the beaker. If a response is detected, you may proceed. If there is no response, a different detection method must be used or the chemical is not volatile enough.
3. Cut the finger (approximately 5 cm long) from a glove used by workers handling the chemical in question. Using the micrometer, take 10 thickness measurements at different locations on the finger.
4. Turn the finger inside-out. Place the open end of the finger onto the ground glass of the inner joint; then place the finer/inner joint into the outer joint.
5. Mount the assembly vertically, outer joint on bottom, onto the ring stand.
6. Place the detector probe into the bottom of the assembly approximately 2 cm from the tip of the finger. Zero the detector, add 1 mL of chemical into the top of the assembly, and monitor the response versus time. Record the elapsed time from the addition of chemical until the first detector response to permeating chemical.
7. Depending on your choice of detectors, make-up air may come in the bottom of the assembly. Care must be taken so that no contaminants enter during the test. It is recommended that fresh make-up air be provided to the bottom of the assembly at a rate greater than or equivalent to that set by the detector.
8. Run the test until the chemical is detected or a prespecified time has elapsed with no chemical breakthrough.

Finger cots have also been analyzed in instances where there was a concern as to the cause of dermatitis. Employees of a telephone company directory assistance office were concerned about the presence of a "shiny-like glitter" in their work area (NIOSH, March 1983). Rubber finger tabs were worn by most operators so they could page through the loose leaf directory assistance listings. The used finger tabs along with one control were ultrasonicated in ethyl alcohol and evaporated onto carbon coated grids for X-ray analysis for particle composition.

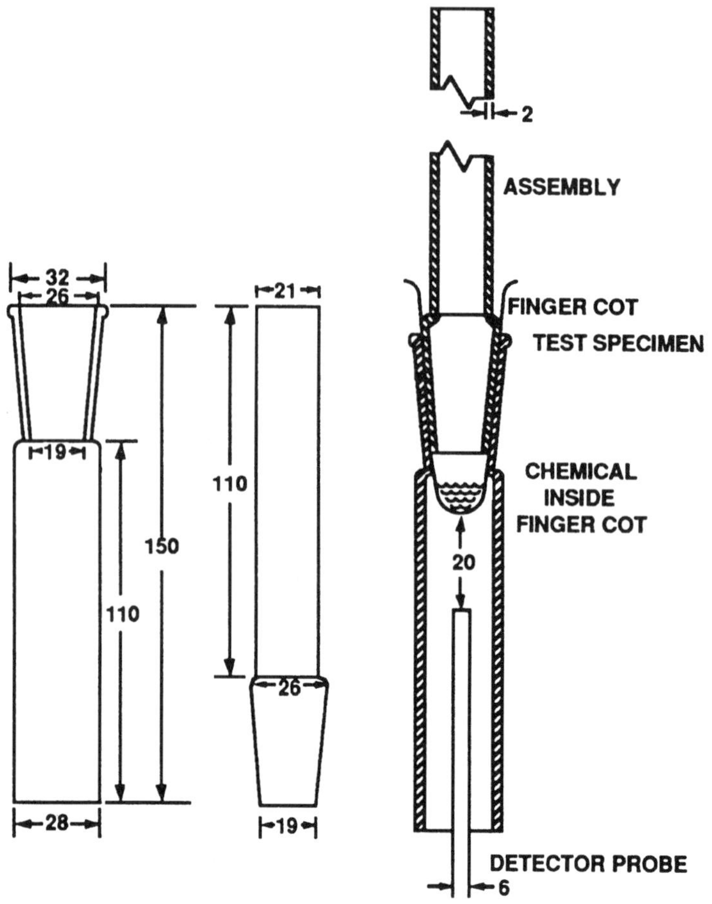

Figure 15-5. Finger cot permeation field test cell. All measurements are in millimeters. Glove material thickness can vary from 0.001 mm to 1.0 mm. Standard glass taper is 24/40.
Source: From NIOSH. 1990. *A Guide for Evaluating the Performance of* CPC. Cincinnati, OH: NIOSH.

Clothing Service Life, CPC Reuse, and Decontamination

Clothing service life is an end user decision depending on the costs and risks associated with clothing decontamination and reuse. CPC can be categorized as reusable or disposable; however, in many cases this distinction is blurred. It is not uncommon to see a disposable suit of Saranex reused several times due to its cost. When CPC is disposed of within the estimated safe use time, the selection process is simple. Disposable garments may, however, not be practical in some cases—their cost may be too great or there may be technical problems in disposing of contaminated products. Doubling up of CPC, one disposable over another, is an option, but the heat stress ramifications and movement difficulties for personnel are significant. CPC for protection against carcinogens should never be targeted for reuse. Reuse of any CPC after decontamination is not recommended unless chemical resistance testing is conducted. The test should evaluate (1) the adverse effect of the decontamination procedure on the CPC material and (2) the effectiveness of the decontamination procedure in removing the chemical from the material.

Sampling can be useful to verify clothing service life, especially if CPC is to be decontaminated and reused or if employees have no specific instructions as to when to dispose of CPC other than when visible contamination is present. A visual examination following use of protective clothing for signs of discoloration, corrosive effects, or any degradation of external materials is the first step as it is very difficult to test every inch of a piece of CPC. Age of CPC is also a factor in determining its resistance. In general, the older the item, the less reliable it is. Even unused CPC may be of poor quality if it has not been stored correctly. Storage at high temperatures (in direct sunlight or in the toolbox of a truck) can deplete plasticizers and lead to embrittlement. Occasional testing of a product that has been in the use/reuse process for a time near the expected product life will provide greater confidence in its effectiveness. In order to be thorough, tests should periodically be performed on unused garments and repeated after a number of exposure and decontamination cycles.

One method consists of decontaminating both site contaminated and laboratory contaminated garments and comparing the results. Site contaminated garments are those that were presumably contaminated during the work. Laboratory contaminated garments are those that were site contaminated but also were contaminated in the laboratory with a known concentration of the most likely contaminant. When this method was used to evaluate PCB exposure to firefighters wearing Nomex, the test concentrations of diluted material—2.4%, 9.0%, 33% (volume-to-volume in dieletric grade mineral oil)—and 100% PCBs were applied via a brush to selected areas on the garments to the point of saturation (NIOSH, February 1987). The volume of PCB applied to the material was approximately 20 mL. The site contaminated garb was decontaminated using a solvent-based dry cleaning system that was designed specifically for decontamination.

The fabric sampling technique consisted of marking an area of the fabric 5 in.^{2} (12.7 cm^2) and within that area marking off five 1 in. squares (2.54 cm^2). Four of these five 1 in. squares were located at the four corners of the larger square, with the fifth located at the center. To determine the precontamination concentration, each of the five 1 in. squares were cut from the larger square to form a composite sample. To determine the postdecontamination concentration within the same area, the remaining fabric within the marked-off section was removed. The purpose of this checkerboard technique was to average out or minimize concentration variations within the sample area. To eliminate variations due to cutting errors and unequal areas of fabric sampled, all results were reported in terms of micrograms of PCB per gram of fabric (μg/g). It was assumed that bulk density variations in the fabric and substrate were minor. To make comparisons between garments more consistent, fabric sections were removed from the same approximate location of each turnout coat and bunker pant sampled. After extraction with toluene and analysis by GC, the removal efficiency of the system was calculated using the following equation:

$$\text{Removal efficiency (\%)} = \frac{(A - B)}{(A)} \times 100$$

where A = initial concentration of contaminant (μg/g) and B = final concentration (μg/g).

Wipes

Wipe samples can be used in the field to determine if CPC is becoming a source of exposure rather than providing protection. OSHA directs its compliance officers to use distilled water only as the solvent for wipe sampling or rinsing CPC that directly contacts the skin (OSHA, 1991). For example, the interiors of respirators can be wiped to determine contaminant breakthrough as well as poor storage or decontamination procedures. Another option recommended by OSHA is to wipe CPC interiors with a *dry* filter. For low-volatile and low-water-soluble chemicals, breakthrough times can be estimated by analyzing periodic wipe samples from the inside surface of the CPC.

Wipe sampling can also be used to measure the effectiveness of decontamination. For example, during a job involving excavation of contaminated soil, workers passing through the decontamination area had the toe of the left boot wiped. After decontamination, the toe of the right boot was wiped and the results were compared (NIOSH, April 1984).

Wipe sampling will also identify if contamination inside a garment has occurred due to sloppy practices during decontamination at other times. If personnel bring contamination with them from other sites—which can occur if several jobs are going on at a time and they do not shower in between—contamination can also get inside a suit or gloves. Many interiors of garments are not smooth, but instead are coated with soft adsorbent materials that do not allow wipe sampling. The usefulness of wipe sampling applications depends heavily on the polymer/chemical construction combination.

Wipe sampling cannot be used as a final indicator that permeation has not occurred; instead it must be used in conjunction with other tests. It is not suitable for CPC materials that may absorb contaminants. Also, the amount of solvent that can be used for wiping is limited in order to minimize any possible interaction between the solvent and the polymer (Stamper et al., 1984). Thus, it is difficult to tell if all the contaminant has been removed. Breakthrough may never be detected if the analytical sensitivity is inadequate and all permeant is removed with each wipe, frequent wipes are taken, and the permeation rate is low. This problem can be minimized if infrequent wipes are taken. However, infrequent wiping decreases the accuracy with which breakthrough time can be defined.

Rinses

Rinses can be done on the exterior of protective gloves using the same methods as for the skin. Rinses have also been done for the interiors of gloves that appeared contaminated. In some cases, both the exteriors and interiors of gloves are rinsed. In one study on grouters, the interiors of the work gloves were suspected as a source of acrylamide exposure (Hills and Greife, 1986). Distilled water was used to rinse the interiors of the gloves. When interior glove contamination is suspected, it is good to do hand rinses as well.

Glove rinses (of the interior) can be useful to determine whether penetration has occurred. It is useful in these instances to know how long the gloves have been in use. It is sometimes difficult to determine whether the contamination was a result of contaminated hands or permeation of the glove material.

Cotton Gloves

Cotton gloves have been used to assess the degree of penetration by a contaminant under protective gloves. They have also been used to compare exposures when no protective gloves were used with what might permeate a neoprene glove (Dubelman et al., 1982). Cotton gloves are prewashed prior to sampling.

Cotton gloves have been used to assess whether a glove with a short breakthrough time could be used for protection against PCBs by workers in transformer maintenance (Perkins and Knight, 1989). The issue here was the high cost of the Viton gloves, which were known to provide good protection against PCBs, and the much lower cost of PVC gloves reported as having a breakthrough time of 0.5 min. Workers wore cotton gloves under the PVC gloves. They were instructed to wash their hands thoroughly before donning the glove. At the end of each task both the PVC and cotton gloves were carefully removed so cross-contamination would not occur. The cotton gloves were then extracted using a standard EPA method for extraction of PCBs from soil. Analyses of the extractant were also performed using EPA methods. In this particular study the results from the cotton gloves were considered low enough that the use of PVC gloves continued. However, additional worker training and good hygiene practices were also instituted in order to further minimize exposures.

Cotton gloves under protective gloves are very useful for detecting breakthrough in situations where a contaminant produces a discoloration. MPDA and methylene dianiline (MDA) are examples. Analysis is not required and the results can be immediately determined in the workplace. Discoloration detection can also be helpful in identifying specific areas of the hand that are exposed due to exerting pressure in various tasks. It is important to spend time observing the workers, what tasks are performed, the length of time required, and how contact with contaminants occurs. For exposure periods, one option is to have the workers change inner gloves with each task.

In another study of exposures to epoxy resins the effective penetration and permeation resistance of the rubber gloves worn by painters was tested in the field (NIOSH, September 1984). Ten sets of cotton inner gloves were taken from painters who had been applying and mixing epoxy surfaces. The gloves were sent to the laboratory for analysis where each glove was cut lengthwise between the ring and middle finger. The middle finger section of one glove and the ring finger section of the other glove pair were combined as one sample and analyzed for MDA. The other halves of each gloved pair were analyzed for diglycidyl ethers of bisphenol A (DGBA). The results are shown in Table 15-3. The hopper-filling and mixing procedures produced the highest exposures to DGBA. The appropriate follow-up would be to either change to a more protective glove or shorten the usage period.

Perma-tec Pads

Perma-tec glove and protective clothing breakthrough indicators are a qualitative system that includes different monitoring media to sample for amines, isocyanates, and solvents. For solvents a patch of charcoal cloth along with a colorimetric microencapsulated indicator next to the charcoal is used to indicate whether breakthrough (of the glove) has occurred. The charcoal cloth can subsequently be analyzed in the laboratory for the solvent of interest. These pads are attached to the hands of a worker before gloving and can be used to assure proper work practice and document protection from dermal exposure.

The current solvent Perma-tec pad had various levels of sensitivity to a wide range of polar solvents. Solvents for which the charcoal cloth has been evaluated include acetone, methyl ethyl ketone, methyl isobutyl ketone, toluene, benzene, methylene chloride, chloroform, hexane, and alcohols. Currently the detection system is nonresponsive to nonpolar solvents such

TABLE 15-3. Grand Gulf Nuclear Power Plant Radiation Waste Area

Glove Pair No.	*Job Description*	*Wear Time (min)*	*DGBA (μg)*	*DGBA Relative Amounts*	*MDA (μg)*	*MDA Relative Amounts*
1	Filling hopper	106	1,100		120	
2	Filling hopper	90	1,000		46	
3	Trowling	168	ND		150	
4	Trowling	90	30		16	
5	Trowling	145	70		5	
6	Trowling	90	90		10	
7	Spraying	90	50		15	
8	Mixing	60	2,000		40	
9	Trowling	90	350		24	
10	Blank	0	ND		ND	

Source: From NIOSH Health Hazard Evaluation. September 1984. Grand Gulf Nuclear Power Plant. HETA 83-132-1508. Cincinnati, OH: NIOSH.
Note: ND = no data.

as naphthas, benzene, and hexane. Research is continuing to extend the range of detection and increase the sensitivity of this indicator system. The charcoal cloth must be removed using care not to contaminate the pad with solvents before or during removal from the worker's hand. The cloth pad should be stored in an airtight container prior to GC analyses. Solvent desorption or thermal desorption with head space analysis can be used. Data comparing permeation testing using automated photoionization systems to detect glove permeation compared to the Perma-tec pads showed that a reasonable correlation existed for the pads as long as the permeation rate was relatively high. However, when the permeation rates were low, the correlation between breakthrough times obtained by the two detection methods was less predictable (Stull and White, 1992).

One method recommended by the manufacturer is to put Perma-tec pads on both hands under the gloves (Fig. 15-6). It is recommended by the manufacturer that the detectors be placed on the thumb, middle finger, and palm, as these represent the areas of highest contact and glove abrasion, which enhance chemical permeation.

The first glove on one hand is removed after 1 hr and the second glove on the other hand is removed after 2 hr. This time period can be increased or decreased until the effective safe use period is determined. As a safety precaution, it is recommended that during the initial evaluation of a new glove, workers should be double gloved and the Perma-tec pads should be worn on the outside of the glove currently in use.

Colorimetric Perma-tec pads of slightly different composition also exist for aromatic amines (MDA, aniline, o-toluidine), aromatic isocyanates (TDI, MDI), aliphatic isocyanates (HDI, HMDI), and hydrazines.

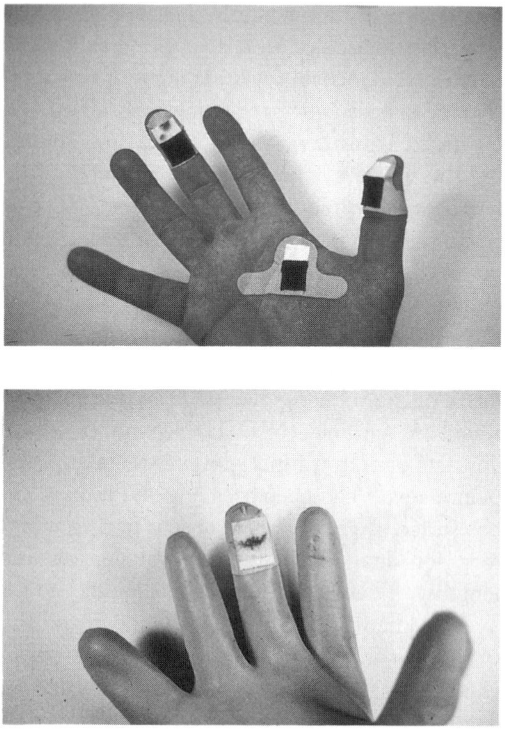

Figure 15-6. *Top:* Perma-tec pads on hands to test for penetration under gloves. Note placement. *Bottom:* A variation is to place pads on glove exteriors.
Source: Both illustrations from CLI Colorimetric Labs, Inc.

Gauze Pads

Gauze and α-cellulose pads have been placed outside of the garments at the back, chest, and shoulders to assess facial, head, and neck exposure as described in Chapter 14. Additional pads placed under the suit at all of these locations as well can be used to monitor the effectiveness of full protective suits. Pads should be centered under seams as well as under unseamed material, since seams are often areas of maximum penetration. Pads may be attached to the suit by using strips of masking or duct tape along two edges of a pad. One study placed gauze pads under and on the exterior of 3M White Cap helmet powered air respirators (Putnam et al., 1983). In Chapter 14 there is a method for cutting patches from Tyvek suits and having them analyzed. Penetration through rubber coats and the underlying cotton clothing was observed in a study where gauze pads were placed beneath two layers of cotton clothing.

Fluorescence

Protective clothing performance has been assessed using a fluorescent tracer during high-volume air blast applications for pesticides (Fenske, 1988). Dermal exposure is measured by illumination of the worker's skin after the protective clothing has been removed with an ultraviolet light (320–400 ηm) in a darkened room and a video imaging system. The fluorescent compound is added to the pesticide solution in the tank of the sprayer. For a more detailed description, see Chapter 13.

The results indicated that material was getting "caught" at openings such as sleeves and the neck and building up in these areas both in front of and under the opening. Hand exposures were due to handling the exteriors of contaminated gloves after removal during breaks.

For PAH contamination, the same examination methods described in Chapter 13 for skin can be used for CPC. In this regard, it is a much safer application. Also, the skin of workers can be monitored after removal of CPC similar to the study described above.

REFERENCES

Abott, I. M., J. L. Bonsall, G. Chester, T. B. Hard, and G. J. Turnbull. 1987. Worker exposure to a herbicide applied with groundsprayers in the United Kingdom. *AIHA J.* **48**(2):167–175.

Bach, E., J. M. Christensen, P. Grandjean, and E. Olsen. 1983. *Indirect and Direct Occupational Lead Exposure* (in Danish). Environmental Projects No. 50. Copenhagen: Danish Agency of Environmental Protection.

Bandara, J. M. R. S., P. C. Kearney, P. G. Vincent, and W. A. Gentner. 1985. Paraquat: A model for measuring exposure. In: *Dermal Exposure Related to Pesticide Use.* Washington, DC: American Chemical Society, pp. 279–285.

Brouwer, D. H., R. Brouwer, G. DeMik, C. L. Maas, and J. J. van Hemmen. 1992. Pesticides in the cultivation of carnations in greenhouses: Part I—Exposure and concomitant health risk. *AIHA J.* **53**(9):575–581.

Chester, G., and R. J. Ward. 1984. Occupational exposure and drift hazard during aerial application of paraquat to cotton. *Arch. Env. Contam. Toxicol.* **13:**551–563.

Davis, J. E., E. R. Stevens, and D. C. Staiff. 1983. Potential exposure of apple thinners to azinphos-methyl and comparison of two methods for assessment of hand exposure. *Bull. Env. Contam. Toxicol.* **31:**631–638.

Davis, J. E., E. R. Stevens, D. C. Staiff, and L. C. Butler. 1982. Potential exposure of apple thinners to Phosalone. *Bull. Env. Contam. Toxicol.* **29:**592–598.

Dubelman, S., R. Lauer, D. D. Arras, and S. A. Adams. 1982. Operator exposure measurements during application of the herbicide Diallate. *J. Agric. Food Chem.* **30:**526–532.

EPA. 1986. *Pesticide Assessment Guidelines Subdivision U, Applicator Exposure Monitoring.* EPA 540/9-87-127. Washington, DC: Office of Pesticide Programs.

EPA. 1988*a*. *Pesticide Hazard Assessment Project: Harvester Exposure Monitoring Studies (1980–1986)*, vol. 1. EPA 540/09-88-036. Washington, DC: EPA.

EPA. 1988*b*. *Pesticide Hazard Assessment Project: Harvester Exposure Monitoring Studies (1980–1986)*, vol. 2. EPA 540/09-88-037. Washington, DC: EPA.

Fenske, R. A. 1988. Comparative assessment of protective clothing performance by measurement of dermal exposure during pesticide applications. *Appl. Ind. Hyg.* **3**(7):207–213.

Fenske, R. A., S. W. Horstman, and R. K. Bentley. 1987. Assessment of dermal exposure to chlorophenols in timber mills. *Appl. Ind. Hyg.* **2:**143–147.

Frank, R., R. A. Campbell, and G. J. Sirons. 1985. Forestry workers involved in aerial application of 2,4-dichlorophenoxy acetic acid (2,4-D): Exposure and urinary excretion. *Arch. Env. Contam. Toxicol.* **14:**427–435.

Hayes, W. J. 1975. *Toxicology of Pesticides.* Baltimore, MD: Williams & Wilkins.

Hills, B. W., and A. L. Greife. 1986. Evaluation of occupational acrylamide exposures. *Appl. Ind. Hyg.* **1**(3):148–151.

Miller, C. S., W. L. Hoover, and W. H. Culver. 1980. Exposure of pesticide applicators to arsenic acid. *Arch. Env. Contam. Toxicol.* **9:**281–288.

NIOSH, Health Hazard Evaluation Report. March 1983. *C&P Telephone Co., Charleston, WV.* HETA 82-275-1285. Cincinnati, OH: NIOSH.

NIOSH, Health Hazard Evaluation Report. April 1984. *Port Authority of NY and NJ, Elizabeth Industrial Park Site, Elizabeth, NJ.* HETA 82-284-1456. Cincinnati, OH: NIOSH.

NIOSH, Health Hazard Evaluation Report. September 1984. *Grand Gulf Nuclear Power Plant, Port Gibson, MS.* HETA 83-132-1508. Cincinnati, OH: NIOSH.

NIOSH, Health Hazard Evaluation Report. February 1987. *Jacksonville Fire Department, Jacksonville, FL.* HETA 84-180-1776. Cincinnati, OH: NIOSH.

NIOSH, Health Hazard Evaluation Report. March 1990. *Chrysler Chemical Division, Trenton, MI.* HETA 87-126-2019. Cincinnati, OH: NIOSH.

OSHA Technical Manual, 2nd ed. 1991. Washington, DC: OSHA.

Perkins, J. L., and V. B. Knight. 1989. Risk assessment of dermal exposure to polychlorinated biphenyls permeating a polyvinyl chloride glove. *AIHA J.* **50:**A-171–A-172.

Popendorf, W. J., R. C. Spear, J. T. Leffingwell, J. Yager, and E. Kahn. 1979. Harvester exposure to Zolone (phosalone) residues in peach orchards. *JOM* **21:**189–194.

Putnam, A. R., M. D. Willis, L. K. Binning, and P. F. Boldt. 1983. Exposure of pesticide applicators to Nitrofen: Influence of formulation, handling systems, and protective garments. *J. Agric. Food Chem.* **31:**645–650.

Rappe, C., M. Nygren, S. Marklund, L. Keller, P. Bergqvist, and M. Hansson. 1985. Assessment of human exposure to polychlorinated dibenzofurans and dioxins. *Env. Health Perspec.* **60:**303–304.

Reed, J. P., F. R. Hall, and J. R. Krueger. 1990. Measurement of ATV applicator exposure to Atrazine using an ELISA method. *Bull. Env. Contam. Toxicol.* **44:**8–12.

Ross, J., T. Thongsinthusak, H. R. Fong, S. Margetich, and R. Krieger. 1990. Measuring potential dermal transfer of surface pesticide residue generated from indoor fogger use: An interim report. *Chemosphere* **20**(3/4):349–360.

Sell, C. R., and J. C. Maitlen. 1983. Procedure for the determination of residues of (2,4-dichlorophenoxy) acetic acid in dermal exposure pads, hand rinses, urine, and perspiration from agricultural workers exposed to the herbicide. *J. Agric. Food Chem.* **31:**572–575.

Stampfer, J. F., M. J. McLeod, M. R. Betts, A. M. Martinez, and S. P. Berardinelli. 1984. Permeation of polychlorinated biphenyls and solutions of these substances through selected protective clothing materials. *AIHA J.* **45**(9):634–641

Stamper, J. H., H. N. Nigg, W. D. Mahon, A. P. Nielson, and M. D. Royer. 1989. Pesticide exposure to greenhouse handgunners. *Arch. Env. Contam. Toxicol.* **18:**515–529.

Stull, J. O., and D. F. White. 1992. A review of overall integrity and material performance tests for the selection of chemical protective clothing. *AIHA J.* **53**(7):455–462.

Taskar, P. K., Y. T. Das, J. R. Trout, S. K. Chattopadhyay, and H. D. Brown. 1982. Measurement of 2,4-dichlorophenoxy acetic acid (2,4-D) after occupational exposure. *Bull. Env. Contam. Toxicol.* **29:**586–591.

Thind, K. S., S. Karmali, and R. A. House. 1991. Occupational exposure of electrical utility linemen to pentachlorophenol. *AIHA J.* **52**(12):547–552.

Vahdat, N., and R. Delaney. 1989. Decontamination of chemical protective clothing. *AIHA J.* **50**(3):152–156.

Ware, G. W., D. P. Morgan, B. J. Estessen, and W. P. Cahill. 1974. Establishment of reentry intervals for organophosphate-treated cotton fields based on human data. II. Azodrin, ethyl and methyl parathion. *Arch. Env. Contam. Toxicol.* **2**(2):117–129.

WHO. 1982. *Field Surveys of Exposure to Pesticides. Standard Protocol: VBC/82.1.* Geneva: Division of Vector Biology and Control/WHO.

WHO. 1986. Field surveys of exposure to pesticides: Standard protocol. Pesticide Development and Safe Use Unit, Division of Vector Biology and Control. *Toxicol. Letters* **33:**223–235.

Winegar, D. A., B. S. Levy, J. S. Andrews, P. J. Landrigan, W. H. Scruton, and M. J. Krause. 1977. Chronic occupational exposure to lead: An evaluation of the health of smelter workers. *JOM* **19**(9):603–606.

Wojeck, G. A., H. N. Nigg, R. S. Braman, J. H. Stamper, and R. L. Rouseff. 1982. Worker exposure to arsenic in Florida grapefruit spray operations. *Arch. Env. Contam. Toxicol.* **11:**661–667.

Wolfe, H. R., W. F. Durham, and G. S. Batchelor. 1961. Health hazards of some dinitro compounds: Effects associated with agricultural usage in Washington state. *Arch. Env. Health* **3:**468–475.

Appendixes

APPENDIX A

Amines

Due to their ability to penetrate the skin and the fact that many are carcinogenic, amines have been the suject of many wipe sampling studies. It is possible that certain isocyanates that use amines such as methylenedianiline (MDA) as a precursor for synthesis may revert to these compounds under certain circumstances. Amines can be very irritating to the skin and often have low vapor pressures that allow them to remain on surfaces for long periods of time. Following a description of two unique methods for sampling amines are examples of sampling for the amines MDA and 4,4'-methylene bis(2-chloroaniline) (MOCA) illustrating the wide variety of methods that can be used.

METHODS

Modified Wet Wipe

The modified wet wipe method allows for on-site screening for contamination due to a variety of different aromatic amines (OSHA, 1991).

Procedure

1. Preload a group of vials with appropriate filters. Make sure the vials have labels.
2. Wear clean nitrile or latex gloves when doing the wipes. Dispose of gloves after each sample to prevent contamination of future samples as well as to oneself.
3. Prepare a diagram of the area or room(s) to be wipe sampled along with locations of key surfaces.
4. Write on the vial label the place where the sample is being collected along with a unique sample number.
5. Withdraw the filter from the vial and wipe approximately 100 cm^2 (3.9 in.) with a cellulose filter that is 7 cm (2.8 in.) in diameter after moistening its center with 5 drops of methanol.
6. After wiping the sample area, apply three drops of fluorescamine (a visualization reagent) to the contaminated area of the filter. Also place a drop of this reagent on an area of the filter that has not contacted the wiped surface. This area becomes a blank, and using the same filter allows for better comparison.
7. Allow 6 min for the reaction, then irradiate the filter with a 366 nm ultraviolet (UV) light. Compare the color development of the contaminated area with the area designated as the blank. A color change to yel-

low is a positive for contamination with the following amines: MOCA, benzidine, 3,3'-dichlorobenzidine, α-naphthylamine, β-naphthylamine, and 4-aminodiphenyl.

8. A discoloration greater than the blank indicates surface contamination, possibly aromatic amines. Repeat wipe sampling of the contaminated areas using the regular surface contamination procedure and send to a laboratory for confirmation. Send a vial containing a blank filter along with the wipe samples.

"Swype" Tests

Surface "swypes" are colorimetric indicators to detect contamination on work surfaces and skin; they are sold by CLI Colorimetric Laboratories. A color indication within 2 min to 3 min is a positive determination. One medium is utilized that changes to a different color depending on what amine has been detected. Table A-1 lists aromatic amines detected by the "swype" test.

Sampling for MDA Exposure

MDA is a light brown or tan crystalline solid with a faint amino-like odor. MDA is slightly soluble in water and very soluble in alcohol and benzene. It is produced commercially by the condensation of aniline and formaldehyde.

TABLE A-1. Aromatic Amines Detected by the "Swype" Test

Amine	*Detection*	*Limit Color*
MDA	3–5 μg	Red
MOCA	3–5 μg	Red
o-Toluidine	3–5 μg	Red
Aniline	3–5 μg	Red
Toluenediamine	3–5 μg	Red
Ethacure 100	10–15 μg	Blue green
Ethacure 300	10–15 μg	Blue green
o-Dichloroamine	3–5 μg	Red
Phenylene diamine	3–5 μg	Purple
Naphthylene diamine	3–5 μg	Purple

Crude MDA (40–60% MDA) is a liquid or hard waxlike substance. Purified (99%) MDA is in the form of either light yellow crystalline flakes or white granules.

Ninety-eight percent of the MDA produced is used in the manufacture of methylenediphenyl diisocyanate (MDI). The remaining 2% is used as a precursor for the manufacture of plastic fibers, antioxidants, dyestuff intermediates, corrosion preventives, and special polymers. The remaining MDA is produced in the pure form for other uses: epoxy resin curing agents, wire coating applications, polyurethane coreactants, pigments and dyes, and defense applications.

The primary industries where workers are exposed to MDA are MDA production, MDI synthesis, reprocessing, filament winding, potting and encapsulation, molding/bonding of tools and specialty small parts, wire coating, application of coating, TGMDA and PACM-20 production, polyurethane curing, advanced composite materials production, and epoxy paints production.

Paints and coatings containing MDA are applied by both spray and roll-on methods. Both these methods pose a risk for airborne and dermal exposure, with spray applications being the most serious. Using the estimate of 2,000 lb/yr usage for a typical painter who spends approximately 10% of the time applying MDA-containing coatings, OSHA (Occupational Safety and Health Administration) calculated that daily airborne exposures would be 2 mg/M^3 and dermal exposure levels would range from 0.50 mg/cm^2/hr for the palms to 0.00134 mg/cm^2/hr for the forearms and upper body. Maintenance workers would most likely experience similar airborne levels of exposure but only one-half of the dermal exposure expected for spray painters. For manual roll-on applications both airborne and dermal exposures decrease. OSHA estimated that airborne and dermal exposures would be comparable to those estimated for the polyurethane curing sector, or 0.160 mg/M^3 and 0.25 mg/cm^2/hr for the palms and 0.00067 mg/cm^2/hr for the forearms and upper body. Other types of work, such as the application by a contractor of epoxy floor coverings at several different sites in a day, are more difficult to assess.

For the most part, finished articles containing MDA have not shown detectable levels on their surfaces, including cured circuit boards and cured epoxies. Swipe samples averaging 0.4 μg per 100 cm^2 were collected during an epoxy putty operation that air cures. Although measurable surface MDA was detected on the epoxy, the relative degree of health hazard was calculated as being much lower. It was estimated that a surface contamination of 2,400 μg per 100 cm^2 would be required in order to pose a health risk equivalent to a 10 ppb airborne exposure (OSHA, 1992).

However, there is little doubt that liquid, powder, granular, or flake mixtures containing MDA in concentrations greater than 0.1% by weight or volume and materials other than finished articles containing MDA in concentrations greater than 0.1% by weight or volume do pose an exposure risk, especially dermal. Due to its low vapor pressure, MDA is more likely to remain on surfaces and pose an exposure hazard over a longer period of time.

MDA is absorbed through the skin at the rate of 2 μg/cm^2/hr. Once deposited on the skin, absorption continues, although the worker may have long since left the workplace and the apparent exposure area. Studies have indicated that absorption of MDA peaks 5 hr after the end of the work shift and that 80% of the substance is cleared from the body within 24 hr of exposure. It is difficult to correlate the amount deposited on the skin with urine biomonitoring because of MDA's rapid elimination from the body.

In its MDA standard, OSHA has chosen to use dermal monitoring as one of the requirements for monitoring exposure. Visual monitoring of exposed skin areas of workers would be required to be performed by their immediate supervisory personnel, including routine inspections of the face, hands, and forearms of employees potentially exposed to MDA. If the inspection reveals yellow staining or other abnormalities associated with MDA, such as red, itchy cracked skin or browning of the fingertips, protection for dermal exposure is required. A visual inspection will not detect all skin exposure, especially that associated with use of sanitary facilities without washing hands. For men, the scrotum area is an important route of exposure due to its high permeability; therefore, medical professionals must be involved in monitoring as well.

A problem with using this method as the only type of monitoring for dermal exposure is that pure MDA does not produce yellow staining, although certain MDA mixtures do. Often meta-phenylene diamine is present in MDA liquid mixtures. While MDA alone does not stain skin or clothing significantly, this compound intensely stains both skin and clothing, more so than other mixtures. Thus, in this case, there may be an overprediction of exposure.

Also concerns have been expressed over the use of soap and detergent to cleanse skin of MDA since it is poorly soluble in water. If the skin is not effectively cleaned and the material remains on the skin of the unknowing worker, exposure could be increased over what is expected. A further complication occurs in plants where MDI is used or synthesized. It is possible that on moist skin (pH 5) or surfaces, MDI will revert to MDA.

If dermal or other worker exposure is occurring, it is imperative that the source of exposure be determined and protective measures be implemented to correct the hazard. Protective measures include the establishment of a regulated area. Employees working in regulated areas are required to wear the appropriate type of chemical protective clothing (CPC) and are prohibited from activities such as smoking and eating. Precautionary signs are posted to designate these areas. By limiting access to only necessary personnel, the number of exposed employees is minimized. A decontamination area should be set up nearby where cleaning of workers, CPC, and equipment can be done. Certain contaminated CPC such as gloves, overboots, and aprons should be disposed of immediately before leaving a regulated area or further contamination of "clean" areas in the plant can occur. Disposal containers should be leaktight and may require lids if contamination is significant enough to generate a vapor pressure over the container.

In addition to regular operations, temporary regulated areas should be set up for other activities where exposure can occur such as maintenance work or spill and leak cleanup. The next step is to identify a mechanism to prevent these exposures from occurring. Industrial hygienists are trained in this type of work. For protective equipment, polyvinyl chloride, natural latex, and polyethylene are currently considered the best choices for protection against MDA.

Dermal and Surface Monitoring for MOCA in an Industrial Facility

MOCA is an example of an aromatic amine that is also a potent animal carcinogen used as a curing agent that is reacted with isocyanate-containing polymers to create a urethane material with a wide variety of uses ranging from industrial products such as gears, gaskets, belts, and rollers to consumer products such as sport boots and skateboard wheels. MOCA is recognized carcinogen in animals and is classified as a potential human carcinogen by the International Agency for Research on Cancer (IARC) and the National Institute of Occupational Safety and Health (NIOSH).

MOCA was originally produced in a flake form in the 1960s that was easily broken down into small inhalable particles. Later, production methods produced soft pellets that reduced the level of dust particles, so this factor should be considered if comparing studies from different periods. Advances have continued to be made with the result that pellets used in the 1990s are more uniform and harder, greatly reducing the presence of dust particles (Polyurethane Manufacturers Association, 1988). These pelletized materials are solids at room temperature and must be melted at 50°C for blending with polyurethane polymers (which are liquids at room temperature). Molten MOCA has a low vapor pressure (<0.000036 mmHg at 100°C) and is, therefore, unlikely to become airborne in the breathing zone of most workers.

A recent study was conducted at a company that manufactures commercial polyurethane products and is a large user of MOCA (NIOSH, May 1986). Process operations are separated within a single building into three major departments: urethane, machine shop, and wood model. The process of interest was the manufacture of MOCA-cured urethane elastomer and its subsequent molding in the molding area of the urethane department. Urethane molds are also often used in high precision aluminum foundries.

Production begins with MOCA-cured urethane from drums of dry pellets that are handled and opened by a worker. The worker whose position is called a mixer, transfers MOCA pellets by hand from the shipping containers to a melting pot, melts the chemical, and dispenses molten MOCA to molders who mix the hot MOCA (either manually in a disposable container with a hand stirrer or using an automatic machine) with an isocyanate propolymer to form a moldable urethane prior to pouring into molds. The urethane mixture is then poured into a heated metal mold and cured at either room temperature or in an oven, depending on product specifications. Trimmers remove the finished urethane part from the molds and then inspect, trim, and prepare the products for shipment. A cleanup person, responsible for sweeping and housekeeping, and supervisors also intermittently pass through the urethane department. All employees in the urethane department wear disposable latex surgical gloves; in addition, the mixers wear Tyvek disposable coveralls and occasionally wear disposable dust masks.

In this study air, surface wipe, and skin pad samples from workers in the urethane department were collected. Both area and personal, full-shift air samples were collected. Personal air samples for MOCA dust were collected in the workers' breathing zones using sampling pumps calibrated at 2 Lpm and worn by the workers; a filter cassette attached at the shirt collar was connected by tubing to the pump. Area samples for MOCA dust were collected using an identical sampling train at some representative locations throughout the department to investigate background concentration of MOCA.

Six of ten area air samples were collected at fixed, nonwork area locations to investigate general background airborne levels. The remaining four area samples were collected directly adjacent to the MOCA melting pot

TABLE A-2. Summary of Air Sampling Results for MOCA

Type	*Number of Samples*	MOCA *Concentration* ($\mu g/M^3$)
Area		
General work area	6	ND
MOCA melting pot (day 1)	1	61
MOCA melting pot (day 2)	1	92
MOCA melting pot (day 3)	1	58
MOCA melting pot (night 1)	1	12
Personal		
Molder A (day)	1	0.70
Molder A (day)	1	0.13
Molder A (day)	1	0.13
Molder A (day)	1	0.06
Molder A (day)	1	0.34
All other samples	35	ND

Notes: ND = None detected.
Limit of detection = 0.015 μg/L.

TABLE A-3. Summary of MOCA Hand Monitor Sampling Results

Job	*Number of Samples*	MOCA *Average Concentration* (*μg/pair*)[a]
Mixer (day)	2	24.6
Molder (day)	13	7.3
Mixer (night)	2	4.7
Molder (night)	6	3.0
Trimmer (day)	2	2.3

Note: Limit of detection varied between 0 μg and 1 μg.
[a]Sum of both palm and back-of-hand pads.

(where large quantities of pure MOCA are handled) to estimate the worst case concentration. Table A-2 summarizes air sampling results for MOCA.

To assess potential skin contamination, each worker wore gauze pads on his most frequently used hand for a full work shift. These "hand monitors" were prepared by attaching elastic straps to two small (1 in.^{2}) surgical cotton gauze pads. The monitors were attached to the outside of latex gloves worn by workers with one pad on the palm and the other pad on the back of the hand. The hand monitor is shown in Chapter 14. This sampling was chosen to simulate worst case conditions (no glove protection). Table A-3 summarizes hand monitoring sampling results for MOCA.

Twenty-four of the 25 sets of hand monitors in the urethane department contained detectable MOCA contamination. In calculating the results the total MOCA detected on both the palm and back-of-the-hand pads were summed to yield a single value for each set of pads. The averaged data indicate that the day mixer, who most directly handled MOCA, had the highest contamination on his gloves (avg. 24.6 μg/set of pads), which confirmed expectations.

Residual material could be contacted by workers brushing against bench tops, opening doors, or handling containers. Wipe samples should include all surfaces in the area where MOCA is stored, used, or handled in its pure form, such as mixing benches, door knobs, and CPC like gloves and aprons (OSHA, 1991). Also, if it is suspected that the employees are not being required to wash after using the material, or that other modes of contamination may be present, the wipes may have to be collected on lunchroom surfaces or other surfaces where other employees may be exposed. It is not uncommon for the mixing area to be separate from the molding area.

Samples were collected by wiping a 100 cm^2 area with dry Whatman filter tabs in a square pattern. Sampling locations were selected from surfaces where workers were predicted to most likely contact settled MOCA dust or condensed vapor, if such contamination was present. For comparison purposes, some wipe samples were collected in areas infrequently touched (tops of storage cabinets) to determine background contamination.

All 23 wipe samples collected indicated low but detectable contamination (Table A-4). MOCA contamination was found in the areas immediately adjacent to the MOCA melting

TABLE A-4. Summary of MOCA Wipe Sampling Results

Location	Number of Samples	MOCA Average Concentration (μg/cm²)
MOCA room near melting pot	3	19.1
Top of standing cabinet, Molding Dept.	2	4.7
MOCA room dispensing counter	3	1.4
Trimmer work table	1	0.1
Molder work table	14	0.5

pot. The average contamination level found on work tables of molders was about 0.5 μg/100 cm^2. Two samples collected on the top of storage cabinets (covered with accumulated dust) did reveal MOCA contamination several times higher than on work tables that were regularly wiped clean. Overall, these results indicate the presence of MOCA contamination throughout the urethane department on most horizontal surfaces where dust could settle.

Urine samples were also collected. All samples collected were spot voids collected at the end of the work shift. Urine samples were also obtained from seven office employees to use as controls. All participants were requested to wash their hands before voiding to minimize direct contamination of the urine samples.

Thirty-eight of 58 samples submitted by exposed workers contained detectable urinary MOCA concentrations. The overall average urinary concentrations for the mixers (61.9 μg/L) was more than four times higher than the overall average for molders (14.8 μg/L) (Table A-5).

From these results it is clear that air sampling inadequately characterizes potential occupational exposures to MOCA. Since MOCA dust rapidly settles to surfaces and since very little vapor is generated during melting, air concentrations are expected to be low. Based on the wipe sampling and dermal monitoring results, the greatest potential for exposures occurs when workers directly contact MOCA or surfaces contaminated with this material. These situations generally involve those required to work in areas where MOCA is stored, transferred, mixed, or melted, and who may not regularly wear gloves, or whose gloves are prone to punctures and tears.

The OSHA standard for MOCA requires that areas where employees may be exposed to this compound be "regulated areas," that is, areas where entry is restricted and where certain controls such as CPC, medical surveillance, and training are required. Once the material is mixed into the urethane, curing should begin, and the exposure to residual isocyanate vapor is a greater concern than the small amounts of catalyst generally used in these mixtures.

TABLE A-5. Urinary MBOCA Results for Molders and Mixers

Job	Number of Participants	Number of Samples	MOCA Average Concentration (μg/pair)[a]	MOCA Maximum Concentration (μg/pair)[a]
Mixer				
Day	1	5	29.9	56.5
Night	1	5	94.0	158.9
Molder				
Day	11	23	9.5	39.3
Night	5	12	20.6	40.0

[a]Adjusted to specific gravity of 1.019 per Cal/OSHA standard practice.

STUDIES

Amine Surface Sampling

Contaminant	*Activity*	*Surface Methods*	*Other Sampling*	*Reference*
3,3'-Dichlorobenzidine (DCB)	Synthesis of dichlorobenzidine and maintenance work	Wipe sampling on surfaces in break room, change room, and laundry room. Wipe samples of CPC including exterior of glove and interior of rubber suit and air helmet with Whatman smear tabs.	Personal breathing zone air samples for DCB Skin pads Urine Bulk sample from well drinking water	NIOSH, November 1985 (HETA 80-35-1635)
DCB	Pigment production	Whatman No. 1 filters wetted with methanol used to wipe surfaces in manufacturing work area, hand tools and locker room	Wipes of workers' hands Personal breathing zone air samples (under air hood) Urine	NIOSH, 1984 (HETA 84-128-1601)
DCB	Pigment manufacture	Gauze pads wetted with isopropanol used to wipe various surfaces routinely contacted by workers (hand tools, locker room, manufacturing area)	Personal breathing zone air samples Area air samples Pads on forearms	NIOSH, May 1986 (HETA 84-58-1700)
DCB	Manufacture of PE and PVC resins where pigment is added and decomposition occurs during extrusion	Wipes of dust settled on the extruder control panel and completed spools of wire using 37 mm GF filters impregnated with sulfuric acid	Area air sampling	Stevenson and Redpath, 1992
DCB	Pigment manufacture	Wipe samples from locker rooms, equipment, and work surfaces	Personal breathing zone air samples Area air samples Urine Gauze pads on forearms	London, Borano, and Lee, 1989

Contaminant	Activity	Surface Methods	Other Sampling	Reference
4,4'-Methylene bis (2-chloroaniline) (MOCA)	Polyurethane product manufacture	Wipe samples with Whatman smear tabs on surfaces routinely contacted by workers	Personal breathing zone air samples Gauze pads on hands Urine	Clapp et al., 1991
MOCA	Urethane casting	Wipes of oven, workbench, floor, tabletop, and refrigerator using Whatman smear tabs	Personal breathing zone air samples Dermal monitors	NIOSH, 1985 (HETA 84-508-1626)
MOCA	Facility manufacturing urethane tracks for snowmobiles	Wipe samples of surfaces in manufacturing area	Personal breathing zone air samples for TDI Area air samples for TDI	Klingner, 1992
MOCA	Maintenance work in a facility using MOCA where employees who did not work in the MOCA area had high urine levels	Wipe samples with colorimetric swypes of tools used for maintenance throughout the facility including the MOCA areas	Urine	Klingner, 1992
MOCA	Office where secretaries had MOCA in their urine adjacent to manufacturing facility where MOCA was used	Wipes with colorimetric swypes of paperwork that followed jobs on the plant floor	Urine	Klingner, 1992
MOCA	Plant using MOCA where urine levels increased after a segregated MOCA production area was built	Wipes of machines and tools with colorimetric swypes	Urine Wipes of shoes Skin wipes	Klingner, 1992
N-Nitrosodiethanolamine	Manufacture of engines and transmissions metal-working shop	Wipe samples of work surfaces	Bulk samples of cutting fluids	NIOSH, October 1982 (HETA 81-317-1202)
Bis-hydroxy ethyltallowamine (BHETA)	Inspection area in facility manufacturing electric panel instruments where employees lifting boxes of parts from conveyor belt developed a rash on arms and hands	Gauze wetted with methanol used to wipe locations where tote boxes (impregnated with BHETA) had been stored and used to see if residual BHETA contamination was present		NIOSH, April 1987 (HETA 85-453-1787)

Amine Dermal Sampling

Contaminant	*Activity*	*Dermal Methods*	*Other Sampling*	*Reference*
3,3'-Dichlorobenzidine (DCB)	Synthesis of dichlorobenzidine and maintenance work	Gauze pads (25 cm^2) with and without aluminum foil backing taped to ventral surface of forearm Skin wipe of palm of worker after removing glove	Personal breathing zone air samples Urine Wipe sampling on surfaces in nonwork areas Bulk sample from well drinking water	NIOSH, November 1985 (HETA 80-35-1635)
DCB	Pigment manufacture	Gauze pads, 2 in. by 2 in. with aluminum backing taped to forearm skin under protective suit and inner clothing	Personal breathing zone air samples (under air hood) Ambient air samples Wipe samples in manufacturing area and changing rooms Urine	NIOSH, May 1986 (HETA 84-58-1700)
DCB	Pigment manufacture	Gauze pads, 2 in. by 2 in., with aluminum backing taped to forearm skin	Personal breathing zone air samples Wipe samples in manufacturing area, hand tools, locker room, and a worker's hand Urine	NIOSH, May 1986 (HETA 84-58-1700)
Metaphenylene diamine	Field testing of glove permeability in a process using epoxy resin and amine hardeners	Cotton gloves under protective gloves inspected for discoloration		Gunderson et al., 1989
4,4'-Methylene bis (2-chloroaniline) (MOCA)	Plant using MOCA where urine levels increased after a segregated production area was built	Skin wipes of plant workers using colorimetric swypes Wipes of exteriors of workers' shoes using colorimetric swypes	Urine Surface wipes	Klingner, 1992
MOCA	Manufacture of MOCA-cured urethane elastomer and molding	1 in. by 1 in. gauze pads with elastic straps over the outside of latex gloves; one pad on dorsal hand, one on palm	Personal breathing zone air samples General work area air samples Wipe samples on surfaces in work areas Urine	Clapp et al., 1991

Contaminant	*Activity*	*Dermal Methods*	*Other Sampling*	*Reference*
MOCA	Urethane casting	Hand monitors of gauze (1 in.^{2}) moistened with glycerine strapped on one hand of workers	Personal breathing zone air samples Surface wipes	NIOSH, 1985 (HETA 84-508-1626)
MOCA	Plant with MOCA and non-MOCA operations where a worker who had transferred to the non-MOCA process had high MOCA urine levels	Wipes of interiors of shoes with colorimetric swypes	Urine	Klingner, 1992
Methylene dianiline (MDA)	Hand application of MDA-containing epoxies and adhesives for aircraft repairs	Hand wipes using colorimetric swypes before and after washing with soap and water	Urine	Groth, Housel, and Klingner, 1992
MDA Diglycidyl ether of bisphenol A	Painters applying epoxy resin surfacers and zinc chromate paints during construction of a power plant	Cotton gloves worn inside of rubber gloves by painters to determine if exterior gloves offered sufficient protection	Personal breathing zone air samples for respirable dust	NIOSH, September 1984 (HETA 83-132-1508)
Isodecanes Polymethacrylate amines	Toner used in platemaking operation	Wipes of hands of employees to determine residual amounts of chemicals following an outbreak of skin irritation when new equipment was installed	Personal breathing zone air samples Wipes of work surfaces Bulk samples of toner	NIOSH, January 1980 (HHE 78-77-659)

REFERENCES

Clapp, D. E., G. M. Piacitelli, D. D. Zaebst, and E. Ward. 1991. Assessing exposure to 4,4'-methylene bis(2-chloroaniline) (MOCA) in the workplace. *Appl. Occup. Env. Hyg.* 6(2):125–130.

Groth, K., T. Housel, and T. Klingner. 1992. Strategy for the Development and Testing of an Effective Dermal Decontamination Procedure for Aromatic Amines. Boston, MA: American Industrial Hygiene Conference, Abstract

Gunderson, E. C., B. A. Kingsley, C. L. Witham, and D. C. Bomberger. 1989. A practical study in laboratory and workplace permeatin testing. *Appl. Ind. Hyg.* 4(12):324–329.

Klingner, T. 1992. New developments in surface contamination monitoring for aromatic amines. In *Proceedings of the Conference on Advanced Composites*, Cincinnati, OH: ACGIH, pp. 43–46.

London, M. A., J. Borano, and S. A. Lee. 1989. 3,3'-Dichlorobenzidene (DCB) at two chemical plants. *Appl. Ind. Hyg.* 4(4):101–104.

NIOSH. 1977. *NIOSH Manual of Analytical Methods*, 2nd ed., vol. 1. Cincinnati, OH: NIOSH.

NIOSH, Health Hazard Evaluation Report. January 1980. *R. L. Polk Co., Cincinnati, OH.* HHE 78-77-659. Cincinnati, OH: NIOSH.

NIOSH, Health Hazard Evaluation. October, 1982. *Harley Davidson Motor Co., Milwaukee, WI.* HETA 81-317-1202. Cincinnati, OH: NIOSH.

NIOSH, Health Hazard Evaluation Report. September 1984. *Grand Gulf Nuclear Power Plant, Port Gibson, MS.* HETA 83-132-1508. Cincinnati, OH: NIOSH.

NIOSH, Health Hazard Evaluation Report. 1984. *Harshaw/Filtrol, Louisville, KY.* HETA 84-128-1601. Cincinnati, OH: NIOSH.

NIOSH, Health Hazard Evaluation Report. 1985. *Steinmetz & Sons, Moscow, PA.* HETA 84-508-1626. Cincinnati, OH: NIOSH.

NIOSH, Health Hazard Evaluation Report. November 1985. *Bofors-Nobel/Lakeway Corporation, Muskegon, MI.* HETA 80-35-1635. Cincinnati, OH: NIOSH.

NIOSH, Health Hazard Evaluation Report. May 1986. *Hilton-Davis Chemical Company, Cincinnati, OH.* HETA 84-58-1700. Cincinnati, OH: NIOSH.

NIOSH, Health Hazard Evaluation Report. April 1987. *Sperry Rand Corp., Great Neck, NY.* HETA 85-453-1787. Cincinnati, OH: NIOSH.

OSHA. 1991. *OSHA Industrial Hygiene Technical Manual*, 2nd ed. Washington, DC, OSHA.

OSHA. August 10, 1992. Occupational exposure to 4,4'-methylenedianiline (MDA). Final rule. Preamble.

Polyurethane Manufacturers Association. March 7, 1988. Submittal by the Polyurethane Manufacturers Association to OSHA regarding the chemical MOCA.

Stevenson, C. S., and D. J. Redpath. 1992. *Respiratory and Dermal Exposure to 3,3'-Dichlorobenzidine as a Thermal Degradation Product during the Extrusion of Polyethylene Insulated Wire.* American Industrial Hygiene Conference, Abstract, Boston.

APPENDIX B

Metals

Metals are an oral hazard as well as an inhalation hazard. Surface buildups can become resuspended and get in the air, and if on a worker's clothing, they can present a hazard to families, including children. In addition to paint, house dust is commonly sampled for metals. Lead paint identification has received a lot of attention recently and the HUD (Department of Housing and Urban Development) criterion for lead paint abatement is unique in that it specifies that surface sampling be done to assure completeness (HUD, 1990). This requirement is essentially the same as for most decontamination situations. HUD has also set specific standards as to what constitutes clean in these situations. Although these standards only apply to residences from a regulatory standpoint, they may also prove useful as guidelines in workplace situations.

There are a number of color change field tests that can be used to identify both surface and skin contamination with metals such as lead, arsenic, and chromium VI. There is also a direct reading instrument that uses X-ray fluorescence (XRF) to detect lead in paint on walls. Although lead is the only current application, this method shows promise for measuring other metallic surface contamination. Wipe samples can be analyzed for both total dust and the specific metal, such as cadmium or lead. It has been found that there is some loss of filter weight due to manipulation of the filter and a correction for this lost weight in the total dust results is required.

METHODS

Wipe Sampling for Lead Paint Abatement

Lead was a major ingredient in many types of paint for years prior to and through World War II. In the early 1950s, other pigment materials became more popular, but lead compounds were still used in some pigments and as drying agents. Federal regulatory efforts began with the Lead Based Paint Poisoning Prevention Act (LBPPPA) in 1971. In 1973, the Consumer Product Safety Commission (CPSC) established a maximum lead content of 0.5% by weight in a dry film of paint newly applied; in 1978, CPSC lowered the definition for lead in paint to 0.06%. However, lead paint is still found on automobiles and heavy duty equipment as well as nonresidential buildings and industrial structures and equipment, bridges, and storage tanks. Concentrations in older paint can be as high as 12% or more.

The action level for lead based paint (LBP) established in the LBPPPA amendments in the 1987 Housing Act is a lead content of 1.0 mg/cm^2 as measured by an XRF analyzer. Some state and local regulations have set a lower level of 0.7 mg/cm^2. Since there is some concern about the reliability of XRF results at these levels, the guidelines recommend backup chemical testing utilizing atomic absorption spectroscopy or inductively coupled plasma atomic emission spectrometry. When using chemical testing, the action level is either 0.5% by weight or 1.0 mg/cm^2.

In any situation where LBP is an issue there are several types of testing that must be done: bulk sampling to determine if lead is present in the paint (as an alternative an XRF analyzer can be used to measure lead directly on the walls); air sampling during abatement to determine the levels of lead dust being generated; and wipe sampling of surfaces for clearance of the abatement job. Testing for lead is conducted before abatement to establish lead levels in surface dust and/or during abatement to determine appropriate lead dust levels for worker protection. Testing must be conducted after abatement to determine whether abatement and cleanup are complete. Laboratories that analyze paint chips, soil samples, and dust samples for lead should participate in the EPA's National Lead Laboratory Accreditation Program.

The following sections describe typical tests required by HUD for paint and surface dust identification. Table B-1 lists typical surfaces tested for lead paint in residences. While currently training is only in the use of XRF instruments, it is likely in the near future that training requirements will be greater for those persons who perform lead paint evaluations and abatement testing.

TABLE B-1. Typical Surfaces Tested for Lead Paint in Residential Housing

Location	*Number of Measurements*
	Interior
Baseboard	One in each area
Ceiling	One in each area
Crown molding	One in each area
Door	Surface of door and one side of the frame on a representative interior door in each area
Fireplace	No specific number
Floor	One in each area
Radiator	No specific number
Shelf	One in each area
Shelf support	One in each area
Stairs	Riser, tread, stringer, newel post, railing cap, balustrade
Wall	Upper wall, lower wall and chair rail in each area
Window	Sash, casing, and sill on a representative window
	Exterior
Bulkhead	No specific number
Ceiling	No specific number
Cornerboard	No specific number
Door	Surface of door and door casing
Fence	No specific number
Floor	No specific number
Joist	No specific number
Lattice	No specific number
Lower railing	No specific number
Painted roofs	No specific number
Porch	No specific number
Railing cap	No specific number
Siding	No specific number
Stairs	Tread, riser, and handrail
Support column	No specific number
Trim	Upper and lower
Window	Sill, casing, and sash of a representative unit (including cellars)

Source: From HUD, 1990. *Lead-based Paint: Interim Guidelines for Hazard Identification and Abatement in Public and Indian Housing*. Washington, DC: U.S. Dept. of Housing and Urban Development, Office of the Secretary for Public and Indian Housing.

X-Ray Fluorescence for Surface Lead Contamination

XRF detectors X-ray the paint on the wall surface, causing lead in the paint, if present, to emit a characteristic frequency of radiation, the intensity of which is measured by the detector and related to the amount of lead in the paint. There are two types of XRF detectors available: direct reading and spectrum analyzers (Fig. B-1). Direct reading XRFs provide the operator with a direct readout of lead concentration in the paint.

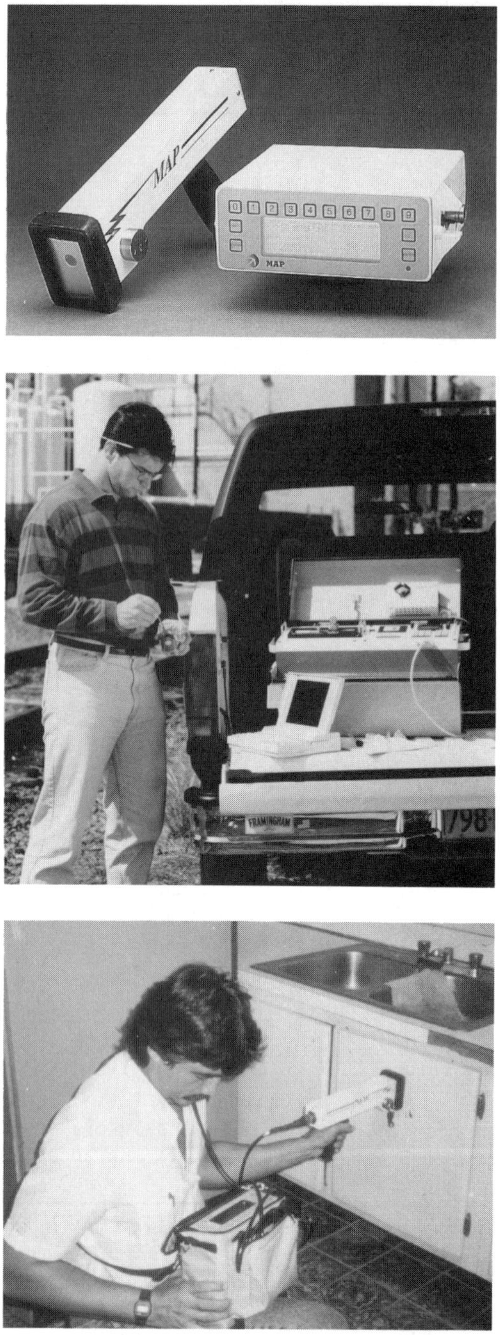

Figure B-1. *Top:* MAP-3 XRF Multichannel Spectrum Analyzer. *Middle:* Model SEFA-P XRF Analyzer from HNU Systems. *Bottom:* Taking a sample using a MAP-3 XRF Multichannel Spectrum Analyzer.
Sources: Top and bottom illustrations courtesy of Scitec Corporation; middle illustration courtesy of HNU Systems, Inc.

Spectrum analyzer XRFs allow a complete radiation spectrum to be analyzed by the instrument's software to improve the accuracy of the lead measurement. No one should operate an XRF instrument unless they have received thorough training in not only the use of the instrument but also radiological safety principles, emergency procedures, and regulation of XRF devices from a source approved by the manufacturer. The instrument must be positioned in such a way that no direct radiation exposure occurs to the eyes or gonads of the operator. While XRFs have been evaluated for paint on typical substrates used in buildings, they are not considered appropriate for detecting lead in paint over metal substrates. XRF is best used in conjunction with other confirmatory testing methods such as bulk sampling and sodium sulfide spot tests.

Direct Reading XRFs

Direct reading XRFs display only a calculated lead concentration. Two different instruments are available: the SK-e, manufactured by Princeton Gamma-Tech, and the Microlead I, manufactured by Warrington Corp. The displayed lead reading when taken on a painted surface is called an apparent concentration because the substrate under the paint and other factors may contribute to the reading. Therefore, a second reading to compensate for the contribution of the substrate is required. This measurement is done by removing the paint from the substrate and taking three XRF readings on the same place where the lead measurement was made. The resulting corrected lead concentration is the difference between the average apparent lead concentration and the average substrate equivalent lead.

For direct reading XRF each instrument has to be routinely tested against the manufacturer's lead standard prior to testing, once an hour during testing, and at the completion of testing. It is usually best to take three measurements at each site to assure that the instrument's variability has not exceeded 0.5 mg/cm^2. Variability can often be corrected by a repeat set of measurements, since the instruments are sensitive to changes in substrate. Curved surfaces usually give higher readings than flat ones.

Corrected XRF results from direct reading XRFs of 1.6 mg/cm^2 are classified as positive, results below 0.5 mg/cm^2 are considered negative, and results between these values are considered inconclusive according to HUD rules.

Spectrum Analyzer XRFs

A spectrum analyzer can display a graph of lead X-ray peak peak intensity relative to the intensity of other interfering radiation, which usually eliminates the need to scrape paint and take substrate measurements. This graph, called an energy spectrum, can be stored for later analysis, analyzed by the instrument's on-board computer, or viewed by the operator when the sample is taken (Fig. B-2). The spectrum analyzer requires more learning time than the direct reading instrument, but can save time in the long run. One commercially available spectrum analyzer is the MAP-3 Spectrum Analyzer from Scitec Corporation.

The MAP-3 Spectrum Analyzer consists of a control console and a scanner that attaches by a 10 ft cable. The 9 lb console contains a dedicated microprocessor system, LCD window, count rate light to indicate the relative number of X-rays detected, and beeper to indicate the end of a measurement cycle. It has a lead-acid battery pack capable of 8–10 hr of continuous use without recharging. It can operate at any angle and has been tested at temperatures between 20°F (–6°C) and 110°F (43°C). It has an RS-232 serial port that allows for downloading of stored data into a computer along with 2 megabytes of operating software and memory capacity, which is sufficient to store up to 2,500 measurements without spectral data or 324 measurements with these data. The readout can be set to show mg/cm^2, parts per million, or percent by weight and the measurement time in seconds.

A graphic spectrum of fluorescence energies is displayed after the measurement of X-ray intensity has been taken. The MAP-3 Spectrum Analyzer will allow up to six different calibrations or sample conditions. The scanner is 13 in.

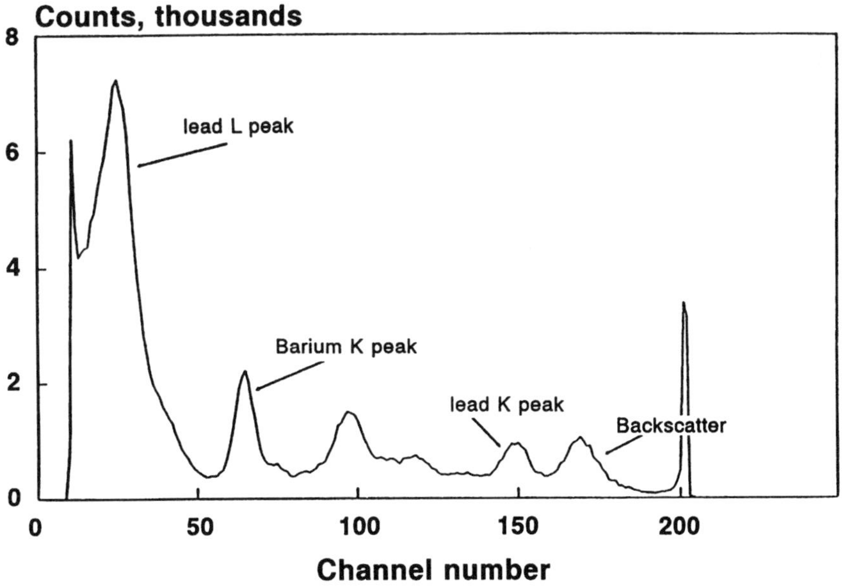

Figure B-2. A spectrum of a paint sample using a MAP-3 Spectrum Analyzer.
Source: Courtesy of Scitec Corporation.

long and weighs 3.5 lb. It is splashproof and has been tested at the same temperature ranges as the controller. Its detector is solid state silicone with a resolution of 170 keV FWHM over an active area of 25 mm^2. The source shutter is designed to house one of three sources: a 40 mCi Co^{57}, a 150 mCi Am^{241}, or an 80 mCi Cd^{109}. The detection limit of this instrument is approximately 0.1 mg/cm^2. Most measurements can be made in 15 sec with a precision of 0.3 mg/cm^2 at the 95% confidence level. The spectrum analyzer is calibrated on typical substrates on which lead paint would be found in residences to HUD lead-in-paint reference standards with a 40 mCi Co^{57} source. An accessory is available that allows the scanner to be attached to a pole and leaned against the wall for "hands-free" measurements. The pole can be extended to make measurements of ceilings, roof overhangs, or other hard-to-reach areas without a ladder.

The unit has two software packages. The AcuTransfer software performs quality control checks on data, monitoring the instrument's performance and comparing it to factory specifications. It compares the lead concentration to the spectral data to assure that measurement precision and accuracy are not affected by "key off," low count, high noise, or "gain shift" conditions. It checks to see that the appropriate calibration was used to make the measurement and prevents changes in downloaded raw data. The Advanced Report Manager can be used to analyze data, sort results, and produce test reports. It classifies measurements as positive, negative, or inconclusive based on the HUD "action level" and the precision of the K-line measurement or the laboratory test results for bulk paint samples and evaluates the L-shell measurements for surface lead. It calculates the weighted average of multiple XRF tests taken on the same spot and uses the precision level of the multiple tests to classify paint conditions as good, satisfactory, poor, and unsatisfactory according to HUD definitions. Finally, it applies HUD's decision rule criteria for single family/scattered site or multifamily testing to determine whether 100% testing or abatement, no further testing, or confirmation testing is required.

A result from a MAP-3 Spectrum Analyzer of 1.3 mg/cm^2 or greater is classified as positive. Results below 0.8 mg/cm^2 are classified as negative and values in between are inconclusive. In general, spectrum analyzer values greater than or equal to 1.3 mg/cm^2 require abatement, while those less than or equal to 0.3 mg/cm^2 indicate no lead is present at or above the regulatory level of 1.0 mg/cm^2. Spectrum analyzer values between 0.4 mg/cm^2 and 1.2 mg/cm^2 require confirmatory laboratory testing.

Interpretation of XRF Measurements

The sampling data from XRFs is then used for each building component tested to determine whether to abate it, test further, or confirm samples by laboratory analysis of bulk paint. There are separate rules for direct reading XRFs and spectrum XRFs. The interpretation of XRF measurements for HUD purposes is as follows:

1. If more than 15% of the component results for direct reading XRF or 11% of the component results for spectrum analyzer XRF are positive, lead is present, and either all such components must be abated or all should be tested to determine which require abatement and which do not. If the testing option is chosen, all inconclusive results must be confirmed.
2. If no XRF results for a component are positive, and 15% of results or less for direct reading XRF or 0% for spectrum analyzer XRF are inconclusive, no abatement or further testing of that component is required.
3. If some XRF results, in the percentages given below, are positive or inconclusive, confirmatory testing is required. All positive XRF results must be confirmed as well as all inconclusive readings above 1.0 mg/cm^2.

Direct Reading XRF: $\leq$ 15% positive
or $>$ 17% inconclusive

Spectrum Analyzer: $\leq$ 11% positive
or $>$ 0% inconclusive

4. If testing under rule number 3 confirms the presence of LBP above the regulated levels, all components of a given type can be abated, or exhaustive testing of the components can be carried out to determine precisely which ones must be abated.

Efforts to remove or encapsulate lead paint or to replace components covered with lead paint can create lead dust. Postabatement cleanup of dust can create additional contamination if not done carefully.

When abatement is conducted only in some rooms of a unit, preabatement wipe sampling outside of the containment area is often done to determine whether the containment is providing sufficient protection against releasing dust. These preabatement samples are compared to postabatement samples in the same areas; if lead levels have risen to unacceptable concentrations, the areas must be cleaned. The number of preabatement wipe samples should be equivalent to the number of postabatement samples.

Visual inspections are performed to ensure that all surfaces requiring abatement have been addressed and that all visible dust and debris have been removed. After visual cleanliness has been confirmed, surface dust sampling must be performed to demonstrate compliance with applicable clearance criteria.

Surface dust sampling should not be conducted if there is a visible accumulation of dust or debris; instead it is deferred until a thorough cleanup has been completed. After selecting the location and number of wipe samples to be collected, the specific area components to be sampled and the specific area sample location on a large component should be selected randomly.

A very large percentage of airborne lead dust is believed to settle out of the air within 24 hr of the completion of postabatement cleanup activities. Therefore, surface dust sampling should not be done any sooner in order for the results to be accurate. Since HUD regulations require that a 1 ft by 1 ft area be wiped, it is helpful to create a variety of plastic templates in different shapes that meet this criterion. One for floors might be square; another should be rectangular to fit a typical window sill.

Procedure

1. Identify and document all areas to be sampled, beginning in one room. Documentation should include location of the sample, surface type, material, and area measurement; abatement status; and abatement method, if known. Figure B-3 shows typical building components that are sampled.
2. Put on a fresh pair of disposable latex gloves to collect each sample. Open up the container of mixed cellulose ester filters and throw the top one away as it is likely to be contaminated. Put the next one inside of a vial as a laboratory blank.
3. Sample areas starting where concentrations are likely to be low and gradually moving up to those expected to contain high lead, if concentrations are known. Usually floors can be assumed to have the highest levels. Place a wipe flat on the surface to be sampled. Rub the wipe in an "S" pattern once over the entire measured area. Fold the wipe in half, folding the dust into the wipe (inside the fold) and rub once over the surface again, at a 90 degree angle to the first "S." Fold the wipe and place it in a vial. Record the sampling information on a form similar to that shown as Figure B-4.
4. Mark the vial with the sample number, location, and surface type and remove and replace gloves.
5. Use the same sampling method each time. Submit one field blank and one preparation blank (total of two) to the lab for each sampling day. The wipe representing the field blank is analyzed directly with no further treatment. The preparation blank is analyzed after it has passed through sample stream, including storage and sample preparation. The field blank represents contamination added in the field; the preparation blank represents contamination added in the field and during storage and sample preparation.

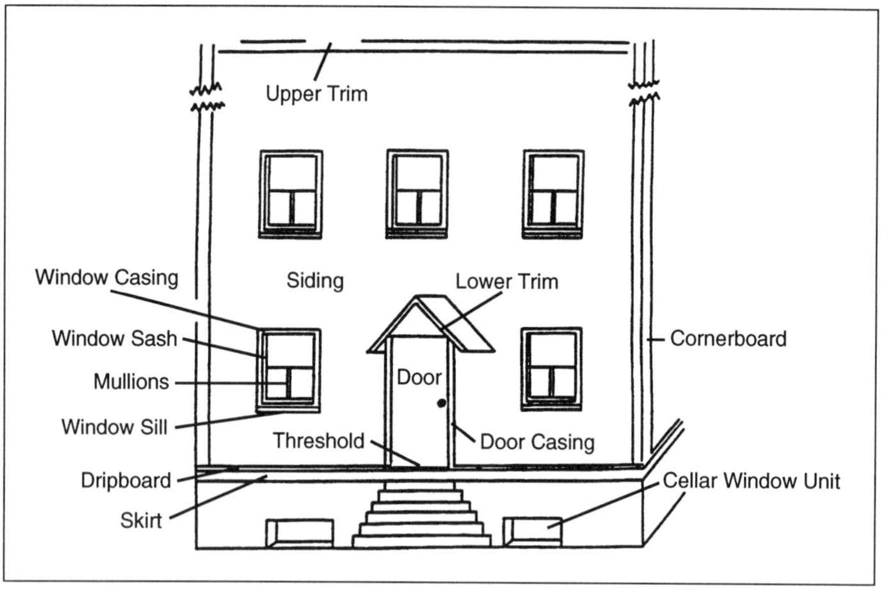

Figure B-3A. Diagram of building components.
Source: From HUD. 1990. *Lead-based Paint: Interim Guidelines for Hazard Identification and Abatement in Public and Indian Housing*. Washington, DC: Department of Housing and Urban Development.

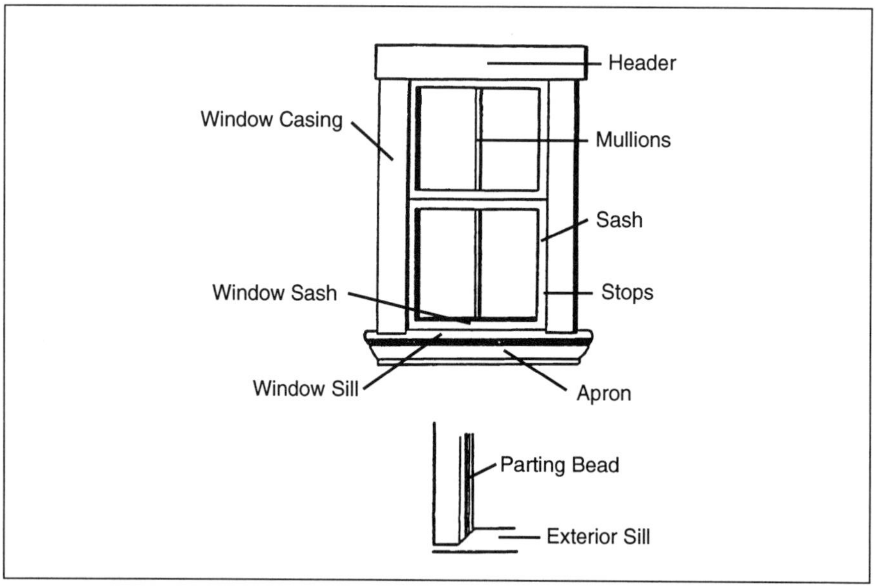

Figure B-3B. Window casing.
Source: From HUD. 1990. *Lead-based Paint: Interim Guidelines for Hazard Identification and Abatement in Public and Indian Housing*. Washington, DC: Department of Housing and Urban Development.

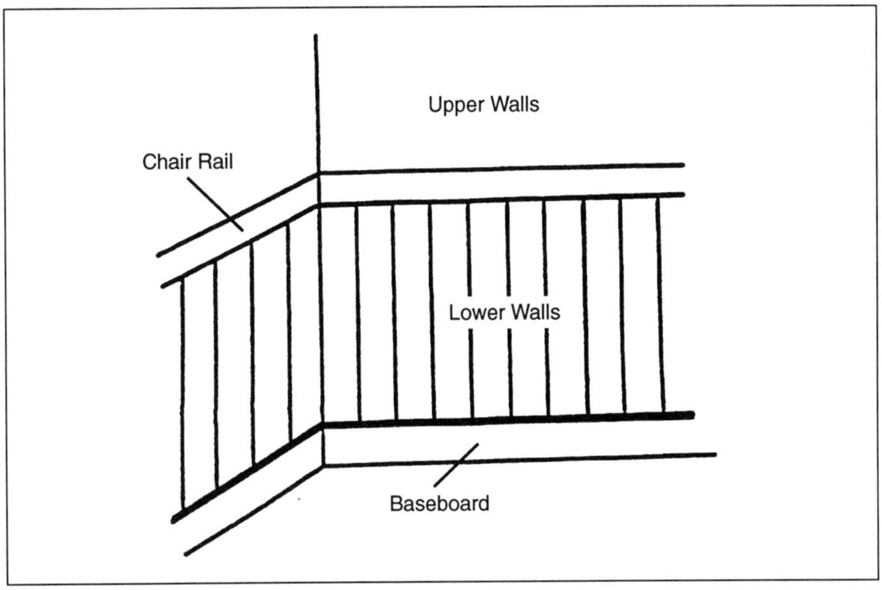

Figure B-3C. Walls.
Source: From HUD. 1990. *Lead-based Paint: Interim Guidelines for Hazard Identification and Abatement in Public and Indian Housing*. Washington, DC: Department of Housing and Urban Development.

Levels of surface lead dust should be stated in weight of lead present per relevant surface area. Lab results for wipe samples should be stated in terms of weight of lead present per wipe. In order to convert laboratory results to weight of lead present per relevant surface area, the surface sampled must be carefully measured and recorded. The wipe sampling procedure must ensure that a very high percentage of the surface dust present is captured on the wipe. Laboratory testing procedures for lead in wipes are the same as for lead in paint film. Laboratory selection is important as there are currently no accreditation programs for laboratories performing lead analysis of wipe samples.

There are no federal standards governing allowable levels of lead in house dust at the present time. The standards established by Maryland and Massachusetts may be used as a guideline:

Floors: 200 $\mu g/ft^2$
Windowsills: 500 $\mu g/ft^2$
Window wells: 800 $\mu g/ft^2$

In each area within an individual unit, compare the residual lead dust level from each wipe sample with the clearance criteria. If any of the lead dust results exceed the criteria, the area must be recleaned. If all residual lead levels for an area meet the clearance criteria, the area is considered ready for reoccupancy. A unit may be cleared for reoccupancy only after all areas within that unit have been cleared according to the criteria.

In the case of exterior abatement, the standard for floors should be applied to porches. In the case of limited abatement, it is important that areas outside the containment area were not contaminated during the abatement work. Therefore, samples should be taken in such areas before and after abatement and the lead levels compared to determine whether an increase attributable to the abatement has occurred. If so, final cleanup and clearance testing must be extended to the affected areas.

Lead-Check Swab

Lead-Check Swabs are self-contained cartridges containing reagents that allow for a rapid screening test to detect lead on surfaces. Ac-

SAMPLE SHEET - ANALYSIS FOR LEAD IN DUST

Date: ______________________ **Lab:** ______________________

Samples Collected By: ______________________

Occupant's Name: ______________________

Address: ______________________

Contractor's Name: ______________________

Address: ______________________

Date and Time Work Completed: ______________________

HEPA Filtration Units Use: No: ______________ **Capacity:** ______________

Sample Type: Initial Test: ______________ **Retest:** ______________

Housing Condition: Good __________ **Substandard** __________ **Grossly Substandard** __________

SAMPLE NO.	LOCATION	SURFACE CODE	MATERIAL CODE	METHOD CODE	AREA IN INCHES (l × w)	LABORATORY RESULTS μg Pb/ft^2	NOTES

Date Received: ______________ **Reported:** ______________ **Analyst:** ______________

Remarks: ______________________

Detection Limit __________ μg/ft^2 **Digestion Method** ______________________

Threshold Limit: Floor: 200 μg/ft^2
Window sill: 500 μg/ft^2
Window well: 800 μg/ft^2

Figure B-4. Documentation form for HUD wipe sampling.
Source: From HUD. 1990. *Lead-based Paint: Interim Guidelines for Hazard Identification and Abatement in Public and Indian Housing.* Washington, DC: Department of Housing and Urban Development.

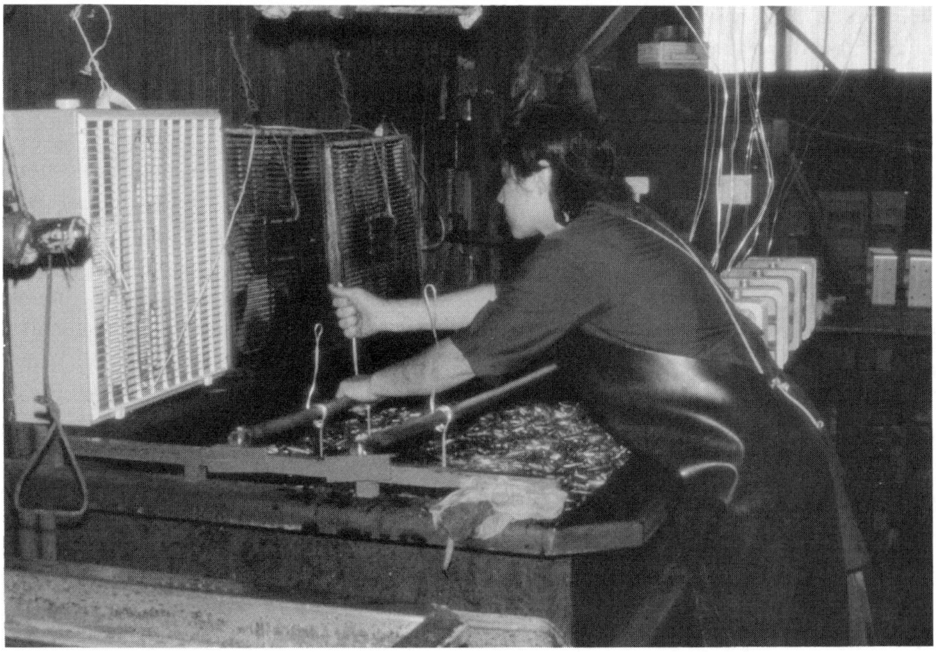

Figure B-5. A chrome electroplating operation. A good place for a chromium VI spot test.

cording to one report, the FDA tested Lead Check Swabs and found they were able to detect the presence or absence of lead in 96.6% of the pieces tested. The National Institute of Standards and Technology found that these swabs were able to detect lead in paint as well as many other testing methods.

Procedure

1. To activate Lead-Check Swabs, squeeze the cartridge at designated spots. Shake well to mix the contents.
2. Rub the test surface with the wet swab.
3. If the swab turns pink within 1 min, lead is present. Use the test confirmation card to compare the color change.

Spot Test for Lead

The sodium sulfide (Na_2S) test allows visual (qualitative) detection of lead on skin and other surfaces. Sodium sulfide reacts with inorganic lead to form a dark brown or black lead sulfide. The materials needed to perform the test are cotton balls, distilled vinegar, a spray bottle of 0.5% Na_2S in water, latex gloves, and 0.5% hydrogen peroxide. Any concentration between 0.5% and 1.5% Na_2S will work, but the lower concentration is preferable since this chemical has a distinct hydrogen sulfide odor. Perform this procedure in a well-ventilated area. It is especially useful for indicating if contamination exists under fingernails. Interferences are other heavy metals that will form sulfides such as nickel, iron, mercury, molybdenum, and copper.

Procedure No. 1 (Askin and Alvarez, 1993)

1. Apply the sodium sulfide solution directly to the hands, forearms, and under the fingernails.
2. If any lead is present, a brown to black color

will appear instantly. The more intense the color, the more lead is present.

3. Note that the lead sulfide stain can be difficult to remove. Washing with vinegar (4% acetic acid), hydrogen peroxide, or certain lead-specific soaps will remove the stain.

Procedure No. 2

This method can test both skin and surfaces and is the preferred one if individuals object to having solution sprayed on them.

1. Use a wipe cotton ball, paper, or gauze soaked in vinegar to clean a surface to be tested for lead.
2. Spray sodium sulfide solution directly onto the wipe and note the extent of the color change.

Surface Contamination Assessment for Arsenic Compounds

Arsenic compounds are of interest in that they not only pose a significant oral toxicity problem but many of these compounds can have adverse effects with skin contact. Arsenic compounds are a common contaminant in most recycling and other foundry operations and have been used as pesticides as well. Thus, the potential for exposure is broad and includes residences. The following wipe test method is appropriate for arsenic and arsenic-containing inorganic compounds (OSHA, 1991).

Procedure

1. Using a clean, disposable glove, remove a 7-cm (2.8-in.)-diameter Whatman 41 filter from the box.
2. Moisten the filter with distilled water. Use a dry filter if sampling for a liquid residue of arsenic trichloride or arsenic trifluoride.
3. Select a sampling area that is at least 100 cm^2.
4. With the leading edge of the filter slightly raised, wipe the surface in a back and forth and up and down motion. A 10 cm by 10 cm template can be used as a guide.
5. Pick up the filter paper, place it on a clean sheet of paper, fold the contaminated side inward, and make one more fold to form a 90 degree angle in the center of the filter.
6. Place the filter, angle first, into a glass vial and close the lid tightly.

Spot Test for Chromium VI

One method of performing a spot test was used to detect chromium VI contamination in an industrial plating operation (Fig. B-5) (NIOSH, 1975).

1. A cotton tipped swab is dipped into a stock solution of 1 normal sulfuric acid and rubbed vigorously on the surface to be tested.
2. One or two drops of a visualizing solution (1% alcoholic solution of diphenylcarbazide) was then placed on the cotton tip.
3. The formation of a blue-violet to red indicates the presence of hexavalent chrome. The visualizing solution is stored in a semi-opaque, dark brown bottle to prevent photodecomposition.

STUDIES

Metals Surface Sampling

Contaminant	*Activity*	*Surface Methods*	*Other Sampling*	*Reference*
Aluminum Chromium Copper Lead Zinc	Aluminum and brass foundry	Whatman filter wipes, both wetted with distilled water and dry, used to wipe (1 ft^2) area on lunchroom table, office desks, lunch boxes, and other employee contact areas	Personal breathing zone air samples for metals, silica, fluorides, oil mist, CTPV, ammonia, aldehydes, ozone, phenol, MDI, cyanide, hexamethylene tetramine, organic vapors, and nitrogen oxides Area air samples for the same Bulk samples of all materials and surface dusts	NIOSH, September 1979 (HHE 79-9-615)
Ammoniacal copper arsenate (as arsenic)	Wood preservative treatment where solution is mixed manually from powders by workers	Wipes of surfaces: finish-cut and rough-cut lumber as well as plywood and telephone poles with Kimwipes	Urine	Rosenberg, Landrigan, and Crowley, 1980
Antimony Bismuth Cadmium Chromium Indium Lead Nickel Tin	Machine shop specializing in tubing fabrication for aircraft equipment: tube bending, milling, furnace brazing, inspection, X-ray, electroplating, welding, and grinding	Gauze (3 in. by 3 in.) wetted with deionized water used to wipe for metal dusts over (100 cm^2) area on workstation tables, desk, and deburring station	Personal breathing zone air samples for solvents, inorganic acids, mineral oil, metal dust, welding fume, and sodium hydroxide	NIOSH, July 1992 (HETA 92-10-2234)
Arsenic Bismuth Lead Mercury	Manufacture of toys and wheel goods (welding, plating, painting, and assembly)	Wipes of (0.5 ft^2) area on presses, control panels, welding booths, and sheet stock in work areas with Whatman 40 filters	Area air sampling Skin wipes Bulk samples of paint	NIOSH, February 1976 (HHE 75-8-263)

Contaminant	*Activity*	*Surface Methods*	*Other Sampling*	*Reference*
Arsenic Beryllium Cadmium Lead Nickel	Evaluation of secondary copper smelter (processing scrap into cathode plates of 99.9% copper) for health concerns (excessive fatigue and skin problems)	Wet wipe samples with Whatman smear tabs for lead contamination in lunchroom Settled dust samples for all metals	Personal breathing zone air samples for all metals	NIOSH, 1984 (HETA 82-24-1428)
Arsenic	Gallium arsenide crystal growing facility	Whatman 42 filters wetted with water used to wipe surfaces in crystal growing area and on grinders and saws in grinding area	Personal breathing zone air samples for particulate and vaporous arsenic compounds General area air samples for particulate and vaporous arsenic compounds	Sheehy and Jones, 1993
Arsenic	Gallium arsenide wafer, field effect transistor, and monolithic microwave integrated circuit manufacture	Whatman 42 filters wetted with water used to wipe inside and outside of puller room and on grinders and saws in grinding area	Personal breathing zone air samples for particulate and vaporous arsenic compounds General area air samples for particulate and vaporous arsenic compounds	Sheehy and Jones, 1993
Arsenic	Manufacture of light emitting diodes	Whatman 42 filters wetted with water used to wipe on grinders and saws in grinding area	Personal breathing zone air samples for particulate and vaporous arsenic compounds General area air samples for particulate and vaporous arsenic compounds	Sheehy and Jones, 1993
Arsenic	Transmission repair shop where owner had developed symptoms of arsenic poisoning	Filter paper used to wipe dust on light fixtures, restroom, and floor surfaces	Area air samples in shop Bulk samples of liquid in shop waste pit and solvent from parts washing tank Urine	NIOSH, August 1985 (HETA 85-120-1616)

Contaminant	Activity	Surface Methods	Other Sampling	Reference
Arsenic	Pollution in residences within 2 miles of a copper smelter using arsenic rich ore (10–15%)	Vacuum samples using a personal air sampling pump of indoor surface dust from undisturbed areas such as the top of a door jamb Grab sample from inside vacuum bag Dustfall samples collected in polyethylene bucket	Personal breathing zone air samples Ambient air samples of indoor and outdoor air for suspended particulate Hand wash Urine Hair Soil Fruit and vegetables Drinking water	Polissar et al., 1990
Beryllium	Beryllium oxide cup used as an insulating case inside rail motor coach power supply	Smear samples collected inside power supply box 2 months and 10 months after normal operation Smear and sticky tape samples on walls, roof, and floor of box after arcing incident	Area air samples	Routledge, 1968
Beryllium	Research laboratory and support facilities	Monthly smear samples collected to evaluate degree of surface decontamination in analytical chemistry, chemical technology, engineering, and mechanical divisions	Personal breathing zone air samples Routine area air samples	Bolton, 1985*a*
Beryllium	Research laboratory and support facilities	Monthly smear samples collected to evaluate housekeeping effectiveness in analytical chemistry, engineering, and mechanical, metallurgy, and reactor chemistry divisions	Area air samples	Bolton, 1985*b*

Contaminant	*Activity*	*Surface Methods*	*Other Sampling*	*Reference*
Beryllium	Boring cores in small cylinders of beryllium oxide in a research lab	Smear samples on top of hood and on floor to determine if dust was escaping from the hood	Area air samples	Bolton, 1985*c*
Beryllium	Changing filters in ventilation system ducts	Smear samples in area following each filter change		Bolton, 1985*d*
Beryllium	Grinding of beryllium oxide blocks	Smear samples on hood and floor near grinder and lathe	Area air samples near machines	Bolton, 1985*d*
Beryllium	Production of lithium compounds from ore in a plant that formerly produced beryllium	Wipe samples of building surfaces	Personal breathing zone air samples for total and respirable dust and hexane Area air samples for respirable dust and beryllium Blood	NIOSH, July 1981 (HHE 80-36-922)
Beryllium	Building on air force base where material was stockpiled that is being decontaminated	Wipe samples collected on concrete floor after first, second, and third wet vacuuming operations and after painting	Personal breathing zone air samples on decontamination personnel Area air samples	NIOSH, 1970 (TA 70-1)
Cadmium Lead	Urban community residences Office buildings Schools Hospitals Supermarkets Chemical laboratories	Settled floor dust collected by vacuuming dust inside a template of 0.5 M by 0.5 M area with a small pump from rugs and nonrug surfaces inside residences and nonresidential buildings	Dust and soil samples from near buildings	Solomon and Hartford, 1976
Cadmium Total dust	Cadmium pigment manufacture	Wipe samples with 0.8 μg 37 mm MCE filters to quantify visible contamination and assess its variation through the milling and shipping areas	Personal breathing zone air samples Blood	Tartre, 1992

Contaminant	*Activity*	*Surface Methods*	*Other Sampling*	*Reference*
Chromated copper arsenate (as copper, chromium VI, arsenic) Ammoniacal copper arsenate (as copper, arsenic)	Treatment of wood with arsenical preservatives using pressure and nonpressure treatments	Wipe samples with filters of dry treated materials to determine the presence of residual salts on the wood surface and the availability for skin contamination Static pressure "touch" samples on wet wood surfaces with filters (10 cm^2)	Area air samples	NIOSH, 1983
Chromated copper arsenate (as arsenic)	Wood preservative treatment using a closed system	Wipes of treated surfaces: finish-cut and rough-cut lumber and telephone poles using Kimwipes	Urine	Rosenberg, Landrigan, and Crowley, 1980
Chromium VI	Radiator condensor dipping operation	Spot tests performed on Whatman smear tabs that have been used to wet wipe work surfaces in the immediate area of the tank and plastic caps that were put into the solution, cleaned, and reused	Personal breathing zone air samples Area air samples Skin wipes Bulk samples	NIOSH, May 1983 (HETA 82-116-1319)
Chromic acid (as chromium VI)	Industrial plating with chromic acid, zinc, cadmium, nickel, and tin	Chemical spot test used to test for the presence of chromium on work room surfaces, work gloves (interior and exterior), and drinking fountain	Personal breathing zone air samples General room air samples Spot test on worker's hands Skin exam	NIOSH, September 1975 (HHE 74-87-221)
Chromic acid (as chromium VI)	Industrial plating operation with nickel, copper, zinc, cadmium, and chromic acid where employees are suffering frequent nosebleeds, nasal sores, blood in nasal mucus, and skin eruptions	Chemical spot test used to test for the presence of chromium on part racks, lunchroom tables, vending machine handles, restroom fixtures, cloth towels, (used) and counters	Area air sampling for chrome, chromium VI, nickel, zinc, phosphate, cyanide, nitrate, and chloride Skin tests PPE tests	NIOSH, December 1973 (HHE 72-118-104)

Contaminant	*Activity*	*Surface Methods*	*Other Sampling*	*Reference*
Chromic acid (as chromium VI)	Industrial plating of automobile parts with chromic acid	Spot tests performed on filters used to wipe work surfaces and lunchroom	Personal breathing zone air samples Area air samples Skin spot tests Bulk sample of masking dip	NIOSH, June 1981 (HETA 81-85-889)
Chromium VI	Fuel pump assembly area in a plant that produces a variety of automobile parts	Wipe samples on work surfaces to determine if chromium VI from the coolant used in the brazing furnace was present	Area air samples for 1,1,1-trichloroethylene and phosgene Skin wipes	NIOSH, September 1977 (HHE 77-12-418)
Cobalt Nickel	Manufacture of hard metal cutting and grinding tools impregnated or studded with industrial diamonds	Whatman smear tabs used to wipe surfaces such as work tables, weigh out, water fountain, floor, telephone handset, and top of exhaust hood in various production areas	Personal breathing zone air samples Area air samples Bulk sample of solvent	NIOSH, November 1987 (HETA 84-288-1847)
Cobalt Copper Nickel Tungsten Zinc	Manufacture of diamond impregnated segments for core drills and gaskets for use in the cement pipe industry: infiltration, furnace and silver brazing	Wipe samples with Whatman filters from the floor and machinery near furnace and inside fume hood (5 cm^2)	Personal breathing zone air samples on furnace operator and silver solderer Area air sampling during silver soldering	NIOSH, August 1982 (HETA 81-212-1169)
Elements (Al, As, Ba, Be, Ca, Cd, Co, Cr, Cu, Fe, Li, Mg, Mn, Mo, Ni, Pb, Pd, K, Pt, Se, Ag, Na, Sn, Te, Th, Ti, W, Va, Yt, Zn, Zr) *See also* Metals	Facility involved in the manufacture of multilayer ceramic capacitors for electronic applications with employee dermatitis problems	Wipe of tables in work area using Whatman smear tabs wetted with distilled water	Area air samples for metals, VOCs, aldehydes, and amines Glove wipes Bulk samples of product, dust and waste fragments	NIOSH, February 1992*b* (HETA 91-51-2177)

Contaminant	*Activity*	*Surface Methods*	*Other Sampling*	*Reference*
Lead	Abrasive blasting to remove LBP from a steel highway bridge	Wipe samples with premoistened baby wipes inside work vehicles and on water coolers to detect surface dust posing an exposure to workers	Personal breathing zone air samples inside and outside of the abrasive blasting hoods Area air samples Bulk samples of used and unused blasting grit Blood Soil	NIOSH, 1991 (HETA 91-6-2193)
Lead	Evaluation of exposures from different methods of lead paint abatement: abrasive blast, heat gun, chemical stripping, setup work, encapsulation of surfaces, and replacement of paint	Surface samples using premoistened baby wipes on porch ballustrade and floor and inside and outside the decontamination structure	Personal breathing zone air samples Area air samples Soil Bulk paint	NIOSH, February 1992*a* (HETA 90-70-2181)
Lead	Radiator repair facility	Wipe sampling of surfaces used to determine exposure to lead from handling soldering wire and lead contaminated radiators	Personal breathing zone air samples General room air samples Blood	NIOSH, 1980 (HETA 80-63-767)
Lead	Small radiator repair facilities where radiators were torn apart and resoldered	Wipes in work and nonproduction areas including office areas using premoistened baby wipes Wipes inside of personal autos of workers using baby wipes	Personal breathing zone air samples Blood Clothing and skin wipes	Piacitelli and Rice, 1993

Contaminant	*Activity*	*Surface Methods*	*Other Sampling*	*Reference*
Lead	Soldering with hand soldering irons in an electronics factory that had recently banned smoking, eating, and drinking in the work area, and wanted to determine any changes in exposure as a result	Surfaces wiped on work benches	Personal breathing zone air samples Area air samples Blood	Courney and Meekin, 1985
Lead	Lead burning on a construction site and evaluation of residences of workers with high blood levels	Wipe samples inside personal autos with premoistened baby wipes	Personal breathing zone air sampling Clothing wipes Blood	Hales et al., 1992
Lead	Manufacture of molded rubber products	Wipes of door knobs, light switches, tables in work area and in lunchroom	Personal breathing zone air samples for lead, antimony oxide, and total dust Area air sampling for lead Skin and PPE wipes Bulk silica flour	NIOSH, December 1980 (HETA 79-75-784)
Lead	Lining steel storage tanks with lead sheeting (grinding, tinning, burning)	Wipe samples using MCE filters and premoistened baby wipes for contamination in lunchroom, the floor of the changing room, and workers' car interiors for surface contamination	Personal breathing zone air samples Blood Clothing wipes	NIOSH, 1991 (HETA 91-290-2131)
Lead	Lining steel storage tanks with lead sheeting (grinding, tinning, burning)	Wipe samples of lunchroom table, water cooler, in change room, inside workers' vehicles, and on workers' shoe soles using premoistened baby wipes	Personal breathing zone air samples Blood	NIOSH, 1992 (HETA 91-391-2174)

Contaminant	*Activity*	*Surface Methods*	*Other Sampling*	*Reference*
Lead	Cleaning prefabricated steel tanks and lining them with either polyvinyl chloride or lead	Wipe samples on surfaces including controls of equipment, restrooms, water fountains, and on floors	Personal breathing zone air samples Blood Bulk sample of dust from vacuum cleaner	NIOSH, December 1991 (HETA 91-393-2171)
Lead	Exterior painting and preparation (abrasive blasting) of an elevated water tower	Premoistened baby wipes used to wipe (1 ft^2) area inside and outside of the containment (walls, exhaust plenum, floor), in the trailer housing office and decontamination areas (water cooler, locker door)	Personal breathing zone air samples during blasting and moving the containment Area air sampling during blasting and inside containment Bulk samples of abrasive blast, soil, and paint	NIOSH, August 1992*b* (HETA 91-209-2249)
Lead	Battery manufacturing facility	Wipes of workbench tops, stacks of production material, tools, unfinished and finished product surfaces	Personal breathing zone air samples Area air samples Hand and face wipes	Chavalitnitkul, Levin, and Chen, 1984
Lead	Battery breaking and recycling operation	Whatman smear tabs used to wipe steering wheel, seat, dashboards and floor in employees' personal autos	Real time area air monitoring Blood	NIOSH, June 1991 (HETA 91-213-2123)
Lead	Manufacturing facility for lead shot, rolled sheet lead, tin-lead solder, pipe, and various other lead products where employees were routinely treated with a chelating agent for lead in blood.	Wipe samples in the lunchroom (bulletin board edge) and locker room (towel dispenser)	Personal breathing zone air samples for respirable and total lead dust Area air sampling for total lead dust Bulk samples of settled dust	NIOSH, 1976 (HHE 73-158-162)
Lead	Police scientific laboratory	Whatman 42 filters used to wipe the wall, floor, and workbench in the weapons testing area	Personal breathing zone air samples for organic vapors Area air samples for ammonia	NIOSH, August 1977 (TA 77-34)

Contaminant	*Activity*	*Surface Methods*	*Other Sampling*	*Reference*
Lead	Firing range	Surface wipes of ($929\ cm^2$) area on table and inside control booth using premoistened baby wipes	Personal breathing zone air samples Area air samples Hand wipes	NIOSH, August 1992*a* (HETA 90-168-2248)
Lead	Firing range	Surface wipes of ($929\ cm^2$) area on a table and desk inside the office/classroom using premoistened baby wipes	Personal breathing zone air samples Area air samples Skin wipes T-shirts	NIOSH, May 1992 (HETA 90-84-2219)
Lead	College with indoor firing range	Wipe of steam pipe in an office of $0.5\ ft^2$ area	Personal breathing zone air sampling on instructors during firing in standing and prone positions Area air samples	NIOSH, January 1979 (HHE 79-1-554)
Lead	Secondary smelting operation reclaiming lead from furnace slag	Wipe samples of office, lunchroom, change room, and water fountain (mouthpiece) surfaces Wipes also collected inside home next to smelting plant and on children's swing set in yard	Area air samples Blood Skin and PPE wipes Bulk samples of dross	NIOSH, February 1979 (TA 78-59)
Lead	Secondary smelting operation reclaiming lead from used batteries	Wipe samples of lunchrooms and inside respirator face pieces	Area air samples Blood	NIOSH, February 1979 (TA 78-59)
Lead	Grinding and polishing of petrified wood	Debris from a carpet sweeper collected and analyzed to determine contamination from flaking wall and ceiling paint	Bulk paint from walls and ceilings	NIOSH, April 1983 (HETA 83-73-1293)

Contaminant	*Activity*	*Surface Methods*	*Other Sampling*	*Reference*
Lead	Steam sterilization in a hospital using lead containing indicators	Whatman smear tabs used to wipe the interior and exterior of the autoclave and of surgical instruments before and after sterilization	Personal breathing zone air samples General area air samples Skin wipes of hands of processing technicians Blood Bulk samples of indicator strips	NIOSH, January 1988 (HETA 87-339-1863)
Lead Metal oxides	Manufacture of glass panels and funnels used in the production of TV picture tubes	Wipe samples using vinyl coated paper tape from lehr belts to compare to metals identified in air samples	Personal breathing zone air samples in burnoff, neck sealer, and furnace areas for lead; in glass press area for CTPV and PAHs Area air samples in burnoff, neck sealer, and furnace areas for lead; in glass press area for sulfur dioxide, CTPV, and PAHs Bulk dust for asbestos	NIOSH, October 1990 (HETA 89-244-2068)
Lead	Manufacture of pewter, bonded porcelain, and ceramic giftware	Wet wipe samples with filters of tabletops of (1 ft^2) area in the lunchroom	Personal breathing zone air samples	NIOSH, March 1980 (HHE 79-132-673)
Lead	Lead in the residential environment	Gauze wipes under beds or over a doorjamb in each house X-ray fluorescence of interior and exterior paint surfaces	Blood Soil samples from top half-inch of soil	Stark et al., 1982
Lead	Residences of workers in a lead storage battery plant	X-ray fluorescence measurements of paint on walls Gauze wipes from the living room, kitchen, and each child's bedroom	Blood of workers and their children Bulk samples of drinking water and paint	Watson, Witherell, and Giguere, 1978

Contaminant	*Activity*	*Surface Methods*	*Other Sampling*	*Reference*
Lead	Office building with excessive dust	Wipes with premoistened baby wipes inside duct work and on various room surfaces	Area air sampling Bulk dust	Giguere et al., 1993
Lead	Abatement of lead containing paint in publicly owned housing using chemical stripping and paint scraping methods	Wipe samples with premoistened baby wipes of surfaces in workers' changing and eating areas	Area air samples	Sussell, Elliott, and Freund, 1991
Lead	Dust inside residences	Prepackaged wet towelettes used to wipe floor and wall surfaces to estimate concentrations to which children might be exposed	Wipe samples of children's hands with prepackaged towels	Vostal et al., 1974
Lead	Children in a high risk residential community	Prepackaged wet towelettes used to wipe a windowsill and uncarpeted floor in areas where the children commonly played inside the home	Hand wipes	Sayre et al., 1974
Lead	Residences of workers with backyard battery repair shops on the same premises	Wipe samples of house dust from the floor of the room where children spent the most time using an aluminum template of 414 $cm+^2$ area and prepackaged moist towelettes	Personal breathing zone air samples Area air samples Soil core samples Bulk paint and drinking water	NIOSH, December 1989 (HETA 87-371-1989)
Lead	Residences where a home lead smelting business was carried out	Premoistened disposable paper towels used to wipe the center of the floor in the room where children spend the most time	Blood Soil sample from yard	Matte et al., 1991

Contaminant	*Activity*	*Surface Methods*	*Other Sampling*	*Reference*
Lead	Residences near a secondary lead smelter	Surface wipes of house dust from floors of rooms where children spent the most time using an aluminum template (414 cm^2) with premoistened towelettes Wipe samples of windowsills and other flat surfaces that are accessible to children using commercial wet towelettes	Soil from yard Bulk paint and drinking water Blood	NIOSH, December 1989 (HETA 87-371-2000)
Lead	Indoor pollution inside residences and comparison with outdoor levels	Dustfall using greased glass plates Vacuum cleaner samples of floor dust over a 1 M^2 area	Area air samples for suspended particulate	Diemel et al., 1981
Lead	Children's exposure to air soil and house dust in their community	Dustfall collected using plastic containers House dust sample collected from vacuum cleaner or using a dust pan	Area air samples (24 hr) at 15 ft elevation at schools in area Blood Soil outside of home (2 in. cores) Bulk samples of drinking water and milk	Angle et al., 1984
Lead	Children's exposure to dust inside houses in inner cities	Wipe samples of floor and wall surfaces inside homes using a commercial wet towelette in a 1 ft^2 area	Wipe samples of children's hands	Vostal et al., 1974
Lead	Homes of secondary lead smelter workers	Wipe samples of floor and wall surfaces inside homes using a commercial wet towelette in a 1 ft^2 area Settled dust over the doorways collected using brushes and glassine envelopes	Blood	Rice et al., 1978

Contaminant	*Activity*	*Surface Methods*	*Other Sampling*	*Reference*
Lead	Evaluation of lead paint abatement practices in residences	Serial wipe measurements of interior dust on house floors, windowsills, and window wells using commercial wet towelettes to wipe surface in a 1 ft^2 area (immediately preabatement, during abatement, after the final cleanup, and 1, 3, and 6–9 months postabatement		Farfel and Chisolm, 1991
Lead	Residential study of children's exposures from birth to 24 months of age	Interior surface dust collected by vacuuming three times over the same area with a personal air sampling pump	Hand wipes Blood	Bornschein et al., 1985
Mercury Mercury oxide	Lighthouses with mercury drive systems	Swab samples from the lens, cupola, motor mount, and window panes using cheesecloth and 1% nitric acid Floor dust collected with a brush	Personal breathing zone air samples Area air samples	van Netten and Teschke, 1988
Metals (30 different)	Soldering	Surface wipe samples with filters at the workstations due to employees' eating, drinking, and smoking at them	Personal breathing zone air samples Area air samples	NIOSH, June 1989 (HETA 87-411-1972)
Metals (30 different)	Incinerator burning municipal waste that disposed of ash on sites directly adjacent to facility	Gauze pads (3 in. by 3 in.) wetted with deionized water used to wipe desktop, floor, lunch table, bulldozer hand controls, and in a hotel room as background	Personal breathing zone air samples for total dust and metals Area air samples for total dust and metals	NIOSH, March 1992 (HETA 88-207-2195)

Contaminant	*Activity*	*Surface Methods*	*Other Sampling*	*Reference*
Metals (26 different)	Scrap metal business with lead contamination in soil	Dry surface wipes using MCE filters collected in the office, warehouse, and from objects in the courtyard to determine the potential for employee exposure	Personal breathing zone air samples Area air samples inside buildings Blood leads	NIOSH, February 1988 (HETA 87-410-1868)
Metals (25 different)	Scrap metal sorting and hide tanning operation with lead contaminated soil from draining acid from scrap batteries onto the property	Dry wipe samples with MCE filters collected in office, warehouse, and on courtyard surfaces	Personal breathing zone air samples Area air samples Blood Soil	NIOSH, February 1988 (HETA 87-410-1868
Metal dusts (Al, Be, Ba, As, Ca, Cd, Co, Cr, Cu, Fe, Li, Mg, Mn, Mo, Ni, Pb, P, Pt, Se, Ag, Na, Sn, Te, Ti, W, Va, Y, Zn, Zr)	Manufacturing facility with contamination from a neighboring zinc recycling company	Wipe samples on surfaces with smear tabs inside offices for elements	Personal breathing zone air samples Area air samples inside buildings Blood leads Bulk samples of furnace filter dust Soil samples	NIOSH, 1991 (HETA 91-73-2165)
Metals, trace	Municipal incineration of waste and conversion to energy	Surface wet wipes with Whatman smear tabs on high skin contact areas (benches, tables, desks, microwave oven) in break and locker rooms and the boiler control room	Personal breathing zone air samples Bulk samples of ash and settled dust	NIOSH, November 1990 (HHE 89-270-2080)
Metals	Office workers with illness symptoms	Wipe samples with Whatman smear tabs in different rooms of all three floors and the basement of the building	Area air sampling for metals and organic vapors	NIOSH, January 1984 (HETA 82-132-1406)

Contaminant	*Activity*	*Surface Methods*	*Other Sampling*	*Reference*
Potassium dichromate (as chromium VI)	Cyanotype printing to transfer photographic prints to fabric in an artist's workshop where the artist developed symptoms of overexposure	Whatman smear tabs wetted with distilled water used to wipe work area surfaces that were treated with spot test chemicals for on site analysis to determine source of artists' skin irritation, burning, and itching Settled dust samples vacuumed with personal air sampling pump Decontamination of board used in process with follow-up spot testing	General area air samples Bulk samples of fabric	NIOSH, May 1981 (HETA 81-171-880)
Thallium	Weighing, melting, and pouring, and cleanup in a research lab operation	Smear samples for work surface contamination	Area air samples	Bolton, 1985*d*
Thallium	Preparation of "buck shots"	Smear samples taken before and after cleanup operations and after subsequent decontamination		Bolton, 1985*e*

Metals Dermal Sampling

Contaminant	Activity	Dermal Methods	Other Sampling	Reference
Arsenic Bismuth Lead Mercury	Manufacture of toys and wheel goods (welding, plating, painting, and assembly)	Wipes of workers' hands with Whatman 40 filters before and after collecting samples	Area air sampling Surface wipes Bulk samples of paint	NIOSH, February 1976 (HHE 75-8-263)
Arsenic Cadmium Lead Manganese	Follow-up study of children living in the vicinity of a primary lead smelter after high lead levels have been found in school playground dust	Hand wash by pouring 500 mL of 0.1 N nitric acid from a bottle slowly over the palm of the dominant hand into a funnel	Continuous ambient air sampling outside on the roof of the school building Blood Bulk samples of dust and dirt from playgrounds	Roels et al., 1980
Arsenic	Pollution in residences within 2 miles of a copper smelter using arsenic rich ore (10–15%)	Hand was using a polyethylene bucket and 500 mL of 0.1 N HCl	Personal breathing zone air samples Ambient air samples of indoor and outdoor air Vacuum samples of indoor surface dust Bulk sample from inside vacuum bag Dustfall samples Urine Hair Soil Fruit and vegetables Drinking water	Polissar et al., 1990
Arsenic	Glassware factory	Hand rinses by pouring 500 mL of 0.1 N nitric acid from a bottle slowly over the palm of the dominant hand into a funnel before and after the shift Mouth rinses using 50 mL of demineralized water over 30 sec with collection in a metal-free funnel/bottle before and after the shift	Personal breathing zone air samples Area air samples for total dust Urine (pre- and postshift)	Roels et al., 1982

Contaminant	*Activity*	*Dermal Methods*	*Other Sampling*	*Reference*
Arsenic acid	Spray tank loading Aerial and ground rig application to cotton	100% cotton overalls with the extract subsequently analyzed	Personal breathing zone air samples	Miller, Hoover, and Culver, 1980
Cadmium	Manufacture of electric condensors	Hand rinses by pouring 500 mL of 0.1 N nitric acid from a bottle slowly over the palm of the dominant hand into a funnel preshift, midmorning, at lunch, midafternoon, and postshift Mouth rinses using 50 mL of demineralized water over 30 sec with collection in a metal-free funnel/bottle on Monday morning and Friday afternoon	Personal breathing zone air samples Area air samples for total dust Bulk samples of dust from workplaces Blood Urine Feces	Roels et al., 1982
Chromic acid (as chromium VI)	Industrial plating with chromic acid, zinc, cadmium, nickel and tin	Chemical spot test used to identify material in orange stains on workers' hands Skin examination for orange discoloration	Personal breathing zone air samples General room air samples Spot tests of work surfaces, PPE	NIOSH, September 1975 (HHE 74-87-221)
Chromic acid (as chromium VI)	Industrial plating operating with nickel, copper, zinc, cadmium and chromic acid where employees are suffering frequent nosebleeeds, nasal sores, blood in nasal mucous and skin eruptions	Chemical spot test used on the finger tips and on exteriors of rubber gloves worn by workers to identify chromium IV contamination	Area air sampling for chrome, chromium VI, nickel, zinc, phosphate, cyanide, nitrate and chloride Surface spot tests	NIOSH, December 1973 (HHE 72-118-104)
Chromic acid (as chromium VI)	Industrial plating of automobile parts	Spot tests performed on filters after wiping workers' hands	Personal breathing zone air samples Area air samples Surface spot tests Bulk sample of masking dip	NIOSH, June 1981 (HETA 81-85-889)

Contaminant	*Activity*	*Dermal Methods*	*Other Sampling*	*Reference*
Chromium VI	Radiator condensor dipping operation where some employees had dermatitis	Spot tests performed on Whatman smear tabs that have been used to wet wipe employees' hands	Personal breathing zone air samples Area air samples Surface wipes Bulk samples	NIOSH, May 1983 (HETA 82-116-1319)
Chromium VI	Erection of a cooling tower using treated lumber	Chemical spot tests on gloves and clothing used to handle treated lumber	Bulk sample of treated lumber	NIOSH, April 1981 (HHE 81-151-862)
Chromium VI	Fuel pump assembly area in a plant that produces a variety of automobile parts	Wipe samples on employees' hands to determine if chromium VI from the coolant used in the brazing furnace was present	Area air samples for 1,1,1-trichloroethylene and phosgene Surface wipes	NIOSH, September 1977 (HHE 77-12-418)
Copper fungicide	Comparison of exposures from high pressure manual spraying and boom spray application to staked tomatoes in fields	Carefree sanitary pads taped to clothing at arms, "V" of neck, forearms, back, chest (left and right), forearms, hands, thighs, legs (front and back), and on shoes		Machado Neto, Matuo, and Matuo, 1992
Copper oxide	Test to determine resuspension of dust and resulting clothing contamination	Double-sided adhesive tape placed at various sites over clothing	Area air sampling	Fish et al., 1965
Elements (Al, As, Ba, Be, Ca, Cd, Co, Cr, Cu, Fe, Li, Mg, Mn, Mo, Ni, Pb, Pd, K, Pt, Se, Ag, Na, Sn, Te, Th, Ti, W, Va, Yt, Zn, Zr)	Facility involved in the manufacture of multilayer ceramic capacitors for electronic applications with employee dermatitis problems	Wipe of glove interior of worker using Whatman smear tabs wetted with distilled water	Area air samples for metals, VOCs, aldehydes and amines Surface wipes Bulk samples of product, dust, and waste fragments	NIOSH, February 1992*b* (HETA 91-51-2177)

Contaminant	*Activity*	*Dermal Methods*	*Other Sampling*	*Reference*
Lead arsenate (0.1%, 0.3%)	Tractor-drawn air blast sprayer on grapefruit; mixing and loading	Gauze pads (10.2 cm by 10.2 cm) 16 ply backed with filter paper attached to forearms, shoulders, thigh fronts, back (center near neck), and chest (upper center near jugular) Cotton gloves (front and back patches were cut for analysis)	Modified respirator with 16 ply gauze backed with filter pads Urine (P.M. postexposure)	Wojeck et al., 1982
Lead	Lining steel storage tanks with lead sheeting (grinding, tinning, burning)	Wipes samples with filters and premoistened baby wipes inside workers' gloves and respirator facepiece, on shirt collars, and on shoes	Personal breathing zone air samples Blood Surface wipes	NIOSH, 1991 (HETA 91-290-2131
Lead	Children living in the vicinity of a large lead smelter	Hand wash with 500 mL 0.1 N nitric acid	Area air sampling of ambient levels Blood Dust and dirt from playgrounds	Roels et al., 1980
Lead	Secondary smelting operation reclaiming lead from furnace slag	Wipe of employee's nose with Whatman filter after removing respirator and of respirator interiors	Area air samples Blood Wipe samples of surfaces in nonwork areas and nearby home Bulk samples of dross	NIOSH, February 1979 (TA 78-59)
Lead	Employees at secondary lead smelter reclaiming lead from plates of old batteries to determine if there was any association between work clothing and exposures to families	Cuff dust from trousers worn under coveralls of workers Cloth samples (2.5 cm^2) from the bottoms of trousers worn under coveralls	Blood lead Hair samples Dust from floor or vacuum cleaner bags	Winegar et al., 1977

Contaminant	*Activity*	*Dermal Methods*	*Other Sampling*	*Reference*
Lead	Small radiator repair shops where radiators are torn apart and reassembled	Wipes of hands (postshift) with premoistened baby wipes of workers before and after washing Forehead wipes Work clothing wipes	Personal breathing zone air samples Area air samples Surface wipes Blood	Piacitelli and Rice, 1993
Lead	Electric cable splicing	Wipe samples on shirt (chest) and pants (left and right thigh) using filters	Personal breathing zone air samples	NIOSH, 1992 (HETA 90-75-2298)
Lead	Manufacture of molded rubber products	Wipes of respirator interior, shoes, and forehead of workers	Personal breathing zone air samples for lead, antimony oxide, and total dust Area air sampling for lead Surface wipes Bulk silica flour	NIOSH, December 1980 (HETA 79-75-784)
Lead	Battery workers	After washing workers were immersed in a bath of 0.0042% sodium sulfide. Brownish to black discoloration indicated the presence of residual lead, which must be removed by further washing.		Lerner and Hogan, 1985
Lead	Japanese battery plant	At the end of the work shift each employee was required to enter a bath of dilute sodium sulfide. If discoloration occurred they were required to wash.		Burton, 1980

Contaminant	*Activity*	*Dermal Methods*	*Other Sampling*	*Reference*
Lead	Test approximating conditions in battery production	Spot test using a few drops of 1% sodium sulfide on premoistened disposable towelette after it has been used to wipe hands 1% sodium sulfide applied directly to skin of hands and observation for dark brown stain		Lerner and Hogan, 1985
Lead	Lead burning evaluation in construction and residences of employees with high blood leads	Wipes with premoistened baby wipes of employees' street shoes and shirt collars	Personal breathing zone air samples Surface wipes in autos Blood	Hales et al., 1992
Lead	Steam sterilization in a hospital using lead containing indicators	Skin wipes of hands of processing technicians with Whatman smear tabs	Personal breathing zone air samples General area air samples Blood from technicians Surface wipes of autoclave and instruments Bulk samples of indicator strips	NIOSH, January 1988 (HETA 87-339-1863)
Lead	Firing range	Hand wipes using premoistened baby wipes	Personal breathing zone air samples Area air samples Surface wipes	NIOSH, August 1992*a* (HETA 90-168-2248)
Lead	Firing range	Hand wipes on police officers using premoistened baby wipes T-shirts	Personal breathing zone air samples Area air samples Surface wipes	NIOSH, May 1992 (HETA 90-84-2219)
Lead	Children in a high risk residential community	Hand wipes with commercial wet paper towelettes	Surface wipe samples in areas where child commonly played	Sayre et al., 1974

Contaminant	*Activity*	*Dermal Methods*	*Other Sampling*	*Reference*
Lead	Children's exposure to dust inside houses in inner cities	Wipe samples of children's hands using commercial wet towelettes. For total lead, one towelette used on hand; for distribution of lead on hand, individual towels were used for every finger and for the palm.	Wipe samples of household floor and wall surfaces	Vostal et al., May 1974
Lead	Residential study of children's exposures from birth to 24 months of age	Hand wipes using six commercial wet towelettes over each hand	Household surface dust vacuumed Blood	Bornschein et al., 1985
Mercury	Shoe manufacturing facility	Clothing of employee with symptoms of mercury poisoning surveyed with direct reading instrument to determine source of mercury	Residential surfaces, furniture, and appliances surveyed	NIOSH, 1972 (HHE 72-38-19)
Mercury	Thermometer manufacturing facility	Direct reading instrument used to sniff workers' clothing and shoes for contamination	Breathing zone air monitoring Area air monitoring Surface monitoring	NIOSH, July 1976 (HETA 76-49-312)
Mercury	Residences of workers at a thermometer manufacturing facility who had children	Direct reading instrument used to sniff workers' clothing and work shoes	General area monitoring in homes and inside closets and washing machines Urine from children	Hudson et al., 1987
Mercury	Thermometer manufacturing facility	Direct reading instrument (JW Lamaire Mercury Vapor Sniffer) used to sniff glass blowers' clothing, work shoes, and respirator interior	Personal breathing zone air samples Urine	NIOSH, November 1977 (TA 77-52)

Contaminant	*Activity*	*Dermal Methods*	*Other Sampling*	*Reference*
Mercury	Dental clinic	Direct reading instrument used to sniff dental assistants' fingers	Personal breathing zone air samples Area air monitoring	NIOSH, 1977 (HETA 76-45-313)
Mercury	Dental clinic	Direct reading instrument used to sniff employees' shoes	Area sampling of surfaces	NIOSH, April 1979 (HHE 79-47-582)
Mercury	Dental clinic	Direct reading instrument used to sniff employees' shoe soles for contamination	Personal breathing zone air samples Ambient air monitoring Surface monitoring	NIOSH, November 1976 (TA 76-108)
Mercury	Dental school clinic	Direct reading instrument (Bachrach MV Mercury Sniffer) used to sniff dental assistants' hands and shoe soles before and after scuffing carpet	Personal breathing zone air samples Area air samples Surface sniffs	NIOSH, March 1978 (TA 78-9)
Silver	Silver reclamation	Photos of faces of workers for the presence of skin discoloration	Blood Urine Feces Hair	Pifer et al., 1989

REFERENCES

Angle, C. R., A. Marcus, I. Cheng, and M. S. McIntire. 1984. Omaha childhood blood lead and environmental lead: A linear total exposure model. *Env. Res.* **35:**160–170.

Askin, D., and B. Alvarez. 1993. Sodium sulfide instantly reveals lead on surfaces. *Occup. Health and Safety*, January, p. 34.

Bolton, N. E. 1985*a*. *Industrial Hygiene, Quarterly Report, 4th Quarter, 1961*. ORNL/TM-9462. Oak Ridge National Lab, TN.

Bolton, N. E. 1985*b*. *Industrial Hygiene, Quarterly Report, 1st Quarter, 1962*. Oak Ridge National Lab, TN.

Bolton, N. E. 1985*c*. *Industrial Hygiene, Quarterly Report, 3rd Quarter, 1963*. Oak Ridge National Lab, TN.

Bolton, N. E. 1985*d*. *Industrial Hygiene, Quarterly Report, 4th Quarter, 1963*. Oak Ridge National Lab, TN.

Bolton, N. E. 1985*e*. *Industrial Hygiene, Quarterly Report, 1st Quarter, 1964*. Oak Ridge National Lab, TN

Bornschein, R. L., P. Succop, K. N. Dietrich, C. S. Clark, S. Que Hee, and P. B. Hammond. 1985. The influence of social and environmental factors on dust lead, hand lead, and blood lead levels in young children. *Env. Res.* **38:**108–118.

Burton, D. J. 1980. An overview of occupational exposure control technology in nonferrous smelting. *Am. J. Ind. Med.* **1:**293–305.

Chavalitnitkul, C., L. Levin, and L. Chen. 1984. Study and models of total lead exposures of battery workers. *AIHA J.* **45**(12):802–808.

Courtney, D., and S. R. Meekin. 1985. Changes in blood lead levels of solderers following the introduction of the control of lead at work regulations (1980). *J. Soc. Occup. Med.* **35:**128–130.

Diemel, J. A. L., B. Brunekreef, J. S. M. Boleu, K. Biersteker, and S. J. Veenstra. 1981. The Arnhem lead study. *Env. Res.* **225:**449–456.

Farfel, M. R., and J. J. Chisolm. 1991. An evaluation of experimental practices for abatement of residential lead-based paint: Report on a pilot project. *Env. Res.* **55:**199–212.

Fish, B. R., R. L. Walker, G. W. Royster, and J. L. Thompson. 1965. Redispersion of settled particulates. In G. W. Royster and B. R. Fish (eds.), *Surface Contamination*. New York: Pergamon Press, p. 80

Giguere, M. T., J. J. Curran, P. D. Morris, K. Williams, and P. Matson. 1993. *Survey of Lead Contamination in an Office Building*. New Orleans, LA: American Industrial Hygiene Conference, Abstract.

Hales, T. R., C. R. McCammon, W. J. Daniels, and S. T. Lee. 1992. *Lead Exposure Among Lead Burners*. Boston, MA: American Industrial Hygiene Conference, Abstract.

HUD. 1990. *Lead-based Paint: Interim Guidelines for Hazard Identification and Abatement in Public and Indian Housing*. Washington, DC: U.S. Dept. of Housing and Urban Development, Office of the Secretary for Public and Indian Housing.

Hudson, P. J., R. L. Vogt, J. Brondum, L. Witherell, G. Myers, and D. C. Paschal. 1987. Elemental mercury exposure among children of thermometer plant workers. *Pediatrics* **79**(60):935–938.

Lerner, S. I., and D. J. Hogan. 1985. Detection of inorganic lead contamination with sodium sulfide. *JOM* **27:**293–294.

Machado Neto, J. G., T. Matuo, and Y. K. Matuo. 1992. Dermal exposure of pesticide applicators in staked tomato *(Lycopersicon esculentum miii)* crops: Efficiency of a safety measure in the application equipment. *Bull. Env. Contam. Toxicol.* **48:**529–534.

Matte, T. D., J. P. Figueroa, S. Ostrowski, G. Burr, L. Jackson-Hunt, and E. L. Baker. 1991. Lead exposure from conventional and cottage lead smelting in Jamaica. *Arch. Env. Contam. Toxicol.* **21:**65–71.

Miller, C. S., W. L. Hoover, and W. H. Culver. 1980. Exposure of pesticide applicators to arsenic acid. *Arch. Env. Contam. Toxicol.* **9:**281–288.

NIOSH, Technical Assistance Report. 1970. TA70-1. *Dental Practice*. Cincinnati, OH: NIOSH.

NIOSH, Health Hazard Evaluation. 1972. *Toxicity Determination Data Sue Co., Inc., Bellcamp, MD.* HHE 72-38-19. Cincinnati, OH: NIOSH.

NIOSH, Health Hazard Evaluation Report. December 1973. *Marsh Plating Corporation, Ypsilanti, MI.* HHE 72-118-104. Cincinnati, OH: NIOSH.

NIOSH, Health Hazard Evaluation Report. September 1975. *Industrial Platers, Inc., Columbus, OH.* HHE 74-87-221. Cincinnati, OH: NIOSH.

NIOSH, Health Hazard Evaluation. 1976. *NL Industries Hoist Plant, Granite City, IL.* HHE 73-158-162. Cincinnati, OH: NIOSH.

NIOSH, Health Hazard Evaluation Report. February 1976. *Hestrom Union Co., Bedford, PA.* HHE 75-8-263. Cincinnati, OH: NIOSH.

NIOSH, Health Hazard Evaluation Report. July 1976. *Jay Instruments and Specialty Co., Cincinnati, OH.* HHE 76-49-312. Cincinnati, OH: NIOSH.

NIOSH, Health Hazard Evaluation Report. November 1976. *Children's Dental Services, Batavia and Cincinnati, OH.* TA 76-108. Cincinnati, OH: NIOSH.

NIOSH, Hazard Evaluation and Technical Assistance Report. August 1977. *New York State Police Scientific Laboratories*, TA 77-34. Cincinnati, OH: NIOSH.

NIOSH, Health Hazard Evaluation Report. 1977. *G. A. Riddell, D. D. S., Cody, WY.* HHE 76-45-313. Cincinnati, OH: NIOSH.

NIOSH, Health Hazard Evaluation Report. September 1977. *Airtex Products, Fairfield, IL.* HHE 77-12-418. Cincinnati, OH: NIOSH.

NIOSH, Health Hazard Evaluation and Technical Assistance Report. November 1977. *Jay Instruments and Specialty Co., Cincinnati, OH.* TA 77-52. Cincinnati, OH: NIOSH.

NIOSH, Health Hazard Evaluation and Technical Assistance Report. March 1978. *Louisiana State University, School of Dentistry, New Orleans, LA.* TA 78-9. Cincinnati, OH: NIOSH.

NIOSH, Health Hazard Evaluation Report. January 1979. *La Salle College, Philadelphia, PA.* HHE 79-1-554. Cincinnati, OH: NIOSH.

NIOSH, Technical Assistance Report. February 1979. *Minerals Reclamation Corporation, Adell and Milwaukee, WI.* TA 78-59. Cincinnati, OH: NIOSH

NIOSH, Technical Assistance Report. February 1979. *Minerals Reclamation Corporation, Adell and Milwaukee, WI.* TA 78-59. Cincinnati, OH: NIOSH.

NIOSH, Health Hazard Evaluation Report. April 1979. *Gladnick Dental Clinic, Wilmington, DE.* HHE 79-47-582. Cincinnati, OH: NIOSH.

NIOSH, Health Hazard Evaluation Report. September 1979. *Arapahoe Aluminum and Brass Foundry, Inc., Englewood, CO.* HHE 79-9-615. Cincinnati, OH: NIOSH.

NIOSH, Health Hazard Evaluation Report. March 1980. *Lance Corp., Hudson, MA.* HHE 79-132-673. Cincinnati, OH: NIOSH.

NIOSH, Health Hazard Evaluation Report. December 1980. *St. Clair Rubber Co., Marysville, MI.* HHE 79-75-784. Cincinnati, OH: NIOSH.

NIOSH, Hazard Evaluation and Technical Assistance Report. 1980. *Rocky Mountain Radiator Service, Boulder, CO.* HETA 80-63-767. Cincinnati, OH: NIOSH.

NIOSH, Health Hazard Evaluation Report. May 1981. *Cyanotype Printing in an Artist's Workshop, Bucyrus, OH.* HETA 81-171-880. Cincinnati, OH: NIOSH.

NIOSH, Health Hazard Evaluation Report, June 1981. *Valley Chrome Platers, Bay City, MI.* HETA 81-85-889. Cincinnati, OH: NIOSH.

NIOSH, Health Hazard Evaluation Report. July 1981. *Lithium Corp. of America, Bessemer City, NC.* HHE 80-36-922. Cincinnati, OH: NIOSH.

NIOSH, Health Hazard Evaluation Report. April 1981. *Spectt, Inc., Cleveland, OH.* HHE 81-151-862. Cincinnati, OH: NIOSH.

NIOSH, Health Hazard Evaluation Report. March 1982. *City of Norwood, Norwood, OH.* HETA 82-17-1067. Cincinnati, OH: NIOSH.

NIOSH, Health Hazard Evaluation Report. August 1982. *N.P.C. Systems, Inc., Milford, NH.* HETA 81-212-1169. Cincinnati, OH: NIOSH.

NIOSH, Health Hazard Evaluatin Report. April 1983. *Russell-Zuhl, Inc., NY.* HETA 83-73-1293. Cincinnati, OH: NIOSH.

NIOSH, Health Hazard Evaluation Report. May 1983. *Modine Manufacturing, McHenry, IL.* HETA 82-116-1319. Cincinnati, OH: NIOSH.

NIOSH, 1983. *Industrial Hygiene Surveys of Occupational Exposure to Wood Preservative Chemicals.* Cincinnati, OH: NIOSH.

NIOSH, Health Hazard Evaluation Report. 1984. *Chemetco, Inc., Alton, IL.* HETA 82-24-1428. Cincinnati, OH: NIOSH.

NIOSH, Health Hazard Evaluation Report. January 1984. *Huntington Alloys, Inc., Huntington, WV.* HETA 82-132-1406. Cincinnati, OH: NIOSH.

NIOSH, Health Hazard Evaluation Report. August 1985. *Dawson Transmission, Gilmore City, IA.* HETA 85-120-1616. Cincinnati, OH: NIOSH.

NIOSH, Health Hazard Evaluation Report. November 1987. *Wheel Trueing Tool Co., Columbia, SC.* HETA 84-288-1847. Cincinnati, OH: NIOSH.

NIOSH, Health Hazard Evaluation Report. January 1988. *St. Francis–St. George Hospital, Cincinnati, OH.* HETA 87-339-1863. Cincinnati, OH: NIOSH.

NIOSH, Health Hazard Evaluation Report. February 1988. *Klotz Brothers, Inc., Staunton, VA.* HETA 87-410-1868. Cincinnati, OH: NIOSH.

NIOSH, Health Hazard Evaluation Report. December 1989. *Technical Assistance to the Jamaican Ministry of Health, Kingston, Jamaica.* HETA 87-371-2000. Cincinnati, OH: NIOSH.

NIOSH, Health Hazard Evaluation Report. June 1989. *Naval Weapons Support Center, Crane, IN.* HETA 87-411-1972. Cincinnati, OH: NIOSH.

NIOSH, Health Hazard Evaluation Report. December 1989. *Technical Assistance to the Jamaican Ministry of Health, Kingston, Jamaica.* HETA 87-371-1989. Cincinnati, OH: NIOSH.

NIOSH, Health Hazard Evaluation Report. October 1990. *Thomson Consumer Electronics, Inc., Circleville, OH.* HETA 89-244-2068. Cincinnati, OH: NIOSH.

NIOSH, Health Hazard Evaluation Report. November 1990. *Harrisburg Steam Generation Facility, Harrisburg, PA.* HETA 89-270-2080. Cincinnati, OH: NIOSH.

NIOSH, Hazard Evaluation and Technical Assistance Report. June 1991. *G. T. Jones Tire & Battery Distributing Inc., Birmingham, AL.* HETA 91-213-2123. Cincinnati, OH: NIOSH.

NIOSH, Health Hazard Evaluation Report. December 1991. *George Metals, Inc., Powder Springs, GA.* HETA 91-393-2171. Cincinnati, OH: NIOSH.

NIOSH, Hazard Evaluation and Technical Assistance Report. 1991. *New England Lead Burning Co. (NELCO), Eaton Metals, Salt Lake City, UT.* HETA 91-290-2131. Cincinnati, OH: NIOSH.

NIOSH, Hazard Evaluation and Technical Assistance Report. 1991. *M&J Painting Company, Covington, KY.* HETA 91-6-2193. Cincinnati, OH: NIOSH.

NIOSH, Health Hazard Evaluation Report. 1991. *Carbonnaire Co., Palmerton, PA.* HETA 91-73-2165. Cincinnati, OH: NIOSH.

NIOSH, Health Hazard Evaluation Report. 1992. HETA 90-075-2298. Cincinnati, OH: NIOSH.

NIOSH, Health Hazard Evaluation Report. 1992. HETA 91-391-2174. Cincinnati, OH: NIOSH.

NIOSH, Health Hazard Evaluation and Technical Assistance Report. January 1992. *New England Lead Burning Co. (NELCO), Eaton Metals, Salt Lake City, UT.* HETA 91-290-2174. Cincinnati, OH: NIOSH.

NIOSH, Health Hazard Evaluation Report. February 1992*a*. *HUD Lead-Based Paint Abatement Demonstration Project.* HETA 90-70-2181. Cincinnati, OH: NIOSH.

NIOSH, Health Hazard Evaluation Report. February 1992*b*. *AVX Corp., Myrtle Beach, SC.* HETA 91-51-2177. Cincinnati, OH: NIOSH.

NIOSH, Health Hazard Evaluation Report. March 1992. *Northwest Incinerator, Philadelphia, PA.* HETA 88-207-2195. Cincinnati, OH: NIOSH.

NIOSH, Health Hazard Evaluation Report. May 1992. *Kansas City Police Department, Kansas City, KS.* HETA 90-84-2219. Cincinnati, OH: NIOSH.

NIOSH, Health Hazard Evaluation Report. July 1992. *Kreisler Industrial Corp., Elmwood Park, NJ.* HETA 92-10-2234. Cincinnati, OH: NIOSH.

NIOSH, Health Hazard Evaluation Report. August 1992*a*. *Independence Police Department, Indoor Range, Independence, MO.* HETA 90-168-2248. Cincinnati, OH: NIOSH.

NIOSH, Health Hazard Evaluation Report. August 1992*b*. *Seaway Painting, Inc., Annapolis, MD.* HETA 91-209-2249. Cincinnati, OH: NIOSH.

OSHA (1991). *OSHA Technical Manual.* Washington, DC: OSHA.

Piacitelli, G., and C. Rice. 1993. Lead contamination in radiator repair shops. *Appl. Occup. Env. Hyg.* **8**(5):434–438.

Pifer, J. W., B. R. Friedlander, R. T. Kintz, and D. K. Stockdale. 1989. Absence of toxic effects in silver reclamation workers. *Scand. J. Work Env. Health* **15:**210–221.

Polissar, L., K. Lowry-Coble, D. A. Kalman, J. P. Hughes, G. van Belle, D. S. Covert, T. M. Burbacher, D. Bolgiano, and N. K. Mottet. 1990. Pathways of human exposure to arsenic in a community surrounding a copper smelter. *Env. Res.* **53:**29–47.

Rice, C., A. Fischbein, R. Lilis, L. Sarkozi, S. Kon, and I. Selikoff. 1978. Lead contamination in the homes of employees of secondary lead smelters. *Env. Res.* **15:**375–380.

Roels, H. A., J. Buchet, R. R. Lauwerys, P. Bruaux, F. Claeys-Thoreau, A. Lafontaine, and G. Verduyn. 1980. Exposure to lead by the oral and the pulmonary routes of children living in the vicinity of a primary lead smelter. *Env. Res.* **22:**81–94.

Roels, H., J. Buchet, J. Truc, F. Croquet, and R. Lauwerys. 1982. The possible role of direct ingestion on the overall absorption of cadmium or arsenic in workers exposed to CdO or As_2O_3 dust. *Am. J. Ind. Med.* **3:**53–65.

Rosenberg, M. J., P. J. Landrigan, and S. Crowley. 1980. Low-level arsenic exposure in wood processing plants. *Am. J. Ind. Med.* **1:**99–107.

Routledge, R. 1968. Possible health risk from beryllium oxide ceramic rectifiers of 1000 H.P. rail motor coaches. *Ann. Occup. Hyg.* **11:**17–21.

Sayre, J. W., E. Charney, J. Vostal, and I. B. Pless. 1974. House and hand dust as a potential source of childhood lead exposure. *Am. J. Dis. Child* **127:**167–170.

Sheehy, J. W., and J. H. Jones. 1993. Assessment of arsenic exposures and controls in gallium arsenide production. *AIHA J.* **54**(2):61–69.

Solomon, R. L., and J. W. Hartford. 1976. Lead and cadmium in dusts and soils in a small urban community. *Env. Sci. and Tech.* **10:**773–777.

Stark, A. D., R. F. Quah, J. W. Meigs, and E. R. DeLouise. 1982. The relationship of environmental lead to blood-lead levels in children. *Env. Res.* **27:**372–383.

Sussell, A. L., L. J. Elliott, and E. Freund. 1991. Occupational hazards of lead-based paint abatement in publicly owned housing. Salt Lake City, UT: American Industrial Hygiene Conference, Abstract.

Tartre, A. 1992. Investigation of surface contamination in a cadmium pigment facility. *Appl. Occup. Env. Hyg.* **7**(5):318–322.

van Netten, C., and K. E. Teschke. 1988. Assessment of mercury presence and exposure in a lighthouse with a mercury drive system. *Env. Res.* **43:**48–57.

Vostal, J. J., E. Taves, J. W. Sayre, and E. Charney. May 1974. Lead analysis of house dust: A method for the detection of another source of lead exposure in inner city children. *Env. Health Perspec* **7:**91–97.

Watson, W. N., L. E. Witherell, and G. C. Giguere. 1978. Increased lead absorption in children of workers in a lead storage battery plant. *JOM* **20**(11):759–761.

Winegar, D. A., B. S. Levy, J. S. Andrews, P. J. Landrigan, W. H. Scruton, and M. J. Krause. 1977. Chronic occupational exposure to lead: An evaluation of the health of smelter workers. *JOM* **19**(9):603–606.

Woject, G. A., H. N. Nigg, R. S. Braman, J. H. Stamper, and R. L. Rouseff. 1982. Worker exposure to arsenic in Florida grapefruit spray operations. *Arch. Env. Contam. Toxicol.* **11:**661–667.

APPENDIX C

PCBs and TCDDs

Polychlorinated biphenyls (PCBs) are chlorinated aromatic hydrocarbons that were manufactured in the United States from 1929 to 1977 and marketed under the trade name Aroclor. PCBs have been used commercially for a wide variety of purposes, including as insulating fluids for electrical equipment, hydraulic fluids, heat transfer fluids, lubricants, plasticizers, and components of surface coatings and inks. Transformer PCBs typically are mixed with tri- and tetrachlorobenzenes. Since the manufacture and use of PCBs in the United States was banned by the Toxic Substances Control Act (TSCA), occupational exposure has been limited almost exclusively to the servicing and repair of transformers and mining machinery that contain PCBs, to leaks from older fluorescent lamp ballasts and certain types of capaciters, and to activities relating to the disposal of PCB contaminated equipment and waste material.

The different PCB mixtures marketed under the Aroclor trade name are often characterized by a four-digit number such as Aroclor 1242. The first two digits denote the type of compound, with "12" indicating biphenyl, and the latter two digits give the weight percentage of chlorine, with the exception of Aroclor 1016, which contains 42% chlorine. Some analytical methods will differentiate the type of PCB that has been sampled. The heights of the five major peaks of the standards are added and those sums are compared to the sums of the peaks in the sample.

Situations where PCBs may require sampling include testing decontamination procedures on waste sites where PCB cleanup is in progress and in offices where leaks of PCB containing ballasts in fluorescent lamps have occurred. Transformer incidents involving the pyrolysis of PCB dielectric fluids may result in the formation of polychlorinated biphenylenes, dibenzofurans, and dibenzo-p-dioxins, which may be widely dispersed in the smoke from the fire (Orris et al., 1986). Transformer incidents involving pressurization of the transformer due to internal arcing have resulted in the release of PCBs as a liquid aerosol. All of these compounds are known for their stability in the environment and ability to persist for years. Typical surfaces of transformers that are sampled include:

Name plate
Low voltage switch
Switch gear case
Main panel
Main switch

Between gauges
Above cooling coils
Circuit breaker
Switch handle
Dike floor and walls
Transformer vault door handle
Top of transformer
Floor with visible stains

Soot formed from the incomplete combustion of PCB askarels in transformer and capacitor fires can contain a complex mixture of potentially toxic chlorinated products. In addition to tetrachlorodibenzofurans (TCDFs) and tetrachlorodibenzodioxins (TCDDs), the soot may contain polychlorinated biphenylenes and polychlorinated nuclear aromatics such as chlorinated pyrenes and chrysenes. The concentrations of these pyrosynthesis products can vary widely depending on the specific conditions of the fire (Hryhorczuk et al., 1986). Soot from PCB-related fires is sometimes sampled by scraping, thus as a bulk sample, and other times using wipes. Table C-1 provides data on levels of TCDFs that have been measured in several different PCB fires.

When a PCB containing ballast fails, proper procedures should be followed to minimize the potential exposure to PCBs such as turning off the light, evacuating the room, venting room air directly outside, removing the failed ballast, cleaning up asphalt residue that may have leaked from the ballast, and wiping down the tops of general contact surfaces such as desks, chairs, and tables. Workers doing the cleanup or equipment removal should wear gloves of neoprene or nitrile and a half mask with an organic vapor cartridge. If additional skin protection is needed, Saranex coveralls should be used. Hard, relatively nonabsorbent surfaces that are contaminated with residue that has leaked from a ballast should be cleaned with an organic solvent such as deodorized kerosenes or mineral spirits. It is important to note that the residue may be concentrated with PCBs and care is needed to prevent skin contact.

General surface cleaning can be done with a solution of octylphenoxypolyethoxyethanol nonionic surfactant detergent in water followed by a water rinse. An application strength of 5% (volume-to-volume) is considered adequate to remove mild surface contamination. The addition of a mild caustic such as trisodium phosphate to the wash solution will help emulsify any thin grease deposits that are on the surfaces prior to the ballast burnout and will also help lift waxes and some furniture polishes that will otherwise absorb PCBs from the air.

There are usually two concerns in these types of incidents: identifying the degree of contamination and providing an adequate decontamination with subsequent verification. In both cases surface sampling is generally the primary

TABLE C-1. Comparison of Tetrachlorodibenzofuran (TCDF) Levels in Wipe Samples from PCB Fires

Sample	*Type*	*PCDF Concentration ($\mu g/M^2$)*	*Other Constituents*
Skovde	PCB + oil fire	1	
Surahammer	PCB + oil fire	1–10	
Stockholm	PCB explosion	1.5	PCBPs (major)
Hallstahmmar	PCB explosion	1–10	
Imatra	PCB explosion	1–3	PCBPs (minor)
Railway locomotive	PCB explosion	1–100	
Kisa	PCB explosion	1–1,000	PCBPs (minor)
Halmstad	PCB explosion	0.1–500	PCBPs (minor)

Source: From Rappe, C., M. Nygren, S. Marklund, L. Keller, P. Bergqvist, and M. Hansson. 1985. Assessment of human exposure to polychlorinated dibenzofurans and dioxins. *Env. Health Perspect.* **60:**303–304.

type of sampling. Cleaning solutions should be analyzed prior to disposal for PCB levels in excess of 50 ppm in order to determine whether they must be disposed of as hazardous wastes. If exposures are suspected, then it is possible that either skin or chemical protective clothing (CPC) samples might be collected. In one study, wipe samples for PCBs were collected using Whatman filter paper saturated with hexane (Hryhorczuk et al., 1986). The area wiped was 1 ft^2. In the case of transformer leaks, vault wipe samples of walls and a bulk sample from the transformer are often collected.

In some cases it is desirable to determine the extent of contamination due to a release or a process that went on for several years, such as transformer manufacturing; for example, a capacitor fire that contained a dielectric fluid with PCBs in it (Rappe et al., 1985). Wipes were collected in the immediate vicinity of the capacitor, on the floor of the capacitor room close to the bank of capacitors, on the wall in the capacitor room, and on a bench on the ground floor. Each of these sites was an increase in the distance from the fire site, demonstrating that high levels of polychlorinated dibenzofurans could only be found in an area close to the fire. Depending on the location of the origin of the release, samples could be collected in concentric circles as well.

Surfaces for sampling in office buildings are often divided into the following categories: floors, vertical surfaces, elevated horizontal surfaces, high skin contact surfaces, and heating, ventilating, and air conditioning (HVAC) interiors. Vertical surfaces include walls, structural columns, and sides of equipment. Elevated horizontal surfaces are higher than 6 ft above the floor; these surfaces include tops of ventilation ducts and pipes, and tops of storage shelves and cabinets. High skin contact surfaces are those with which a person would probably have frequent and/or prolonged direct dermal contact. Typical high skin contact surfaces include desks, tables, counters, file cabinets, mail handling equipment, and miscellaneous work surfaces. The HVAC interior samples are usually obtained by removing a duct ceiling diffuser and wiping the surface toward the duct.

The standards used for decontamination of PCB-contaminated surfaces have varied in different situations. Usually separate levels are set for TCDDs and TCDFs if the situation has involved a fire. Tables C-2 and C-3 provide data on various cleanup levels that have been set, as well as the basis for setting them. Where different categories of exposure concern exist for different areas, the standards also vary.

METHODS

Wipe Test Using Gauze (NIOSH, 1985)

1. Use 3 in. by 3 in. cotton gauze pads that have been Soxhlet extracted with hexane. Prior to sampling, wet each pad with 8 mL pesticide grade hexane.
2. Put on a phthalate-free glove prior to each sample.
3. Mark off a surface area of 0.25 M^2 and wipe the surface with the hexane saturated pad initially in a horizontal direction using a forward and backward motion. Do a second wiping of the surface using a clean portion of the same gauze pad in a vertical direction with the same forward and backward motion.
4. Place the gauze pad in a brown glass sample container equipped with a Teflon-lined lid.
5. In some cases samples are composited. To do this, wipe four different areas of the same size using a fresh pad for each. Then combine all four pads in the same container.
6. An alternative approach is to use gauze pads that are 2 in. by 2 in. and wet them with 4 mL hexane, and then wipe an area 100 cm^2 (0.01 M^2).

For a variation of this method (NIOSH, March 1986), a surface is marked into 0.25 M^2 areas using a galvanized steel template or a metal tape measure. Using a 3 in. by 3 in. Soxhlet extracted cotton gauze pad wetted with 8 mL pesticide grade hexane, each 0.25 M^2 area is wiped with a freshly gloved hand. The surface is wiped in two directions with the second direction at a 90 degree angle to the first direction.

TABLE C-2. PCB Decontamination Criteria Used for Various Transformer Fires

Decontamination Site	*Standard Accepted for Decontamination* Surface	Air	Dose Basis for Development of Risk Assessment
Binghamton, NY			
TCDD/TCDF	3.3–28 ηg/M^2	10 ρg/M^3	2 ρg/kg
PCBs	1.0 μg/100 cm^2	1.0 μg/M^3	
San Francisco, CA			
TCDD/TCDF	3ηg/M^2 above background	10 ρg/M^3	2 ρg/kg
PCBs	1.0 μg/100 cm^2		
Columbus, OH			
TCDD/TCDF	20 ηg/M^2 high contact surfaces	10 ρg/M^3	2 ρg/kg
PCBs	1.0 μg/100 cm^2	1.0 μg/M^3	
Sante Fe, NM			
TCDD/TCDF	3 ηg/M^2		2 ρg/kg
PCBs	0.5 μg/10 cm^2		
Tulsa, OK			
TCDD/TCDF	3.3–38 ηg/M^2	10 ρg/M^3	2 ρg/kg
PCBs	1.0 μg/100 cm^2	1.0 μg/M^3	
Canada			
TCDD/TCDF	25 ηg/M^2 high contact surfaces	10 ρg/M^3	0.2–1.0 ρg/kg/day (model dependent)
PCBs	1.25 μg/100 cm^2		

Source: From Wade, R. L. 1986. Development of decontamination guidelines for PCB/PCDF and PCDD decontamination in areas of high exposure potential. In J. P. Crine (ed.), *Hazards, Decontamination, and Replacement of PCB, A Comprehensive Guide*. New York: Plenum Press.

Each gauze pad is used to wipe only one 0.25 M^2 area. The gauze pad is then placed in a glass sample container equipped with a Teflon-lined lid. This same method has been applied using 2 in. by 2 in. cotton gauze pads wetted with 4 mL hexane with the wipe sampling area decreased to 0.01 M^2 (100 cm^2).

Cotton puffs saturated with a mixture of petroleum ether and acetone (4:1) have been used to sample for PCBs on work tables, tools, and other surfaces (Maroni et al., 1981). The plugs were prewashed with hexane and then extracted with petroleum ether and analyzed.

Surface samples for TCDFs and TCDDs can be collected using Soxhlet extracted cotton gauze pads (3 in. by 3 in.) wetted with 8 mL pesticide grade hexane (Kominsky, 1989). The sampling procedure consisted of marking off a surface into a 0.25 M^2 area using a galvanized steel template or a metal tape measure. Each 0.25 M^2 area was wiped, with a gauze pad held with a gloved hand, in two directions; the second direction was performed at a 90 degree angle to the first direction. The gauze pad sample was then placed in a glass sample container equipped with a Teflon-lined lid.

Another variation used to perform wipe sampling for PCBs and TCDDs uses a swab. This method was applied during the Seveso, Italy, incident, where a chemical factory released a cloud of toxic chemicals that contaminated the surrounding community with TCDD and other pollutants, to determine the extent of contamination, although subsequently vegetation and soil sampling replaced this approach (EPA, 1985). The plant produced trichlorophenol,

TABLE C-3. Some Commonly Cited Standards for PCB Decontamination

Limit	*Agency*	*Date*	*Exposure Scenario*	*Applicability and Restriction*
<100 μg/100 cm²	Consensus	5/17/85	Restricted access areas	For spills of fluid of 10 lb or more PCB weight
<100 μg/100 cm²	Concensus	5/17/85	Nonrestricted access areas	For spills of 1 lb or more of PCB by weight; utility poles and asphaltic materials considered constituent PCBs
10 μg/100 cm²	Concensus	5/17/85	High contact areas; residential yards, sidewalks, playgrounds, and roadways	Spills of PCBs onto solid surfaces, asphalt, metal, concrete, wood poles
100 μg/100 cm²	Concensus	8/23/85	Reduced public access areas; industrial facilities, rural roadways, rural fields, and oil fields; also, restricted access electrical substations	Spills of PCB materials onto solid surfaces or electrical equipment and machinery prior to redistribution in commerce
0.5 μg/100 cm²	NIOSH	11/10/83	Presumably inferior surfaces	Based on upper background limit in nonmanufacturing facilities
1 μg/100 cm²	Dept. of Public Health, City, and County, San Francisco	11/17/83	General occupancy. Safe reentry levels for decontaminated areas, office building.	Agency health-based cleanup criteria determined by risk assessment for One Market Plaza
10 μg/100 cm²			Restricted access, transformer vault (assumes 2 hr/month occupancy)	
1 μg/100 cm²	NY Dept. of Health	1981	Office building, general exposure. PCB value used as indicator for presence of TCDD/TCDF.	Agency health-based cleanup criteria determined by risk assessment

Sources: Adapted from Woodyard, J. P. 1986 State-of-the-art-Technology for PCB decontamination of concrete. In J. P. Crine (ed.). *Hazards, Decontamination, and Replacement of PCB; A Comprehensive Guide*. New York: Plenum Press, pp. 117–133.

which was used as the starting material in the manufacture of hexachlorophene at a second facility. The procedure involved partially hydrolyzing tetrachlorobenzene to sodium trichlorophenate with sodium hydroxide in a mixed solvent of xylene and ethylene glycol. Unreacted glycol was subsequently recovered by distillation. When the distillation was complete, water was introduced into the reaction vessel and the entire mass was transferred to a second reactor. Trichlorophenate was then transformed to trichlorophenol by acidification with hydrochloric acid. TCDD is formed as an unwanted by-product during the synthesis of trichlorophenol by thermal condensation of trichlorophenate at temperatures above 180°C.

During the tetrachlorobenzene hydrolysis reaction process at the Seveso facility, batch temperatures were maintained at 140°–150°C. Whenever reactor temperatures approached the danger threshold, further increases were limited by manually opening a valve to introduce water into a cooling coil. This plant was not equipped with automatic alarm devices to signal unusual events in the production cycle or safety devices to halt the cycle if necessary. The explosion occurred on a Saturday as workers were shutting down the production cycle for the weekend. At that point, distillation of the ethylene glycol solvent was only one-third complete and interrupting the cycle at this point was a breech of normal operating procedures. Midday there was an exothermic reaction that raised the temperature and pressure in the reactor, which caused a safety valve rupture disk to open. The explosion contaminated nearby homes, farmland, and animals as well as the manufacturing plant.

The sampling method is as follows (EPA, 1985): A square sampling area of 0.25 M^2 was wiped back and forth, vertically and horizontally, with a 10 g degreased cotton swab saturated with 20–30 mL of a 1:4 acetone:hexane mixture. The cotton swabs were preextracted with hexane before use. Before changing wiping directions, the swab was turned over to present a clean surface for wiping. The cotton swab was held in a clean metal clamp while sampling was performed and stored in a glass-stoppered jar prior to extraction. The jars, normally of dark glass, were cleaned by repeated washing with purified hexane. Used cotton swabs were extracted three times with 200 mL of the acetone: hexane solvent and the extracts were pooled for analysis.

Wipe Method with Smear Tabs

Surface wipe samples for PCBs have been collected by applying moderate pressure to the backs of pesticide-quality cyclohexane-moistened Whatman No. 50 smear tabs and wiping a unit area of approximately 100 cm^2. A fresh, disposable, polyvinyl chloride glove was worn for each wipe sample to prevent cross-contamination of the samples. After wiping the surface, the smear tab was folded face-inward, then folded inward once more, and sealed in a 20 mL glass vial with a Teflon-lined screw cap.

INTERPRETATION OF RESULTS

The ratio of PCBs to total TCDFs/TCDDs is useful in assessing the extent of TCDF/TCDD contamination. Once the range of these ratios has been established for a given fire, these ratios can permit the use of PCB analysis as a crude surrogate for TCDF/TCDD analysis. the PCD:TCDF/TCDD ratio in the Chicago fire was 183:1, which falls between the ratios in the San Francisco fire (300:1) and the Binghamton fire (16:1). 2,3,7,8-TCDF comprised 3% of the total TCDFs in the Chicago fire compared to 2% in the San Francisco fire and 175 in the Binghamton fire. A comparison of the PCB:TCDF/TCDD ratio and relative distribution of TCDF cogeners in the unburned Askarel with those in soot demonstrates the pyrosynthesis of TCDFs.

Results of several investigations of PCB surface contamination in office buildings with no known releases indicated that a "background" level of surface contamination exists, in the range of 50–100 $\mu g/M^2$ (NIOSH, 1987*a*). Therefore, for surfaces in the occupational environment that may be routinely contacted with the unprotected skin, NIOSH investigators have recommended that PCB contamination not exceed 100 $\mu g/M^2$, which is the lowest feasible level considering background contamination.

A variety of action levels have been set in different incidents involving transformer accidents (Table C-4). The EPA has stated that the level of oncogenic risk associated with dermal exposures to 50 $\mu g/M^2$ of PCBs on hard, indoor, high contact surfaces is between 1×10^{-5} and 1×10^{-6}. The EPA's cleanup criteria for high contact indoor surfaces is 1,000 $\mu g/M^2$. The EPA has also stated that surface standards of 10,000 $\mu g/M^2$ for indoor low contact surfaces (and vaults) and high contact surfaces in a restricted access industrial facility would not present significant risks to workers or the general population. However, the EPA has also stated that high contact surfaces such as manually operated machinery may require surface standards more stringent than 1,000 $\mu g/M^2$.

Sampling results for TCDDs and TCDFs are often expressed as 2,3,7,8-TCDD equivalents. Toxicity equivalency factors are defined as the

TABLE C-4. Action Levels Developed for Cleanup in Different Transformer Accidents

Location	*Surface Concentration*
Finland	5 ηg (2,3,7,8-TCDF/m²)
Sweden	50 ηg/m²
Binghamton	14 ηg/m² TCDD equivalent
San Francisco	1 ηg/m² TCDD equivalent
Santa Fe	2 ηg/m² TCDD equivalent

Source: From H. Buser, C. Rappe, and P. Bergqvist. 1985. Analysis of TCDFs, dioxins, and related compounds in environmental samples. *Env. Health Perspec.* **60:**293–302.

TABLE C-5. Toxicity Equivalency Factors (TEFs)

Compound	*EPA-TEFs/ 1987*	*EPA-TEFs/ 1989 (Revised)*
Mono-, Di, and TriCDDs	0	0
2,3,7,8-TCDD	1	1
Other TCDDs	0.01	0
2,3,7,8-PeCDD	0.5	0.5
Other PCDDs	0.005	0
2,3,7,8-HxCDDs	0.04	0.1
Other HxCDDs	0.0004	0
2,3,7,8-HpCDDs	0.001	0.01
Other HpCDDs	0.00001	0
OCDD	0	0.001
Mono-, Di-, and TriCDFs	0	0
2,3,7,8-TCDF	0.1	0.1
Other TCDFs	0.001	0
1,2,3,7,8-PeCDF	0.1	0.05
2,3,4,7,8-PeCDF	0.1	0.5
Other PeCDFs	0.001	0
2,3,7,8-HxCDFs	0.01	0.1
Other HxCDFs	0.0001	0
2,3,7,8-HpCDFs	0.001	0.01
Other HpCDFs	0.00001	0
OCDF	0	0.001

Source: From *Health Hazard Evaluation Report*. August 1992. Metropolitan Sewer District, Mill Creek Facility, Cincinnati, OH. HETA 91-261-2245. Cincinnati, OH: NIOSH.

concentration of 2,3,7,8-tetrachlorodibenzo-p-dioxin, which by itself is believed to exhibit the same biological potency as a mixture of structurally related compounds (TCDF/TCDD) actually present in a sample. The procedure was developed by the New York State Department of Health for estimating the total toxicity of a mixture of TCDFs and TCDD as part of the development of reoccupancy criteria for the Binghamton State Office Building. The building experienced a PCB transformer fire in 1981 and TCDD contamination spread throughout it. This procedure calculates the amount of 2,3,7,8-TCDD that would have to be present to exhibit the same toxicity as the measured quantities of each of the various other TCDFs and TCDDs that are present, and adds these calculated amounts of 2,3,7,8-TCDD to obtain an estimate of the TCDD equivalent toxicity of the mixture. The procedure assumes certain ratios of toxicities (termed weighting factors) between 2,3,7,8-TCDD and the other TCDFs and TCDDs.

However, calculation methods vary. The method used in New York is less conservative than the California method, which assigns an equal potency to all tetra- to hepta-2,3,7,8 chlorine substituted dioxins and dibenzofurans rather than weighting downward the higher chlorinated TCDDs and TCDFs (Schecter, 1986). The EPA adopted a set of weighting factors in 1987 and in 1989 adopted the international toxicity equivalency factors (Table C-5). Tables C-6 and C-7 provide comparisons between EPA, New York, and California methods.

An 8 hr occupational exposure limit (OEL) of 0.2 ηg/M³ has been proposed for 2,3,7,8-TCDD along with a 15 min short term exposure limit of 0.27 μg/M³ using a basic risk assessment approach (Leung, Murray, and Paustenbach, 1988). These limits were established to be "cancer-safe."

TABLE C-6. A Comparison of Calculations of 2,3,7,8-TCDD Equivalents Using New York and California Methods

Best Estimate of Average Concentration	×	*Relative Activity of Compound Class vs Dibenzodioxins*	×	*Relative Activity Due to Chlorine Substitution*	=	*New York Calculation* 2,3,7,8-TCDD Equivalents	*California Calculation* 2,3,7,8-TCDD Equivalents
2,3,7,8-TCDF / 8 pg/M³	×	1/3	×	1	=	2.7 pg/M³	8 pg/M³
Penta CDFs: 1,2,3,7,8 + 1,2,3,4,8 + 2,3,4,7,8 / 14 pg/M³	×	1/3	×	1	=	4.7 pg/M³	14 pg/M³
Hexa CDFs: 9 pg/M³	×	1/3	×	1/30	=	0.1 pg/M³	18 pg/M³

Source: From Schecter, A. 1986. The Binghamton state office building PCB, dioxin and dibenzofuran electrical transformer incident: 1981–1986. *Chemosphere* **15**(9/12):1273–1280.

TABLE C-7. A Comparison of EPA and New York Calculations for 3,3,7,8-TCDD Equivalents

Compound	*CDD/F (ηg/g)*	*EPA TEFs*	*EPA TEs (ηg/g)*	*New York TEFs*	*New York TEs (ηg/g)*
2,3,7,8-TCDDs	0.0	1.00000	0.000	1.00000	0.000
Other TCDDs	0.3	0.01000	0.003	0.00000	0.000
2,3,7,8-PeCDDs	1.3	0.50000	0.650	1.00000	1.300
Other PeCDDs	4.8	0.00500	0.024	0.00000	0.000
2,3,7,8-HxCDDs	23.0	0.04000	0.920	0.03000	0.690
Other HxCDDs	75.0	0.00040	0.030	0.00000	0.000
2,3,7,8-HpCDDs	394.0	0.00100	0.394	0.00000	0.000
Other HpCDDs	330.0	0.00001	0.003	0.00000	0.000
OCDD	5890.0	0.00000	0.000	0.00000	0.000
2,3,7,8-TCDFs	7.1	0.10000	0.710	0.33000	2.343
Other TCDFs	139.0	0.00100	0.139	0.00000	0.000
2,3,7,8-PeCDFs	4.8	0.10000	0.480	0.33000	1.584
Other PeCDFs	11.2	0.00100	0.011	0.00100	0.011
2,3,7,8-HxCDFs	2.4	0.01000	0.024	0.01000	0.024
Other HxCDFs	19.6	0.00010	0.002	0.00000	0.000
2,3,7,8-HpCDFs	15.2	0.00100	0.015	0.00000	0.000
Other HpCDFs	34.8	0.00001	0.000	0.00000	0.000
OCDF	36.0	0.00000	0.000	0.00000	0.000
Total 2,3,7,8-TCDD equivalents			3.406		5.952

Source: From Deutsch, D. G., and T. D. Goldfarb. 1988. PCDD/PCDF contamination following a plastics fire in a university lecture hall building. *Chemosphere* **17**(12):2423–2431.

STUDIES

PCBs and TCDDs Surface Sampling

Contaminant	*Activity*	*Surface Methods*	*Other Sampling*	*Reference*
PCBs	Distribution house with crates of catalogues received from a publishing company that had a transformer fire and spill	Wipes of gray-white residue on catalogues	Bulk sample of residue	NIOSH, March 1983*b* (HETA 82-370-1270)
PCBs	Residue from fire 5 years previous in switching center of Telephone Co. building	Wipe samples of residue on ledges and piping from several floors		NIOSH, December 1980 (HETA 80-155-776)
PCBs	School where capacitor containing PCBs overheated in a basement storage room	Wet wipe samples ($100\ cm^2$) with Whatman smear tabs on books, desks, walls, floors, ceilings, and other surfaces in the room where the capacitor overheated and in other areas as background	Area air samples	NIOSH, July 1981 (HETA 81-237-915)
PCBs	Auto parts facility that had worked on scrap transformers	Wet wipe samples ($100\ cm^2$) of desks, sinks, tools, and hand controls Wipe samples in control (nonexposed) areas	Skin wipes Bulk samples of soil, dirt, and soot Blood	NIOSH, March 1983*a* (HETA 82-246-1275)
PCBs	Glassworks facility with fires and leaks from fluorescent light ballasts as well as suspected underground contamination	Wipes with Whatman No. 50 smear tabs of dusty surfaces and top of soda machine, wall, and ceiling.	Area air samples for PCBs and formaldehyde Blood Bulk samples of cinder block for pesticides	NIOSH, May 1983 (HETA 82-206-1306)

Contaminant	Activity	Surface Methods	Other Sampling	Reference
PCBs	Company involved in rewinding electric motors, repairing transformers, performing spill cleanups of transformer fluid, and retrofitting transformers with PCB containing fluid	Wet wipes with Whatman smear tabs of tabletops, machine handles, toolbox surfaces, equipment surfaces, and floors in work areas, break room, and office	Area air samples Skin and PPE wipes Blood	NIOSH, April 1984*a* (HETA 83-281-1457)
PCBs	Repair of electrical transformers	Dry wipes (100 cm^2) with Whatman smear tabs in the office, assembly area, and equipment surfaces	Personal breathing zone air samples Area air samples Blood Skin wipes Bulk transformer fluid	NIOSH, August 1982 (HETA 81-204-1160
PCBs	Workers performing maintenance on electrical transformers	Dry wipe samples using MCE filters on counters, desks, barrels, and consoles inside the maintenance shop	Bulk samples of transformer fluid and waste oil	NIOSH, July 1982 (HETA 81-46-1144)
PCBs	Storage area of utility company for out-of-service transformers where PCB containing transformers were stored	Wet wipes with gauze of forklift hoist, truck and oil filtering equipment	Area air samples Bulk transformer fluid Soil	NIOSH, September 1986 (HETA 86-224-1732)
PCBs	Employees for a utility involved in the removal of capacitors and transformers and in removing PCB containing fluid from transformers	Surface wipe samples of lunchroom surfaces, work surfaces such as forklifts, barrels, and hand-held tools and fences (75–100 cm^2) collected with wet Whatman smear tabs	Personal breathing zone air samples Area air samples Blood Soil Skin wipes	NIOSH, June 1984*a* (HETA 80-212-1474)
PCBs	Employees for a utility working at a facility that receives PCB contaminated equipment	Surface wipe samples of work surfaces and handheld tools (75–100 cm^2) collected with wet Whatman smear tabs	Personal breathing zone air samples Area air samples Blood Skin wipes	NIOSH, June 1984*a* (HETA 80-212-1474)

Contaminant	*Activity*	*Surface Methods*	*Other Sampling*	*Reference*
PCBs	Employees for a utility involved in PCB fires, explosions, spills, and/or incidences that require cleanup	Surface wipe samples of work surfaces and handheld tools (75–100 cm^2) collected with wet Whatman smear tabs	Personal breathing zone air samples Area air samples Blood Skin wipes	NIOSH, June 1984*a* (HETA 80-212-1474)
PCBs	Electrical fire inside an underground transformer vault	Wipe samples from surfaces near the fire scene collected with wet sterile cotton pads (100 cm^2). Other surfaces thought to be less contaminated wiped with dry Whatman smear tabs.	PPE wipes Bulk soot scraped from transformer surface	NIOSH, July 1983 (HETA 82-224-1336)
PCBs	Railroad maintenance facility where PCB-contaminated capacitors were repaired that contained a waste liquid pit	Wet wipe samples using gauze of surfaces in lunchrooms, work areas, and on tools	Personal breathing zone air samples Soil Floor scrapings Bulk liquid from pit	NIOSH, August 1986 (HETA 86-184-1719)
PCBs	Releases (venting) repair of inverter-converters containing 22 PCB containing capacitors for railroad cars	Wet wipes (100 cm^2) with gauze of windows, cabinet, generator, and inverter-converter in work area	Bulk sample of vacuum cleaner dust	NIOSH, March 1985 (HETA 84-533-1565)
PCBs	Maintenance electricians in large office buildings with PCB containing transformers who inspect and repair leading transformers	Wet and dry wipes with Whatman No. 40 filters on surfaces inside work trucks and vault	Personal breathing zone air samples Area air samples inside and outside of transformer vaults Blood Urine Skin and PPE wipes Bulk transformer fluid (for TCDD/TCDF)	NIOSH, October 1984 (HETA 80-7-1520)

Contaminant	Activity	Surface Methods	Other Sampling	Reference
PCBs	Two office buildings with no history of experiencing an electrical transformer fire or failure to develop background data for cleanup standards	Wet wipes with gauze of high skin contact building surfaces (desks, cabinets), floors and walls, elevated horizontal surfaces and on the interior surface of the air handling units	Area air samples	NIOSH, September 1987*b* (HETA 86-472-1832)
TCDDs TCDFs	Two office buildings with no history of experiencing an electrical transformer fire or failure to develop background data for cleanup standards	Wet wipes with gauze of elevated horizontal surfaces, high skin contact surfaces, and the interiors of air handling units	Area air samples	NIOSH, September 1987*b* (HETA 86-472-1832
PCBs	Office buildings with no reported history of having experienced an electrical transformer fire or failure	Wipes (0.25 m^2) using gauze of high skin contact surfaces (desks, tables, and counters) and the interior surface of the fresh air intake plenums	Area air samples	NIOSH, July 1987 (HETA 86-112-1819)
TCDDs TCDFs	Office buildings with no reported history of having experienced an electrical transformer fire or failure	Wipes (0.25 m^2) using gauze of high skin contact surface (desks, tables, and counters)	Area air samples	NIOSH, July 1987 (HETA 86-112-1819)
Polychlorinated biphenylenes TCDFs TCDDs Polychlorinated pyrenes	Electrical power station	Wipe sample to identify by-products of a PCB containing capacitor explosion		Rappe et al., 1985

Contaminant	*Activity*	*Surface Methods*	*Other Sampling*	*Reference*
Polychlorinated biphenylenes TCDFs TCDDs Polychlorinated pyrenes	High frequency casing operation	Floor wipes next to the capacitor bank, on the wall 2 M away, on a bench 10 M away to identify extent of contamination from a PCB containing capacitor fire		Rappe et al., 1985
Polychlorinated biphenylenes TCDFs TCDDs Polychlorinated pyrenes	Steel mill oven explosion	Wipes to identify surface contamination following a PCB containing capacitor fire		Rappe et al., 1985
Polychlorinated biphenylenes TCDFs TCDDs Polychlorinated pyrenes	Foundry	Wipe samples before and after cleaning operations associated with capacitor explosion		Rappe et al., 1985
Polychlorinated biphenylenes TCDFs TCDDs Polychlorinated pyrenes	Railway locomotive	Wipe samples following PCB containing capacitor explosion inside locomotive		Rappe et al., 1985
Polychlorinated biphenylenes TCDFs TCDDs Polychlorinated pyrenes	Debarking in a saw mill	Wipe samples following explosion of PCB containing capacitor explosion		Rappe et al., 1985
PCBs	Office building	Wipe to identify residual contamination in basement of building after contamination through air shafts during PCB containing transformer fire	Area air samples	Schecter and Tiernan, 1985
PCBs	Transformer maintenance and repair	Wipes using Whatman smear tabs of work surfaces frequently contacted by workers	Personal breathing zone air samples	Lees, Corn, and Brysse, 1987

Contaminant	*Activity*	*Surface Methods*	*Other Sampling*	*Reference*
PCBs	Elementary school	Wet wipe samples with Whatman smear tabs (cyclohexane) of leaking fluorescent lamp ballasts to identify PCBs in material	Area air samples	NIOSH, 1982 (HETA 82-068-1111)
PCBs	Electric capacitor manufacture and testing	Wet wipe samples with cotton balls (petroleum ether/acetone) from work tables, tools, capacitor baskets, conveyors	Personal breathing zone air samples Wipes of palms of hands Blood	Maroni et al., 1981
PCBs	Maintenance and repair of distribution transformers at an electric utility	Wipes of tabletops and floor of test area, tools, and pieces of equipment	Personal breathing zone air samples Wipes of hands and faces of workers	Smith et al., 1982
TCDDs TCDFs	Plastics fire in a university lecture hall	Wipes of desks, podium, walls, table, bookcases, floors and walls	Area air samples Bulk samples of soot and carpet	Deutsch and Goldfarb, 1988
PCBs TCDFs TCDDs	Transformer fire in a large office building in Chicago	Wipe samples of surfaces on several floors to determine the extent of contamination	Area air samples Bulk samples of filters from the ventilation system	Hryhorczuk et al., 1986
PCBs TCDFs TCDDs	Electrical fire in basement caused a transformer to fail and release fluid, which burned; smoke from fire contaminated parts of the building	Initial wet and dry wipe samples of soot on several floors and inside the ventilation system to determine the extent of contamination Ongoing wipe tests of cleaned areas	Area air samples inside and outside building Air sampling of air released from air pollution control system Bulk samples of treated wastewater Bulk soot from remote areas	Stephens, 1986 EPA, 1985

Contaminant	*Activity*	*Surface Methods*	*Other Sampling*	*Reference*
PCBs TCDDs	Fire in a transformer vault in a federal office building in Tulsa in which smoke entered the ventilation system of the building	Contamination assessment associated with 27 air handling systems. Gauze wet (hexane) wipes (0.25 m^2 area). Side-by-side sampling PCBs/TCDD on interior of ventilation systems and in office interiors.	Area air samples	NIOSH, 1985 (HETA 85-289-1738)
PCBs	Overheated transformer vented 50 gallons PCB fluid	Surface wipes of firefighters PPE (SCBA, helmets, boots) and of the vault surface	Area air samples Blood	Orris et al., 1986
PCBs	Office buildings with no known PCB problems, some containing PCB transformers and others without; a laboratory; and schools	Wipe samples to determine background levels of PCBs	Area air samples	Oatman and Roy, 1986
TCDFs TCDDs	Remediation of a manufacturing facility that had used PCB fluids	Composite wipe samples on walls, floors, ceilings to determine the extent of contamination; single samples for "hot spots"	Bulk samples of building materials Bulk samples of water, sludge, soil, and oil	Clark, 1991
PCBs	Gear manufacturing company operating in a building where transformers were previously manufactured	Swab samples of walls, ceiling, floor, and work surfaces inside the building	Area air samples Soil and sediment	Christiani et al., 1986
TCDDs	Sontag road area that was sprayed with contaminated oil for dust control	Surface dust samples from building interiors were collected from household vacuum cleaners and with portable Dustbusters	Soil	EPA, 1985

Contaminant	*Activity*	*Surface Methods*	*Other Sampling*	*Reference*
PCBs	Ballast burnouts in fluorescent lights in junior high school	Wipe samples of high dermal contact surfaces		NIOSH, 1991 (HHE 89-183-2101)
PCBs TCDDs/TCDFs	Fire in underground transformer vault underneath bank building Evaluation of exposures to firefighters and maintenance personnel	Filter papers used to wipe the interior of the vault for PCBs and PCDDs/PCDFs. Wipes for PCBs used to evaluate the spread of materials to adjacent areas: ventilation shafts, parking garage, exterior of building. Samples also collected to determine background surface concentrations in uninvolved adjacent buildings.	Area air samples Air filters from the ventilation system Bulk sample of transformer fluid Blood	NIOSH, December 1985 (HETA 84-006-1639)
PCBs	Ballast burnout in corridor of office building	Wet wipe samples using Whatman smear tabs on corridor and nearby office surfaces	General area air samples	NIOSH, April 1982 (HETA 82-063-1095)
PCBs	Servicing and maintaining electrical power distribution equipment	Wet wipe samples using Whatman smear tabs on horizontal surfaces in maintenance and warehouse areas and the exteriors of respirator facepieces to determine if contamination exists	General area air samples Blood of maintenance workers	NIOSH, October 1983 (HETA 81-415-1385)

Contaminant	*Activity*	*Surface Methods*	*Other Sampling*	*Reference*
PCBs TCDD/TCDF	Power transformer relief valve release of fluid into transformer vault in high school	Wipe samples using Whatman smear tabs on building surfaces inside vault, hallways, cafeteria, and classrooms before and after decontamination	Area air samples Blood from firefighters Bulk transformer fluid	NIOSH, June 1984*b* (HETA 82-310-1475)
PCBs	Occupants in building previously occupied by a manufacturer of PCB containing electrical components	Wipe samples using gauze of building interior surfaces such as light fixtures, walls, and floor	General area air samples	NIOSH, March 1986 (HETA 85-334-1676)
PCBs	Extrusion press operation that used hydraulic fluids containing PCBs	Wipes using gauze on work and building surfaces, tools, and lunch tables	Personal breathing zone air samples General area air samples Blood of operators Floor and wall scrapings Bulk hydraulic and coolant fluids	NIOSH, September 1987*a* (HETA 86-445-1831)
PCBs	Electrical capacitor manufacturing plant in which the use of PCBs has been discontinued	Wipe samples using Whatman filters of workplace surfaces (stairwells, basement, manufacturing floors) to determine the need for decontamination	Blood	Acquavella et al., 1986
PCBs	Cleanup of abandoned building complex in steel mill where leaks of PCB transformer fluid had occurred and were stored in drums	Surface wipes of basement surfaces	Bulk groundwater and samples of drum contents Blood	NIOSH, June 1991 (HETA 91-27-2117)

Contaminant	*Activity*	*Surface Methods*	*Other Sampling*	*Reference*
PCBs	Office building where fire occurred in electrical transformer containing PCBs in basement; soot from fire carried up ventilation ducts	Wipes with 3 in. by 3 in. cotton gauze, hexane of 0.25 M^2 area of building surfaces including ceilings, desks, floors, tables, cabinets, and interior of HVAC	Area air samples	NIOSH, February 1988*a* (HETA 86-92-1870)
PCDDs	Office building where fire occurred in electrical transformer containing PCBs in basement; soot from fire carried up ventilation ducts	Wipes with 3 in. by 3 in. cotton gauze, hexane of 1.0 M^2 area (4 pad composite) of building surfaces including ceilings, desks, floors, tables, cabinets, and interior of HVAC	Area air samples	NIOSH, February 1988*a* (HETA 86-92-1870)
PCBs	Commercial hazardous waste incinerator	Wipes with 3 in. by 3 in. cotton gauze, hexane of 0.25 M^2 area marked out with tape measure on floors, benches, inside lockers in change room, sole of street shoe, furniture in offices, and on lunchroom surfaces	Personal breathing zone air samples on warehouse-workers, drum pumpers and crushers, sludge handler, load shredder, mechanic, and operators General area air samples Blood	NIOSH, February 1988*b* (HETA 86-519-1874)
TCDDs TCDFs	Commercial hazardous waste incinerator	Wipes with 3 in. by 3 in. cotton gauze, hexane of 1.0 M^2 area (4 pad composite) marked out with tape measure on floors		NIOSH, February 1988*b* (HETA 86-519-1874)

Contaminant	*Activity*	*Surface Methods*	*Other Sampling*	*Reference*
PCBs	School with fluorescent lamps with PCB containing ballasts where there had been burnouts—Ingraham	Wipes with 2 in. by 2 in. cotton gauze and hexane using template or tape measure in classrooms with and without ballast burnouts on work counters, storage and file cabinets, and desks.	General area air samples	NIOSH, November 1987 (HETA 85-72-1850)
PCBs	School with fluorescent lamps with PCB containing ballasts where there had been burnouts—Bryant	Wipes with 2 in. by 2 in. cotton gauze and hexane using template or tape measure in classrooms with and without ballast burnouts on desks, wall clock, HVAC ducts, and bookshelves	General area air samples	NIOSH, November 1987 (HETA 85-72-1850)
PCBs	School with fluorescent lamps with PCB containing ballasts where there had been burnouts—Seward	Wipes with 2 in. by 2 in. cotton gauze and hexane using template or tape measure in classrooms with and without ballast burnouts on desks, HVAC ducts, and fire sprinkler pipe	General area air samples	NIOSH, November 1987 (HETA 85-72-1850)
PCBs	School with fluorescent lamps with PCB containing ballasts where there had been burnouts—Catherine Blane	Wipes with 2 in. by 2 in. cotton gauze and hexane using template or tape measure in classrooms with and without ballast burnouts on window ledges, walls, desks, beams, floors, wall clock, work counter, and fire extinguishers	General area air samples	NIOSH, November 1987 (HETA 85-72-1850)

Contaminant	*Activity*	*Surface Methods*	*Other Sampling*	*Reference*
PCBs	Post office to determine concentration of PCBs present as normal levels of background contamination to use as a standard for comparison of buildings with known PCB contamination	Wipes with 3 in. by 3 in. cotton gauze and hexane over 0.25 M^2 area with template or measured off on floors, high skin contact surfaces, vertical and elevated horizontal surfaces on all floors and in basement	General area air sampling inside building	NIOSH, September 1987*c* (HETA 87-166-1835)
PCBs	High school with fluorescent lamps with PCB containing ballasts and high frequency of burnouts	Wipes with 3 in. by 3 in. cotton gauze, hexane of 0.25 M^2, 0.5 M^2, and 1.0 M^2 areas on teacher and student desktops, storage cabinets in rooms where teachers experienced symptoms, and in reference rooms with no reported symptoms	Area air samples in same rooms as wipes	NIOSH, August 1987 (HETA 87-288-1828)
PCBs	Office building with electrical transformers (leaking) located at roof level	Wipes with 3 in. by 3 in. cotton gauze, hexane of 0.25 M^2 area inside office areas of the building on desktops, floors, walls, supply room air grille, air ducts, and tabletops.	Area air samples inside building	NIOSH, March 1988 (HETA 87-122-1881)
PCBs	Electrical transformer leak inside vault next to mechanical room containing an air handling unit for the office building	Wipes with 3 in. by 3 in. cotton gauze, hexane on 0.25 M^2 areas on interior surfaces in vault (floors, dike walls) and areas outside of vault (floors, mat, hallway, doors) on same floor	Area air samples inside and outside of vault	NIOSH, November 1988 (HETA 88-54-1936)

Contaminant	*Activity*	*Surface Methods*	*Other Sampling*	*Reference*
PCBs	Maintenance employees who are responsible for inspecting transformer vaults for leaks in military stations—Fort Meyers	Wipes with 3 in. by 3 in. cotton gauze, hexane of 0.25 M^2 marked off areas of transformer surfaces, break room lunch table, electric shop benchtop	Personal breathing zone air sampling on maintenance employees during inspection of vaults General area air sampling on top of transformer	NIOSH, May 1989 (HETA 88-328-1961)
PCBs	Maintenance employees who are responsible for inspecting transformer vaults for leaks in military stations—Fort McNair	Wipes with 3 in. by 3 in. cotton gauze, hexane of 0.25 M^2 marked off areas of transformer surfaces, van steering wheel and tools	Personal breathing zone air sampling on maintenance employees during inspection of vaults General area air sampling on top of transformer	NIOSH, May 1989 (HETA 88-328-1961)
PCBs	Maintenance employees who are responsible for inspecting transformer vaults for leaks in military stations—Cameron Station	Wipes with 3 in. by 3 in. cotton gauze, hexane of 0.25 M^2 marked off areas of transformer surfaces, tools, truck steering wheel and driver's seat, and electric shop floor and benchtop	Personal breathing zone air sampling on maintenance employees during inspection of vaults General area air sampling on top of transformer	NIOSH, May 1989 (HETA 88-328-1961)
TCDDs	Incinerator used for sludge from municipal sewer processing plant	Wipes with 3 in. by 3 in. cotton gauze, hexane after marking boundaries of 100 cm^2 area in dewatering building and incinerator building	Personal breathing zone air samples of metals and inorganic acids Area air samples of organic vapors, inorganic gases and acids, silica and metals Bulk samples of dewatered sludge, debris from wall, dust from stair well and under conveyor belt	NIOSH, August 1992 (HETA 91-261-2245)

Contaminant	*Activity*	*Surface Methods*	*Other Sampling*	*Reference*
TCDDs TCDFs	Incinerator burning municipal waste that disposed of ash on sites directly adjacent to facility	Surface wipes with 3 in. by 3 in. cotton gauze pads and hexane (0.25 M^2) and four pads composited per sample (1.0 M^2) on desktop, floor, lunch table, change room bench, and in a hotel room as background	Area air samples for PCDD/PCDF, respirable dust and silica inside and outside of building	NIOSH, March 1992 (HETA 88-207-2195)
PCBs	Spill of transformer fluid inside transformer vault located within the confines of an open office area in a large building	Wipe with 3 in. by 3 in. cotton gauze wetted with hexane on areas where boundaries were marked out on surface to create 0.25 M^2 area. In vault, floors and walls were wiped, and in offices, carpet, file cabinet, desktop, tabletop, wall, and mail room floor were wiped.	Area air samples inside vault and in office areas	NIOSH, 1992 (HETA 90-78-2095)
PCBs	Elementary school	Wipe samples for surface contamination resulting from ballast burnouts on fluorescent lamps	Area air samples	NIOSH, 1987*b* (HETA 85-414-1805)
PCBs	Private utility company during routine maintenance of PCB containing transformers in underground vaults (collecting samples, overhauling, inspecting)	Wipes of tools, transformers, switchboxes, filter press, tables, and floors with MCE filters (100 cm^2)	Personal breathing zone air samples Skin wipes Blood Urine	NIOSH, May 1978 (HHE 77-7A-7B-486)

Contaminant	*Activity*	*Surface Methods*	*Other Sampling*	*Reference*
PCBs	Turnkey environmental service in PCB management including draining and disposal of PCB containing transformers at facility	Cotton gauze (3 in. by 3 in.) with hexane used to wipe 0.25 M^2 on floors, stair rails, drain and flush pad, forklift, bottom of leather boots, lunchroom, lab and office surfaces	Personal breathing zone air samples General area air samples Blood	NIOSH, April 1990 (HETA 86-510-2032)
TCDDs TCDFs	Turnkey environmental service in PCB management including draining and disposal of PCB containing transformers at facility	Cotton gauze (3 in. by 3 in.) with hexane used to wipe 0.25 M^2 (4 pad composite for 1.0 M^2) on drain and flush pad and floors	General area air samples	NIOSH, April 1990 (HETA 86-510-2032)

PCBs and TCDDs Dermal Sampling

Contaminant	*Activity*	*Dermal Methods*	*Other Sampling*	*Reference*
PCBs	Manufacture of electric capacitors	Palms of workers' hands swabbed with cotton plugs soaked with solvent	Area air samples Wipes of tools and worktable Blood	Maroni et al., 1981
PCBs	Electrical equipment manufacturing including large power capacitors and maintenance operations	Skin wipes using Whatman smear tabs No. 50 of forehead, nose, and cheek areas	Personal breathing zone air samples Blood	Smith et al., 1982
PCBs	Company involved in rewinding electric motors, repairing transformers, performing spill cleanups of transformer fluid, and retrofitting transformers with PCB containing fluid	Wet wipe samples of workers' palms and the interiors of work gloves with Whatman smear tabs	Area air samples Surface wipes Blood	NIOSH, April 1984*a* (HETA 83-281-1457)
PCBs	Private utility company during inspection of transformers in underground vaults	Skin wipes using Whatman smear tabs No. 50 of face and hands of workers	Personal breathing zone air samples Surface wipes of work area Blood	Smith et al., 1982
PCBs	Private utility company during routine maintenance of PCB containing transformers in underground vaults (collecting samples, overhauling, inspecting)	Hand and face wipes with MCE filter or its backup pad of employees' hands and faces before and after washing	Personal breathing zone air samples Wipes in work area Blood Urine	NIOSH, May 1978 (HHE 77-7A-7B-486)
PCBs	Repair of electrical transformers	Dry wipes of palm and inner finger area of worker using Whatman smear tabs	Personal breathing zone air samples Area air samples Blood Surface wipes Bulk transformer fluid	NIOSH, August 1982 (HETA 81-204-1160)

Contaminant	*Activity*	*Dermal Methods*	*Other Sampling*	*Reference*
PCBs	Electrical fire inside an underground transformer vault	Whatman smear tab wet and dry wipes of firefighter's clothing: sleeves and front of turnout coat, top of boot, helmet interior and face shield, and SCBA facepiece	Surface wipes Bulk soot scraped from transformer surface	NIOSH, July 1983 (HETA 82-224-1336)
PCBs	Fire inside a tunnel involving a 7-car subway train with electrical components containing PCBs	Samples of turnout coats analyzed to determine if they are contaminated	Area air samples in tunnel Blood	NIOSH, July 1985 (HETA 82-319-1569)
PCBs	Fire at a transformer oil reclamation facility	5 in.^{2} fabric samples cut from some of the contaminated Nomex garments worn by the firefighters after being dry cleaned and compared to fabric samples from laboratory contaminated garments that had also been cleaned to determine the effectiveness of decontamination		NIOSH, February 1987 (HETA 84-180-1776)
PCBs	Auto parts facility that had worked on scrap transformers	Wet wipe samples of workers' right palms (75 cm^2) using Whatman smear tabs	Surface wipes Bulk samples of soil, dirt, and soot Blood	NIOSH, March 1983*a* (HETA 82-246-1275)
PCBs	Employees for a utility working at a facility that receives PCB contaminated equipment	Skin wipe samples of hands and foreheads of workers (70–100 cm^2) collected with wet Whatman smear tabs Wipes of shoes and boots with wet Whatman smear tabs	Personal breathing zone air samples Area air samples Blood Surface wipes Soil	NIOSH, June 1984*a* (HETA 80-212-1474)

Contaminant	*Activity*	*Dermal Methods*	*Other Sampling*	*Reference*
PCBs	Employees for a utility working at a facility that receives PCB contaminated equipment	Skin wipe samples of hands and foreheads of workers (75–100 cm^2) collected with wet Whatman smear tabs	Personal breathing zone air samples Area air samples Blood Surface wipes	NIOSH, June 1984*a* (HETA 80-212-1474)
PCBs	Employees for a utility involved in PCB fires, explosions, spills, and/or incidences that require cleanup	Skin wipe samples of hands and foreheads of workers (75–100 cm^2) collected with wet Whatman smear tabs	Personal breathing zone air samples Area air samples Blood Surface wipes	NIOSH, June 1984*a* (HETA 80-212-1474)
PCBs	Maintenance electricians in large office buildings with PCB containing transformers who inspect and repair leaking transformers	Wet and dry wipes with Whatman No. 40 filters of hands of workers and respirator and safety goggle interiors	Personal breathing zone air samples Area air samples inside and outside of transformer vaults Blood Urine Surface wipes Bulk transformer fluid (for TCDD/TCDF)	NIOSH, October 1984 (HETA 80-7-1520)
PCBs Organic Vapors	PCB contaminated landfill cleanup activities	Wet wipe samples collected using Whatman smear tabs from the toe of the left work boot prior to decontamination and from right work boot toe after decontamination to verify the effectiveness of cleaning.	Personal breathing zone air samples Area air samples at site boundaries	NIOSH, April 1984*b* (HETA 82-284-1456)
TCDDs TCDFs	Incinerator burning municipal waste that disposed of ash on sites directly adjacent to facility	Surface wipes with cotton gauze (3 in. by 3 in.) pads and hexane (0.25 M^2). Four pads composited per sample (1.0 M^2 total area). Collected on desktop, floor, lunch table, change room bench, and in a hotel room as background	Area air samples for PCDD/PCDF, respirable dust and silica inside and outside of building	NIOSH, March 1992 (HETA 88-207-2195)

REFERENCES

Acquavella, M. S., N. J. Hanis, M. J. Nicolich, and S. C. Phillips. 1986. Assessment of clinical, metabolic, dietary and occupational correlations with serum polychlorinated biphenyl levels among employees at an electrical capacitor manufacturing plant. *JOM* **28**(11):1177–1180.

Christiani, D. C., D. Kriebel, N. J. Fox, and E. L. Baker. 1986. Persistently elevated polychlorinated biphenyl levels from residual contamination of workplace surfaces. *Am. J. Ind. Med.* **10:**143–151.

Clark, A. N. 1991. Results of an investigation of an old manufacturing facility for levels of polychlorinated dibenzofurans and polychlorinated dibenzodioxins. *Chemosphere* **23**(8/10):1001–1008.

Deutsch, D. G., and T. D. Goldfarb. 1988. PCDD/PCDF contamination following a plastics fire in a university lecture hall building. *Chemosphere* **17**(12):2423–2431.

EPA. 1985. Guide for decontaminating building, structures and equipment at superfund sites. EPA 600/2-85-028. Washington, DC: EPA.

Fenske, R. A., S. W. Horstman and R. K. Bentley. 1987. Assessment of dermal exposure to chlorophenols in timber mills. *Appl. Ind. Hyg.* **2**(4):143–147.

Hryhorczuk, D. O., P. Orris, J. R. Kominsky, J. Melius, W. Burton, and D. L. Hinkamp. 1986. PCB, PCDF, and PCDD exposure following a transformer fire: Chicago. *Chemosphere* **15**(9/12):1297–1303.

Kominsky, J. R. 1989. Background concentrations of polychlorinated dibenzofurans (PCDFs) and polychlorinated dibenzo-p-dioxins in office buildings in Boston, MA. *Chemosphere* **18**(1/6):599–608.

Lees, P. S. J., M. Corn, and F. N. Brysse. 1987. Evidence for dermal absorption as the major route of body entry during exposure of transformer maintenance and repairmen to PCBs. *AIHA J.* **48**(3):257–264.

Leung, H. W., F. J. Murray, and d. J. Paustenbach, 1988. A proposed occupational exposure limit for 2,3,7,8-tetrachlorodibenzo-p-dioxin. *AIHA J.* **49**(9):466–474.

Maroni, M., A. Colombi, S. Cantoni, E. Ferioli, and V. Foa. 1981. Occupational exposure to polychlorinated biphenyls in electrical workers. I. Environmental and blood polychlorinated biphenyl concentrations. *Brit. J. Ind. Med.* **38:**49–54.

NIOSH, Health Hazard Evaluation Report. May 1978. *Union Electric Co., St. Louis,* MO. HHE 77-7A-7B-486. Cincinnati, OH: NIOSH.

NIOSH, Technical Assistance Report. December 1980. *The New York Telephone Co., New York.* HHE 80-155-776. Cincinnati, OH: NIOSH.

NIOSH, Health Hazard Evaluation Report. July 1981. *Our Lady of Visitation Elementary School, Cincinnati, OH.* HETA 81-237-915. Cincinnati, OH: NIOSH.

NIOSH, Health Hazard Evaluation Report. April 1982. *Hamilton County Health Department, Cincinnati, OH.* HETA 82-063-1095. Cincinnati, OH: NIOSH.

NIOSH, Health Hazard Evaluation Report. 1982. *Miamitown Grade School, Cincinnati, OH.* HETA 82-068-1111. Cincinnati, OH: NIOSH.

NIOSH, Health Hazard Evaluation Report. July 1982. *Long Island Lighting Co., Hicksville, NY.* HETA 81-46-1144. Cincinnati, OH: NIOSH.

NIOSH, Health Hazard Evaluation Report. August 1982. *Mowbray Engineering Co., Greenville, AL.* HETA 81-204-1160. Cincinnati, OH: NIOSH.

NIOSH, Health Hazard Evaluation Report. March 1983*a*. *Swissvale Auto Surplus Parts, Inc., Pittsburgh, PA.* HETA 82-246-1275. Cincinnati, OH: NIOSH.

NIOSH, Health Hazard Evaluation Report. March 1983*b*. *Kistler Communications, Inc., Denver, CO.* HETA 82-370-1270. Cincinnati, OH: NIOSH.

NIOSH, Health Hazard Evaluation Report. May 1983. *New Renaissance Glass Works, Oakland, CA.* HETA 82-206-1306. Cincinnati, OH: NIOSH.

NIOSH, Health Hazard Evaluation Report. July 1983. *Miami Fire Dept., Miami, FL.* HETA 82-224-1336. Cincinnati, OH: NIOSH.

NIOSH, Health Hazard Evaluation Report. October 1983. *High Voltage Maintenance Corporation, Mentor, OH.* HETA 81-415-1385. Cincinnati, OH: NIOSH.

NIOSH, Health Hazard Evaluation Report. April 1984*a*. *Holley Electric Corporation, Jesup, GA.* HETA 83-281-1457. Cincinnati, OH: NIOSH

NIOSH, Health Hazard Evaluation Report. April 1984*b*. *Port Authority of NY and NJ, Elizabeth Industrial Park Site, Elizabeth, NJ.* HETA 82-284-1456. Cincinnati, OH: NIOSH.

NIOSH, Health Hazard Evaluation Report. June 1984*a*. *Pacific Gas and Electric Company, San Francisco,* CA. HETA 80-212-1474. Cincinnati, OH: NIOSH.

NIOSH, Health Hazard Evaluation Report. June 1984*b*. *Hill-Murray High School, Maplewood, MN.* HETA 82-310-1475. Cincinnati, OH: NIOSH.

NIOSH, Health Hazard Evaluation Report. October 1984. *GSA Switchgear Shop, Washington, DC.* HETA 80-7-1520. Cincinnati, OH: NIOSH.

NIOSH, Health Hazard Evaluation Report. 1985. *Page Belcher Federal Building, Tulsa, OK.* HETA 85-289-1738. Cincinnati, OH: NIOSH.

NIOSH, Health Hazard Evaluation Report, March 1985. *Long Island Rail Road, Jamaica, NY.* HETA 84-533-1565. Cincinnati, OH: NIOSH.

NIOSH, Health Hazard Evaluation Report. July 1985. *International Association of Firefighters, NJ.* HETA 82-319-1569. Cincinnati, OH: NIOSH.

NIOSH, Health Hazard Evaluation Report. December 1985. *First National Bank, Chicago, IL*. HETA 84-006-1639. Cincinnati, OH: NIOSH.

NIOSH, Health Hazard Evaluation Report. 1986. *Page Belcher Federal Building, Tulsa, OK*. HETA 85-289-1738. Cincinnati, OH: NIOSH.

NIOSH, Health Hazard Evaluation Report. March 1986. *Olin Corp., Marion, IL*. HETA 85-334-1676. Cincinnati, OH: NIOSH.

NIOSH, Health Hazard Evaluation Report. August 1986. *Amtrack, Long Island City, NY*. HETA 86-184-1719. Cincinnati, OH: NIOSH.

NIOSH, Health Hazard Evaluation Report. September 1986. *Colorado River Agency, Parker, AZ*. HETA 86-224-1732. Cincinnati, OH: NIOSH.

NIOSH, 1987*a*. PCB exposures following fluorescent light ballast burnout. *Appl. Ind. Hyg.* 3(2):R-24.

NIOSH, Health Hazard Evaluation Report. 1987*b*. *New Mexico State Highway Dept. General Office Building*. HETA 85-414-1805. Cincinnati, OH: NIOSH.

NIOSH, Health Hazard Evaluation Report. February 1987. *Jacksonville Fire Department, Jacksonville, FL*. HETA 84-180-1776. Cincinnati, OH: NIOSH.

NIOSH, Health Hazard Evaluation Report. July 1987. *Commercial Office Buildings, Sante Fe, NM*. HETA 86-112-1819. Cincinnati, OH: NIOSH.

NIOSH, Health Hazard Evaluation Report. August 1987. *Henry Ford High School, Detroit, MI*. HETA 87-288-1828. Cincinnati, OH: NIOSH.

NIOSH, Health Hazard Evaluation Report. September 1987*a*. *Aluminum Company of America, Lafayette, IN*. HETA 86-445-1831. Cincinnati, OH: NIOSH.

NIOSH, Health Hazard Evaluation Report. September 1987*b*. *Commercial Office Buildings, Boston, MA* HETA 86-472-1832. Cincinnati, OH: NIOSH.

NIOSH, Health Hazard Evaluation Report. September 1987*c*. *U.S. Post Office Building, Oklahoma City, OK*. HETA 87-166-1835. Cincinnati, OH: NIOSH.

NIOSH, Health Hazard Evaluation Report. November 1987. *Seattle Public Schools, Seattle, WA*. HETA 85-72-1850. Cincinnati, OH: NIOSH.

NIOSH, Health Hazard Evaluation Report. February 1988*a*. *50 Staniford Street Office Building, Boston, MA*. HETA 86-92-1870. Cincinnati, OH: NIOSH.

NIOSH, Health Hazard Evaluation Report. February 1988*b*. *ENSCO, El Dorado, AR*. HETA 86-519-1874. Cincinnati, OH: NIOSH.

NIOSH, Health Hazard Evaluation Report. March 1988. *General Dynamics, Airforce Plant #19, San Diego, CA*. HETA 87-122-1881. Cincinnati, OH: NIOSH.

NIOSH, Health Hazard Evaluation Report. November 1988. *U.S. Customs Service, Washington, DC*. HETA 88-54-1936. Cincinnati, OH: NIOSH.

NIOSH, Health Hazard Evaluation Report. May 1989. *U.S. Army Corps of Engineers, Arlington, VA*. HETA 88-328-1961. Cincinnati, OH: NIOSH.

NIOSH, Health Hazard Evaluation Report. April 1990. *National Electric (Aptus), Inc., Coffeyville, KS*. HETA 86-510-2032. Cincinnati, OH: NIOSH.

NIOSH, Health Hazard Evaluation Report. 1991. *Andrew Jackson Jr. High, Crosslands, WV*. HETA 89-183-2101. Cincinnati, OH: NIOSH.

NIOSH, Health Hazard Evaluation Report. 1992. *Office Building Evaluation*. HETA 90-78-2095. Cincinnati, OH: NIOSH.

NIOSH, Health Hazard Evaluation Report. June 1991. *LTV Steel Company, East Chicago, IN*. HETA 91-27-2117. Cincinnati, OH: NIOSH.

NIOSH, Health Hazard Evaluation Report. March 1992. *Northwest Incinerator, Philadelphia, PA*. HETA 88-207-2195. Cincinnati, OH: NIOSH.

NIOSH, Health Hazard Evaluation Report. August 1992. *Metropolitan Sewer District, Mill Creek Facility, Cincinnati, OH*. HETA 91-261-2245. Cincinnati, OH: NIOSH.

Oatman, L., and R. Roy. 1986. Surface and indoor air levels of polychlorinated biphenyls in public buildings. *Bull. Env. Contam. Toxicol.*- **37**:461–466.

Orris, P., J. R. Kominsky, D. Hryhorczuk, and J. Melius. 1986. Exposure to polychlorinated biphenyls from an overheated transformer. *Chemosphere* **15**(9/12):1305–1311.

Rappe, C., S. Marklund, L. Kjeller, P. Bergqvist, and M. Hansson. 1985. Strategies and techniques for sample collection and analysis: Experience from the Swedish PCB accidents. *Env. Health Perspect.* **60**:279–292.

Schecter, A. 1986. The Binghamton State Office PCB, dioxin and dibenzofuran electrical transformer incident: 1981–1986. *Chemosphere* **15**(9/10):1273–1280.

Schecter, A., and T. Tiernan. 1985. Occupational exposure to polychlorinated dioxins, polychlorinated furans, polychlorinated biphenyls, and biphenylenes after an electrical panel and transformer accident in an office building in Binghamton, NY. *Env. Health Perspect.* **60**:305–313.

Smith, A. B., J. Schloemer, L. K. Lowry, A. W. Smallwood, R. N. Ligo, R. Stanaka, W. Stringer, M. Jones, R. Hervin, and C. J. Glueck. Metabolic and health consequences of occupational exposure to polychlorinated biphenyls. *Brit. J. Ind. Med.* **39**:361–369.

Stephens, R. D. 1986. Transformer fire, Spear Street Tower, One Market Plaza, San Francisco, CA. *Chemosphere* **15**:1281–1289.

APPENDIX D

Pesticides

METHODS

Application

Subdivision U is one of a series of the EPA's Pesticide Assessment Guidelines whose purpose is to aid pesticide registrants and others in designing and carrying out field studies that measure, using personal monitoring techniques, potential dermal and respiratory exposure to pesticides when used according to widespread and commonly recognized practice. These guidelines address direct exposure encountered during any pesticide application operation and related occupational activities including weighing and mixing the concentrated chemical and loading the material into the application equipment. These guidelines also include indoor testing procedures to measure postapplication exposure to people as a result of indoor use of pesticides. In general, monitoring of exposure during application of pesticides at indoor sites involves the same considerations as monitoring during outdoor applications.

If a pesticide is being studied for registration, the EPA's protocols must be followed. Most applicator dermal exposure data have been collected using α-cellulose and multilayered gauze pads for the past 30 years. Due to concerns regarding comparison of these data with new data, the EPA has a preference for these pads. For other materials an appropriate demonstration of the comparability or superiority of that method must be done first. The EPA also has specific preferences for pad locations. These are described in Chapter 14. In addition to the standard external patches, if the pesticide is to be used only when workers are wearing specific protective clothing, extra pads are required to assess penetration. Even if the label specifies that protective gloves must be worn, hand exposure under the gloves must be assessed. Hand exposure is to be assessed using the bag rinse method described in Chapter 12.

Tests must be carried out at label application rates using the actual formulation and packaging that will be commercially available. The EPA may require the estimation of exposure to active ingredient(s), inerts or contaminants, any other chemicals present in the formulation, any degradation or transformation product(s), or any combination of these. Outside applications must be performed under weather conditions that are consistent with label restrictions or that are generally recognized as acceptable for spraying.

Quality control requirements include field fortified samples and blanks. There should be at least one field fortified sample per worker per monitoring period for each fortification level.

Sampling During Reentry Following a Pesticide Application

Postapplication to workers as a result of outdoor uses is covered in the EPA's Subdivision K—Reentry Guidelines. Reentry is usually performed to do harvesting of crops and is of great concern because of the potential for poisoning large groups of workers. Reentry levels are required by the EPA only for highly toxic pesticides that have uses likely to result in high dermal and inhalation exposure to people entering pesticide treated fields. In general, reentry intervals are required when an exposure or risk assessment procedure indicates the potential for adverse chronic effects on people entering a treated site, including neurotoxic, teratogenic, reproductive, and carcinogenic effects. The exposures can vary widely depending on whether the crops are ground cover, in bushes, or on trees.

A number of factors affect the extent of a reentry hazard. The most important factors are the surface and airborne residue levels of the parent compound and its toxic alteration products, the amount of these residues transferred to people, the absorbed dose, and the toxicological response to the absorbed residues. Many variables have direct impact on these key factors. Residue levels at a treated site are affected by climate, formulation, rate and frequency of application, conditions during application, type of crop, and the length of time since application. The transfer of residues to people may be influenced by the type of work such as pruning or thinning, duration and frequency of activity, and type of clothing worn.

In Subdivision K, the section on Human Exposure Monitoring Data describes needed use practice information; explains exposure data requirements; provides procedures for measurement of inhalation and dermal exposure; and suggests standards for reporting the data (see, e.g., Fig. D-1). Activities to be described include the nature of the activity, principal sources of exposure, unusual environmental conditions such as high temperatures or humidity, level of physical exertion, and expected frequency and duration of activity. Measurement of dermal exposure to a pesticide during reentry into leafy crops should be combined with measurement of dislodgeable foliar residues. If significant exposure from soil borne residues is expected, these measurements should be combined with quantification of soil residues.

Similar to applicator studies, reentry studies also are done primarily with α-cellulose or multilayered gauze pads. Hand exposure is assessment using light cotton gloves.

Five peach orchards were harvested each for three days at decreasing postapplication intervals (Popendorf et al., 1979). Both aerosol and dermal exposure measurements were performed for the organophosphate pesticide Zolone plus its metabolite Zoloxon. Low levels of Guthion, also an organophosphate, were present in some of the orchards from prior applications. Aerosol samples were collected at 1.7 Lpm for 1–2 hr during the workday from near the breathing zone of each worker. Respiratory doses were calculated from the airborne concentrations and estimated respiratory volumes of 24 M^3 during each three day work sequence. Dermal doses to pickers were estimated using 4 in. by 4 in. gauze patches taped to the skin. A knit nylon glove backed by a pad was used to monitor hand exposure. At the end of each week, the patches from each location were pooled for extraction and analysis. The results were adjusted for exposure time and patch area at each location and then multiplied by the proportionate body surface area; these results, as shown in Table D-1, were summed to estimate the whole body dermal dose of each compound for each week.

Approximately 98–99% of the total dose thus calculated were attributed to the dermal rather than respiratory route. These calculations do not account for possible variations in the rate of chemical absorption at different skin locations.

Figure D-1. Applicator exposure survey form.

Sampling Date ________________ Monitoring Times: ___________ to ___________

Compound Identification

☐ Fungicide ☐ Herbicide ☐ Insecticide ☐ Fumigant
☐ Plant growth inhibitor

Formulation:
Liquid (lb ai/gal) ________________ or Solid (% ai by wgt) ________________
☐ Emulsifiable concentrate ☐ Wettable powder
☐ Suspension (aqueous) ☐ Dry-flowable
☐ Microencapsulated ☐ Dust
☐ Solution ☐ Granule
☐ Liquid (undiluted; fumigant) [ai = active ingredient]

Site Data

Location (state/province and country) ________________________________
Crop conditions: ☐ Indoor ☐ Outdoor
Height ________________ Row spacing (ft) ________________

Application Information

Method of Application:
☐ Groundboom rail car ☐ Aerial rotary wing ☐ Shank injection
☐ Groundboom tractor ☐ Aerial fixed wing ☐ Fumigation
☐ Groundboom truck ☐ High pressure hand wand ☐ Backpack
☐ Solid broadcast spreader ☐ Low pressure hand wand ☐ Air blast
☐ Liquid broadcast spreader
Other (describe): ________________________________
Rate: (lb ai/acre) ___________ and (gal/acre) __________ Total lb ai applied ___________
Total Number of Acres Treated ________________
Final Mix Concentration (lb ai/gal Diluent) ________________
Total Number of Gallons Sprayed ________________
Number of Tank Applications Monitored ________________
Vehicle Make and Model ________________

Cab Type:
☐ Open cab (cockpit) ☐ Closed cab (cockpit)/window closed
☐ Closed cab (cockpit)/window open ☐ Closed cab (cockpit)/window closed/filtered air
Ground Speed ________________
Applicator Make and Model ________________________________
Disc No. ________________ No. Nozzles ________________
Nozzle: Type/Mfr. ________________ Model No. ________________
Nozzle Pressure (psi) ________________ Boom Height Aboveground (ft) ________________
Sheath Width (ft) ________________ Boom Length (ft) ________________
Shank/Probe Type: ☐ Knives ☐ Sweeps ☐ Other

Figure D-1. *(Continued)*

Depth of Injection/Incorporation (inches) ________________
Describe Application Procedure ____

____

Weather Data

% Relative Humidity: High ________________ Low ________________
Temperature (°F): High ________________ Low ________________
Wind Speed: ☐ 0–5 mph ☐ 6–10 mph ☐ >10 mph
Wind Direction Relative to Travel: ☐ Parallel ☐ Perpendicular
Other (describe) ________________________________

Personal Information

Is Study Participant a:
☐ Private applicator ☐ Commercial applicator ☐ Noncertified applicator
☐ Certified applicator Other ________________________________
Years of Experience: ☐ <1 ☐ 1–5 ☐ 6–10 ☐ 11–15 ☐ 16–20 ☐ >20

Personal Clothing

Pants: ☐ None ☐ Long-legged ☐ Short-legged
Shirt: ☐ None ☐ Long-sleeved
Jacket: ☐ No ☐ Yes
Shoes/Boots: ☐ None ☐ Rubber ☐ Fabric ☐ Leather

Chemical Protective Clothing

Protective Suit/Coveralls: Type of Material ________________________________
Clean or Contaminated ________________
Style ________________________________
Eye/Face Protection: Type ________________________________
Hat/Hood: Type of Material ________________________________
Style ________________________________
Gloves: Type of Material ________________________________
Clean or Contaminated ________________
Style ________________________________

Airborne Exposure Data

Air Sampling Time (hr) ________________

Method of measuring airborne exposure:
(1) Filter on respirator
(2) Personal air sampling pump and media. Describe media ________________________

____

(3) Area monitoring. Describe method and location ________________________________

____

Quantification Limit (μg) ________________

Figure D-1. *(Continued)*

Concentration Collected (μg) ______________ Air Volume Collected (L) ______________

Flow Rate (L/min): Initial ____________ Final ____________ Avg ____________

Dermal Exposure Data

Dermal Sampling Time (hr) ______________

Method of Measuring Dermal Exposure Excluding Hands:

(1) Pad. Describe pad construction ______________________________

____

(2) Solvent rinse. Type of solvent ______________________________

(3) Clothing. Describe clothing ______________________________

____

(4) Other. Describe ______________________________

Method of Measuring Hand Exposure:

(1) Hand rinse. Type of solvent ______________________________

(2) Gloves. Describe ______________________________

(3) Other. Describe ______________________________

Dermal Exposure Values Excluding Hands (μg/cm²)

	Inside Clothing		Outside Clothing	
Head	______________		______________	
Neck front	______________		______________	
Neck back	______________		______________	
Upper arms	(R)____	(L)____	(R)____	(L)____
Shoulders	(R)____	(L)____	(R)____	(L)____
Chest	(R)____	(L)____	(R)____	(L)____
Back	(R)____	(L)____	(R)____	(L)____
Forearms	(R)____	(L)____	(R)____	(L)____
Hips	(R)____	(L)____	(R)____	(L)____
Thighs	(R)____	(L)____	(R)____	(L)____
Shins	(R)____	(L)____	(R)____	(L)____
Calves	(R)____	(L)____	(R)____	(L)____
Ankles	(R)____	(L)____	(R)____	(L)____
Feet	(R)____	(L)____	(R)____	(L)____

Average Quantification Limit (μu/cm²): ______________

Hand Exposure Values (μg): (R) __________ (L) __________ Both __________

Average Quantification Limit (μg): ______________

If incidental contact with the pesticide was observed, please circle the response(s) that best describe(s) the situation:

(1) Observed hand contact

(2) Observed face contact

(3) Observed contact with other body parts

Please provide a brief description of the incidental exposure situation: ______________

____

TABLE D-1. Integrated Dermal Dose to Each Location (mg)

Zolone	*Week 1*	*Week 2*	*Week 3*	*Week 4*
Hands	95.0	116.1	84.2	158.0
Forearms	9.8	17.6	12.2	12.3
Upper arms	4.3	14.5	13.4	13.1
Head	7.3	11.6	23.0	24.1
Neck	1.6	2.4	2.4	2.6
Shoulders	0.4	1.7	1.4	0.7
Chest	1.0	1.8	1.1	2.5
Back	0.6	1.7	2.0	3.8
Hips	0.2	0.2	0.6	1.3
Thighs	0.7	1.0	2.3	5.1
Calves	1.4	0.3	0.5	7.9
Feet	0.2	0.1	0.1	0.9
Total without hands	27.3	52.9	58.9	74.3
Overall	122.3	169.0	143.1	232.1

	Guthion[a]	*Zoloxon*	*Zoloxon*	*Zoloxon*
Hands	20.8	2.17	1.82	1.39
Forearms	2.82	0.28	0.29	0.08
Upper arms	0.57	0.17	0.35	0.11
Head	1.38	0.17	0.68	0.22
Neck	0.30	0.03	0.05	0.04
Shoulders	0.06	0.04	0.04	0.01
Chest	0.24	<0.01	0.03	0.03
Back	0.06	<0.01	0.05	0.10
Hips	0.04	<0.01	0.02	0.07
Thighs	0.14	<0.01	0.06	0.07
Calves	<0.02	<0.01		0.01
Feet		<0.01		0.01
Total without hands	5.62	0.69	1.56	0.74
Overall	26.4	2.86	3.38	2.13

Source: From Popendorf, W. J., R. C. Spear, J. T. Leffingwell, J. Yager, and E. Kahn. 1979. Harvester exposure to Zolone® (Phosalone) residues in peach orchards. *JOM* **21**(3):189–194.

[a]Total dose of 2.6 mg Zoloxon (2.5 to the hands) in week 1 is not listed.

STUDIES

Pesticide Surface Sampling

Contaminant	Activity	Surface Methods	Other Sampling	Reference
Atrazine Azodrin Bidrin Bladex Ciodrin Nudrin Trimethyl phosphite Vapona	Synthesis and formulation plant	Whatman filters, dry or moist, used to wipe lunchroom tables, forklift truck steering wheel, pesticide containers ready for shipment, handrails and process equipment likely to be touched by hands	Personal breathing zone air samples for organic vapors and some pesticides Area air samples for organic vapors and some pesticides Skin wipes	NIOSH, December 1979 (HHE 77-126-646)
Aldicarb	Pesticide manufacturing plant	Wipes of surfaces in clinic, lab, control room, lunchrooms, and drumming area with Whatman smear tabs	Personal breathing zone air samples Blood CPC wipes	NIOSH, 1985 (HETA 78-4-1511)
Azodrin	Synthesis and formulation plant	Dry filters used to wipe lunch table and forklift	Personal breathing zone air samples Area air samples Skin wipes on workers	NIOSH, July 1982 (HETA 80-137-1145)
Carbaryl	Power sprayer and garden pump application to tree boles	Samples for spray fallout and drift using plastic petri dishes circling the tree bole	Paper dosimetry samples on personnel	Haverty et al., 1983
Chlorpyrifos	Application to corn via an overheat irrigation system	Polyurethane pads stationed at selected sites outside the treatment area to identify drift Foliage residue	Dermal pads Cotton gloves	Brady et al., 1991
DEF	Aerial spray application to cotton fields	Mylar sheets (6 in. by 18 in.) on ground inside and at edge of field to collect drift	Area air samples 25 ft from sheets	Kilgore et al., 1984

Contaminant	*Activity*	*Surface Methods*	*Other Sampling*	*Reference*
DEF	Cotton picking	Wet wipes on tractor surfaces with Whatman smear tabs	Personal breathing zone air samples Area air samples Skin wipes Blood Bulk cotton	NIOSH, July 1984 (HETA 81-463-1477)
DEF	Cotton gin	Wet wipes inside gin with Whatman smear tabs	Personal breathing zone air samples Area air samples Skin Blood Bulk cotton Settled dust	NIOSH, July 1984 (HETA 81-463-1477)
DEF	Ground spray from vehicle of cotton fields	Mylar sheets taped to pressed hardboard placed between rows, away from the spray area and on the spray rig Petri dishes glued to pressed hardboard	Scaleless chickens in cages located 400 M offsite, onsite, in between rows, and on the spray rig—held for observation for symptoms for 29 days following spraying	Wilson et al., 1980.
Dibrom	Pesticide manufacture	Wipes of surfaces in clinic, lab, control room, lunchrooms, and drumming area with Whatman smear tabs	Personal breathing zone air samples Blood PPE wipes	NIOSH, 1985 (HETA 78-4-1511)
Disulfoton	Granular application using tractor-drawn gravity feed or broadcast application	Greased glass slides set at different heights in the working area to collect fallout for particle sizing	Dermal pads Personal air samples Area air samples for particle sizing Bulk samples of granules for pesticide concentration	Lloyd and Bell, 1967
2,4-Dichlorophenoxy acetic acid	Mixing Aerial application of 2,4-D by forestry workers	Wet cotton swabs of helicopters, vehicles, workplace, and living and eating quarters to identify source of continuing exposure once spraying had stopped	Disposable suits urine	Frank, Campbell, and Sirons, 1985

Contaminant	*Activity*	*Surface Methods*	*Other Sampling*	*Reference*
Ethylene dibromide (EDB)	Forest service workers developed rash after removing plastic covering from piles of wood that had been used as a cover during spraying to kill beetles and one month "cure" period following	Wipes with filter paper (36 in.^{2}) of wet underside of plastic.	Bulk sample of condensate on plastic and bulk of plastic material	NIOSH, November 1983 (HETA 83-408-1389)
Ethyl parathion (10%)	Hand spraying on pea, bean, and tomato plants inside a greenhouse	Petri dishes placed on the floors, walls, and ceiling to collect spray fallout Foliage residue	Area air samples Blood	Culver et al., 1958
Fenitrothion	Forest spraying for spruce budworm control	Glass plates set out in nearby blueberry fields at intervals to determine spray drift		Wood and Stewart, 1976
Fenthion	Aerial application for mosquito control near estuary water	Filter papers to identify drift placed on a raft and a dock Culture dishes with water to determine amount deposited on water surface		Wang, Lenahan, and Tucker, 1987
Heptachlor Lindane	Pesticide formulating facility	Filter wipes on desk, floor, and first aid kit in locker room	Personal breathing zone air samples during mixing and loading	NIOSH, July 1978 (TA 77-66)
Lorsban	Cotton picking	Wet wipes of tractor surfaces with Whatman smear tabs	Personal breathing zone air samples Area air samples Skin wipes Blood Bulk cotton	NIOSH, July 1984 (HETA 81-463-1477)
Lorsban	Cotton gin	Wet wipes inside gin with Whatman smear tabs	Personal breathing zone air samples Area air samples Skin Blood Bulk cotton Settled dust	NIOSH, July 1984 (HETA 81-463-1477)

Contaminant	*Activity*	*Surface Methods*	*Other Sampling*	*Reference*
Malathion	Park service employees who became ill after a pesticide was applied around the visitor center to control ants	Cotton gauze wetted with hexane used to wipe flat surfaces (countertops, floors, shelves, tile floors, and patio) inside and outside the building and the bottom of the investigator's shoe	General area air samples inside building Blood Bulk pesticide	NIOSH, June 1986 (HETA 85-527-1704)
Methyl parathion	Spray application to cotton	Aluminum foil (1 ft^2) placed in a horizontal position on top of cotton to collect spray fallout Foliage residue	Clothing of workers Gauze pads Hand washes Personal breathing zone air samples	Ware et al., 1973
Nudrin	Synthesis and formulation plant	Dry wipe samples with filters of lunch table and control panel	Personal breathing zone air samples Area air samples Skin wipes on workers	NIOSH, July 1982 (HETA 80-137-1145)
Pesticides	Fire and explosion in a warehouse used to store pesticides	Wipe samples of exteriors of nearby buildings	General area air samples Foilage from trees in area Weeds Bulk sample of runoff water from the site	NIOSH, December 1986 (HHE 84-484-1754)
Phorate	Granular application using tractor-drawn gravity feed or broadcast application	Greased glass slides set at different heights in the working area to collect fallout for particle sizing	Dermal pads Personal air samples Area air samples for particle sizing Bulk samples of granules for pesticide concentration	Lloyd and Bell, 1967
Phosdrin	Pesticide manufacture	Wipes of surfaces in clinic, lab, control room, lunchrooms, and drumming area with Whatman smear tabs	Personal breathing zone air samples Blood PPE wipes	NIOSH, 1985 (HETA 78-4-1511)

Contaminant	*Activity*	*Surface Methods*	*Other Sampling*	*Reference*
Pydrin	Cotton picking	Wet wipes of tractor with Whatman smear tabs	Personal breathing zone air samples Area air samples Skin wipes Blood Bulk cotton	NIOSH, July 1984 (HETA 81-463-1477)
Pydrin	Cotton gin	Wet wipes inside gin with Whatman smear tabs	Personal breathing zone air samples Area air samples Skin Blood Bulk cotton Settled dust	NIOSH, July 1984 (HETA 81-463-1477)
2,4,5-T	Helicopter spraying, tractor mist blower, backpack spraying of rice fields or forests	Mylar sheets to determine the width of the helicopter spray pattern and to obtain information on drift	Dermal pads Modified respirator	Lavy, Shepard, and Bouchard, 1980
Terbufos	Formulation and packaging	Wipe samples with Whatman smear tabs of work area, lunchroom, and locker room surfaces	Personal breathing zone air samples Area air samples	NIOSH, 1984 (HETA 82-465-1323)
Thionzin	Granular application using tractor-drawn gravity feed or broadcast application	Greased glass slides set at different heights in the working area to collect fallout for particle sizing	Dermal pads Personal air samples Area air samples for particle sizing Bulk samples of granules for pesticide concentration	Lloyd and Bell, 1967
Vapona	Pesticide manufacture	Wipes of surfaces in clinic, lab, control room, lunchrooms, and drumming area with Whatman smear tabs	Personal breathing zone air samples Blood PPE wipes	NIOSH, 1985 (HETA 78-4-1511)

Pesticide Dermal Sampling

Contaminant	*Activity*	*Dermal Methods*	*Other Sampling*	*Reference*
Abamectin	Hand wand spray application	Fabric-covered gauze pad with aluminum foil backing Cotton gloves Hand wash with water and Surten	Personal breathing zone air samples	Rech, Bissel, and del Valle, 1988 (HS-1491)
Abamectin Dodemorph Bupirimate	Cutting, sorting and bundling of treated flowers	Cotton gloves that covered hands and forearms changed after each 1 hr of exposure along with an assessment of work rate		Brouwer et al., 1992*b*
Acephate	Mixing/loading in a closed system to determine its effectiveness Ground application	Unwashed cotton cloth and rayon:polyester pads (4 in. by 4 in.) attached to the exterior of the clothing at shoulder, chest, waist, and knee	Area air samples around mixing/loading sites and on tractors Blood Urine (spot; pre-job, 3 wk intervals)	Knaak et al., 1980
Acephate	Hand harvesting tobacco	Tyvek jacket with 8-ply gauze pads (2 in. by 2 in.) with glassine paper backing attached to the exterior at forearms, breasts, shoulders, and back Cotton gloves with an 8-ply gauze pad (2 in. by 2 in.) with glassine backing attached to the back	Personal breathing zone air samples Urine High volume area air samples Foliage residue Soil	EPA, 1988a (Study 5)
Alachlor	Application	Gauze pads (10 cm by 10 cm) attached to cap, and clothing at back, chest, forearm of dominant arm, thigh, and under clothing on undershirt at chest	Urine (12 hr)	Dubelman and Cowell, 1989

WP = Wettable powder
EC = Emulsifiable concentrate

Contaminant	*Activity*	*Dermal Methods*	*Other Sampling*	*Reference*
Alachlor	Application	Gauze pads (10 cm by 10 cm) on cap (near forehead), back, chest (over and under shirt), forearm sleeve on dominant arm and thigh	Urine (12 hr) Photographs and videotaping of workers	Dubelman and Cowell, 1989
Alachlor (EC) and microencapsulated	Closed system loading and spray application	12-ply gauze pads (4 in. by 4 in.) pinned to exterior of clothing on the cap, chest, back, forearm, and thigh and underneath on the undershirt	Urine (12 hr)	Cowell et al., 1987
Aldicarb	Hand harvesting peas	Gauze pads (4 in. by 4 in.) with a glassine backing attached to arm bands and pinned to the outside of workers' clothing at knee level Cotton gloves followed by 95% ethanol hand rinses	Personal breathing zone air samples Foliage residue Soil	EPA, 1988*a* (Study 2)
Aldicarb	Pesticide manufacture	Wipes of gloves used for drumming, sampling, and in lab with Whatman smear tabs	Personal breathing zone air samples Blood Surface wipes	NIOSH, 1985 (HETA 78-4-1511)
Aldrin	Spray applications for borers in subfloor areas of buildings already erected or spray on foundations for buildings not yet erected	Pairs of filter papers pinned to hat, shoulder, back, chest, arm, wrist, and thigh on top of overalls	Blood Modified respirator with prefilters	Simpson and Shandar, 1972
Aldrin	Spray applications for termites in subfloor areas of buildings already erected or spray on foundations for buildings not yet erected	Pairs of filter papers pinned to hat, shoulder, back, chest, arm, wrist, and thigh on top of overalls	Blood Modified respirator with prefilters	Simpson and Shandar, 1972

WP = Wettable powder
EC = Emulsifiable concentrate

Contaminant	*Activity*	*Dermal Methods*	*Other Sampling*	*Reference*
Aluminum tris-o-ethyl phosphonate	Mixing/loading Backpack spraying application of ornamentals in greenhouses	Standardized work clothing with 12-ply gauze pads (3 in. by 3 in.) in custom-aluminized holder with 5.6 cm circle exposed, placed outside clothing at shoulder tops, forearms, chest, back, thighs, lower legs, and front of baseball cap; second set (excluding cap) placed inside clothing, nonoverlapping Pre- and postexposure hand rinses with 250 mL 10% isopropanol in distilled water (3 repetitions) (workers wore latex gloves)	Personal breathing zone air samples	Fenske, Hamburger, and Guyton, 1987
Atrazine	Mixing/loading, boom application, and spray gun application	Tyvek coveralls worn during each operation. Patches cut from the suits at the thigh, forearm, and chest for analysis.	Respirators with filter paper discs placed behind cartridges	Reed, Hall, and Krueger, 1990
Atrazine Azodrin Bidrin Bladex Ciodrin Nudrin Trimethyl phosphite Vapona	Synthesis and formulation plant	Whatman filter wipes of employees' hands after removal of their gloves	Personal breathing zone air samples for organic vapors and some pesticides Area air samples for organic vapors and some pesticides Surface wipes	NIOSH, December 1979 (HHE 77-126-646)
Azinphos-ethyl	Spraying in orchards	Filter paper (12.5 cm) pinned on clothing at hat, arm (top), wrist, shoulder, back, chest, thigh	Respirator pads	Simpson, 1965

Contaminant	*Activity*	*Dermal Methods*	*Other Sampling*	*Reference*
Azinphos-methyl	Checking cotton for the presence of insects after pesticide application by ground or airplane spraying	Cotton shirt sleeves Cotton T-shirts Cotton gloves	Modified respirator with pads	Quinby, Walker, and Durham, 1958
Azinphos-methyl	Hand harvesting cucumbers	Gauze pads (103.2 cm^2), one on each forearm outside the shirt and one on each forearm inside the shirt	Personal breathing zone air samples Urine Foliage residue Soil	EPA, 1988*b* (Study 9)
Azinphos-methyl	Ultra-low-volume air blast spraying of orchards	Gauze pads (6.35 cm by 6.35 cm, exposed) in cardboard lantern slide mounts backed with impermeable plastic pinned to the underside of cotton clothing (2 layers) so that backing is against skin at chest, back, upper and lower arms, upper and lower legs. In some cases rubber coats and/or pants were also worn. Fluorescent tracer added to spray, skin fluorescence evaluation of participants	Personal breathing zone air samples Urine (24 hr pre- and post-exposure) Blood	Franklin et al., 1981
Azinphos-methyl	Reentry into citrus groves to pick fruit	Pads on arms and head Cotton (?) gloves	Personal breathing zone air samples Blood Fruit Foliage residue	Lamb, 1980

WP = Wettable powder
EC = Emulsifiable concentrate

Contaminant	*Activity*	*Dermal Methods*	*Other Sampling*	*Reference*
Azinphos-methyl	Mixing/loading in a closed system to determine its effectiveness Ground application	Unwashed cotton cloth and rayon:polyester pads (4 in. by 4 in.) attached to the exterior of the clothing at shoulder, chest, waist, and knee	Area air samples around mixing/ loading sites and on tractors Blood Urine (spot; Prejob, 3 week intervals)	Knaak et al., 1980
Azinphos-methyl (0.05%)	Air blast spraying fruit orchards	32 ply gauze pads (11.4 cm by 11.4 cm) attached to shoulders, back of neck, "V" of chest, and forearms Bag hand rinse or swab with 95% ethanol	Modified respirator with filter pads	Wolfe, Durham, and Armstrong, 1967
Azinphos-methyl (450 ppm)	Mixing/loading High pressure spraying with tractors in apple and peach orchards	Pads of heavy blotter paper (α-cellulose) placed at back (center) inside and outside of clothing, near collar outside, upper arm (right), thigh (right)	Modified respirators with cotton filter pads Urine (4 hr during application, 1 hr postapplication) Foliage residue	Hansen et al., 1978
Azinphos-methyl (WP)	Hand harvesting apples	Tyvek jackets with combination α-cellulose (4 in. by 4 in.) with 9 ply gauze (2 in. by 2 in.) centers stapled to the exterior of the jacket at the arms, chest, and back. Pads of 4 in. by 4 in. α-cellulose were stapled to the interior of the jacket adjacent to the exterior pads. Cotton gloves	Personal breathing zone air samples Urine Foliage residue Soil Apple rinse water	EPA, 1988*a* (Study 13)
Azinphos-methyl (WP)	Thinning apples 1, and 2, and 6, and 9 days after spray application	Gauze pads on forearms Cotton or nylon gloves Ethanol (95%) hand rinse	Personal breathing zone air samples	Davies, Stevens, and Staiff, 1983

Contaminant	*Activity*	*Dermal Methods*	*Other Sampling*	*Reference*
Azinphos-methyl (WP)	Air blast spray application to orchards	Standardized work clothing with pads of gauze (6.35 cm by 6.35 cm, exposed) in cardboard lantern slide mounts backed with impermeable plastic with 6 pads pinned under clothing so that backing is against skin at chest, back, upper and lower arms, upper and lower legs and 4 pinned outside at chest, back, arms, and legs Cotton gloves to measure penetration through protective gloves	Urine (pre- and postexposure, 24 hr)	Franklin, Muir, and Moody, 1986
Azinphos-methyl (WP)	Aerial spraying (pilots) Air blast spraying of orchards (tractor operators)	Strips of α-cellulose (3 ply) wrapped around the forehead (2 in. by 10 in.) and wrists (2 in. by 6 in.)	Personal breathing zone air samples Modified respirators with filter pads	Jegier, 1964*b*
Azinphos-methyl (WP)	Formulating and air blast spraying of apple orchards	Strips of α-cellulose (3 ply) wrapped around the forehead (2 in. by 10 in.) and wrists (2 in. by 6 in.)	Personal breathing zone air samples Modified respirators with filter pads Blood	Jegier, 1964*a*
Azodrin	Reentry into treated fields to inspect cotton	Blue jeans and cotton T-shirts were extracted Hand and wrist rinse with 125 mL distilled water	Personal breathing zone air samples Blood Urine (24 hour) Foliage residue	Ware et al., 1974
Azodrin	Synthesis and formulation plant	Dry filter wipe samples on workers' hands, neck, and forehead for skin contamination	Personal breathing zone air samples Area air samples Surface wipes in work area	NIOSH, July 1982 (HETA 80-137-1145)

WP = Wettable powder
EC = Emulsifiable concentrate

Contaminant	*Activity*	*Dermal Methods*	*Other Sampling*	*Reference*
Benlate	Mixing/loading Crop harvest and spraying for home use	12 ply gauze pads (4 in. by 4 in.) with filter paper backing Applicators: taped at shoulders, upper center of chest and forearms Hand harvesting: forearms, shoulders, chest, upper thighs, and lower legs Home use: forearms, shoulders, back of neck, chest, upper thighs, and lower legs Cotton gloves	Modified respirators with gauze pads stapled to the filters	Everhart and Holt, 1982
Benlate	Hand harvesting blackberries and raspberries	12 ply surgical sponges (3 in. by 3 in.) with polyethylene backings inside glassine envelopes with a circular opening (60 mm diam). Pads were fastened to a headband or brim of a cap for the face and stapled to a tightly fitting cotton T-shirt at the chest, back, and upper arm. Pads were attached to lower arms and legs with surgical tape. and/or Cotton gloves	Personal breathing zone air samples High volume area air samples Urine Foliage residue Soil	EPA, 1988*b* (Study 7)
Benlate	Mixing/loading Airblast application on apple orchards from tractors some with spray cabs (with charcoal air filters) and others without	16 ply gauze pads (4 in. by 4 in.) with aluminum foil backings taped on chest, back and left leg at knee Cotton gloves		Spittler and Bourke, 1985

Contaminant	*Activity*	*Dermal Methods*	*Other Sampling*	*Reference*
Benlate (WP)	Mixing, application with high pressure low boom and low pressure low boom sprayers, harvesting and scouting of green beans	16 ply gauze pads (4 in. by 4 in.) with aluminum foil backings taped on chest, back and left leg at knee Cotton gloves		Spittler and Bourke, 1985
Benomyl	Hand harvesting grapes	Gauze pads (3 in. by 3 in.) with glassine paper backings stapled to gabardine forearm/thigh bands Cotton gloves followed by 95% ethanol hand rinses	Personal breathing zone air samples Urine Foliage residue Soil	EPA, 1988*a* (Study 3)
Benomyl	Hand harvesting blueberries	Tyvek jacket with 8 ply gauze pads (2 in. by 2 in.) with glassine paper backing attached to the exterior at forearms, breasts, and shoulders and back Cotton gloves with an 8 ply gauze pad (2 in. by 2 in.) with glassine backing attached to the back	Personal breathing zone air samples Urine High volume area air samples Foliage residue Soil	EPA, 1988*a* (Study 7)
Benomyl	Hand harvesting strawberries	12 ply gauze pads (3 in. by 3 in.) with polyethylene backing in a glassine paper envelope with a circular (60 mm diameter) opening taped to the wrist Cotton gloves	Foliage residue	EPA, 1988*b* (Study 4)

WP = Wettable powder
EC = Emulsifiable concentrate

Contaminant	*Activity*	*Dermal Methods*	*Other Sampling*	*Reference*
Benomyl (WP)	Hand harvesting grapes	Gauze pads (3 in. by 3 in.) with glassine paper backings stapled to gabardine forearm bands and pinned to the outside of workers' clothing at chest and shoulders Cotton gloves followed by 95% ethanol hand rinses	Personal breathing zone air samples Urine Foliage residue Soil	EPA, 1988*a*, Study 3
Benomyl Bifenox Captan Chlorothalonil Chlorpyrifos DCNA Diazinon Diphenamid Fenvalerate Glyphosate Metaxyl Triadimefon	Conifer tree nursery work: weeders, scouts, packers	8-layer cotton gauze pads stapled to filter paper pinned at ankles (1 outside, 1 inside clothing), forearms (2 on the outside of the shirt sleeve and 2 on the inside), upper chest, upper back and hat of personal clothing Bag hand rinse with 10% ethanol in water	Urine, spot and 24 hr	Lavy et al., 1993
Benomyl Chlorothalonil Chlorpyrifos DCNA Fenvalerate Metalaxyl	Conifer tree nursery work: weeders, scouts, packers	8-layer cotton gauze pads stapled to filter paper pinned at ankles (1 outside, 1 inside clothing), forearms (2 on the outside of shirt sleeve and 2 on the inside), upper chest, upper back and hat of personal clothing Bag hand rinse with 10% ethanol in water	Urine, spot and 24 hr	Lavy et al., 1993

Contaminant	*Activity*	*Dermal Methods*	*Other Sampling*	*Reference*
Benomyl Chlorothalonil Chlorpyrifos Diphenamid Napropamid	Conifer tree nursery work: weeders, scouts, packers	8-layer cotton gauze pads stapled to filter paper pinned at ankles (1 outside, 1 inside clothing), forearms (2 on the outside of shirt sleeve and 2 on the inside), upper chest, upper back and hat of personal clothing Bag hand rinse with 10% ethanol in water	Urine, spot and 24 hr	Lavy et al., 1993
Benomyl Bifenox Captan Carbaryl Chlorothalonil Diazinon Glyphosate Oxyfluorfen Sethoxydim Triadimefon	Conifer tree nursery work: weeders, scouts, packers	8-layer cotton gauze pads stapled to filter paper pinned at ankles (1 outside, 1 inside clothing), forearms (2 on the outside of shirt sleeve and 2 on the inside), upper chest, upper back and hat of personal clothing Bag hand rinse with 10% ethanol in water	Urine, spot and 24 hr	Lavy et al., 1993
Chlorothalonil Maneb	Conifer tree nursery work: weeders, scouts, packers	8-layer cotton gauze pads stapled to filter paper pinned at ankles (1 outside, 1 inside clothing), forearms (2 on the outside of shirt sleeve and 2 on the inside), upper chest, upper back and hat of personal clothing Bag hand rinse with 10% ethanol in water	Urine, spot and 24 hr	Lavy et al., 1993

WP = Wettable powder
EC = Emulsifiable concentrate

Contaminant	*Activity*	*Dermal Methods*	*Other Sampling*	*Reference*
Benthiocarb (granular)	Mixing/loading (dumping) Airplane with open cockpit application (pilot)	Fabric covered gauze pad with aluminum foil backing Hand wash with water	Personal breathing zone air samples	Maddy et al., 1982*c* (HS-898)
Binapacryl (0.3%)	Tractor drawn air blast spraying fruit orchards	α-Cellulose pads (10.2 cm by 10.2 cm) with filter paper backings placed on the shins, thigh fronts, forearms, shoulders, back of neck, and upper chest near "V" of neck	Modified respirator with filter pads	Wolfe et al., 1972
Bravo	Mixing, application with low pressure, low boom; high pressure low boom; and drop nozzle sprayers, harvesting, and scouting of cabbage and onions	16 ply gauze pads (4 in. by 4 in.) with aluminum foil backings taped on chest, back and left leg at knee Cotton gloves		Spittler and Bourke, 1985
Captan	Hand harvesting strawberries	12 ply gauze pads (3 in. by 3 in.) with polyethylene backing in a glassine paper envelope with a circular (60 mm diameter) opening taped to the wrist Cotton gloves	Foliage residue	EPA, 1988*b* (Study 4)
Captan	Mixing/loading High pressure spraying with tractors in apple and peach orchards	Pads of heavy blotter paper (α-cellulose) placed at back (center) inside and outside of clothing, near collar outside, upper arm (right), thigh (right)	Modified respirators with cotton filter pads Urine (4 hr during application, 1 hr postapplication) Foliage residue	Hansen et al., 1978

Contaminant	*Activity*	*Dermal Methods*	*Other Sampling*	*Reference*
Captan	Hand harvesting strawberries and weeding	12 ply surgical sponges (3 in. by 3 in.) with a polyethylene backing inside a glossy paper envelope with a circular (60 mm diameter) opening. Pads were mounted on a headband or side of a cap, stapled to a tightly fitting cotton T-shirt over the chest sternum, center back, and upper arms. Pads were taped to the skin of lower arms and legs. Cotton gloves, some with the tips of the thumb and first two fingers of one hand removed.	Personal breathing zone air samples Foliage residue Soil	EPA, 1988*b* (Study 1)
Captan	Hand harvesting strawberies	12 ply gauze pads (3 in. by 3 in.) with polyethylene backings inside glassine envelopes with a circular opening (60 mm diameter). Pads were fastened to a headband or brim of a cap for the face and stapled to a tightly fitting cotton T-shirt at the chest, back, and upper arm. Pads were attached to lower arms and legs with surgical tape. Cotton gloves	Foliage residue Soil	EPA, 1988*b* (Study 5)

WP = Wettable powder
EC = Emulsifiable concentrate

Contaminant	*Activity*	*Dermal Methods*	*Other Sampling*	*Reference*
Captan	Strawberry harvesting (some with protective gloves, others without)	100% cotton tight fitting long underwear that was later analyzed Hand washes (400 mL of 1% Surten solution)	Foliage residue Urine (24 hr)	Maddy et al., 1989
Captan	Strawberry harvesting	Cotton sleeves (shoulder to wrist) and cotton leggings (thigh to ankle) Cotton gloves	Foliage residue Strawberries	Ritcey et al., 1987
Captan	Seed potato treatment: filling hoppers of dusting machines with pesticide, cutting and sorting potatoes, planting treated seed potatoes with tractor, and planter observers riding behind a planter containing treated seed potatoes	32 ply gauze pads (11.4 cm by 11.4 cm) with filter paper backings attached to shoulders and upper centers of back and chest outside clothing Bag hand rinse with 95% ethanol	Modified dust respirator	Stevens and Davies, 1981
Captan	Mixing/loading Tractor mounted boom spray application	Muslin fabric (4 in. by 4 in.) attached to outside of clothing at chest, back, forearms (inside), thighs, and shins Rinse of exteriors of latex gloves	Personal breathing zone air samples Respirator filters Urine (spot, postshift and preshift) Foliage residue Fruit Bulk samples of spray tank formulation	Winterlin et al., 1984
Captan	Hand picking strawberries and collecting foliage and fruit samples	Muslin (4 in. by 4 in.) fabric attached to outside of clothing at chest, back, forearms, thighs, and shins Rinse of exteriors of latex gloves	Area air samples Urine (spot, postshift and preshift) Foliage residue Fruit	Winterlin et al., 1984

Contaminant	*Activity*	*Dermal Methods*	*Other Sampling*	*Reference*
Captan	Mixing/loading Application and workers engaged in thinning and harvesting grapes	Muslin cloth patches (10 cm by 10 cm) attached to white disposable scrub apparel (pants, tunic top and gown sleeves) slipped over the outer garment of the workers. Patches were placed at the chest, back, forearms, thighs, and shins. Cotton gloves	Area air samples Respirator filter pads Urine, spot collected pre-exposure, 4 hr postexposure and day after exposure Dislodgeable residues on foliage and grapes	Winterlin et al., 1986
Captan (WP)	Apple orchard spraying from tractors	Cellulose pads attached to shoulders, back, and chest	Modified respirator for inhalation exposure	McJilton, Berckman, and Deer, 1983
Captan (WP)	Hand harvesting apples	Tyvek jackets with combination α-cellulose (4 in. by 4 in.) and 9 ply gauze (2 in. by 2 in.) centers stapled to the exterior of the jacket at the arms, chest, and back. Pads of α-cellulose (4 in. by 4 in.) were stapled to the interior of the jacket adjacent to the exterior pads Cotton gloves	Personal breathing zone air samples Urine Foliage residue Soil Apple rinse water	EPA, 1988*a* (Study 13)
Captan (WP)	Boom spray application to chrysanthemums in greenhouses	α-Cellulose pads (10.16 cm by 10.16 cm) with glassine backings taped to outside of clothing at back (middle), shoulders, fore-arms, thigh (fronts), and shins Bag hand wash with 200 mL 95% ethanol	Personal breathing zone air samples	Stamper et al, 1989*b*; Nigg, Stamper, and Mahon, 1988

WP = Wettable powder
EC = Emulsifiable concentrate

Contaminant	*Activity*	*Dermal Methods*	*Other Sampling*	*Reference*
Captan (WP)	Span spray application to chrysanthemums in greenhouses	α-Cellulose pads (10.16 cm by 10.16 cm) with glassine backing taped to outside of clothing at back (middle), shoulders, forearms, thighs (fronts), and shins Bag hand wash with 200 mL 95% ethanol	Personal breathing zone air samples	Stamper et al., 1989*b*; Nigg, Stamper, and Mahon, 1988
Captan + Benomyl	Hand harvesting of strawberries	12 ply gauze pads (3 in. by 3 in.) inside special holders with a 28 cm^2 opening taped to forearms Cotton gloves	Foliage	Zweig, Gao, and Popendorf, 1983
Captofol	Hand harvesting of blueberries	Tyvek jacket with 9 ply gauze (4 in. by 4 in.) on top of α-cellulose pads stapled to the exterior at forearms, shoulders, and breasts, and center of back. Pads of α-cellulose were also attached to the inner surface of the jacket at right forearm, chest, and back. Cotton gloves	Personal breathing zone air samples Urine High volume area air samples Soil	EPA, 1988*a* (Study 12)
Carbaryl	Urban application: homeowner, gardener, golf course greenskeeper, commercial structural pest control operator, orchardsmen, and truck farmers	Standardized jump suits with short sleeves issued. Pads (10.2 cm by 10.2 cm) of 8 ply gauze over chromatography paper (0.16 mm) with glassine paper backing. Four pads fastened to outside clothing or skin (if uncovered) and four pads placed beneath clothing (but offset). Hand wash (ethanol:water, 50:50)	Personal breathing zone air samples Blood	Gold et al., 1982

Contaminant	Activity	Dermal Methods	Other Sampling	Reference
Carbaryl (WP)	Power spray application to trees by commercial pesticide applicator	Standardized jumpsuits with short sleeves issued. Pads (10.2 cm by 10.2 cm) of 8 ply gauze over chromatography paper (0.16 mm) with glassine paper backing were fastened above wrist on skin. Pads were attached outside and underneath suits at lower leg, chest, and back and were offset. Hand wash with 200 mL of ethanol:water (50:50).	Personal breathing zone air samples Blood (pre- and postexposure)	Leavitt et al., 1982
Carbaryl (WP)	Power spray application to trees, lawns, and gardens by commercial pesticide applicator	Pads (10.2 cm by 10.2 cm) of 8 ply gauze over chromatography paper (0.16 mm) with glassine paper backing were fastened to the outside of clothing at chest, back, wrist, leg; beneath the clothing at chest, back, leg Hand wash with 200 mL of ethanol:water (50:50)	Personal breathing zone air samples Blood (pre- and postexposure)	Leavitt et al., 1982

WP = Wettable powder
EC = Emulsifiable concentrate

Contaminant	*Activity*	*Dermal Methods*	*Other Sampling*	*Reference*
Carbaryl (10% dust)	Hand harvesting of cucumbers	Tyvek jackets with α-cellulose pads (4 in. by 4 in.) with glassine backings attached to the exterior at forearms, chest (each side), shoulders, and one on the center of the upper back Cotton gloves	Personal breathing zone air samples Foliage residue Soil	EPA, 1988*a* (Study 1)
Carbaryl	Hand harvesting of peas	Tyvek jackets with α-cellulose pads (4 in. by 4 in.) with glassine backings attached to the exterior at forearms, chest (each side), shoulders, and one on the center of the upper back Cotton gloves	Personal breathing zone air samples Foliage residue Soil	EPA, 1988*a* (Study 1)
Carbaryl	Hand harvesting of cucumbers	Gauze pads (4 in. by 4 in.) with a glassine backing attached to elastic arm bands and pinned to the outside of workers' clothing at knee level Cotton gloves followed by 95% ethanol hand rinses	Personal breathing zone air samples Foliage residue Soil	EPA, 1988*a* (Study 2)
Carbaryl	Spraying in orchards	Filter paper (12.5 cm by 12.5 cm) pinned on clothing at hat, arm (top), wrist, shoulder, back, chest, thigh	Respirator pads	Simpson, 1965
Carbaryl	Hand harvesting of strawberries	12 ply gauze pads (3 in. by 3 in.) inside special holders with 28 cm^2 opening taped to skin of forearms and lower legs Cotton gloves	Foliage residue	EPA, 1988 (Study 2); Zweig et al., 1985

Contaminant	*Activity*	*Dermal Methods*	*Other Sampling*	*Reference*
Carbaryl	Hand harvesting of blueberries	12 ply gauze pads (3 in. by 3 in.) with polyethylene backings inside glassine envelopes with a circular opening (60 mm diameter). Pads were fastened to a headband or brim of a cap for the face and were stapled to a tightly fitting cotton T-shirt at the chest, back, and upper arm. Pads were attached to lower arms and legs with surgical tape. Cotton gloves	Foliage residue Soil	EPA, 1988*b* (Study 5)
Carbaryl	Collecting foliage samples in an okra field	Gauze pads (100 cm2) located on the outside and inside sleeves and on the chest pockets of cotton chambray work shirts	Urine Foliage residue	EPA, 1988*b* (Study 8)
Carbaryl	Mixing/loading Aerial flagging Hand gun spraying Bystanders Apple orchard thinners	8 ply gauze (10 cm by 10 cm) pads with filter paper/cardboard backings attached to disposable jackets at shoulders, chest, back, and on forearms Hand rinse with 150 mL of 95% ethanol	Foliage residue	Maitlen, Sell, and McDonough, 1982

WP = Wettable powder
EC = Emulsifiable concentrate

Contaminant	*Activity*	*Dermal Methods*	*Other Sampling*	*Reference*
Carbaryl	Power sprayer and garden pump application to trees	Whatman chromatography (14.5 cm^2) paper (grade 3 MM) taped to the worker at forearms, thighs, and lower legs	Surface samples for spray fallout and drift	Haverty et al., 1983
Carbaryl	Formulation of 4% and 5% dust Air blast application to fruit orchards (0.045%–0.06%)	α-Cellulose pads (10.2 cm by 10.2 cm) with filter paper backings placed on the shins, thigh fronts, forearms, shoulders, back of neck, and upper chest near "V" of neck for spray 32 ply gauze pads (11.4 cm by 11.4 cm) for dust backed with filter paper attached to shoulders, back of neck, "V" of chest, shins, thigh (fronts), and forearms.	Modified respirator with filter Urine	Comer et al., 1975
Carbaryl (WP)	Aerial spraying (pilots) Air blast spraying of orchards (tractor operators)	Strips of 3 ply α-cellulose wrapped around the forehead (2 in. by 10 in.) and wrists (2 in. by 6 in.)	Personal breathing zone air samples Modified respirators with filter pads	Jegier, 1964*b*
Carbofuran	Hand harvesting sugar cane	Tyvek jackets with α-cellulose pads (4 in. by 4 in.) with glassine backings attached to the exterior at forearms, chest (each side), shoulders, and one on the center of the upper back Cotton gloves	Personal breathing zone air samples Foliage residue Soil	EPA, 1988*a* (Study 1)

Contaminant	*Activity*	*Dermal Methods*	*Other Sampling*	*Reference*
Carbofuran	Mixing-loading Ground-rig spray application for grasshopper control over grain	Tegaderm plastic film taped on skin beneath work clothing at neck, shoulders, chest, back, upper arms, forearms, hips, thighs, calves, ankles, and wrists; placed on forehead and side of head; and outside of clothing at forearm (right), chest, and back. Tyveks worn over work clothing during mixing. Hand rinse with 400 mL isopropyl alcohol	Personal breathing zone air samples Urine (postexposure, 24 hr) Blood (pre- and postexposure)	Hussain et al., 1990
Carbophenothion (0.3%)	Tractor drawn air blast spraying of fruit orchards	α-Cellulose pads (10.2 cm by 10.2 cm) with filter paper backings placed on the shins, thigh fronts, forearms, shoulders, back of neck, and upper chest near "V" of neck	Modified respirator with filter pads	Wolfe et al., 1972
Carboxin-thiram	Commercial seed treating with liquid application using barrel or mist treaters	α-Cellulose pads (12.5 cm by 12.5 cm) over chromatography filter paper (100 cm2) over glassine paper with brown wrapping paper backings taped to the outside of clothing at upper arm and chest (opposite arm with pad) Hand wash with 95% ethanol	Gauze (12 ply) over α-cellulose over filter paper in modified respirators	Grey, Marthre, and Rogers, 1983

WP = Wettable powder
EC = Emulsifiable concentrate

Contaminant	*Activity*	*Dermal Methods*	*Other Sampling*	*Reference*
Chlordane	Application via subslab injection for termite control Residential exposure (airborne)	12 ply gauze pads (10.2 cm by 10.2 cm), with chromatographic paper midlayers and glassine paper backing attached to outside of clothing at shoulders, forearms, ankles, chest, and back. Pads inside clothing (offset) at chest, back, shoulders, and ankles. Hand wash (200 mL hexane)	Personal breathing zone air samples Area air samples (residents)	Kamble et al., 1992
Chlordane	Spray applications for borers in subfloor areas of buildings already erected or spray on foundations for buildings not yet erected	Pairs of filter papers pinned to hat, shoulder, back, chest, arm, wrist, and thigh on top of overalls	Blood Modified respirator with prefilters	Simpson and Shandar, 1972
Chlordane Dieldrin	Farmer with long lasting residue Pest control operators with long lasting residue Former pest control operator with a skin disorder	Hand rinse with 30 mL hexane poured over them up to several days after last usage	Blood	Kazen et al., 1974
Chlordimeform (WS bags, liquid)	Mixing/loading with closed system (liquid) or adding intact bags Aerial spray application	Fabric covered gauze pad with aluminum foil backing Hand wash with water	Personal breathing zone air samples	Maddy et al., 1983*a* (HS-1063)
Chlordimeform (WS packets)	Mixing/loading Aerial spray application	Fabric covered gauze pad with aluminum foil backing Hand wash with water	Personal breathing zone air samples	Maddy et al, 1982*d* (HS-1067)

Contaminant	*Activity*	*Dermal Methods*	*Other Sampling*	*Reference*
Chlorobenzilate	Mixing/loading Airblast spraying of orange trees	α-Cellulose pads (4 in. by 4 in.) with a surgical sponge on front and glassine paper backings were pinned inside shirt on back, chest, shoulders, upper arms, and forearms; inside pants at shins Bag hand rinse (95% ethanol)	Urine (spot samples) Foliage residue Fruit	Nigg, Stamper, and Queen, 1986
Chlorobenzilate (liquid)	Mixing/loading (pouring) Boom oscillator application and hand wand spray application	Fabric covered gauze pad with aluminum foil backing Hand wash with water	Personal breathing zone air samples	Maddy et al., 1983c (HS-903)
Chlorobenzilate (1.08 g/L)	Mixing/loading Airblast spraying from canopied tractors in citrus groves	α-Cellulose pads on shins and thighs under rubber aprons and on outside clothing at shoulders, chest, upper back, forearms, wrists (mixer/loader) α-Cellulose pads on outside of disposable coveralls at shoulders, chest, back, wrists, shins, and under disposable coveralls on clothing at thighs and forearms (applicator)	Personal breathing zone air samples Urine	Nigg and Stamper, 1983

WP = Wettable powder
EC = Emulsifiable concentrate

Contaminant	Activity	Dermal Methods	Other Sampling	Reference
Chlorobenzilate (liquid)	Citrus harvesting (reentry)	Cotton T-shirts with combination α-cellulose (4 in. by 4 in.) and 16 ply surgical sponge pads (top) with glassine backings pinned inside on both shoulders, chest, back, both forearms, and both upper arms. Thigh and shin pads were taped outside work clothing.	Urine, noon and after an unexposed weekend Foliage residue Fruit	Nigg, Stamper, and Queen 1984
Chlorothalonil	Spraying pesticide using handheld lances or spray guns	Long-sleeve cotton gloves	Personal breathing zone air samples	Brouwer et al., 1992
Chlorothalonil	Hand harvesting tomatoes	Gauze pads (103.2 cm^2) placed near the ankles and on the inner forearm Cotton twill gloves Hand towel wash of hands		EPA, 1988*b* (Study 10)
Chlorothalonil	Dusting with knapsack dust blowers and subsequent reentry into greenhouses to do cutting and sorting/bundling of carnations	Long-sleeve cotton gloves	Personal breathing zone air samples	Brouwer et al., 1992
Chlorothalonil (WP)	Boom spray application to chrysanthemums in greenhouses	α-Cellulose pads (10.16 cm by 10.16 cm) with glassine backing taped to outside of clothing at back (middle), shoulders, forearms, thighs (fronts), and shins Bag hand wash with 200 mL 95% ethanol	Personal breathing zone air samples	Stamper et al., 1989*b*; Nigg, Stamper, and Mahon, 1988

Contaminant	*Activity*	*Dermal Methods*	*Other Sampling*	*Reference*
Chlorothalonil (75% WP) Chlorpyrifos (50% WP) Ethazol (30% WP) Fluvalinate (22.3% EC)	Drench application with a handgun in an opensided greenhouse where chrysanthemums and African violets were grown	α-Cellulose pads (10.16 cm by 10.16 cm) with glassine paper backings attached at the chest, each forearm, thigh fronts, and shins on top of their work clothing Hand wash	Personal breathing zone air samples	Stamper et al., 1989*c*
Chlorpyrifos	Greenhouse handgun spraying of violets and chrysanthemums using coarse and fine sprays	α-Cellulose pads (10.16 cm by 10.16 cm) with glassine paper backing placed on back (middle), chest, shoulders, forearms (dorsal), thighs (ventral), shins (ventral) on outside of clothing. If CPC (Tyvek coveralls, butyl rubber aprons, boots) was worn, pad was outside of it. Pads placed inside coveralls adjacent to position of outside pad at chest, forearms, thighs, and shins. Bag hand wash (200 mL of 95% ethanol)	Personal breathing zone air samples	Stamper et al., 1989*a*; Nigg, Stamper, and Mahon, 1988

WP = Wettable powder
EC = Emulsifiable concentrate

Contaminant	*Activity*	*Dermal Methods*	*Other Sampling*	*Reference*
Chlorpyrifos	Pulse fogging with handgun to chrysanthemums and violets in greenhouses	α-Cellulose pads (10.16 cm by 10.16 cm) with glassine paper backing placed on back (middle), chest, shoulders, forearms (dorsal), thighs (ventral), shins (ventral) on outside of clothing. If CPC (Tyvek coveralls, butyl rubber aprons, boots) was worn, pad was outside of it. Pads placed inside coveralls adjacent to position of outside pad at chest, forearms, thighs, and shins. Bag hand wash (200 mL of 95% ethanol)	Personal breathing zone air samples Urine	Stamper et al., 1988; Nigg, Stamper, and Mahon, 1988
Chlorpyrifos	Application to corn via an overhead irrigation system	Polyurethane foam (6 mm thick) pads on hat, at shoulders, forearms, chest (mid), thigh (front), and ankle Cotton gloves	Area pads for drift Foliage residue	Brady et al., 1991
Chlorpyrifos (WP)	Boom spray application to chrysanthemums in greenhouses	α-cellulose pads (10.16 cm by 10.16 cm) with glassine backing taped to outside of clothing at back (middle), shoulders, fore-arms, thighs (fronts), and shins Bag hand wash with 200 mL 95% ethanol	Personal breathing zone air samples	Stamper et al., 1989*b*; Nigg, Stamper, and Mahon, 1988

Contaminant	*Activity*	*Dermal Methods*	*Other Sampling*	*Reference*
Chlorpyrifos (WP)	Span spray application to chrysanthemums in greenhouses	α-Cellulose pads (10.16 cm by 10.16 cm) with glassine backing taped to outside of clothing at back (middle), shoulders, fore-arms, thighs (fronts), and shins Bag hand wash with 200 mL 95% ethanol	Personal breathing zone air samples	Stamper et al., 1989*b*; Nigg, Stamper, and Mahon, 1988
Chlorthion	Operating aerosol machine against mosquitoes	α-Cellulose pads (1.5 in. by 16 in.) as head-bands and bands (1.5 in. by 8 in.) on ankle over socks, pads (4 in. by 4 in.) at forearms, neck (back and front) Cotton knit glove (one hand)	Personal breathing zone air samples Modified respirator with filter over cartridge Blood	Culver, Caplan, and Batchelor, 1956
Cypermethrin	Pesticide spraying on tea plants	6 ply gauze pads stapled to filter backing attached to front of work jackets on the chest and abdomen, and to thigh and ankle Cotton gloves	Gauze filters in respirators for respirable exposure	Wan, 1990
Cypermethrin	Mixing/loading Aerial application of an ultra low volume formulation to cotton	Tyvek overalls and hoods that were subsequently analyzed Cotton gloves Acrylic nylon socks	Urine (24 hr)	Chester et al., 1987

WP = Wettable powder
EC = Emulsifiable concentrate

Contaminant	Activity	Dermal Methods	Other Sampling	Reference
2,4-D Amine salt	Tractor ground rig boom spraying	Standardized clothing issued. Glass fiber filters (47 mm diameter) impregnated with ethylene glycol mounted with gauze in front, cardboard backing, with 4 pads pinned to outside of clothing at chest, back, arms, and legs and 9 placed underneath the work clothing at chest (left side), upper arms, wrists, knees, and ankles Hand rinse with 750 mL (1%) sodium bicarbonate (postexposure)	Urine (24 hr)	Grover et al., 1986*b*
2,4-D Amine salt	Tractor drawn ground rig application (with and without cabs)	Standardized set of clothing issued. Glass fiber filters (47 mm diameter) impregnated with ethylene glycol mounted with gauze in front, cardboard backing, placed under the work clothing at chest (left side), upper arms, wrists, knees, and ankles; pads placed over clothing at neck, near left elbow, on cap, chest (left side). Hand rinse with 750 mL (1%) sodium carbonate	Personal breathing zone air samples Urine (24 hr)	Grover et al., 1986*a*
2,4-D	Mixing/loading Aerial application of 2,4-D by forestry workers	Disposable Tyvek suits with hoods; cut into portions for analysis (hood, arms, torso, legs)	Urine Swabs of helicopters, vehicles, workplace, and living and eating quarters	Frank, Campbell, and Sirons, 1985

Contaminant	*Activity*	*Dermal Methods*	*Other Sampling*	*Reference*
2,4-D	Handgun spray application to aquatic weeds from airboats	α-Cellulose (10 cm by 10 cm) pads attached to wrists, forearms, shoulders, back (center near neck), chest (near neck), and thighs (front) on outside of clothing Cotton gloves (square cut from palm and back)	Personal breathing zone air samples Urine (24 hr)	Nigg and Stamper, 1983
2,4-D	Hand spraying of weeds	Gauze pads (0.67 ft^2) attached to back and chest; paper cap covering head	Personal breathing zone air samples Blood (pre- and postexposure) Urine (pooled, pre-, during, and 4–7 hr postexposure) Vegetation residue Soil	Taskar et al., 1982
2,4-D	Filling of pesticide sprayers Application with tractor powered hydraulic sprayers Manual spraying from backpack sprayers	Disposable body suits, gauntlets, and hoods Nylon socks	Personal breathing zone air sampling	Abbott et al., 1987
2,4-D	Mixing/loading Application	8 ply gauze (10 cm by 10 cm) pads with filter paper/ cardboard backings attached to disposable jackets at shoulders, chest, back, and on forearms Hand rinse with 150 mL of 95% ethanol Perspiration adsorbed onto cotton T-shirts	Urine	Sell and Maitlen, 1983

WP = Wettable powder
EC = Emulsifiable concentrate

Contaminant	*Activity*	*Dermal Methods*	*Other Sampling*	*Reference*
2,4-D	Aerial application and ground spray	Denim patches attached to clothing near bare skin areas: shirt cuff, collar, hat band	Personal breathing zone air samples Urine (12 hr)	Lavy et al., 1982
DDT	Indoor and outdoor house spraying	α-Cellulose pads with glassine paper backings on tops of the shoulders, the back, upper chest near the jugular notch, back of forearms and neck, front of thighs, and over the nose and mouth (if no respirator used).	Air samples Modified respirator with filter pads Urine	Wolfe et al., 1959
DDT (50% WP)	Formulation plant—mixing, bag filling, bag top closure (sewing), and packing filled bags	Gauze pads, 32 ply (11.4 cm^2), for dust backed with filter paper attached to shoulders, back of neck, "V" of chest, and fore-arms outside clothing	Modified respirator with filter pads Urine (postshift)	Wolfe and Armstrong, 1971
DDT and BHC in combination (5% & 1%; 15% & 50%; 20% & 3%)	Forest spraying with a tractor, hand carried boom, and airplane	Pads attached to shoulders, forearm, and front of neck	Personal breathing zone air samples	Wasserman et al., 1960
DEF Lorsban Pydrin	Cotton gin	Skin wipes of palms, wrists, and forehead of workers with Whatman smear tabs	Personal breathing zone air samples Area air samples Work surface wipes Blood Bulk cotton Settled dust	NIOSH, July 1984 (HETA 81-463-1477)
DEF	Cotton ginning (ginner, press-man, janitor)	Flannel (4 in. by 4 in.) pads pinned at chest, back, and thigh fronts outside clothing	Area air samples Urine Bulk samples of cotton before and after ginning	Kilgore et al., 1984

Contaminant	*Activity*	*Dermal Methods*	*Other Sampling*	*Reference*
DEF	Mixing/loading with closed system Aerial spray application to cotton (pilot, flagger)	Flannel (4 in by 4 in.) cloth pads pinned at chest and back outside clothing (flagger, mixer/loader)	Parts of clothing from flagger mannequin High volume area air samples Personal breathing zone air samples (pilot, flagger) Drift samples Urine (preshift)	Kilgore et al., 1984
DEF	Cotton picking	Skin wipes of palms, wrists, and forehead of workers with Whatman smear tabs	Personal breathing zone air samples Area air samples Work surface wipes Blood Bulk cotton	NIOSH, July 1984 (HETA 81-463-1477)
DEF (S,S,S-tributylphosphorotrithioate) Merphos	Mixing/loading Aerial application as a cotton defoliant	Dacron/cotton 65/35 cloth pads (10.5 cm by 10.5 cm) over 12 ply gauze with backings of aluminum foil and stiff paper attached or Dacron cotton 65/35 cloth pads (10.5 cm by 10.5 cm) with a stiff paper backing attached to exterior of regular work clothing at thigh, upper chest, upper arms, and neck (posterior). If disposable coveralls worn, pad was placed underneath at these positions. Hand rinse with 100 mL of 95% ethanol.	Personal breathing zone air samples Blood	Lotti et al., 1983

WP = Wettable powder
EC = Emulsifiable concentrate

Contaminant	Activity	Dermal Methods	Other Sampling	Reference
DEF	Harvesting cotton with tractor (operator inside cab)	Flannel (4 in. by 4 in.) pads pinned at chest, back, and thigh fronts outside clothing	Personal breathing zone air samples inside and outside cab Urine Foliage residue	Kilgore et al., 1984
Deildrin (0.03%)	Power hand gun spraying fruit orchards from portable machine	Gauze pads, 32 ply, (11.4 cm by 11.4 cm) for spray attached to shoulders, back of neck, "V" of chest, and forearms Bag hand rinse or swab with 95% ethanol	Modified respirator with filter pads	Wolfe, Durham, and Armstrong, 1967
Deltamethrin	Spray application to cotton fields using sprayers with a single pressure nozzle	Gauze pads (5 cm by 5 cm) attached to the head, chest, back, forearms, thighs, legs, hands, and feet. An additional pair of gauze pads was placed underneath and on top of polyester trousers to determine pesticide absorption.	Personal breathing zone air samples Area air samples for particle size distributions Urine (prework, and at various hour intervals following application) Blood	Zhang et al., 1991
Deltamethrin	Vaporizer application to french beans inside of greenhouses	Gauze pads (100 cm^2) on top of clothing at "V" of neck, shoulders, back, upper arms, forearms, thighs, lower legs Cotton gloves	Area air samples Foliage residue	Mestres et al., 1985

Contaminant	*Activity*	*Dermal Methods*	*Other Sampling*	*Reference*
Deltamethrin Methamidophos	Spray application to cotton fields using sprayers with a single pressure nozzle	Gauze pads (5 cm by 5 cm) attached to the head, chest, back, forearms, thighs, legs, hands, and feet. An additional pair of gauze pads was placed underneath and on top of polyester trousers to determine pesticide absorption.	Personal breathing zone air samples Area air samples for particle size distributions Urine (prework, and at various hour intervals following application) Blood	Zhang et al., 1991
Demeton O Demeton S	Mixing/loading in a closed system to determine its effectiveness Ground application	Unwashed cotton cloth and rayon:polyester pads (4 in. by 4 in.) attached to the exterior of the clothing at shoulder, chest, waist, and knee	Area air samples around mixing/ loading sites and on tractors Blood Urine (spot; Prejob, 3 week intervals)	Knaak et al., 1980
Dialifor Phosalone	Evaluation of illnesses in 118 out of 120 workers who became ill during hand harvesting of grapes after treatment with these pesticides	Trousers worn during the work Skin swabs from a 5 cm to 10 cm area of the inside arm at the elbow	Blood Foliage residues	Knaak et al., 1978
Diallate	Tank filling, spray application	Gauze pads (4 in. by 4 in.) attached to hat (front and back), shoulders, chest, and back pads attached to disposable jackets or coveralls Cotton gloves	Personal breathing zone air samples Area air samples Soil	Dubelman et al., 1982

WP = Wettable powder
EC = Emulsifiable concentrate

Contaminant	*Activity*	*Dermal Methods*	*Other Sampling*	*Reference*
Diazinon	Mixing/loading in a closed system to determine its effectiveness Ground application	Unwashed cotton cloth and rayon:polyester pads (4 in. by 4 in.) attached to the exterior of the clothing at shoulder, chest, waist, and knee	Area air samples around mixing/ loading sites and on tractors Blood Urine (spot; prejob, 3 week intervals)	Knaak et al., 1980
Diazinon (0.06%)	Tractor drawn air blast spraying fruit orchards	α-Cellulose pads (10.2 cm by 10.2 cm) with filter paper backings placed on the shins, thigh fronts, forearms, shoulders, back of neck, and upper chest near "V" of neck	Modified respirator with filter pads	Wolfe et al., 1972
Diazinon	Mixing/loading Truck mounted tank and handheld sprayer (liquid) application to lawns for insect control Rotary type spreader for granule application	Monitoring under clothing with surgipads (289 cm^2) placed at wrists, ankles, and inner thighs; and 12 ply gauze sponges (10.2 cm by 10.2 cm) placed on chest (upper and lower) and back (upper and lower)	Personal breathing zone air samples	Freeborg, Daniel, and Konopinski, 1985

Contaminant	*Activity*	*Dermal Methods*	*Other Sampling*	*Reference*
Diazinon (WP)	Tractor powered air blast spray application to pear orchards	Fluorescent tracer (4-methyl-7-diethylamino-coumarin) added to spray formulation. Pre- and postexposure video images under UV light of hands, forearms, upper arm, head, upper torso (neck to breast), and lower torso (breast to waist) 12 ply gauze pads (3 in. by 3 in.) with polyethylene backings placed in an envelope with a circular opening. Two pads attached to outside of coverall at left breast and right shoulder blade and two attached inside coverall on T-shirt at right breast and left shoulder blade.	Personal breathing zone air samples Area gauze pads on top of spray rig	Fenske, Leffingwell, and Spear, 1985
Diazinon granules	Ground application to eradicate Japanese beetle larvae	Gauze pads taped together with a backing of aluminum foil and paper placed on the outside of coveralls on the right and left chest and the center back. Pads were also placed on the front of the right and left boot, underneath the coveralls. Hand rinse with 100 mL of 95% ethanol at breaks and end of shift	Personal breathing zone air samples Area air samples inside truck enclosure Urine (pre- and postshift)	Weisskopf et al., 1988

WP = Wettable powder
EC = Emulsifiable concentrate

Contaminant	*Activity*	*Dermal Methods*	*Other Sampling*	*Reference*
Dibrom	Pesticide manufacture	Wipes of gloves used for drumming, sampling, and in lab with Whatman smear tabs	Personal breathing zone air samples Blood Surface wipes	NIOSH, 1985 (HETA 78-4-1511)
Dicofol	Airblast application to citrus to determine penetration of coveralls by pesticides	Bag handwash with 10% methanol in water. α-Cellulose pads (10.16 cm by 10.16 cm) with glassine paper backings attached to disposable polypropylene Duraguard coveralls at the chest, each forearm, thigh fronts, and shins on top and underneath (offset) the material.		Nigg et al., 1990
Dicofol	Airblast application to citrus to determine penetration of coveralls by pesticides	α-Cellulose pads (10.16 cm by 10.16 cm) with glassine paper backings attached to disposable polypropylene SMS coveralls at the chest, each forearm, thigh fronts, and shins on top and underneath (offset) the material.		Nigg et al., 1990
Dicofol	Airblast application to citrus to determine penetration of coveralls by pesticides	α-Cellulose pads (10.16 cm by 10.16 cm) with glassine paper backings attached to untreated 65/35 cotton/poly twill coveralls at the chest, each forearm, thigh fronts, and shins on top and underneath (offset) the material.		Nigg et al., 1990

Contaminant	*Activity*	*Dermal Methods*	*Other Sampling*	*Reference*
Dicofol	Airblast application to citrus to determine penetration of coveralls by pesticides	α-Cellulose pads (10.16 cm by 10.16 cm) with glassine paper backings attached to fluorocarbon treated 65/35 cotton/poly twill coveralls at the chest, each forearm, thigh fronts, and shins on top and underneath (offset) the material.		Nigg et al., 1990
Dicofol	Greenhouse handgun spraying of violets and chrysanthemums with coarse and fine sprays	α-Cellulose pads (10.16 cm by 10.16 cm) with glassine paper backings placed on back (middle), chest, shoulders, forearms (dorsal), thighs (ventral), shins (ventral), on outside of clothing. If CPC (Tyvek coveralls, butyl rubber aprons, boots) was worn, pad was outside of it. Pads placed inside coveralls adjacent to position of outside pad at chest, forearms, thighs, and shins. Bag hand wash (200 mL of 95% ethanol)	Personal breathing zone air samples	Stamper et al., 1989*a*; Nigg, Stamper, and Mahon, 1988

WP = Wettable powder
EC = Emulsifiable concentrate

Contaminant	Activity	Dermal Methods	Other Sampling	Reference
Dicofol	Mixing/loading Airblast application to citrus with canopied tractor	α-Cellulose pads (4 in. by 4 in.) with glassine paper backings taped to outside of workers' clothing at the left side of the chest, upper arms, shoulders, back, thighs, shins on the outside of coveralls; on the work shirt underneath coveralls at chest pocket and forearms; and pinned on the inside of the shirt at chest and forearms; three layers of pads, all pads were nonoverlapping Bag hand rinse with 95% ethanol	Urine (24 hr)	Nigg et al., 1991
Dicofol	Mixing/loading Airblast application to citrus with canopied tractor	α-Cellulose pads (4 in. by 4 in.) with glassine paper backings taped to outside of clothing at the left side of the chest, upper arms, shoulders, back, thighs, shins on the outside of coveralls; on the work shirt underneath coveralls at chest pocket and forearms; and pinned on the inside of the shirt at chest and forearms; three layers of pads, all pads were nonoverlapping Bag hand rinse with 95% ethanol	Polyurethane foam mask	Nigg, Stamper, and Queen, 1986

Contaminant	*Activity*	*Dermal Methods*	*Other Sampling*	*Reference*
Dicofol	Mixing/loading Airblast application to citrus with canopied tractor	α-Cellulose pads (4 in. by 4 in.) with glassine paper backings pinned and taped to the left front chest pocket of work shirt, forearms, shoulders, back, thighs, and shins on the outside of pants. Inside normal work clothing pinned at chest and forearms (nonoverlapping) of work shirt. Hand rinse with 95% ethanol	Polyurethane foam mask	Nigg, Stamper, and Queen, 1986
Dicofol	Pneumatic disc harrow application to lemon trees inside of plastic greenhouses	Gauze pads (100 cm^2) on top of clothing at "V" of neck, shoulders, back, upper arms, forearms, thighs, lower legs Cotton gloves	Area air samples Foliage residue	Mestres et al., 1985
Dicofol (0.04%)	Tractor drawn air blast spraying fruit orchards	α-Cellulose pads (10.2 cm by 10.2 cm) with filter paper backings placed on the shins, thigh fronts, forearms, shoulders, back of neck, and upper chest near "V" of neck	Modified respirator with filter pads	Wolfe et al., 1972
Dieldrin (0.02%-0.03%)	Air blast spraying fruit orchards	32 ply gauze pads (11.4 cm by 11.4 cm) attached to shoulders, back of neck, "V" of chest, and forearms Bag hand rinse or hand swab with 95% ethanol	Modified respirator with filter pads	Wolfe, Durham, and Armstrong, 1967

WP = Wettable powder
EC = Emulsifiable concentrate

Contaminant	*Activity*	*Dermal Methods*	*Other Sampling*	*Reference*
Dieldrin	Spraying pear orchards	32 ply gauze pads (11.4 cm^2) for dust with filter paper backings attached to shoulders, back of neck, "V" of chest, and forearms outside clothing Hand swab with 95% ethanol impregnated gauze swabs	Respirator filter pads	Wolfe, Durham, and Armstrong, 1963
Dieldrin	House spraying for control of disease vectors	Postlip filter paper pads (10 cm by 10 cm) secured with elastic sticking plaster or zinc oxide tape to clothing on one side of the body on the back of the neck, shoulder, back of wrist and outside of ankle under clothing on skin on the other side of the body at the shoulder, back of wrist, ankle, cheek (5 cm by 5 cm) and stomach		Fletcher, Press, and Wilson, 1959
Dieldrin	House spraying for control of disease vectors	Lanolin impregnated Postlip filter paper pads (10 cm by 10 cm) secured with elastic sticking plaster or zinc oxide tape to clothing on one side of the body on the back of the neck, shoulder, back of wrist and outside of ankle under clothing on skin on the other side of the body at the shoulder, back of wrist, ankle, cheek (5 cm by 5 cm) and stomach		Fletcher, Press, and Wilson, 1959

Contaminant	*Activity*	*Dermal Methods*	*Other Sampling*	*Reference*
Dilan (0.08%)	Tractor drawn air blast spraying fruit orchards	α-Cellulose pads (10.2 cm by 10.2 cm) with filter paper backings placed on the shins, thigh fronts, forearms, shoulders, back of neck, and upper chest near "V" of neck	Modified respirator with filter pads	Wolfe et al., 1972
Dimethoate	Knapsack spraying inside plastic greenhouses with tomatoes	12 ply gauze sponges (10 cm by 10 cm) impregnated with ethylene glycol backed with aluminum foil and flexible cardboard pinned to the outside of clothing on chest, back, shoulders, upper arms, forearm near wrist, upper legs	Personal breathing zone air samples Blood	Al-Jaghbir, Salhab, and Hamarsheh, 1992
Dimethoate	Oscillating boom spraying of citrus (open tractor, tractor with open windows on cab or closed windows)	12 ply gauze sponges (10 cm by 10 cm) impregnated with ethylene glycol backed with aluminum foil and flexible cardboard pinned to the outside of clothing on chest, back, shoulders, upper arms, forearm near wrist, upper legs	Personal breathing zone air samples Urine (pre- and postshift)	Carman et al., 1982
Dimethoate	Knapsack mist blower and duster application	α-Cellulose pads (10 cm by 10 cm) over clothing or on skin at upper surface of left forearm, front of left leg (above ankle and midthigh), sternum, between shoulder blades, headdress, skin of upper abdomen	Blood	Copplestone et al., 1976

WP = Wettable powder
EC = Emulsifiable concentrate

Contaminant	*Activity*	*Dermal Methods*	*Other Sampling*	*Reference*
Dimethoate	Mixing/loading in a closed system to determine its effectiveness Ground application	Unwashed cotton cloth and rayon:polyester pads (4 in. by 4 in.) attached to the exterior of the clothing at shoulder, chest, waist, and knee	Area air samples around mixing/ loading sites and on tractors Blood Urine (spot; prejob, 3 week intervals)	Knaak et al., 1980
Dimethoate (0.2%)	Greenhouse tomato spraying operations	12 ply gauze pads (10 cm diameter) attached to the head, chest, "V" of neck, shoulders, elbows, thighs, and legs Cotton gloves	Personal breathing zone air samples	Adamis et al., 1985
Dimethoate Benomyl	Harvesting of roses in greenhouses following fumigation	Cotton gloves	Foliage residues	Liesivuori, Liukkonen, and Pirhonen, 1988
Dinitro-o-cresol (DNOC) (19% slurry)	Apple thinning spraying	α-Cellulose pads with glassine paper backings on forearms, shoulders, thighs, and back and front of neck.	Respirator filters Urine (spot samples) Blood	Batchelor, Walker, and Elliott, 1956
Dinobuton (0.06%)	Tractor drawn air blast spraying fruit orchards	α-Cellulose pads (10.2 cm by10.2 cm) with filter paper backings placed on the shins, thigh fronts, forearms, shoulders, back of neck, and upper chest near "V" of neck	Modified respirator with filter pads	Wolfe et al., 1972
Dinoseb	Hand harvesting potatoes	8 ply gauze pads (2 in. by 2 in.) attached to the outside of workers' clothing at forearms, thighs, and calfs Cotton gloves with an 8 ply gauze pad (2 in. by 2 in.) with a glassine backing attached to the back	Personal breathing zone air samples Urine High volume area air samples Soil	EPA, 1988*a* (Study 8)

Contaminant	*Activity*	*Dermal Methods*	*Other Sampling*	*Reference*
Dioxathion	Citrus harvesting (reentry)	Gauze pads placed on upper arms and calves	Personal breathing zone air samples Foliage residue	Popendorf, 1980
Dioxathion	Contaminated road dust near ochard where workers were picking oranges	Arms and hands washed in dilute detergent solution with brushing (5 replications)	Personal breathing zone air samples Foliage residue Tree washings Soil	Westlake, Gunther, and Carman, 1973
Diquat (1.76%)	Mixing/loading Spraying weeds from airboats	α-Cellulose pads (10 cm by 10 cm) on back (center), chest, shoulders, forearms, thigh (front), shin (front) on outside of clothing Hand rinse with water or cotton gloves	Urine (PM)	Wojeck et al., 1983
Disulfoton (5%)	Granular application using tractor drawn gravity feed or broadcast application	α-Cellulose pads (10.2 cm by 10.2 cm) with filter paper backings placed on the shins, thigh fronts, forearms, shoulders, back of neck, and upper chest near "V" of neck attached to the outside of workers' clothing including hat	Personal breathing zone air samples Modified respirator with filter Particle size measurements using air and surface samples Bulk samples of granules for pesticide concentration	Lloyd and Bell, 1967
Disulfoton (10%)	Pelletized fertilizer mixing with granular pesticide in a rotating drum, dumping of materials into hopper Liquid injection of concentrate pesticide into mixing drum Filling bags with mix, stacking bags onto pallets	Gauze pads 32 ply, (11.4 cm^2) for dust backed with filter paper attached to shoulders, back of neck, "V" of chest, and forearms outside clothing Hand wash	Area air samples Modified respirator with filter pads Blood Urine	Wolfe et al., 1978

WP = Wettable powder
EC = Emulsifiable concentrate

Contaminant	*Activity*	*Dermal Methods*	*Other Sampling*	*Reference*
Dithiopyr	Mixing/loading Application to turfgrass	12 ply gauze pads (4 in. by 4 in.) pinned to outside of clothing at back, chest, shoulders, forearms, thighs, lower legs Hand wash using 200 mL of 2% Igepal	Personal breathing zone air samples Urine (prework and postwork 72 hr)	Cowell, Lottman, and Manning, 1991
DNOC (0.02%–0.04%)	Air blast spraying fruit orchards	32 ply gauze pads (11.4 cm by 11.4 cm) attached to shoulders, back of neck, "V" of chest, and forearms. Bag hand rinse or swab with 95% ethanol	Modified respirator with filter pads	Wolfe, Durham, and Armstrong, 1967
DNOC (0.02%–0.04%)	Chemical thinning of apple blossoms by power hand gun spraying	32 ply gauze pads (11.4 cm by 11.4 cm) attached to shoulders, back of neck, "V" of chest, and forearms Bag hand rinse or swab with 95% ethanol	Respirator filter pads	Wolfe, Durham, and Armstrong, 1967
Endosulfan	Mixing/loading in a closed system to determine its effectiveness Ground application	Unwashed cotton cloth and rayon:polyester pads (4 in. by 4 in.) attached to the exterior of the clothing at shoulder, chest, waist, and knee	Area air samples around mixing/loading sites and on tractors Blood Urine (spot; prejob, 3 week intervals)	Knaak et al., 1980
Endosulfan	Hand harvesting peas	Gauze pads (3 in. by 3 in.) with glassine paper backings stapled to gabardine forearm/thigh bands Cotton gloves followed by 95% ethanol hand rinses	Personal breathing zone air samples Urine Foliage residue Soil	EPA, 1988*a* (Study 3)

Contaminant	*Activity*	*Dermal Methods*	*Other Sampling*	*Reference*
Endosulfan	Hand harvesting corn	Gauze pads (3 in. by 3) with glassine paper backings stapled to gabardine forearm/thigh bands and pinned to the outside of workers' clothing at chest and shoulders and pinned to each side of a cap worn by the worker Cotton gloves followed by 95% ethanol hand rinses	Personal breathing zone air samples Urine Foliage residue Soil	EPA, 1988*a* (Study 3)
Endosulfan	Hand harvesting tomatoes	8 ply gauze pads (2 in. by 2 in.) attached to the outside of workers' clothing at forearms, thighs, and calfs Cotton gloves with an 8 ply gauze pad (2 in. by 2 in.) with a glassine backing attached to the back	Personal breathing zone air samples High volume area samples	EPA, 1988*a* (Study 9)
Endosulfan (0.06%)	Tractor drawn air blast spraying fruit orchards	α-Cellulose pads (10.2 cm by 10.2 cm) with filter paper backings placed on the shins, thigh fronts, forearms, shoulders, back of neck, and upper chest near "V" of neck	Modified respirator with filter pads	Wolfe et al., 1972
Endrin	Aerial spraying (pilots) Airblast spraying of orchards (tractor operators)	Strips of 3 ply α-cellulose wrapped around the forehead (2 in. by 10 in.) and wrists (2 in. by 6 in.)	Personal breathing zone air samples Modified respirators with filter pads	Jegier, 1964*b*

WP = Wettable powder
EC = Emulsifiable concentrate

Contaminant	*Activity*	*Dermal Methods*	*Other Sampling*	*Reference*
Endrin (1% in dust)	Spraying apple orchard cover crops for mouse control; dusting potatoes	α-Cellulose pads (10.2 cm by 10.2 cm) with filter paper backings for dust; 32 ply gauze pads (11.4 cm by 11.4 cm) for spray; attached to shoulders, back of neck, "V" of chest and forearms outside clothing Bag hand rinse with 95% ethanol	Modified respirator with filter pads Residue on apples Grass	Wolfe, Durham, and Armstrong, 1963
Endrin (0.05%)	High pressure power hand gun spraying or operating power air blast or boom sprayers on orchard cover crops for mouse control	23 ply gauze pads (11.4 cm by 11.4 cm) attached to shoulders, back of neck, "V" of chest, and forearms Bag hand rinse or swab with 95% ethanol	Modified respirator with filter pads	Wolfe, Durham, and Armstrong, 1967
	Aerial and ground rig application to cotton: pilots, loader, flagman	Denim cloth pads (10 cm by 10 cm) attached with safety pins to clothing at the chest, abdomen, upper and lower back, knees, forearms, and shoulders Hand rinses with acetone:distilled water (1:1)	Personal breathing zone air samples	Atallah, Cahill, and Whitacre, 1982
EPTC GENEP 7EC	Mixing/loading Tractor driven power take-off sprayer application	Gauze (23.75 cm^2) pads, 10 placed on outside of clothing and one inside; chest at throat, back, shoulders, forearms, chest (inside), thighs, shins Hand wash (800 mL water + surfactant)	Personal breathing zone air samples Urine	Knaak et al., 1989

Contaminant	*Activity*	*Dermal Methods*	*Other Sampling*	*Reference*
Ethazol	Greenhouse handgun spraying of violets and chrysanthemums with coarse and fine sprays	α-Cellulose pads (10.16 cm by 10.16 cm) with glassine paper backings placed on back (middle), chest, shoulders, forearms (dorsal), thighs (ventral), shins (ventral) on outside of clothing. If CPC (Tyvek coveralls, butyl rubber aprons, boots) was worn, pad was outside of it. Pads placed inside coveralls adjacent to position of outside pad at chest, forearms, thighs, and shins. Bag hand wash (200 mL of 95% ethanol)	Personal breathing zone air samples	Stamper et al., 1989*a*; Nigg, Stamper, and Mahon, 1988
Ethazol	Pulse fogging with handgun to chrysanthemums and violets in greenhouses	α-Cellulose pads (10.16 cm by 10.16 cm) with glassine paper backings placed on back (middle), chest, shoulders, forearms (dorsal), thighs (ventral), shins (ventral) on outside of clothing. If CPC (Tyvek coveralls, butyl rubber aprons, boots) was worn, pad was outside of it. Pads placed inside coveralls adjacent to position of outside pad at chest, forearms, thighs, and shins. Bag hand wash (200 mL of 95% ethanol)	Personal breathing zone air samples; Urine	Stamper et al., 1988; Nigg, Stamper, and Mahon, 1988

WP = Wettable powder
EC = Emulsifiable concentrate

Contaminant	*Activity*	*Dermal Methods*	*Other Sampling*	*Reference*
Ethion (WP)	Formulation work: mixing, bag filling, stacking bags on pallets, packing bags into cartons	α-Cellulose pads ($10.2\ cm^2$) backed with filter paper placed on the shins, thigh fronts, forearms, shoulders, back of neck, and upper chest near "V" of neck	Modified respirator with filters	Wolfe, Staiff, and Armstrong, 1978*a*
Ethion	Mixing/loading Airblast spray application to citrus	α-Cellulose (10 cm by 10 cm) pads attached to fore-arms, shoulders, back (center near neck), chest (near neck), and thighs (front) outside of clothing Cotton gloves (square from palm and back)	Modified respirator with pad Blood Urine	Wojeck et al., 1981
Ethion	Mixing/loading Application to citrus	α-Cellulose pads attached to the interior and exterior on opposing sides of a work shirt. Different types of fabrics evaluated for permeation.	Urine	Davies et al., 1982*a*
Ethion	Mixing/loading including refilling of spray tank after field was freshly sprayed Application to citrus groves using an air blast blower	α-Cellulose pads with glassine paper backings attached to front (chest) of coverall, one on exterior, the other offset underneath next to skin to determine the effectiveness of different clothing worn by workers: normal working clothes, 100% cotton denim coveralls, and 100% cotton denim coveralls coated with Scotchgard™.	Urine (daily at specific intervals)	Davies et al., 1982c

Contaminant	*Activity*	*Dermal Methods*	*Other Sampling*	*Reference*
Ethion	Airblast application to citrus to determine penetration of coveralls by pesticides	α-Cellulose pads (10.16 cm by 10.16 cm) with glassine paper backings attached to disposable polypropylene SMS coveralls at the chest, each forearm, thigh fronts, and shins on top and underneath (offset) the material		Nigg et al., 1990
Ethion	Airblast application to citrus to determine penetration of coveralls by pesticides	α-Cellulose pads (10.16 cm by 10.16 cm) with glassine paper backings attached to fluorocarbon treated 65/35 cotton/poly twill coveralls at the chest, each forearm, thigh fronts, and shins on top and underneath (offset) the material		Nigg et al., 1990
Ethion (0.06%)	Tractor drawn air blast spraying of fruit orchards	α-Cellulose pads (10.2 cm by10.2 cm) with filter paper backings placed on the shins, thigh fronts, forearms, shoulders, back of neck, and upper chest near "V" of neck	Modified respirator with filter pads	Wolfe et al., 1972

WP = Wettable powder
EC = Emulsifiable concentrate

Contaminant	*Activity*	*Dermal Methods*	*Other Sampling*	*Reference*
Ethion in an oil-water formulation	Handgunning young citrus trees while walking or riding on the back of a truck	α-Cellulose pads (4 in. by 4 in.) with glassine backing on the outside of clothing on the front of the hat, on the upper middle of the back, on the chest near the pectoral region, facing the front on each shoulder, on the forearm, on the front of each thigh Hand wash using 250 mL of 95% ethanol (3 rinses)		Nigg, Stamper, and Mahon, 1990
Ethyl parathion (WP)	Formulation work: mixing, bagging, stacking bags on pallets; sealing bag tops/packing bags in cartons for shipment	α-Cellulose pads ($10.2\ cm^2$) backed with filter paper placed on the shins, thigh fronts, forearms, shoulders, back of neck and upper chest near "V" of neck	Modified respirator with filters	Wolfe, Staiff, and Armstrong, 1978
Ethyl parathion	Spraying low volume concentrated materials (0.24%–0.36%) and high volume diluted (0.03%) materials in orchards	α-Cellulose pads attached to shoulders, "V" of chest, back of neck, forearms on the worker's body or clothing Hand rinse with ethanol or hand swabbing with ethanol impregnated gauze	Modified respirator with filter pads	Wolfe, Armstrong, and Durham, 1966
Ethyl parathion	Knapsack spraying of tomato bushes	Filter paper (12.5 cm by 12.5 cm), two layers, pinned to clothing at the back near neck base, chest center, wrist, arm near elbow, shoulders, hat	Personal breathing zone air samples Modified respirator with cotton pads	Simpson and Beck, 1964

Contaminant	*Activity*	*Dermal Methods*	*Other Sampling*	*Reference*
Ethyl parathion	Hand harvesting blueberries	Tyvek jacket with 8 ply gauze pads (2 in. by 2 in.) with glassine paper backing attached to the exterior at forearms, breasts, and shoulders and back Cotton gloves with an 8 ply gauze pad (2 in. by 2 in.) with glassine backing attached to the back	Personal breathing zone air samples Urine High volume area air samples Foliage residue Soil	EPA, 1988*a* (Study 7)
Ethyl parathion	Citrus harvesting (reentry)	Gauze pads placed on upper arms and calves	Personal breathing zone air samples Foliage residue	Popendorf, 1980
Ethyl parathion	Oscillating boom spraying of citrus (open tractor, tractor with open windows on cab or closed windows)	12 ply surgical sponges (10 cm by 10 cm) impregnated with ethylene glycol with aluminum foil and flexible cardboard backings pinned to the outside of clothing on chest, back, shoulders, upper arms, forearm near wrist, upper legs	Personal breathing zone air samples Urine (pre- and postexposure)	Carman et al., 1982
Ethyl parathion	Mixing/loading Application with low pressure, low boom; high pressure, high boom; high pressure, low boom; and drop nozzle sprayers, harvesting, and scouting of cabbage and onions	16 ply gauze pads (4 in. by 4 in.) with aluminum foil backings taped on chest, back and left leg at knee Cotton gloves		Spittler and Bourke, 1985
Ethyl parathion	Air blast spray application with filtered air cab	Fabric covered gauze pad with aluminum foil backing Hand wash with water and Surten	Personal breathing zone air samples	Wang, Lenahan, and Tucker, 1987

WP = Wettable powder
EC = Emulsifiable concentrate

Contaminant	*Activity*	*Dermal Methods*	*Other Sampling*	*Reference*
Ethyl parathion	Hand harvesting onions by youth and adult field workers	Nylon gloves	High volume area air samples Urine Foliage residue Soil	EPA, 1988*a* (Study 11); Munn, Keefe, and Savage, 1985
Ethyl parathion	Aerial spray application: pilots and ground crew	Filter paper wetted with ethylene glycol attached to shirt Hand wash with hexane	Area air samples	Richter et al., 1980
Ethyl parathion	Mixing/loading Application with high pressure, low boom; and low pressure, low boom sprayers and harvesting of green beans	16 ply gauze pads (4 in. by 4 in.) with aluminum foil backings taped on chest, back and left leg at knee Cotton gloves		Spittler and Bourke, 1985
Ethyl parathion	Boom oscillator application	Cotton T-shirt and leggings under coveralls Hand wash with water Analysis of cotton glove liners	Personal breathing zone air samples	Maddy et al., 1984 (HS-1059)
Ethyl parathion (0.33%)	Power airblast spraying on fruit orchards	α-Cellulose pads on top of clothing at shoulders, back, chest ("V" of neck)	Urine (24 hr) Modified respirator with pads	Durham and Wolfe, 1962
Ethyl parathion (WP)	Aerial spraying (pilots) Airblast spraying of orchards (tractor operators)	Strips of 3 ply α-cellulose wrapped around the forehead (2 in by 10 in.) and wrists (2 in. by 6 in.)	Personal breathing zone air samples Modified respirators with filter pads	Jegier, 1964*b*
Ethyl parathion	Reentry into treated fields to inspect cotton	Blue jeans and cotton T-shirts Hand and wrist rinse with 125 mL hexane or Hand rinse with 125 mL benzene	Personal breathing zone air samples Blood Urine (24 hr) Foliage residue	Ware et al., 1974
Ethyl parathion	Mixing/loading in a closed system to determine its effectiveness Ground application	Unwashed cotton cloth and rayon:polyester pads (4 in. by 4 in.) attached to the exterior of the clothing at shoulder, chest, waist, and knee	Area air samples around mixing/loading sites and on tractors Blood Urine (spot; pre-job, 3 week intervals)	Knaak et al., 1980

Contaminant	*Activity*	*Dermal Methods*	*Other Sampling*	*Reference*
Ethyl parathion	Reentry into orange grove to pick after spraying	16 ply gauze pads with polyethylene backings taped to the skin of each worker at various locations and pads of shirt material (3 in. by 3 in.) were attached to the exterior of work clothing adjacent to skin pads	Personal breathing zone air samples Blood Urine (24 hr) Foliage residues	Spear et al., 1977
Ethyl parathion (10%)	Tying up mature pea plants and bean plants after they had been sprayed with pesticide inside a greenhouse	Headbands of absorbent paper Forearms and hand swabs with cotton balls and 95% ethanol	Blood Foliage residue	Culver et al., 1958
Ethyl parathion (10%)	Handling harvested beans, peas, or tomatoes Planting peas Transplanting bean and pea plants Watering beans All activities inside a greenhouse where pesticide has been sprayed	Forearms and hand swabs with cotton balls and 95% ethanol	Blood Foliage residue	Culver et al., 1958
Paraoxon	Citrus harvesting (reentry)	Gauze pads placed on upper arms and calves	Personal breathing zone air samples Foliage residue	Popendorf, 1980
Ethyl parathion Endosulfan	Mixing/loading in a closed system to determine its effectiveness Ground application	Unwashed cotton cloth and rayon:polyester pads (4 in. by 4 in.) attached to the exterior of the clothing at shoulder, chest, waist, and knee.	Area air samples around mixing/loading sites and on tractors Blood Urine (spot; prejob, 3 week intervals)	Knaak et al., 1980
Ethylene dibromide	Mixing and loading in closed system Soil injection application	Hand wash	Personal breathing zone air samples	Maddy et al., 1979 (HS-593)

WP = Wettable powder
EC = Emulsifiable concentrate

Contaminant	*Activity*	*Dermal Methods*	*Other Sampling*	*Reference*
Fenamiphos	Mixing/loading using closed transfer system to formulate Spray application with tractor	32 ply gauze pads (11.4 cm by 11.4 cm) for dust with filter paper backings attached to shoulders, back of neck, "V" of chest, shins, thigh (fronts), and forearms Hand wash with distilled water		Knaak, Jacobs, and Wang, 1986
Fenamiphos (liquid)	Mixing/loading in closed system Soil injection application	Fabric covered gauze pad with aluminum foil backing Hand wash with water	Personal breathing zone air samples	Wang, Fredrickson, and Jacobs, 1983 (HS-1033)
Fenitrothion	Spray application on tea plants	Gauze (6 ply) pads stapled to filter backing attached to front of work jackets on the chest and abdomen, and to thigh and ankle Cotton gloves	Gauze filters in respirators for respirable exposure	Wan, 1990
Fenthion (granular, 1%)	Hand dispersal of granules	32 ply gauze pads (11.4 cm by 11.4 cm) for dust with filter paper backings attached to shoulders, back of neck, "V" of chest, and forearms outside clothing Bag hand rinse with 95% ethanol	Modified respirator with filter Blood Cigarettes (half-smoked)	Wolfe, Armstrong, and Durham, 1974
Fenthion (liquid, 0.06%)	Hand gun power spray application for mosquito control	α-Cellulose pads (10.2 cm by 10.2 cm) with filter paper backings placed outside clothing on the shins, thigh fronts, forearms, shoulders, back of neck, and upper chest near "V" of neck Bag hand rinse with 95% ethanol	Modified respirator with filter Blood Cigarettes (half-smoked)	Wolfe, Armstrong, and Durham, 1974

Contaminant	*Activity*	*Dermal Methods*	*Other Sampling*	*Reference*
Fenthion (liquid, 0.06%)	Backpack hand pressure spray application for mosquito control	α-Cellulose pads (10.2 cm by 10.2 cm) with filter paper backings placed outside clothing on the shins, thigh fronts, forearms, shoulders, back of neck, and upper chest near "V" of neck Bag hand rinse with 95% ethanol	Modified respirator with filter Blood Cigarettes (half-smoked)	Wolfe, Armstrong, and Durham, 1974
Fenvalerate	Spray application to cotton fields using sprayers with a single pressure nozzle	Gauze pads (5 cm by 5 cm) attached to the head, chest, back, forearms, thighs, legs, hands, and feet. An additional pair of gauze pads was placed underneath and on top of polyester trousers to determine pesticide absorption.	Personal breathing zone air samples Area air samples for particle size distributions Urine (prework, and at various hour intervals following application) Blood	Zhang et al., 1991
Fenvalerate Methamidophos	Spray application to cotton fields using sprayers with a single pressure nozzle	Gauze pads (5 cm by 5 cm) attached to the head, chest, back, forearms, thighs, legs, hands, and feet. An additional pair of gauze pads were placed underneath and on top of polyester trousers to determine pesticide absorption.	Personal breathing zone air samples Area air samples for particle size distributions Urine (prework, and at various hour intervals following application) Blood	Zhang et al., 1991
Fluazifop-butyl	Backpack and vehicle spraying	Disposable "Corovin" overalls Cotton gloves	Personal breathing zone air samples Urine (24 hr) "Aseptex" face mask	Chester and Hart, 1986

WP = Wettable powder
EC = Emulsifiable concentrate

Contaminant	*Activity*	*Dermal Methods*	*Other Sampling*	*Reference*
Fluorescent tracer	Air blast spraying of citrus	Fluorescent tracer (4-methyl-7-diethylamino-coumarin) added to spray tanks. Evaluation of workers' skin under UV light at head/neck, hands, forearms, upper arms, upper and lower legs, and torso with video imaging system before and after application while wearing either cotton/polyester 50/50 shirts and pants, cotton/polyester 65/35 coveralls, or Tyvek coveralls to determine the degree of protection.		Fenske, 1988*a*
Fluvalinate	Greenhouse handgun spraying of violets and chrysanthemums using coarse and fine sprays	α-Cellulose pads (10.16 cm by 10.16 cm) with glassine paper backing placed on back (middle), chest, shoulders, forearms (dorsal), thighs (ventral), and shins (ventral) on outside of clothing. If CPC (Tyvek coveralls, butyl rubber aprons, boots) was worn, pad was outside of it. Pads placed inside coveralls adjacent to position of outside pad at chest, forearms, thighs, and shins. Bag hand wash (200 mL of 95% ethanol)	Personal breathing zone air samples	Stamper et al., 1989*a*; Nigg, Stamper, and Mahon, 1988

Contaminant	*Activity*	*Dermal Methods*	*Other Sampling*	*Reference*
Fluvalinate	Pulse fogging with handgun to chrysanthemums and violets in greenhouses	α-Cellulose pads (10.16 cm by 10.16 cm) with glassine paper backings placed on back (middle), chest, shoulders, forearms (dorsal) thighs (ventral), and shins (ventral) on outside of clothing. If CPC (Tyvek coveralls, butyl rubber aprons, boots) was worn, pad was outside of it. Pads placed inside coveralls adjacent to position of outside pad at chest, forearms, thighs, and shins. Bag hand wash (200 mL of 95% ethanol)	Personal breathing zone air samples Urine	Stamper et al., 1988; Nigg, Stamper, and Mahon, 1988
Fluvalinate (EC)	Boom spray application to chrysanthemums in greenhouses	α-Cellulose pads (10.16 cm by 10.16 cm) with glassine paper backings taped to outside of clothing at back (middle), shoulders, forearms, thighs (fronts), and shins. Bag hand wash with 200 mL 95% ethanol	Personal breathing zone air samples	Stamper et al., 1989*b*; Nigg, Stamper, and Mahon, 1988

WP = Wettable powder
EC = Emulsifiable concentrate

Contaminant	*Activity*	*Dermal Methods*	*Other Sampling*	*Reference*
Fluvalinate (EC)	Span spray application to chrysanthemums in greenhouses	α-Cellulose pads (10.16 cm by 10.16 cm) with glassine paper backings taped to outside of clothing at back (middle), shoulders, forearms, thighs (fronts), and shins. Bag hand wash with 200 mL of 95% ethanol	Personal breathing zone air samples	Stamper et al., 1989*b*; Nigg, Stamper, and Mahon, 1988
Glyphosate	Mixing/loading Spray application	Treated glass fiber pads mounted in 35 mm plastic slide mounts pinned to clothing at hands, shoulders, chest, thighs, and shoes	Personal breathing zone air samples	NIOSH, 1985 (HETA 83-341-1557)
Glyphosate	Tractor drawn spraying and hand spraying application to weeds and hand weeding	8-layer cotton gauze (7.5 cm by 7.5 cm) pads stapled to filter paper pinned to ankle (1 inside and 1 outside clothing), thigh front (1 inside and 1 outside pant leg), lower forearms (2 inside and 2 outside shirt-sleeve) or attached with a velcro bracelet if short sleeve shirt worn, upper chest, upper back (near neck) and hat Some workers only had pads on clothing exteriors at same places.	Urine	Lavy et al., 1992

Contaminant	*Activity*	*Dermal Methods*	*Other Sampling*	*Reference*
Guthion	Mixing/loading Airblast application on apple orchards from tractors, some with spray cabs (with charcoal air filters) and others without	16 ply gauze pads (4 in. by 4 in.) with aluminum foil backings taped on chest, back, and left leg at knee Cotton gloves		Spittler and Bourke, 1985
Heptachlor	Application via subslab injection for termite control Residential exposure (airborne)	Gauze pads (10.2 cm by 10.2 cm), 12 ply with chromatographic paper midlayers and glassine paper backing attached to outside of clothing at shoulders, forearm, ankles, chest, and back. Pads inside clothing (offset) at chest, back, shoulders, and ankles. Hand wash (200 mL hexane)	Personal breathing zone air samples Area air samples (residents)	Kamble et al., 1992
Heptachlor	Spray applications for termites in subfloor areas of buildings already erected or spray on foundations for buildings not yet erected	Pairs of filter papers pinned to hat, shoulder, back, chest, arm, wrist, and thigh on top of overalls	Blood Modified respirator with prefilters	Simpson and Shandar, 1972
Herbicides	Manual boom spraying from backpack sprayers	Water sensitive paper strips mounted with elastic bands around the ankle, calf, thigh, and forearm on the right side of body; clipped to waist and chest pockets		Lengerich and Burroughs, 1989

WP = Wettable powder
EC = Emulsifiable concentrate

Contaminant	*Activity*	*Dermal Methods*	*Other Sampling*	*Reference*
Imidan	Mixing/loading Airblast application on apple orchards from tractors, some with spray cabs (with charcoal air filters) and others without	16 ply gauze pads (4 in. by 4 in.) with aluminum foil backings taped on chest, back, and left leg at knee Cotton gloves		Spittler and Bourke, 1985
Imidan (WP)	Hand harvesting apples	Tyvek jackets with combination α-cellulose (4 in. by 4 in.) and 9 ply gauze pad (2 in. by 2 in.) centers stapled to the exterior of the jacket at the arms, chest, and back. Pads of α-cellulose (4 in. by 4 in.) were stapled to the interior of the jacket adjacent to the exterior pads. Cotton gloves	Personal breathing zone air samples Urine Foliage residue Soil Apple rinse water	EPA, 1988*a* (Study 13)
Isopropanolamine salts of dinitro-o-secondary butylphenol (DNOSBP)	Spray application in corn and pea fields with boom ground sprayers	α-Cellulose pads (10.2 cm by 10.2 cm) with filter paper backings placed on the shins, thigh fronts, forearms, shoulders, back of neck, and upper chest near "V" of neck Cotton work clothing (pants, shirt) T-shirt Socks Inspection of workers and pads for visible staining of skin, clothing, and pads Bag hand rinse with water	Respirator with modified filter pads Urine	Wolfe, Durham, and Batchelor, 1961

Contaminant	*Activity*	*Dermal Methods*	*Other Sampling*	*Reference*
Lindane	Manual seed treatment	12 ply gauze (3 in. by 3 in.) inside custom envelope with round opening pinned outside clothing at chest, back, shoulders, forearms, thighs, lower legs, with a second set taped to skin under clothing in same places but offset from outside pads Hand wash with 10% isopropanol in distilled water	Personal breathing zone air samples	Fenske et al., 1990
Lorsban	Mixing Application using low pressure sprayer from an open tractor on green beans	Tyvek suits along with 16 ply gauze pads (4 in. by 4 in.) with aluminum foil backings placed outside and underneath at chest, back, and left leg at knee Cotton gloves		Spittler and Bourke, 1985
Lorsban	Cotton picking	Skin wipes of palms, wrists, and forehead of workers with Whatman smear tabs	Personal breathing zone air samples Area air samples Blood Work surface wipes Bulk cotton	NIOSH, July 1984 (HETA 81-463-1477)
Malathion (0.04%–0.08%)	Air blast spraying fruit orchards	32 ply gauze pads (11.4 cm by 11.4 cm) attached to shoulders, back of neck, "V" of chest, and forearms. Bag hand rinse or swab with 95% ethanol	Modified respirator with filter pads	Wolfe, Durham, and Armstrong, 1967

WP = Wettable powder
EC = Emulsifiable concentrate

Contaminant	*Activity*	*Dermal Methods*	*Other Sampling*	*Reference*
Malathion (2.5%, 5%)	Operating aerosol machine to kill mosquitoes	α-Cellulose pads (1.5 in. by 16 in.) as headbands and bands (1.5 in. by 8 in.) on ankle over socks, pads (4 in. by 4 in.) at forearms, neck (back and front) Cotton knit glove (one hand)	Personal breathing zone air samples Modified respirator with filter over cartridge Blood	Culver, Caplan, and Batchelor, 1956
Malathion	Hand harvesting blueberries	Tyvek jacket with 8 ply gauze pads (2 in. by 2 in.) with glassine paper backing attached to the exterior at forearms, breasts, and shoulders and back Cotton gloves with a 8 ply gauze pad (2 in. by 2 in.) with a glassine backing attached to the back	Personal breathing zone air samples Urine High volume area air samples Foliage residue Soil	EPA, 1988*a* (Study 7)
Malathion	Hand harvesting blueberries	Tyvek jacket with 8 ply gauze pads (2 in. by 2 in.) with glassine paper backing attached to the exterior at forearms, breasts, and shoulders and back Cotton gloves with an 8 ply gauze pad (2 in. by 2 in.) with a glassine backing attached to the back	Personal breathing zone air samples Urine High volume area air samples Soil	EPA, 1988*a* (Study 10)
Malathion	Hand harvesting onions by youth and adult field workers	Nylon gloves	High volume area air samples Urine Foliage residue Soil	EPA, 1988*a* (Study 11); Munn, Keefe, and Savage, 1985

Contaminant	*Activity*	*Dermal Methods*	*Other Sampling*	*Reference*
Malathion	Hand harvesting blueberries	Tyvek jacket with 9-ply gauze (4 in. by 4 in.) on top of α-cellulose pads stapled to the exterior at forearms, shoulders, and breasts, and center of back. Pads of α-cellulose were also attached to the inner surface of the jacket at right forearm, chest, and back. Cotton gloves	Personal breathing zone air samples Urine High volume area air samples Soil	EPA, 1988*a* (Study 12)
Malathion	Mixing/loading Application with high volume air blast from tractor to citrus	Fluorescent tracer (4-methyl-7-diethylamino-coumarin) added to pesticide formulation during mixing; examination of workers' skin under (320–440 ηm) UV pre- and postshift with video images recorded of head, hands, forearms, upper arms, and torso Standardized CPC with 12 ply gauze pads (3 in. by 3 in.) attached to outside of workers' clothing at head, shoulders, back, chest, forearms, thighs, and lower legs	Urine (preshift, spot; during and postshift, 8 hr)	Fenske, 1988*b*

WP = Wettable powder
EC = Emulsifiable concentrate

Contaminant	Activity	Dermal Methods	Other Sampling	Reference
Malathion (5% dust)	Formulation work: mixing, bag filling, stacking bags on pallets, packing bags into cartons	α-Cellulose pads (10.2 cm^2) backed with filter paper placed on the shins, thigh fronts, forearms, shoulders, back of neck, and upper chest near "V" of neck	Modified respirator with filters	Wolfe, Staiff, and Armstrong, 1978
Malathion	Mixing/loading in a closed system to determine its effectiveness Ground application	Unwashed cotton cloth and rayon:polyester pads (4 in. by 4 in.) attached to the exterior of the clothing at shoulder, chest, waist, and knee	Area air samples around mixing/loading sites and on tractors Blood Urine (spot; prejob, 3 week intervals)	Knaak et al., 1980
Malathion (WP)	Aerial spraying (pilots) Airblast spraying of orchards (tractor operators)	Strips of 3 ply α-cellulose wrapped around the forehead (2 in. by 10 in.) and wrists (2 in. by 6 in.)	Personal breathing zone air samples Modified respirators with filter pads	Jegier, 1964*b*
Maleic hydrazide	Hand harvesting of flue cured tobacco	Combination pads with 4 ply gauze on the front over α-cellulose (10 cm by 10 cm) with glassine paper backing placed outside of clothing at forearms, back, ribs (left and right), and thighs Hand rinse with 299 mL of 95% ethanol (2 replicates)	Modified respirator with gauze pad over filter Urine (during and postexposure, 48 hr) Foliage residue	Herman, Hunt, and Sheets, 1985
Maleic hydrazide	Spray application to tobacco using high and low clearance tractors	Pads of α-cellulose (10.2 cm by 10.2 cm) attached by tape or pinned to outside of clothing at the chest, back, thighs, and calves. Pads sewn to elastic wrist bands on forearms.	Modified respirator with gauze/cellulose pad over filter Urine (preexposure, spot; during and postexposure, 36 hr)	Hunt, Wojeck, and Sheets, 1985

Contaminant	*Activity*	*Dermal Methods*	*Other Sampling*	*Reference*
Mancozeb ETU	Mixing/loading Aerial application	Gauze pads (10.16 cm by 10.16 cm) stapled to clothing outside and underneath clothing at chest, back, forearms Cotton gloves	Modified respirator with collecting pads (7.01 cm) Urine (pre- and postapplication)	Mumma, Brandes, and Gordon, 1985
Mancozeb ETU	Mixing/loading Tractor application using an air blast sprayer	Gauze pads (10.16 cm by 10.16 cm) stapled to clothing outside and underneath clothing at chest, back, forearms Cotton gloves	Modified respirator with collecting pads (7.01 cm) Urine (pre- and postapplication)	Mumma, Brandes, and Gordon, 1985
Maneb	Mixing/loading in a closed system to determine its effectiveness Ground application	Unwashed cotton cloth and rayon:polyester pads (4 in. by 4 in.) attached to the exterior of the clothing at shoulder, chest, waist, and knee	Area air samples around mixing/ loading sites and on tractors Blood Urine (spot; pre-job, 3 week intervals)	Knaak et al., 1980
Maneb (as Mn)	Weighing out Application to pine nurseries from tractor pulled tank sprayers with cabs	Pad samplers (10 cm by 10 cm) attached to clothing	Personal breathing zone air samples for maneb and ethylenethiourea (ETU) Urine (postshift) for ETU	Savolainen et al., 1989
Maneb-lindane	Commercial seed-treating with dust application using auger or barrel treaters	Pads of α-cellulose (12.5 cm by 12.5 cm) over chromatography filter paper (100 cm^2) over glassine paper with brown wrapping paper backing taped to the outside of clothing at upper arm and chest (opposite arm with pad) Hand wash with 95% ethanol	Gauze (12 ply) over α-cellulose over filter paper in modified respirators	Grey, Marthre, and Rogers, 1983

WP = Wettable powder
EC = Emulsifiable concentrate

Contaminant	Activity	Dermal Methods	Other Sampling	Reference
Maneb	Mixing/loading Application with low pressure, low boom; high pressure, low boom; high pressure, high boom; and drop nozzle sprayers, harvesting, and scouting of onions	16 ply gauze pads (4 in. by 4 in.) with aluminum foil backings taped on chest, back, and left leg at knee Cotton gloves		Spittler and Bourke, 1985
MCPA Mecoprop Dichlorprop	Tractor boom spray application to fields	Pads of Whatman filter paper (10 cm by 10 cm) taped to the exterior of clothing on the back, chest, thigh, forearm, and on the skin of forearm	Urine (postwork and next morning)	Manninen et al., 1986
MCPA	Clearing saw use in forest	Tablecloth paper sheets (27 cm by 23 cm) affixed to arms and breast of clothing	Disposable mask Cages of rats to identify acute effects Swab samples of cages for residue	Hattula, Wasenius, and Arstila, 1979
MCPA	Filling and tractor spray application of fields	Workers issued white Tyveks and fluoresceine added to pesticide mixture. Workers' Tyvek coveralls examined and photographed for evidence of yellow staining.	Personal breathing zone air samples Urine (preshift, midshift, and postshift) Bulk samples of sprayed liquid for chlorophenol contamination	Kolmodin-Hedman, Hoglund, and Akerblom, 1983
MCPA (5%) 2,4-D (25%)	Bush killing with a bush saw with a built-in herbicide spray applicator	32 ply gauze pads (11.4 cm by 11.4 cm) with filter paper backings on the inside and outside of protective clothing on the chest, back, leg, and arm to determine the effectiveness of six different types of protective suits	Urine	Ojanen et al., 1992

Contaminant	*Activity*	*Dermal Methods*	*Other Sampling*	*Reference*
MCPA (15%) 2,4-D (7.5%)	ULV spraying of bushes	32 ply gauze pads (11.4 cm by 11.4 cm) with filter paper backings on the inside and outside of protective clothing on the chest, back, leg, and arm to determine the effectiveness of six different types of protective suits	Urine	Ojanen et al., 1992
Methidathion	Citrus harvesting (reentry)	Gauze pads placed on upper arms and calves	Personal breathing zone air samples Foliage residue	Popendorf, 1980
Methidaxon	Citrus harvesting by hand (reentry)	Gauze pads placed on upper arms and calves	Personal breathing zone air samples Foliage residue	Popendorf, 1980
Methiocarb	Hand harvesting of blueberries	Tyvek jacket with 9 ply gauze (4 in. by 4 in.) on top of α-cellulose pads stapled to the exterior at forearms, shoulders, breasts, and center of back. Pads of α-cellulose were also attached to the inner surface of the jacket at right forearm, chest, and back. Cotton gloves	Personal breathing zone air samples Urine High volume area air samples Soil	EPA, 1988*a* (Study 12)

WP = Wettable powder
EC = Emulsifiable concentrate

Contaminant	*Activity*	*Dermal Methods*	*Other Sampling*	*Reference*
Methiocarb	Hand harvesting of blueberries	12 ply gauze pads (3 in. by 3 in.) with polyethylene backings inside glassine envelopes with a circular opening (60 mm diameter). Pads were fastened to a headband or brim of a cap for the face and were stapled to a tightly fitting cotton T-shirt at the chest, back, and upper arm. Pads were attached to lower arms and legs with surgical tape. Cotton gloves	Foliage residue Soil	EPA, 1988*b* (Study 5)
Methiocarb	Hand harvesting of blueberries	12 ply surgical sponges (3 in. by 3 in.) with polyethylene backings inside glassine envelopes with a circular opening (60 mm diameter). Pads were fastened to a headband or brim of a cap for the face and were stapled to a tightly fitting cotton T-shirt at the chest, back, and upper arm. Pads were attached to lower arms and legs with surgical tape. and/or Cotton gloves	Personal breathing zone air samples High volume area air samples Urine Foliage residue Soil	EPA, 1988*b* (Study 7)
Methomyl	Mixing/loading in a closed system to determine its effectiveness Ground application	Unwashed cotton cloth and rayon:polyester pads (4 in. by 4 in.) attached to the exterior of the clothing at shoulder, chest, waist, and knee	Area air samples around mixing/loading sites and on tractors Blood Urine (spot; prejob, 3 week intervals)	Knaak et al., 1980

Contaminant	*Activity*	*Dermal Methods*	*Other Sampling*	*Reference*
Methomyl	Hand harvesting of cucumbers	Gauze pads (103.2 cm^2) placed near the ankles and on the inner forearm. Cotton twill gloves Hand towel wash of hands		EPA, 1988*b* (Study 11)
Methomyl	Reentry into greenhouses 3–7 days following application of insecticide to cucumbers and tomatoes	Bag rinse of the hand of preference with 360 mL distilled water	Personal breathing zone air samples Area air samples Foliage residue Soil	Boleij et al., 1991
Methyl demeton	Knapsack spraying of tomato bushes	2 ply filter paper (12.5 cm by 12.5 cm), pinned to clothing at the back near neck base, chest center, wrist, arm near elbow, shoulders, hat	Personal breathing zone air samples Modified respirator with cotton pads	Simpson and Beck, 1964
Methyl parathion	Reentry into treated cotton fields	Gauze pads (3 in. by 2.5 in.) taped onto denim jeans at shins, thighs, hips, and on skin of forearms Blue jeans and T-shirts were extracted Hand rinse with 250 mL hexane	Personal breathing zone air samples Blood Urine (24 hr) Foliage residue Spray deposition samples	Ware et al., 1973
Methyl parathion Endosulfan	Mixing/loading in a closed system to determine its effectiveness Ground application	Unwashed cotton cloth and rayon:polyester pads (4 in. by 4 in.) attached to the exterior of the clothing at shoulder, chest, waist, and knee	Area air samples around mixing/ loading sites and on tractors Blood Urine (spot; prejob, 3 week intervals)	Knaak et al., 1980

WP = Wettable powder
EC = Emulsifiable concentrate

Contaminant	*Activity*	*Dermal Methods*	*Other Sampling*	*Reference*
Methyl parathion	Hand harvesting of peanuts	Gauze pads (4 in. by 4 in.) with a glassine backing attached to elastic arm bands and pinned to the outside of workers' clothing at knee level Cotton gloves followed by 95% ethanol hand rinses	Personal breathing zone air samples Foliage residue Soil	EPA, 1988*a* (Study 2)
Methyl parathion	Hand harvesting of onions by youth and adult field workers	Nylon gloves	High volume area air samples Urine Foliage residue Soil	EPA, 1988*a* (Study 11); Munn, Keefe, and Savage, 1985
Methyl parathion	Simulated worst case exposure to dislodgeable residues of insecticide	Cotton gloves	Modified respirator with filters Foliage residue	Davies et al., 1981
Methyl parathion	Mixing/loading Air blast application on apple orchards from tractors, some with spray cabs (with charcoal air filters) and others without	16 ply gauze pads (4 in. by 4 in.) with aluminum foil backings taped on chest, back, and left leg at knee Cotton gloves		Spittler and Bourke, 1985
Methyl parathion	Mixing/loading in a closed system to determine its effectiveness Ground application	Unwashed cotton cloth and rayon:polyester pads (4 in. by 4 in.) attached to the exterior of the clothing at shoulder, chest, waist, and knee	Area air samples around mixing/loading sites and on tractors Blood Urine (spot; prejob, 3 week intervals)	Knaak et al., 1980
Methyl parathion Ethyl parathion	Reentry into treated cotton fields	Blue jeans and cotton T-shirts Hand rinse with 250 mL hexane	Blood Urine (24 hr) Foliage residue	Ware et al., 1973
Methyl parathion	Checking cotton for the presence of insects after pesticide application by ground or airplane spraying	Cotton shirt sleeves Cotton T-shirts Cotton gloves	Modified respirator with pads	Quinby, Walker, and Durham, 1958

Contaminant	*Activity*	*Dermal Methods*	*Other Sampling*	*Reference*
Methyl parathion	Reentry into treated fields to inspect cotton	Blue jeans and cotton T-shirts Hand and wrist rinse with with 125 mL hexane	Personal breathing zone air samples Blood Urine (24 hr) Foliage residue	Ware et al., 1974
Methyl parathion	Reentry into treated fields to inspect cotton	Blue jeans and cotton T-shirts Rinse of arms, from wrist bone to shoulder, with 125 mL acetone Swabs of torso skin with ethanol saturated gauze pads (2 in. by 2 in.) Hand rinse with 125 mL acetone	Personal breathing zone air samples Blood Urine (24 hr) Foliage residue	Ware et al., 1974
Mevinphos	Hand harvesting turnips and mustard greens	Gauze pads (103.2 cm^2) placed on the inner forearm Cotton twill gloves	Personal breathing zone air samples Foliage residue Soil	EPA, 1988*b* (Study 12)
Mevinphos	Mixing/loading in a closed system to determine its effectiveness Ground application	Unwashed cotton cloth and rayon:polyester pads (4 in. by 4 in.) attached to the exterior of the clothing at shoulder, chest, waist, and knee	Area air samples around mixing/loading sites and on tractors Blood Urine (spot; prejob, 3 week intervals)	Knaak et al., 1980
Mevinphos (liquid)	Mixing/loading Aerial spray application	Fabric covered gauze pad with aluminum foil backing Hand wash with water	Personal breathing zone air samples	Maddy et al., 1981 (HS-876)
Mevinphos (liquid)	Mixing/loading in closed system Aerial spray application	Fabric covered gauze pad with aluminum foil backing Hand wash with water	Personal breathing zone air samples	Maddy et al., 1982*b* (HS-889)

WP = Wettable powder
EC = Emulsifiable concentrate

Contaminant	*Activity*	*Dermal Methods*	*Other Sampling*	*Reference*
Mevinphos	Manual spray application to flowers inside greenhouses Reentry for flower collection and handling inside greenhouse that had been treated using manual spray, mist blower, or automatic fogger	Filter paper (11 cm by 11 cm) taped outside and inside of CPC or work clothing of sprayers in the same position at both forearms, chest, upper back, and both thighs and in same places of work clothing of plant handlers Hand rinse of individual hands with ethanol	Personal breathing zone air samples Area air samples Blood Foliage	Kangas et al., 1993
Molinate (granular)	Loading (dumping) Airplane with closed, airconditioned cockpit used for application	Fabric covered gauze pad with aluminum foil backing Hand wash with water	Personal breathing zone air samples	Maddy et al., 1982*a* (HS-887)
Molinate (liquid and granular)	Mixing/loading Flagman Aerial application to rice	Gauze pads (10.2 cm by 10.2 cm) attached to coveralls at right chest, left back, shoulders, forearms, and thighs and two additional pads taped under coveralls at left chest and right back of T-shirt. Bag hand wash in 200 mL ethanol (postshift)	Personal breathing zone air samples	Knarr et al., 1985
Monocrotophos	Reentry into treated fields to inspect cotton	Blue jeans and cotton T-shirts Hand rinse with 125 mL acetone	Personal breathing zone air samples Blood Urine (24 hr) Foliage residue	Ware et al., 1974
Naled	Mixing/loading in a closed system to determine its effectiveness Ground application	Unwashed cotton cloth and rayon:polyester pads (4 in. by 4 in.) attached to the exterior of the clothing at shoulder, chest, waist, and knee	Area air samples around mixing/loading sites and on tractors Blood Urine (spot; prejob, 3 week intervals)	Knaak et al., 1980

Contaminant	*Activity*	*Dermal Methods*	*Other Sampling*	*Reference*
Nitrofen (WP and EC)	Mixing, loading, spraying	Gauze pads (10.2 cm by 10.2 cm, 5.1 cm by 5.1 cm) with foil backing. Larger pads attached to chest, lower leg, forearm inside and outside of protective suit and inside respirator helmet. Smaller pads attached inside and outside of rubber gloves.	Area air sampling (tractor cab) Air samples inside and outside of respirator helmet	Putnam et al., 1983
Nitrofen (WP and liquid)	Mixing/loading (pouring from bulk bags) Boom spray application	Fabric covered gauze pads with aluminum foil backing on outside of clothing Hand wash with water and ivory detergent	Personal breathing zone air samples collected inside and outside of respirators	Maddy et al., 1980 (HS-745)
Orthene	Mixing/loading Application with high pressure, low boom; and low pressure, low boom sprayers; harvesting and scouting of green beans	16 ply gauze pads (4 in. by 4 in.) with aluminum foil backings taped on chest, back, and left leg at knee Cotton gloves	Area air sampling inside and outside of spray cab	Spittler and Bourke, 1985
Oxydemeton-methyl (liquid)	Mixing/loading with closed system	Fabric covered gauze pad with aluminum foil backing Cotton gloves Hand wash with water and Surten	Personal breathing zone air samples	Oshita, Schneider, and Margetich, 1988 (HS-1398)

WP = Wettable powder
EC = Emulsifiable concentrate

Contaminant	*Activity*	*Dermal Methods*	*Other Sampling*	*Reference*
Oxydemetonmethyl	Mixing/loading in a closed system to determine its effectiveness Ground application	Unwashed cotton cloth and rayon:polyester pads (4 in. by 4 in.) attached to the exterior of the clothing at shoulder, chest, waist, and knee	Area air samples around mixing/ loading sites and on tractors Blood Urine (spot; pre-job, 3 week intervals)	Knaak et al., 1980
Paraquat	Tractor mounted, low boom spray on orchards	α-Cellulose pads (10.2 cm by 10.2 cm) with filter paper backings placed on the shins, thigh fronts, forearms, shoulders, back of neck, and upper chest near "V" of neck Hand rinse with water	Modified respirator with filters Urine	Staiff et al., 1975
Paraquat	Cannabis harvesting	100% white cotton cloth patches (28 cm by 30 cm) over arms and legs Leather gloves (over rubber) Disposable plastic boots	Foliage residue	Bandara et al., 1985
Paraquat	Aerial application to cotton (pilots)	Polyethylene backed Whatman 542 filter paper (100 cm^2) atttached to skin or clothing at forehead, "V" of neck, back of neck, left forearm, right thigh, right lower leg White cotton T-shirts and elasticized support bandage on left leg (ankle to thigh) Bleached cotton gloves	Personal breathing zone air samples	Chester and Ward, 1984

Contaminant	*Activity*	*Dermal Methods*	*Other Sampling*	*Reference*
Paraquat	Aerial application to cotton (flagger)	Polyethylene backed Whatman 542 filter paper (100 cm^2) atttached to skin or clothing exterior at forehead, shoulders, back of neck, abdomen, left forearm, left or right thigh, left or right lower leg White cotton T-shirts and elasticized support bandage under clothing on left leg (ankle to thigh) Bleached cotton gloves	Personal breathing zone air samples 3M disposable respirator	Chester and Ward, 1984
Paraquat	Mixing/loading	Polyethylene backed Whatman 542 filter paper (100 cm^2) atttached to skin or clothing exterior at forehead, back of neck, "V" of neck, left upper arm, right thigh White cotton T-shirts and elasticized support bandage under clothing on left leg (ankle to thigh) Bleached cotton gloves	Personal breathing zone air samples	Chester and Ward, 1984

WP = Wettable powder
EC = Emulsifiable concentrate

Contaminant	*Activity*	*Dermal Methods*	*Other Sampling*	*Reference*
Paraquat	Knapsack spraying for weed control application Carriers (no pad under sprayer)	Polyethylene backed Whatman 542 filter paper (80 cm^2) atttached to skin or clothing on forehead, left arm (mid forearm), mid upper arm, mid lower leg (left), or if boots worn below knee at mid thigh; beneath clothing at sternum, "V" of neck, lower back beneath sprayer	Personal breathing zone air samples Urine (spot, postspray)	Chester and Woolen, 1981
Paraquat	Knapsack spraying for weed control application	Elasticized support bandages under clothing on either left leg (thigh to ankle) or both legs (thigh to ankle) Cotton gloves	Personal breathing zone air samples	Chester and Woolen, 1981
Paraquat	Rubber tappers working in previously sprayed areas (reentry)	Polyethylene backed Whatman 542 filter paper (80 cm^2) attached to skin or beneath clothing on forehead, "V" of neck, sternum, mid-left forearm, mid-left thigh, and mid-left lower leg		Chester and Woolen, 1981
Paraquat	Rubber tappers working at the same time as spray application occurred	Polyethylene backed Whatman 542 filter paper (80 cm^2) attached to skin or beneath clothing on forehead, "V" of neck, sternum, mid-left forearm, mid-left thigh, and mid-left lower leg Elasticized support bandages under clothing on right leg (thigh to ankle)	Personal breathing zone air samples	Chester and Woolen, 1981

Contaminant	*Activity*	*Dermal Methods*	*Other Sampling*	*Reference*
Paraquat (0.05%, 0.07%)	Tractor drawn spray application with drop boom	α-Cellulose pads (10 cm by 10 cm) on back (center), chest, shoulders, forearms, thigh (front), shin (front) on outside of clothing Hand rinse with water or cotton gloves	Urine (PM)	Wojeck et al., 1983
Permethrin	Greenhouse tomato spray application	12 ply gauze pads (10 cm diameter) attached to the head, chest, "V" of neck, shoulders, elbows, thighs, and legs. Cotton gloves	Personal breathing zone air samples	Adamis et al., 1985
Perthane (0.12%)	Tractor drawn air blast spraying fruit orchards	α-Cellulose pads (10.2 cm by 10.2 cm) with filter paper backings placed on the shins, thigh fronts, forearms, shoulders, back of neck, and upper chest near "V" of neck	Modified respirator with filter pads	Wolfe et al., 1972
Pesticides	Farmers with long lasting residues in their bodies	Hand rinse with 30 mL hexane poured over them twice up to several days after last usage	Blood	Kazen et al., 1974
Pesticides, organophosphates (liquid)	Mixing/loading with closed system	Fabric covered gauze pads with aluminum foil backings Hand wash with water	Personal breathing zone air samples	Alcoser, 1988 (HS-1406)
Phorate	Mixing/loading in a closed system to determine its effectiveness Ground application	Unwashed cotton cloth and rayon:polyester pads (4 in. by 4 in.) attached to the exterior of the clothing at shoulder, chest, waist, and knee	Area air samples around mixing/ loading sites and on tractors Blood Urine (spot; pre-job, 3 week intervals)	Knaak et al., 1980

WP = Wettable powder
EC = Emulsifiable concentrate

Contaminant	*Activity*	*Dermal Methods*	*Other Sampling*	*Reference*
Phorate (10%)	Granular application using tractor drawn gravity feed or broadcast application	α-Cellulose pads (10.2 cm by 10.2 cm) with filter paper backings placed on the shins, thigh fronts, forearms, shoulders, back of neck, and upper chest near "V" of neck attached to outside of workers' clothing including hat	Personal breathing zone air samples Modified respirator with filter Particle size measurements using air and surface samples Bulk samples of granules for pesticide concentration	Lloyd and Bell, 1967
Phosalone	Reentry into sprayed citrus groves to trim and prune trees	Cotton chambray fabric (prewashed or unwashed) pads (4 in. by 4 in.) backed with 9 ply cheesecloth over 2 ply aluminum foil pinned to exterior clothing at chest, shoulder, thigh, and back	Urine (postshift) Blood (postshift) Foliage residue	Knaak et al., 1978
Phosalone	Reentry into sprayed citrus groves to trim and prune trees	Cotton knit jersey fabric (prewashed or unwashed) pads (4 in. by 4 in.) backed with 9 ply cheesecloth over 2 ply aluminum foil pinned to exterior clothing at chest, shoulder, thigh, and back	Urine (postshift) Blood (postshift) Foliage residue	Knaak et al., 1978
Phosalone	Reentry into sprayed citrus groves to trim and prune trees	Rayon/polyester (1:1) fabric (prewashed or unwashed) pads (4 in. by 4 in.) backed with 9 ply cheesecloth over 2 ply aluminum foil pinned to exterior clothing at chest, shoulder, thigh, and back	Urine (postshift) Blood (postshift) Foliage residue	Knaak et al., 1978

Contaminant	*Activity*	*Dermal Methods*	*Other Sampling*	*Reference*
Phosalone	Hand harvesting of peaches	16 ply gauze pads with polyethylene backings taped to the skin of each worker at two locations selected from a daily rotating schedule. Pads of shirt material (3 in. by 3 in.) were attached to the exterior of work clothing adjacent to skin pads. Nylon glove backed by a pad for hands	Personal breathing zone air samples Blood (prework, daily) Foliage residues	Popendorf et al., 1979
Phosalone (WP)	Apple thinning	32 ply gauze pads (11.4 cm by 11.4 cm) with filter paper backings attached to shoulders, upper center of the chest and back, and outside of forearms Cotton or nylon gloves	Personal breathing zone air samples Foliage residue	Davies et al., 1982*a*
Phosphamidon	Mixing/loading in a closed system to determine its effectiveness Ground application	Unwashed cotton cloth rayon:polyester pads (4 in. by 4 in.) attached to the exterior of the clothing at shoulder, chest, waist, and knee	Area air samples around mixing/loading sites and on tractors Blood Urine (spot; prejob, 3 week intervals)	Knaak et al., 1980
Pirimiphosmethyl	Greenhouse tomato spraying operations	12 ply gauze pads (10 cm diameter) attached to the head, chest, "V" of neck, shoulders, elbows, thighs, and legs Cotton gloves	Personal breathing zone air samples	Adamis et al., 1985

WP = Wettable powder
EC = Emulsifiable concentrate

Contaminant	*Activity*	*Dermal Methods*	*Other Sampling*	*Reference*
Plictran	Mixing/loading Air blast application on apple orchards from tractors, some with spray cabs (with charcoal air filters) and others without	16 ply gauze pads (4 in. by 4 in.) with aluminum foil backings taped on chest, back and left leg at knee Cotton gloves		Spittler and Bourke, 1985
Premerge	Mixing/loading Application using low pressure sprayer from an open tractor on green beans	Tyvek suits along with 16 ply gauze pads (4 in. by 4 in.) with aluminum foil backings placed outside and underneath at chest, back, and left leg at knee Cotton gloves		Spittler and Bourke, 1985
Pydrin	Mixing/loading Application with low pressure, low boom and drop nozzle sprayers to cabbage Scouting cabbage	16 ply gauze pads (4 in. by 4 in.) with aluminum foil backings taped on chest, back, and left leg at knee Cotton gloves		Spittler and Bourke, 1985
Pydrin	Cotton picking	Skin wipes of palms, wrists, and forehead of workers with Whatman smear tabs	Personal breathing zone air samples Area air samples Work surface wipes Blood Bulk cotton	NIOSH, July 1984 (HETA 81-463-1477)
Randox	Mixing/loading Application with low pressure, low boom and drop nozzle sprayers and scouting of onions	16 ply gauze pads (4 in. by 4 in.) with aluminum foil backings taped on chest, back, and left leg at knee Cotton gloves		Spittler and Bourke, 1985
S-Ethyl-N,N-dipropyl thiocarbamate	Mixing/loading Application	Gauze pads (23.75 cm^2) attached to clothing at chest, back, shoulders, forearm, back, thighs, and shin and inside clothing at chest Hand rinse with 200 mL water containing surfactant	Personal breathing zone air samples Urine	Knaak et al., 1989

Contaminant	*Activity*	*Dermal Methods*	*Other Sampling*	*Reference*
Sevin	Harvesting and scouting of green beans	16 ply gauze pads (4 in. by 4 in.) with aluminum foil backings taped on chest, back, and left leg at knee Cotton gloves		Spittler and Bourke, 1985
Sodium salt of DNOC	Spray thinning apples	α-Cellulose pads (10.2 cm by 10.2 cm) with filter paper backings placed outside clothing on the shins, thigh fronts, forearms, shoulders, back of neck, and upper chest near "V" of neck Cotton work clothing (pants, shirt) T-shirt Socks Bag hand rinse with water	Respirator filter pads Urine	Wolfe, Durham, and Batchelor, 1961
Pyrethroid, synthetic (25 g/L)	ULVA spray application to cotton	Aluminum foil on forearm (left), shin (left), thigh front (left), sternum, back, on top of clothing and forehead, and upper abdomen taped to skin. Impact sensitive chart recorder paper at chest and back	Breathing zone air samples Urine	Prinsen and van Sittert, 1980
Systox	Harvesting and scouting of cabbage	16 ply gauze pads (4 in. by 4 in.) with aluminum foil backings taped on chest, back, and left leg at knee Cotton gloves		Spittler and Bourke, 1985

WP = Wettable powder
EC = Emulsifiable concentrate

Contaminant	*Activity*	*Dermal Methods*	*Other Sampling*	*Reference*
2,4,5-T	Herbicide spraying by backpack, tractor mist blower, helicopter	Gauze pads (10 cm by 10 cm) with cellulose backings attached to clothing on the chest, back, upper arms, and upper thighs	Personal breathing zone air samples Urine (12 hr on 3 different days)	Lavy, Shephard, and Mattice, 1980
2,4,5-T	Helicopter spraying, tractor mist blower, backpack spraying of rice fields or forests	9 ply gauze pads (100 cm^2) backed with two layers of Whatman No. 1 filter paper attached to the outer garments at the upper back and chest, bicep of arm, upper front of thigh	Surface sampling for drift, spray pattern Modified respirator with polyurethane filter	Lavy, Shepard, and Mattice, 1980
Terbufos	Application with planter mounted granular applicators during corn planting	Gauze pads pinned both inside and outside of coveralls at chest (midpoint), between shoulder blades, right lower leg (front), right thigh, right forearm (back), right upper arm (front), all pads offset	Personal breathing zone air samples Urine (pre- and postexposure, 24 hr) Blood	Devine et al., 1986
Tetradifon (0.03%)	Tractor drawn air blast spraying fruit orchards	α-Cellulose pads (10.2 cm by 10.2 cm) with filter paper backings placed on the shins, thigh fronts, forearms, shoulders, back of neck, and upper chest near "V" of neck	Modified respirator with filter pads	Wolfe et al., 1972
Thiodan	Mixing Application with drop nozzle sprayers to cabbage Scouting cabbage	16 ply gauze pads (4 in. by 4 in.) with aluminum foil backings taped on chest, back, and left leg at knee Cotton gloves		Spittler and Bourke, 1985

Contaminant	*Activity*	*Dermal Methods*	*Other Sampling*	*Reference*
Thionazin (10%)	Granular application using tractor drawn gravity feed or broadcast application	α-Cellulose pads (10.2 cm by 10.2 cm) with filter paper backings placed on the shins, thigh fronts, forearms, shoulders, back of neck, and upper chest near "V" of neck attached to outside of workers' clothing including hat	Personal breathing zone air samples Modified respirator with filter Particle size measurements using air and surface samples Bulk samples of granules for pesticide concentration	Lloyd and Bell, 1967
Thiophanate-methyl (liquid)	Spraying pesticide using handheld lances or spray guns	Long sleeve cotton gloves	Personal breathing zone air samples	Brouwer et al., 1992
Thiram	Dusting with knapsack dust blowers and subsequent reentry into greenhouses to do cutting and sorting/bundling of carnations	Long sleeve cotton gloves	Personal breathing zone air samples	Brouwer et al., 1992
Toxaphene	Hand harvesting peanuts	Gauze pads (4 in. by 4 in.) with a glassine backing attached to elastic arm bands and pinned to the outside of workers' clothing at knee level Cotton gloves followed by 95% ethanol hand rinses	Personal breathing zone air samples Foliage residue Soil	EPA, 1988*a* (Study 2)
Toxaphene	Hand harvesting onions by youth and adult field workers	Nylon gloves	High volume area air samples Urine Foliage residue Soil	EPA, 1988*a* (Study 11); Munn, Keefe, and Savage, 1985

WP = Wettable powder
EC = Emulsifiable concentrate

Contaminant	*Activity*	*Dermal Methods*	*Other Sampling*	*Reference*
Toxaphene	Hand harvesting peas	Tyvek jackets with α-cellulose pads (4 in. by 4 in.) with glassine backing attached to the exterior at forearms, chest (each side), shoulders, and one on the center of the upper back Cotton gloves	Personal breathing zone air samples Foliage residue Soil	EPA, 1988*a* (Study 1)
Toxaphene	Mixing/loading in a closed system to determine its effectiveness Ground application	Unwashed cotton cloth and rayon:polyester pads (4 in. by 4 in.) attached to the exterior of the clothing at shoulder, chest, waist, and knee	Area air samples around mixing/ loading sites and on tractors Blood Urine (spot; prejob, 3 week intervals)	Knaak et al., 1980
Toxaphene (liquid)	Mixing/loading (pouring) Aerial spray application	Cloth covered gauze pad with aluminum foil backing Hand wash with water	Personal breathing zone air samples	Wang, Fredrickson, and Jacobs, 1983 (HS-1053)
Treflan	Hand harvesting peas	Tyvek jackets with α-cellulose pads (4 in. by 4 in.) with glassine backings attached to the exterior at forearms, chest (each side), shoulders, and one on the center of the upper back Cotton gloves	Personal breathing zone air samples Foliage residue Soil	EPA, 1988*a* (Study 1)
Treflan	Harvesting of green beans	16 ply gauze pads (4 in. by 4 in.) with aluminum foil backings taped on chest, back, and left leg at knee Cotton gloves		Spittler and Bourke, 1985
Triadimefon (WS packets)	Mixing/loading Boom spray application	Cloth covered gauze pads with aluminum foil backings Hand wash with water and soap	Personal breathing zone air samples	Maddy et al., 1983*b* (HS-1034)

Contaminant	*Activity*	*Dermal Methods*	*Other Sampling*	*Reference*
Tributyl phosphorotrithioate (liquid)	Mixing/loading in closed system Aerial spray application and washdown of airplane Flagging airplane	Fabric covered gauze pads placed under and outside of protective clothing Hand wash with ethanol	Personal breathing zone air samples	Peoples et al., 1981 (HS-676)
Trichlorfon (WP)	Mixing/loading Spray application to lawns for insect control by commercial pesticide company	Monitoring under clothing with surgipads (289 cm^2) placed at wrists, ankles, and inner thighs; and 12 ply gauze sponges (10.2 cm by 10.2 cm) placed on chest (upper and lower) and back (upper and lower)	Personal breathing zone air samples	Freeborg, Daniel, and Konopinski, 1985
Triethanolamine (DNOC)	Spray thinning apples	α-Cellulose pads (10.2 cm by 10.2 cm) with filter paper backings placed outside clothing on the shins, thigh fronts, forearms, shoulders, back of neck, and upper chest near "V" of neck Cotton work clothing (pants, shirt) T-shirt Socks Bag hand rinse with water	Respirator filter pads Urine	Wolfe, Durham, and Batchelor, 1961

WP = Wettable powder
EC = Emulsifiable concentrate

Contaminant	*Activity*	*Dermal Methods*	*Other Sampling*	*Reference*
Vinclozolin	Hand harvesting blueberries	12 ply gauze pads (3 in. by 3 in.) with polyethylene backings inside glassine envelopes with a circular opening (60 mm diameter). Pads were fastened to a headband or brim of a cap. They were stapled to a tightly fitting cotton T-shirt at the chest, back, and upper arm. Pads were attached to lower arms and legs with surgical tape. Cotton gloves	Foliage residue Soil	EPA, 1988*b* (Study 5)
Vinclozolin	Hand harvesting strawberries	Gauze pads Cotton gloves	Foliage residue	EPA, 1988*b* (Study 3)
Zineb	Dusting with knapsack dust blowers Reentry into greenhouses to do cutting and sorting/bundling of carnations	Long sleeve cotton gloves	Personal breathing zone air samples	Brouwer et al., 1992
Zineb	Mixing/loading in a closed system to determine its effectiveness Ground application	Unwashed cotton cloth and rayon:polyester pads (4 in. by 4 in.) attached to the exterior of the clothing at shoulder, chest, waist, and knee	Area air samples around mixing/loading sites and on tractors Blood Urine (spot; prejob, 3 week intervals)	Knaak et al., 1980

REFERENCES

Abbott, I. M., J. L. Bonsall, G. Chester, T. B. Hard, and G. J. Turnbull. G. 1987. Worker exposure to a herbicide applied with groundsprayers in the United Kingdom. *AIHA J.* **48**(2): 167–75.

Adamis, Z., A. Antal, I. Fuzesi, J. Molnar, L. Nagy, and M. Susan. 1985. Occupational exposure to organophosphorus insecticides and synthetic pyrethroid. *Int. Arch. Occup. Env. Health* **56:**299–305.

Al-Jaghbir, M. T., A. S. Salhab, and F. A. Hamarsheh. 1992. Dermal and inhalation exposure to methoate. *Arch. Env. Contam. Toxicol.* **22:**358–361.

Alcoser, D. 1988. *A Study of Dermal and Inhalation Exposure of Mixer/Loaders to Pesticides While Using a Closed Mixing and Loading System.* Worker Health and Safety Branch Report HS-1406. Sacramento, CA: Department of Pesticide Regulation, CalEPA.

Atallah, Y. H., W. P. Cahill, and D. M. Whitacre. 1982. Exposure of pesticide applicators and support personnel to O-ethyl O-(4-nitrophenyl) phenylphosphonothioate (EPN). *Arch. Env. Contam. Toxicol.* **11:**219–225.

Bandara, J. M. R. S., P. C. Kearney, P. G. Vincent, and W. A. Gentner. 1985. Paraquat: A model for measuring exposure. In R. C. Honeycutt, G. Zweig, and N. N. Ragsdale (eds.), *Dermal Exposure Related to Pesticide Use.* Washington, DC: American Chemical Society, pp. 279– 285.

Batchelor, G. S., K. C. Walker, and J. W. Elliott. 1956. Dinitroorthocresol exposure from apple-thinning sprays. *Arch. Ind. Health* **13:**593–596.

Boleij, J. S. M., H. Kromhout, M. Fleuren, W. Tieleman, and G. Verstappen. 1991. Reentry after methomyl application in greenhouses. *Appl. Occup. Environ. Hyg.* **6**(8):672–676.

Brady, U. E., R. Tippins, J. Perry, J. R. Young, and R. D. Wauchope. 1991. Chlorpyrifos exposure of workers entering sweet corn after chemigation. *Bull. Env. Contam. Toxicol.* **46:**343–350.

Brouwer, D. H., R. Brouwer, G. DeMik, C. L. Maas, and J. J. van Hemmen. 1992*a*. Pesticides in the cultivation of carnations in greenhouses: Part I—Exposure and concomitant health risk. *AIHA J.* **53**(9): 575–581.

Brouwer, R., H. Marqurt, G. de Mik, and J. van Hemmen. 1992*b*. Risk assessment of dermal exposure of greenhouse workers to pesticides after reentry. *Arch. Env. Contam. Toxicol.* **23:**273–280.

Carman, G. E., Y. Iwata, J. L. Pappas, J. R. O'Neal, and F. A. Gunther. 1982. Pesticide applicator exposure to insecticides during treatment of citrus trees with oscillating boom and airblast units. *Arch. Env. Contam. Toxicol.* **11:**651–659.

Chester, G. and T. B. Hart. 1986. Biological monitoring of a herbicide applied though backpack and vehicle spraying. *Toxicol. Letters* **33:**137–149.

Chester, G. and R. J. Ward. 1984. Occupational exposure and drift hazard during aerial application of Paraquat to cotton. *Arch. Env. Contam. Toxicol.* **13:**551–563.

Chester, G. and B. H. Woolen. 1981. Studies of the occupational exposure of Malaysian plantation workers to Paraquat. *Brit. J. Ind. Med.* **38:**23–33.

Chester, G., L. D. Hatfield, T. B. Hart, B. C. Leppert, H. Swaine, and O. J. Tummon. 1987. Worker exposure to, and absorption of, cypermethrin during aerial application of an "ultra low volume" formulation to cotton. *Arch. Env. Contam. Toxicol.* **16:**69–78.

Comer, S. W., D. C. Staiff, J. F. Armstrong, and H. R. Wolfe. 1975. Exposure of workers to carbaryl. *Bull. Env. Contam. Toxicol.* **13**(4):385–391.

Copplestone, J. F., Z. I. Fakhri, J. W. Miles, C. A. Mitchell, Y. Osman, and H. R. Wolfe. 1976. Exposure to pesticides in agriculture: A survey of spraymen using dimethoate in the Sudan. *Bull. WHO* **54:**217–223.

Cowell, J. E., C. M. Lottman, and M. J. Manning. 1991. Assessment of lawn care worker exposure to dithiopyr. *Arch. Env. Contam. Toxicol.* **21:**195–201.

Cowell, J. E., R. G. Danhaus, J. L. Kuntsman, A. G. Hackett, M. E. Oppenhuizen, and J. R. Steinmetz. 1987. Operator exposure from closed system loading and application of alachlor herbicide. *Arch. Env. Contam. Toxicol.* **16:**327–332.

Culver, D., P. Caplan, and G. W. Batchelor. 1956. Studies of human exposure during aerosol application of malathion and chlorthion. *Arch. Ind. Health* **13:**37–50.

Culver, D., J. Kinosian, W. Thielen, and R. Graul. 1958. A study of exposure to parathion in a greenhouse. *Arch. Ind. Health* **18:**235–247.

Davies, J. E., E. R. Stevens, and D. C. Staiff. 1983. Potential exposure of apple thinners to azinphosmethyl and comparison of two methods for assessment of hand exposure. *Bull. Env. Contam. Toxicol.* **31:**631–638.

Davies, J. E., D. C. Staiff, L. C. Butler, and E. R. Stevens. 1981. Potential exposure to dislodgable residues after application of two formulations of methyl parathion to apple trees. *Bull. Env. Contam. Toxicol.* **27:**95–100.

Davies, J. E., H. F. Enos, A. Barquet, C. Morgade, and V. H. Freed. 1982*a*. Protective clothing studies in the field: An alternative to reentry. In J. R. Plimmer (ed.), *Pesticide Residues and Exposure.* Washington, DC: American Chemical Society, 168–182.

Davies, J. E., E. R. Stevens, D. C. Staiff, and L. C. Butler. 1982*b*. Potential exposure of apple thinners to phosalone. *Bull. Env. Contam. Toxicol.* **29:**592, 598.

Davies, J. E., V. H. Freed, H. F. Enos, R. C. Duncan, A. Barquet, C. Morgade, L. J. Peters, and J. X. Danauskas. 1982*c*. Reduction of pesticide exposure with protective clothing for applicators and mixers. *JOM* **24:**464–468.

Devine, J. M., G. B. Kinoshita, R. P. Peterson, and G. L. Picard. 1986. Farm worker exposure to terbufos (phosphorodithioic acid, S-(tert-burylthio) methyl O,O-diethyl ester) during planting operations of corn. *Arch. Env. Contam. Toxicol.* **15:**113–119.

Dubelman, S. and J. E. Cowell. 1989. Biological monitoring technology for measurement of applicator exposure. In R. G. M. Wang, C. A. Franklin, R. C. Honeycutt, and J. C. Reinert (eds.), *Biological Monitoring for Pesticide Exposure.* Washington, DC: American Chemical Society, pp. 240–250.

Dubelman, S., R. Lauer, D. D. Arras, and S. A. Adams. 1982. Operator exposure measurements during application of the herbicide Diallate. *J. Agric. Food Chem.* **30:**528–532.

Durham, W. F., and H. R. Wolfe. 1962. Measurement of the exposure of workers to pesticides. *Bull. Wld. Hlth. Org.* **26:**75–91.

EPA Pesticide Hazard Assessment Project. 1988*a*. Harvestor exposure monitoring studies (1980–1986), vol. I, 13 studies. EPA 540/09-88-036. Washington, DC: EPA.

EPA Pesticide Hazard Assessment Project. 1988*b*. Harvestor exposure monitoring studies (1980–1986), vol. II, 12 studies. EPA 540/09-88-037. Washington, DC: EPA.

Everhart, L. P. and R. F. Holt. 1982. Potential benlate fungicide exposure during mixer/loader operations, crop harvest, and home use. *J. Agric. Food Chem.* **30:**222–227.

Fenske, R. A. 1988*a*. Comparative assessment of protective clothing performance by measurement of dermal exposure during pesticide applications. *Appl. Ind. Hyg.* **3**(7):207–213.

Fenske, R. A. 1988*b*. Correlation of fluorescent tracer measurements of dermal exposure and urinary metabolite excretion during occupational exposure to malathion. *AIHA J.* **49**(9):438–444.

Fenske, R. A., S. J. Hamburger, and C. L. Guyton. 1987. Occupational exposure to fosetyl-al fungicide during spraying of ornamentals in greenhouses. *Arch. Env. Contam. Toxicol.* **16:**615–621.

Fenske, R. A., J. T. Leffingwell, and R. C. Spear. 1985. Evaluation of fluorescent tracer methodology for dermal exposure assessment. In R. C. Honeycutt, G. Zweig, and N. N. Ragsdale (eds.), *Dermal Exposure Related to Pesticide Use.* Washington, DC: American Chemical Society, pp. 377–393.

Fenske, R.A., A. M. Blacker, S. J. Hamburger, and G. S. Simon. 1990. Worker exposure and protective clothing performance during manual seed treatment with lindane. *Arch. Env. Contam. Toxicol.* **19:**190–196.

Fletcher, T. E., J. M. Press, and D. B. Wilson. 1959. Exposure of spray-men to dieldrin in residual spraying. *Bull. Wld. Hlth Org.* **20:**15–25.

Frank, R., R. A. Campbell, and G. J. Sirons. 1985. Forestry workers involved in aerial application of 2,4-dichlorophenoxyacetic acid (2,4-D) exposure and urinary excretion. *Arch. Env. Contam. Toxicol.* **14:**427–435.

Franklin, C. A., N. J. Muir, and R. P. Moody. 1986. The use of biological monitoring in the estimation of exposure during the application of pesticides. *Toxicol. Letters* **33:**127–136.

Franklin, C. A., R. A. Fenske, R. Greenhalgh, L. Mathieu, H. V. Dnldy, J. J. Liffingwell, and R. C. Spear. 1981. Correlation of urinary pesticide metabolite excretion with estimated dermal contact in the course of occupational exposure to guthion. *J. Toxicol. Env. Health* **7:**715–731.

Freeborg, R. P., W. H. Daniel, and V. J. Konopinski. 1985. Applicator exposure to pesticides applied to turfgrass. In R. C. Honeycutt, G. Zweig, and N. N. Ragsdale (eds.), *Dermal Exposure Related to Pesticides.* Washington, DC: American Chemical Society, pp. 287–295.

Gold, R. E., J. R. C. Leavitt, T. Holcslaw, and D. Tupy. 1982. Exposure of urban applicators to carbaryl. *Arch. Env. Contam. Toxicol.* **11:**63–67.

Grey, W. E., D. E. Marthre, and S. J. Rogers. 1983. Potential exposure of commercial seed-treating applicators to the pesticides carboxin-thiram and lindane. *Bull. Env. Contam. Toxicol.* **31:**244–250.

Grover, R., A. J. Cessna, N. I. Muir, D. Riedel, C. A. Franklin, and K. Yoshida. 1986*a*. Factors affecting the exposure of ground-rig applicators to 2,4-D dimethylamine salt. *Arch. Env. Contam. Toxicol.* **15:**677–686.

Grover, R., C. A. Franklin, N. I. Muir, A. J. Cessna, and D. Riedel. 1986*b*. Dermal exposure and urinary metabolite excretion in farmers repeatedly exposed to 2,4-D amine. *Toxicol. Letters* **33:**73–83.

Hansen, J. D., B. A. Schneider, M. Olive, and J. J. Bates. 1978. Personnel safety and foliage residue in an orchard spray program using azinphos-methyl and captan. *Arch. Env. Contam. Toxicol.* **7:**63–71.

Hattula, M. L., V. Wasenius, and A. U. Arstila. 1979. The exposure to MCPA in the use of clearing saw. *Chemosphere* **7:**473–476.

Haverty, M. I., M. Page, P. J. Shea, J. B. Hoy, and R. W. Hall. 982. Drift and worker exposure resulting from two methods of applying insecticides to pine bark. *Bull. Env. Contam. Toxicol.* **30:**223–228.

Herman, N. D., T. W. Hunt, and T. J. Sheets. 1985. Hand harvester exposure to maleic hydrazide (MH) in flue-cured tobacco. *Bull. Env. Contam. Toxicol.* **34:**469–475.

Hunt, T. W., G. W. Wojeck, and T. J. Sheets. 1985. Applicator exposure to maleic hydrazide (MH) in flue-cured tobacco. *Bull. Env. Contam. Toxicol.* **34:**403–406.

Hussain, M., K. Yoshida, M. Atiemo, and D. Johnston. 1990. Occupational exposure of grain farmers to carbofuran. *Arch. Env. Contam. Toxicol.* **19:**197–204.

Jegier, Z. 1964*a*. Exposure to guthion during spraying and formulating. *Arch. Env. Health* **8:**565–569.

Jegier, Z. 1964*b*. Health hazards in insecticide spraying of crops. *Arch. Env. Health* **8:**670–674.

Kamble, S. T., C. L. Ogg, R. E. Gold, and A. D. Vance. 1992. Exposure of applicators and residents to chlordane and heptachlor when used for subterranean termite control. *Arch. Env. Contam. Toxicol.* **22:**253–259.

Kangas, J., S. Laitinen, A. Jauhiainen, and K. Savolainen. 1993. Exposure of sprayers and plant handlers to mevinphos in Finnish greenhouses. *AIHA J.* **2:**150–153.

Kazen, C., A. Bloomer, R. Welch, A. Oudbier, and H. Price. 1974. Persistence of pesticides on the hands of some occupationally exposed people. *Arch. Env. Health* **29:**315–318.

Kilgore, W., C. Fischer, J. Rivers, N. Akesson, J. Wicks, W. Winters, and W. Winterlin. 1984. Human exposure to DEF/merphos. *Res. Rev.* **91:**71–101.

Knaak, J. B., K. C. Jacobs, and G. M. Wang. 1986. Estimating the hazard to humans applying Nemacur 3EC with rat dermal-dose ChE response data. *Bull. Env. Contam. Toxicol.* **37:**159–163.

Knaak, J. B., S. A. Peoples, T. J. Jackson, A. S. Fredrickson, R. Enos, K. T. Maddy, J. B. Bailey, M. E. Dusch, F. A. Gunther, and W. L. Winterlin. 1978. Reentry problems involving the use of dialifor on grapes in the San Joaquin Valley of California. *Arch. Env. Contam. Toxicol.* **7:**465–481.

Knaak, J. B., K. T. Maddy, M. A. Gallo, D. T. Lillie, E. M. Craine, and W. F. Serat. 1978. Worker reentry study involving phosalone application to citrus groves. *Toxicol. Appl. Pharm.* **46:**363–374.

Knaak, J. B., T. Jackson, A. S. Fredrickson, L. Rivera, K. T. Maddy, and N. B. Akesson. 1980. Safety effectiveness of closed-transfer, mixing-loading, and application equipment in preventing exposure to pesticides. *Arch. Env. Contam. Toxicol.* **9:**231–245.

Knaak, J. B., M. A. Al-Bayati, O. G. Raabe, J. L. Wiedmann, J. W. Pensyl, J. H. Ross, A. P. Leber, and P. Jones. 1989. Mixer-loader-applicator exposure and percutaneous absorption studies involving EPTC herbicide. In R. G. M. Wang, C. A. Franklin, R. C. Honeycutt, and J. C. Reinert (eds.), *Biological Monitoring for Pesticide Exposure*. Washington, DC: American Chemical Society, pp. 288–303.

Knarr, R. D., G. L. Cooper, E. A. Brian, M. G. Kleinschmidt, and D. G. Graham. 1985. Worker exposure during aerial application of a liquid and a granular formulation of ordram selective herbicide to rice. *Arch. Env. Contam. Toxicol.* **14:**523–527.

Kolmodin-Hedman, B., S. Hoglund, and M. Akerblom. 1983. Studies on phenoxy acid herbicides. I. Field study of occupational exposure to phenoxy acid herbicides (MCPA, dichlorprop, mecoprop and 2,4-D) in agriculture. *Arch. Toxicol.* **54:**257–265.

Lamb, D. W. 1980. Early studies with azinphos methyl to determine re-entry times for citrus pickers. In W. F. Tordoir and E. A. H. van Heemstra (eds.), *Field Worker Exposure During Pesticide Application*. Amsterdam: Elsevier, pp. 121–127.

Lavy, T. L., J. S. Shepard, and D. C. Bouchard. 1980. Field worker exposure and helicopter spray pattern of 2,4,5-T. *Bull. Env. Contam. Toxicol.* **24:**90–96.

Lavy, T. L., J. S. Shepard, and J. D. Mattice. 1980. Exposure measurements of applicators spraying (2,4,5-trichlorophenoxy) acetic acid in the forest. *J. Agric. Food Chem.* **28:**626–630.

Lavy, T. L., J. D. Walstad, R. R. Flynn, and J. D. Mattice. 1982. (2,4-Dichlorophenoxy) acetic acid exposure received by aerial application crews during forest spray operations. *J. Agric. Food Chem.* **30:**375–381.

Lavy, T. L., J. E. Cowell, J. R. Steinmetz, and J. H. Massey. 1992. Conifer seedling nursery worker exposure to glyphosate. *Arch. Env. Contam. Toxicol.* **22:**6–13.

Lavy, T. L., J. D. Mattice, J. H. Massey, and B. W. Skulman. 1993. Measurements of year-long exposure to tree nursery workers using multiple pesticides. *Arch. Env. Contam. Toxicol.* **24:**123–144.

Leavitt, J. R. C., R. E. Gold, T. Holcslaw, and D. Tupy. 1982. Exposure of professional pesticide applicators to carbaryl. *Arch. Env. Contam. Toxicol.* **11:**57–62.

Lengerich, S. K., and F. G. Burroughs. 1989. Near real-time monitoring of potential dermal exposure during backpack herbicide spraying. *AIHA J.* **50**(10):516–519.

Liesivuori, J., S. Liukkkonen, and P. Pirhonen. 1988. Reentry intervals after pesticide application in greenhouses. *Scand. J. Work. Env. Health* **14**(suppl 1):35–36.

Lloyd, G. A., and G. J. Bell. 1967. The exposure of agricultural workers to pesticides used in granular form. *Ann. Occup. Hyg.* **10:**97–104.

Lotti, M., C. E. Becker, M. J. Aminoff, J. E. Woodrow, J. N. Seiber, R. E. Talcott, and R. J. Richardson. 1983. Occupational exposure to the cotton defoliants DEF and Merphos. *JOM* **25:**517–522.

Machado Neto, J. G., T. Matuo, and Y. K. Matuo. 1992. Dermal exposure of pesticide applicators in staked tomato (*Lycopersicon esculentum miii*) crops: Efficiency of a safety measure in the application equipment. *Bull. Env. Contam. Toxicol.* **48:**529–534.

McJilton, C. E., G. E. Berckman, and H. M. Deer. 1983. Captan exposure in apple orchards. *AIHA J.* **44**(3):209–210.

Maddy, K. T., and D. Richmond. 1987. *Monitoring the Effectiveness of an Enclosed Air-Conditioned Cab in Mitigating the Potential Exposure Hazard of Organophosphate Insecticides to Applicators During Applications to Row Crops*. Worker Health and Safety Branch Report HS-1381. Sacramento, CA: Department of Pesticide Regulation, CalEPA.

Maddy, K. T., B. Cusick, A. S. Fredrickson, D. Richmond, M. Mazza, and R. Beall. 1979. *Ethylene*

Dibromide During Soil Injection. Worker Health and Safety Branch Report HS-593. Sacramento, CA: Department of Pesticide Regulation, CalEPA.

Maddy, K. T., L. Johnston, C. Smith, F. Schneider, and T. Jackson. 1980. *A Study of Mixer/Loaders and Applicators to Nitrofen (TOK) in Monterey and Santa Barbara Counties of California*. Worker Health and Safety Branch Report HS-745. Sacramento, CA: Department of Pesticide Regulation, CalEPA.

Maddy, K. T., C. Winter, S. Cepello, and A. S. Fredrickson. 1981. *Monitoring of Potential Occupational Exposures of Mixer/Loaders and Pilots During Application of Mevinphos (Phosdrin) in Monterey County in 1981*. Worker Health and Safety Branch Report HS-876. Sacramento, CA: Department of Pesticide Regulation, CalEPA.

Maddy, K. T., F. Schneider, J. Lowe, and S. A. Fredrickson. 1982*a*. *A Study of the Dermal and Inhalation Exposure of Loaders, Pilots and Flaggers to Molinate (Ordram) in Colusa County in May, 1981*. Worker Health and Safety Branch Report HS-887. Sacramento, CA: Department of Pesticide Regulation, CalEPA.

Maddy, K. T., C. Winter, S. Cepello, and S. A. Fredrickson. 1982*b*. *Monitoring of Potential Occupational Exposure of Mixer/Loaders, Pilots and Flaggers During Application of Mevinphos (Phosdrin) in Imperial County in 1981*. Worker Health and Safety Branch Report HS-889. Sacramento, CA: Department of Pesticide Regulation, CalEPA.

Maddy, K. T., F. Schneider, H. R. Fong, J. Lowe, and N. Siani. 1982*c*. *A Study of Dermal and Inhalation Exposure of Mixer/Loaders Applicators and Flaggers to Bendicarb (Bolero) in Colusa County in California*. Worker Health and Safety Branch Report HS-898. Sacramento, CA: Department of Pesticide Regulation, CalEPa.

Maddy, K. T., D. Gibons, L. O'Connell, D. Meinders, C. Cooper, and M. Wroe. 1982*d*. *Potential Exposure to Chlordimeform During Application to Cotton in Imperial Valley in 1982*. Worker Health and Safety Branch Report HS-1067. Sacramento, CA: Department of Pesticide Reglation, CalEPA.

Maddy, K. T., D. Gibbons, L. O'Connell, D. Meinders, C. Cooper, and M. Wroe. 1983*a*. *Potential Exposure of Workers to Chlordimeform During Application to Cotton in Imperial County in 1982 Trial Application*. Worker Health and Safety Branch Report HS-1063. Sacramento, CA: Department of Pesticide Regulation, CalEPA.

Maddy, K. T., R. G. Wang, C. M. Au, and N. Siani. 1983*b*. *Monitoring of Occupational Exposures of Mixer/Loaders and Applicators to Bayleton 50% WP in Kern County in 1982*. Worker Health and Safety Branch Report HS-1034. Sacramento, CA: Department of Pesticide Regulation, CalEPA.

Maddy, K. T., L. P. O'Connell, C. K. Winter, and S. Margetich. 1983*c*. *Monitoring of the Potential Exposure of Ground Applicators and Mixer/Loaders to Chlorobenzilate During Application to Lemon Orchards*. Worker Health and Safety Branch Report HS-903. Sacramento, CA: Department of Pesticide Regulation, CalEPA.

Maddy, K. T., D. Gibbons, S. L. Kilgore, and S. Margetich. 1984. *Potential Exposure of Applicators to Parathion When Treating Citrus in Riverside County*. Worker Health and Safety Branch Report HS-1059. Sacramento, CA: Department of Pesticide Regulation, CalEPA.

Maddy, K. T., R. I. Krieger, L. O'Connell, M. Bisbiglia, and S. Margetich. 1989. Use of biological monitoring data from pesticide users in making pesticide regulatory decisions in California. In R. G. M. Wang, C. A. Franklin, R. C. Honeycutt, and J. C. Reinert (eds.), *Biological Monitoring for Pesticide Exposure*. Washington, DC: American Chemical Society, pp. 338–353.

Maitlen, J. C., C. R. Sell, and L. M. McDonough. 1982. Workers in the agricultural environment. In J. R. Plimmer (ed.), *Pesticide Residues and Exposure*. Washington, DC: American Chemical Society, pp. 83–103.

Manninen, A., J. Kangas, T. Klen, and H. Savolainen. 1986. Exposure of Finnish farm workers to phenoxy acid herbicides. *Arch Env. Contam. Toxicol.* **15**:107–111.

Mestres, R., C. Francois, C. Causse, L. Vian, and G. P. Winnett. 1985. Survey of exposure to pesticides in greenhouses. *Bull. Env. Contam. Toxicol.* **35**:750–756.

Mumma, R. O., G. A. Brandes, and C. F. Gordon. 1985. Exposure of applicators and mixer-loaders during the application of mancozeb by airplanes, airblast sprayers, and compressed-air backpack sprayers. In R. C. Honeycutt, G. Zweig, and N. N. Ragsdale (eds.), *Dermal Exposure Related to Pesticide Use*. Washington, DC: American Chemical Society, pp. 201–219.

Munn, S., T. J. Keefe, and E. P. Savage. 1985. A comparative study of pesticide exposures in adults and youth migrant field workers. *Arch. Env. Health* **40**(4):215–220.

Nigg, H. N., and J. H. Stamper. 1983*a*. Exposure of Florida airboat aquatic weed applicators to 2,4-dichlorophenoxyacetic acid (2,4-D). *Chemosphere* **12**(2):209–215.

Nigg, H. N., and J. H. Stamper. 1983*b*. Exposure of spray applicators and mixer-loaders to chlorobenzilate miticide in Florida citrus groves. *Arch. Env. Contam. Toxicol.* **12**:477–482.

Nigg, H. N., J. H. Stamper, and W. D. Mahon. 1988. *Pesticide Exposure to Florida Greenhouse Applicators*. EPA 600/2-88/033. Washington, DC: EPA

Nigg, H. N., J. H. Stamper, and W. D. Mahon. 1990. Handgun applicator exposure to ethion in Florida citrus. *Arch. Env. Contam. Toxicol.* **45**:463–468.

Nigg, H. N., J. H. Stamper, and R. M. Queen. 1984. The development and use of a universal model to

predict tree crop harvester pesticide exposure. *AIHA J.* **45**(3):182–186.
Nigg, H. N., J. H. Stamper and R. M. Queen. 1986. Dicofol exposure to Florida citrus applicators: Effects of protective clothing. *Arch. Env. Contam. Toxicol.* **15:**121–134.
Nigg, H. N., J. H. Stamper, E. P. Easter, W. D. Mahon and J. O. DeJonge. 1990. Protection afforded citrus pesticide applicators by coveralls. *Arch. Env. Contam. Toxicol.* **19:**635–639.
Nigg, H. N., J. H. Stamper, S. N. Deshmukh, and R. M. Queen. 1991. 4,4'-Dichlorobenzilic acid urinary excretion by Dicofol pesticide applicators. *Chemosphere* **22**(3/4):365–373.
NIOSH, Hazard Evaluation and Technical Assistance Report. July 1978. *Platte Chemical Co., Fremont, NH.* TA 77-66. Cincinnati, OH: NIOSH.
NIOSH, Health Hazard Evaluation Report. December 1979. *Shell Chemical Company, Rocky Mountain Arsenal, Denver,* CO. HHE 77-126-646. Cincinnati, OH: NIOSH.
NIOSH, Health Hazard Evaluation Report. January 1980. *R. L. Polk Company, Cincinnati, OH.* HHE 78-77-659. Cincinnati, OH: NIOSH.
NIOSH, Health hazard Evaluation Report. September 1981. *Boehringer Ingelheim, Ltd., Ridgefield, CT.* HETA 81-247-958. Cincinnati, OH: NIOSH.
NIOSH, Health Hazard Evaluation Report. July 1982. *Shell Chemical Company, Denver,* CO. HHE 80-137-1145. Cincinnati, OH: NIOSH.
NIOSH, Health Hazard Evaluation Report. November 1983. *U.S. Forest Service, Dillon District, Frisco,* CO. HETA 83-408-1389. Cincinnati, OH: NIOSH.
NIOSH, Health Hazard Evaluation Report. 1984. *Universal Formulations, Inc., Cleveland, OH.* HHE 82-465-1323. Cincinnati, OH: NIOSH.
NIOSH, Health Hazard Evaluation Report. July 1984. *Colorado River Indian Reservation, Parker, AZ.* HETA 81-463-1477. Cincinnati, OH: NIOSH.
NIOSH, Health Hazard Evaluation Report. 1985. *Shell Chemical Co., Axis, AL.* HETA 78-4-1511. Cincinnati, OH: NIOSH.
NIOSH, Health Hazard Evaluation Report. January 1985. *Bureau of Reclamation, U.S. Dept. of the Interior, Denver,* CO. HETA 83-341-1557. Cincinnati, OH: NIOSH.
NIOSH, Health Hazard Evaluation Report. June 1986. *Canyon de Chelly National Monument, Chinle, AZ.* HETA 85-527-1704. Cincinnati, OH: NIOSH.
NIOSH, Health Hazard Evaluation Report. December 1986. *Detroit Fire Fighters, Detroit, MI.* HETA 84-484-1754. Cincinnati, OH: NIOSH
Ojanen, K., R. Sarantilla, T. Klen, A. Lotjonen, and J. Kangas. 1992. Evaluation of the efficiency and comfort of protective clothing during herbicide spraying. *Appl. Occup. Env. Hyg.* **7**(12):815–819.
Oshita, C. M., F. A. Schneider, and S. Margetich. 1988. *An Exposure Study of Mixer/Loaders and Applicators Using Oxydemeton-Methyl (Metasystox-R) in the Salinas and Santa Maria Valleys of California in 1986.* Worker Health and Safety Branch Report HS-1398. Sacramento, CA: Department of Pesticide Regulation, CalEPA.
Peoples, S. A., K. T. Maddy, P. R. Datta, L. Johnston, C. Smith, D. Conrad, and C. Cooper. 1981. *Monitoring of potential Exposures of Mixer/Loaders, Pilots and Flaggers During Application of Tributyl Phosphorotrithioate (DEF) and Tributyl Phosphorothrithioite (Folex) to Cotton Fields in the San Joaquin Valley of California in 1979.* Worker Health and Safety Branch Report HS-676. Sacramento, CA: Department of Pesticide Regulation, CalEPA.
Popendorf, W. 1980. Exploring citrus harvesters' exposure to pesticide contaminated foliar dust. *AIHA J.* **41:**652–659.
Popendorf, W. J., R. C. Spear, J. T. Leffingwell, J. Yager, and E. Kahn. 1979. Harvester exposure to Zolone® (Phosalone) residues in peach orchards. *JOM* **21**(3):189–194.
Prinsen, G. H., and N. J. van Sittert. 1980. Exposure and medical monitoring study of a new synthetic pyrethroid after one season of spraying on cotton in Ivory Coast. In W. F. Tordoir and E. A. H. van Heemstra (eds.), *Field Worker Exposure During Pesticide Application.* Amsterdam: Elsevier, pp. 105–120.
Putnam, A. R., M. D. Willis, L. K. Binning, and P. F. Boldt. 1983. Exposure of pesticide applicators to nitrofen: Influence of formulation, handling systems, and protective garments. *J. Agric. Food Chem.* **31:**645–650.
Quinby, G. E., K. C. Walker and W. F. Durham. 1958. Public health hazards involved in the use of organic phosphorus insecticides in cotton culture in the delta area of Mississippi. *J. Econ. Entomol.* **51:**831–838.
Rech, C., S. Bissel, and J. del Valle. 1988. *Potential Dermal and Respiratory Exposure to Abamectin During Greenhouse Applications.* Worker Health and Safety Branch Report HS-1491. Sacramento, CA: Department of Pesticide Regulation, CalEPA.
Reed, J. P., F. R. Hall, and H. R. Krueger. 1990. Measurement of ATV applicator exposure to attrazine using an ELISA method. *Bull. Env. Contam. Toxicol.* **44:**8–12.
Richter, E. D., B. Cohen, M. Luria, J. Schoenberg, E. Weisenberg, and M. Gordon. 1980. Exposures of aerial spray workers to parathion. *Israel J. Med. Sci.* **16:**96–100.
Ritcey, G., R. Frank, F. L. McEwen, and H. E. Braun. 1987. Captan residues on strawberries and estimates of exposure to pickers. *Bull. Env. Contam. Toxicol.* **38:**840–846.
Savolainen, K., P. Kurttio, T. Vartiainen, and J. Kangas. 1989. Ethylenethiourea as an indicator of

exposure to ethylenebisdithiocarbamate fungicides. *Arch. Toxicol. Suppl.* **13:**120–123.

Sell, C. R., and J. C. Maitlen. 1983. Procedure for the determination of residues of (2,4-dichlorophenoxy)acetic acid in dermal exposure pads, hand rinses, urine, and perspiration from agricultural workers exposed to the herbicide. *J. Agric. Food Chem.* **31:**572–575.

Simpson, G. R. 1965. Exposure to orchard residues, dermal and inhalation exposures. *Arch. Env. Health.* **10:**884–885.

Simpson, G. R., and A. Beck. 1964. Exposure to parathion. *Arch. Env. Health* **11:**784–786.

Simpson, G. R., and A. Shandar. 1972. Exposure to chlorinated hydrocarbon pesticides by pest control operators. *Med. J. Aust.* **8:**1060–1063.

Spear, R. C., W. J. Popendorf, J. T. Leffingwell, T. H. Milby, J. E. Davies, and W. F. Spencer. 1977. Fieldworkers' response to weathered residues of parathion. *JOM* **19**(6):406–410.

Spittler, T. D., and J. B. Bourke. 1985. Potential exposure in the application of pesticides to orchard and field crops. In R. C. Honeycutt, G. Zweig, and N. N. Ragsdale (eds.), *Dermal Exposure Related to Pesticide Use*. Washington, DC: American Chemical Society, pp. 297–310.

Staiff, D. C., S. W. Comer, J. W. Armstrong, and H. R. Wolfe. 1975. Exposure to the herbicide, paraquat. *Bull. Env. Contam. Toxicol.* **14:**334–340.

Stamper, J. H., H. N. Nigg, and R. M. Queen. 1986. Prediction of pesticide dermal exposure and urinary metabolite level of tree crop harvesters from field residues. *Bull. Env. Contam. Toxicol.* **36:**693–700.

Stamper, J. H., H. N. Nigg, W. D. Mahon, A. P. Nielson, and M. D. Royer. 1988. Pesticide exposure to greenhouse handgunners. *Chemosphere* **17**(5):1007–1023.

Stamper, J. H., H. N. Nigg, W. D. Mahon, A. P. Nielsen, and M. D. Royer. 1989*a*. Pesticide exposure to greenhouse handgunners. *Arch. Env. Contam. Toxicol.* **18:**515–529.

Stamper, J. W., H. N. Nigg, W. D. Mahon, A. P. Nielsen, and M. D. Boyer. 1989*b*. Applicator exposure to fluvalinate, chlorpyrifos, captan, and chlorothalonil in Florida ornamentals. *J. Agric. Food Chem.* **37:**240–244.

Stamper, J. H., H. N. Nigg, W. D. Mahon, A. P. Nielsen, and M. D. Royer. 1989*c*. Pesticide exposure to a greenhouse drencher. *Bull. Env. Contam. Toxicol.* **42:**209–217.

Stevens, E. R., and J. E. Davies, 1981. Potential exposure of workers during seed potato treatment with Captan. *Bull. Env. Contam. Toxicol.* **26:**681–688.

Taskar, P. K., Y. T. Das, J. R. Trout, S. K. Chattopadhyay, and H. D. Brown. 1982. Measurement of 2,4-dichlorophenoxyacetic acid (2,4-D) after occupational exposure. *Bull. Env. Contam. Toxicol.* **29:**586–591.

Wan, H. 1990. Pesticide exposure of applicators working in tea plantations. *Bull. Env. Contam. Toxicol.* **45:**459–462.

Wand, R., F. Schneider, D. Alcoser, S. Siaz, C. Cooper and M. Bisbiglia. 1987. *Pesticide Exposure to Applicators During Dormant Spraying of Trees While in an Enclosed Cab Equipped with a Charcoal Air Filtration System in California, January, 1986*. Worker Health and Safety Branch Report HS-1390. Sacramento, CA: Department of Pesticide Regulation, CalEPA.

Wang, R. G., S. Fredrickson, and K. C. Jacobs. 1983. *A Study of Dermal and Inhalation Exposure of a Mixer/Loader, Pilot, and Two Flaggers to Toxaphene in Fresno County California*. Worker Health and Safety Branch Report HS-1053, Sacramento, CA: Department of Pesticide Regulation, CalEPA.

Wang, R. G., K. C. Jacobs, and S. A. Fredrickson. 1983. *A Study of Dermal and Inhalation Exposure of Mixer/Loaders and Applicators to Nemacur in Fresno and Tulare Counties of California*. Worker Health and Safety Branch Report HS-1033. Sacramento, CA: Department of Pesticide Regulation, CalEPA.

Wang, T. C., R. A. Lenahan, and J. W. Tucker. 1987. Deposition and persistence of aerially-applied fenthion in a Florida estuary. *Bull. Env. Contam. Toxicol.* **38:**226–231.

Ware, G. W., D. P. Morgan, B. J. Estesen, W. P. Cahill, and D. M. Whitacre. 1973. Establishment of reentry intervals for organophosphate-treated cotton fields based on human data: I. Ethyl- and methyl parathion. *Arch. Env. Contam. Toxicol.* **1**(1):48–59.

Ware, G. W., D. P. Morgan, B. J. Estesen, and W. P. Cahill. 1974. Establishment of reentry intervals for organophosphate-treated cotton fields based on human data. II. Azodrin, ethyl and methyl parathion. *Arch. Env. Contam. Toxicol.* **2**(2):117–129.

Ware, G. W., D. P. Morgan, B. J. Estesen, and W. P. Cahill. 1975. Establishment of reentry intervals for organophosphate-treated cotton fields based on human data. III. 12 to 72 hours post-treatment exposure to monocrotophos, ethyl- and methyl parathion. *Arch. Env. Contam. Toxicol.* **3:**289–299.

Wasserman, M., S. Iliescu, G. Mandric, and P. Horvath. 1960. Toxic hazards during DDT and BHC-spraying of forests against *Lymantria monacha*. *Arch. Ind. Health* **21:**503–508.

Weisskopf, C. P., J. N. Seiber, N. Maizlish, and M. Schenker. 1988. Personnel exposure to diazinon in a supervised pest eradication program. *Arch. Env. Contam. Toxicol.* **17:**210–212.

Westlake, W. E., F. A. Gunther, and G. E. Carman. 1973. Worker environment research: Dioxathion residues on and in orange fruits and leaves, in dislodgeable particulate matter, and in the soil beneath sprayed trees. *Arch. Env. Contam. Toxicol.* **1:**60–83.

Wilson, B. W., C. M. Cisson, W. R. Randall, J. E. Woodrow, J. N. Sieber, and J. B. Knaak. 1980. Organophosphate risk assessment. Field testing of DEF with the scaleless chicken. *Bull. Env. Contam. Toxicol.* **24:**921–928.

Winterlin, W. L., W. W. Kilgore, C. R. Mourer, and S. R. Schoen. 1984. Worker reentry studies for captan applied to strawberries in California. *J. Agric. Food Chem.* **32:**664–672.

Winterlin, W. L., W. W. Kilgore, C. R. Mourer, G. Hall, and D. Hodapp. 1986. Worker reentry into captan-treated grape fields in California. *Arch. Env. Contam. Toxicol.* **15:**301–311.

Wojeck, G. A., H. N. Nigg, J. H. Stamper, and D. E. Bradway. 1981. Worker exposure to ethion in Florida citrus. *Arch. Env. Contam. Toxicol.* **10:**725–735.

Wojeck, G. A., J. F. Price, H. N. Nigg, and H. J. Stamper. 1983. Worker exposure to paraquat and diquat. *Arch. Env. Contam. Toxicol.* **12:**65–70.

Wolfe, H. R., and J. F. Armstrong. 1971. Exposure of formulating plant workers to DDT. *Arch. Env. Health* **23:**169–176.

Wolfe, H. R., J. F. Armstrong, and W. F. Durham. 1966. Pesticide exposure from concentrate spraying. *Arch. Env. Health* **13:**340–344.

Wolfe, H. R., J. F. Armstrong, and W. F. Durham. September 1974. Exposure of mosquito control workers to fenthion. *Mosquito News*, pp. 263–267.

Wolfe, H. R., W. F. Durham, and J. F. Armstrong. 1963. Health hazards of the pesticides endrin and dieldrin: Hazards in some agricultural uses in the Pacific Northwest. *Arch. Env. Health* **6:**458–464.

Wolfe, H. R., W. F. Durham, and J. F. Armstrong. 1967. Exposure of workers to pesticides. *Arch. Env. Health* **14:**622–633.

Wolfe, H. R., W. F. Durham, and G. S. Batchelor. 1961. Health hazards of some dinitro compounds: Effects associated with agricultural usage in Washington state. *Arch. Env. Health* **3:**468-475.

Wolfe, H. R.., D. C. Staiff, and J. F. Armstrong. 1978. Exposure of pesticide formulation workers to parathion. *Bull. Env. Contam. Toxicol.* **20:**340–343.

Wolfe, H. R., K. C. Walker, J. W. Elliott, and W. F. Durham. 1959. Evaluation of the health hazards involved in house spraying with DDT. *Bull. WHO* **20:**1–14.

Wolfe, H. R., J. F. Armstrong, D. C. Staiff, and S. W. Comer. 1972. Exposure of spraymen to pesticides. *Arch. Env. Health* **25:**29–31.

Wolfe, H. R., D. C. Staiff, J. F. Armstrong, and J. E. Davies. 1978. Exposure of fertilizer mixing plant workers to disulfoton. *Bull. Env. Contam. Toxicol.* **20:**79–86.

Wood, G. W., and D. K. R. Stewart. 1976. Fenitrothion residues in blueberry fields after aerial forest spraying. *Bull. Env. Contam. Toxicol.* **15**(5):623–629.

Zhang, Z., J. Sun, S. Chen, Y. Wu, and F. He. 1991. Levels of exposure and biological monitoring of pyrethroids in spraymen. *Brit. J. Ind. Med.* **48:**82–86.

Zweig, G., R. Gao, and W. Popendorf. 1983. Simultaneous dermal exposure to captan and benomyl by strawberry harvesters. *J. Agric. Food Chem.* **31:**1109–1113.

Zweig, G., R. Gao, J. M. Witt, W. J. Popendorf, and K. T. Bogen. 1985. Exposure of strawberry harvesters to carbaryl. In R. C. Honeycutt, G. Zweig, and N. N. Ragsdale (eds.), *Dermal Exposure Related to Pesticide Use*. Washington, DC: American Chemical Society, pp. 123–138.

Index

Note: For specific contaminants, the reader is also referred to the tabular material on pages 21–26, 27, 28, 37, 38, 73–87, 101–114, 131–133, 138–157, 219–225, 245–246, 280–284, 316–317, 366, 371–374, 387–410, 422–439, 448–537.